Understanding Medical Terminology

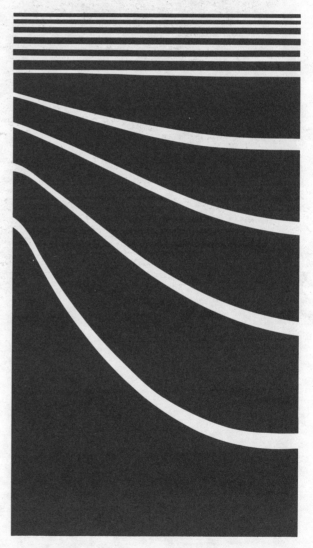

EIGHTH EDITION

Understanding Medical Terminology

Sr. Agnes Clare Frenay, FSM, RN, MS
deceased

Sr. Rose Maureen Mahoney, FSM, RRA, MA
Healthcare Consultant
Franciscan Sisters of Mary
St. Louis, MO

Illustrations by
Christopher J. Burke, MS, AMI
University of Michigan
Ann Arbor, MI

The Catholic Health Association of the United States

St. Louis, MO 63134-0889

Copyright © 1989
by
The Catholic Health Association of the United States
4455 Woodson Road
St. Louis, MO 63134-0889

First Edition published 1958. Eighth Edition 1989.

Library of Congress Cataloging-in-Publication Data

Frenay, Agnes Clare.
    Understanding medical terminology/Agnes Clare Frenay, Rose Maureen
Mahoney.—8th ed.
        p. cm.
    Includes bibliographical references.
    ISBN 0-87125-157-4 : $21.50
    1. Medicine—Terminology. I. Mahoney, Rose Maureen. II. Title.
R123.F7 1989
610'.4—dc20   89-17427
                                                                  CIP

Printed in the United States of America.

Contents

Illustrations vii

Tables ix

Foreword xi

Preface xiii

Introduction xv

PART ONE

1. Orientation to Medical Terminology 3
2. Disorders of the Skin and Breast 25
3. Musculoskeletal Disorders 39
4. Neurologic and Psychiatric Disorders 65
5. Cardiovascular Disorders 99
6. Disorders of the Blood and Blood-Forming Organs 139
7. Respiratory Disorders 159
8. Digestive Disorders 179
9. Urogenital Disorders 211
10. Gynecologic Disorders 233
11. Obstetrical, Fetal, and Neonatal Conditions 251
12. Endocrine and Metabolic Disorders 271
13. Disorders Pertaining to the Sense Organ of Vision 293
14. Disorders Pertaining to the Sense Organ of Hearing 317
15. Multisystem Disorders 331

PART TWO

16. Selected Terms Pertaining to Anesthesiology 369
17. Selected Terms Pertaining to Gerontology 379
18. Selected Terms Pertaining to Oncology 399
19. Selected Terms Pertaining to the Clinical Laboratory 421
20. Selected Terms Pertaining to Radiology, Diagnostic Ultrasound, and Magnetic Resonance Imaging 463
21. Selected Terms Pertaining to Nuclear Medicine 495
22. Selected Terms Pertaining to Physical Therapy 515

PART THREE

Review Guide 531

Answers to multiple choice questions in review guide 582

Index 583

Illustrations

1. Anatomic division of abdomen 22
2. Clinical division of abdomen... 22
3. Posterior view of body.. 23
4. Directional planes of body 23
5. Skin-coloring process... 26
6. Various types of simple epithelium and glands.. 29
7. Skeleton, anterior view... 40
8. Skeleton, posterior view 41
9. Mature femur, posterior view 45
10. Transverse diaphyseal fracture... 45
11. Green-stick fracture... 45
12. Comminuted fracture 45
13. Immature fracture, longitudinal section 45
14. Intertrochanteric fracture repaired by nail and side plate 45
15. Insertion of femoral head prosthesis 45
16. Medullary nailing of femur 45
17. Acetabular component with socket for prosthetic head of femoral component... 51
18. Anterior/posterior view of hip after hip replacement arthroplasty 51
19. Lateral view of knee after total knee replacement arthroplasty..................... 51
20. Anterior/posterior view of knee after total knee replacement arthroplasty 51
21. Muscles, anterior view 54
22. Muscles, posterior view 55
23. Motor neuron (efferent)... 67
24. Sensory neuron (afferent) 67
25. Formation of spinal nerve 67
26. Structure of neuron... 67
27. Transverse section of spinal cord at level of origin of third lumbar nerve 72
28. Median section of brain and spinal cord 72
29. Location of extracranial or intracranial lesions in cerebrovascular disease 74
30. Occlusive lesion of the bifurcation of the common carotid artery extending
    into the carotid artery 74
31. Subclavian steal syndrome 74
32. Anterior view of heart 100
33. Schematic diagram of conduction system of heart....................................100
34. Ventricular fibrillation: life-threatening arrhythmia 104
35. Terminal ventricular fibrillation and ventricular standstill—asystole 104
36. Direct myocardial revascularization by triple aortocoronary bypass 110
37. Internal mammary artery bypass grafts for myocardial revascularization,
    anterior view..110
38. Normal electrocardiographic cycle..125
39. Developmental phases of neutrophils..140
40. Main lymphatics and lymph nodes 150
41. Larynx, anterior view 161
42. Larynx, right lateral view...161
43. Trachea, bronchi, lungs, and pleural sacs..165
44. Lobes of lung 166

45. Bronchopulmonary segments of lungs 166
46. Salivary glands 183
47. Scheme of digestive tract...195
48. Longitudinal section of kidney..212
49. Structure of renal corpuscle 212
50. Diagram of nephron 212
51. Hypospadias 219
52. Cystoscope used to examine interior of urinary bladder.............................221
53. Male reproductive organs...225
54. Uterus, uterine tubes, and ovaries (schematic) 236
55. Normal ovulatory cycle 236
56. Clinical stages of cervical cancer..237
57. Bimanual compression of uterus for uterine atony 255
58. Incomplete inversion of uterus...255
59. Placental types...256
60. Amniocentesis...262
61. Manual delivery of placenta...262
62. Right occipitoanterior (ROA) fetal position 263
63. Left sacroposterior (LSP) fetal position 263
64. Right scapuloposterior (RScP) fetal position.......................................263
65. Hormones of adenohypophysis; direct and indirect effect on target organs........272
66. Chromosomes from normal human male cell 281
67. Human sex chromosomes, normal pattern and chromosomal aberrations 281
68. Karyotype or idiogram of normal human male 285
69. Horizontal section of eyeball through the optic nerve..............................294
70. Lacrimal apparatus 303
71. Schematic section through middle and inner ear 318
72. Distribution of vestibulocochlear nerve to inner ear 318
73. Approaches for ablative procedures for treatment of vertigo 323
74. Different frequencies creating different wave patterns in basilar membrane
    within the cochlea 325
75. Some selected organisms 344
76. Broca's area and Wernicke's area of the brain 389
77. Normal artery, arterial coats, and lumen 393
78. Atheromatous plaques in intima, capillary bleeding, and early mural
    thrombosis 393
79. Rupture of ulcerated, intimal plaque, mural thrombosis, and occlusion 393
80. Stages of atherosclerosis...393
81. Three methods of ultrasound imaging..477
82. Stable nuclides and radioactive nuclides 499
83. Radioiodine and the thyroid gland...506
84. Cerebral hemorrhage resulting in right-sided hemiplegia 525

Tables

1. Some conditions of the skin and breast amenable to surgery 34
2. Some orthopedic conditions amenable to surgery 59
3. Some conditions amenable to neurosurgery 93
4. Coronary risk factors of prime importance according to Framingham study 113
5. Some cardiovascular conditions amenable to surgery 128
6. Modified Schilling's hemogram—differential leukocyte count 145
7. Rye histopathologic classification of Hodgkin's disease (Modified from Lukes and Butler Classification) 151
8. Modified Ann Arbor Staging Classification for Hodgkin's disease 151
9. Some disorders of the blood and blood-forming organs amenable to surgery 156
10. Some respiratory conditions amenable to surgery 174
11. Gastric types in relation to architectural structures of individuals 188
12. Some digestive conditions amenable to surgery....................................203
13. Some urogenital conditions amenable to surgery..................................228
14. Some gynecologic conditions amenable to surgery................................246
15. Some obstetric and neonatal conditions amenable to surgery 266
16. Cytogenetic studies 286
17. Some endocrine conditions amenable to surgery..................................288
18. Some eye conditions amenable to surgery 310
19. Some ear conditions amenable to surgery 327
20. Laboratory tests for major infectious diseases 345
21. Causes of arterial hypotension encountered during anesthesia 370
22. Evaluation of response intensity 373
23. Classification of selected general anesthetics 377
24. Comparison of FIGO and TNM staging systems for carcinoma of the ovary 404
25. Classification of common neoplasms 404
26. Environmental causes of human cancer 416
27. Measurements of the metric system..422
28. Traditional measurements...423
29. Selected hematologic findings in disease 425
30. Compatibility of blood for transfusion...427
31. Characteristic reference values of arterial blood gases.............................433
32. Serum enzyme activity postmyocardial infarction..................................438
33. Liver function tests 452
34. Ultrasonic findings related to ovarian lesions......................................480
35. Some radionuclides in diagnosis 507
36. Some radionuclides in therapy..509

Foreword

Sr. Rose Maureen Mahoney, FSM, and her mentor and coauthor, the late Sr. Agnes Clare Frenay, FSM, have drawn on their lifelong experiences in healthcare to provide assistance to those who would improve their understanding of the language of medicine.

This up-to-date treatise can benefit not only those who seek an introduction to the understanding of medical terms, but also those who choose to refine their medical language—and, of course, those who instruct others.

In this revised and expanded eighth edition of *Understanding Medical Terminology,* Sr. Mahoney continues and complements the work of Sr. Frenay, with careful attention to current developments in the ever unfolding drama of medical practice.

Previous editions of *Understanding Medical Terminology* have been translated into a seven-volume braille edition by the American Printing House for the Blind in Louisville, KY. Similar transcriptions have been produced by the New York Association for the Blind. The Library of Congress has been given permission to transcribe this text into large type in connection with its program for the visually impaired.

Sr. Rose Maureen Mahoney, building upon the pioneering scholarship of Sr. Agnes Clare Frenay, has produced a highly practical and comprehensive text that is current and authoritative. This work will serve well students, instructors, and others seeking an understanding of medical terminology.

Vallee L. Willman, MD
Professor of Surgery
St. Louis University
School of Medicine and
Chairman
Department of Surgery
The University Hospital
St. Louis, MO

Preface

The eighth edition of *Understanding Medical Terminology* offers a structured approach to the learning of medical terms. The text design provides insight into the construction of words as well as definitions of words common to this specialized vocabulary. A working vocabulary must include terms that are both *remembered* and *understood*. There are few specialized vocabularies in our culture as important as that of medical terminology, given the life-and-death complexity of modern medicine.

Concentrated research by the author over the past four years underlies the revised and updated contents of each chapter; the text addresses relatively new or changing terms and usage, such as those found in the clinical laboratory, radiology, ultrasound, magnetic resonance imaging, and other rapidly developing medical technologies, as well as enduring standard terms. The tables, figures, and illustrations appearing in this edition reinforce the learning process.

Special appreciation is extended to the late Sr. Agnes Clare Frenay, FSM, for her contributions to the development and structure of the text, including past editions and the present edition.

Recognition and gratitude is extended to those physicians, professors, and healthcare professionals who reviewed chapters or gave individual consultation. Physicians included the following: Todd Gavin, MD, professor of urology, Washington University School of Medicine, and staff urologist, Barnes Hospital, St. Louis; Kevin B. Herbert, PhD, professor and chairman of the Classical Language Department, Washington University; V. Yaeger, MD, professor of anatomy, St. Louis University School of Medicine; John G. Gregory, MD, professor of urology, St. Louis University School of Medicine, and staff urologist, St. Mary's Health Center, St. Louis; Vallee Willman, MD, professor of surgery, St. Louis University School of Medicine, and chairman of the Department of Surgery, The University Hospital, St. Louis; Eugene F. Tucker, MD, associate professor of pathology, St. Louis University School of Medicine, and director of Medical Laboratories, St. Mary's Health Center, St. Louis; Ella Swierkosz, PhD, associate professor of pediatric/adolescent medicine, St. Louis University School of Medicine, and director of Virology and Microbiology Laboratory Departments, Cardinal Glennon Children's Hospital, St. Louis; Neil Gallagher, MD, associate professor of medicine and director of the Oncology Department, St. Mary's Health Center, St. Louis; Munir Ahmad, MD, associate professor of internal medicine, St. Louis University School of Medicine, and director of the Nuclear Medicine Department, St. Mary's Health Center, St. Louis.

The following individuals from St. Mary's Health Center, St. Louis, assisted in reviewing terms: Thomas E. Reh, MD, director of radiology; John J. McNamara, MD, staff radiologist; William Nalesnik, PhD, radiation physicist, Nuclear Medicine Department; Sadat Ayata, MD, director of anesthesiology; E.S. Rader, MD, chief of urology; and Morey Gardner, MD, director of infectious diseases and medical education. Healthcare professionals included Sr. Marie Duchesne Herold, FSM, author of the book, *New Life: Preparation of Religious for Retirement,* for her helpful consultation regarding the chapter on gerontology; and Sr. Mary Leo Rita Volk, FSM, for her assistance in the area of cytogenetic studies. Special thanks for assistance in proofreading goes to Sr. Anna Hillenbrand, CSJ, RRA.

A very special debt of gratitude is extended to the Governing Board of the Franciscan Sisters of Mary for appointing the author to the mission of researching and developing the eighth edition of the text, *Understanding Medical Terminology.*

Sr. Rose Maureen Mahoney, FSM

Introduction

The eighth edition of *Understanding Medical Terminology* represents a revised and enlarged text that introduces the student to terms widely used in the medical sciences and in the field of healthcare.

Chapter Organization—General

The text is divided into three major parts: chapters 1 through 15 provide background and context; chapters 16 through 22 concentrate on terms and exercises related to specialty areas; and the remaining chapter contains review materials. We will examine these three major parts in detail, particularly the first, which lays the foundation for much of what we wish to accomplish in this book.

Chapter Organization—Details

Part One. The first section of the text, Background and Context, introduces the student to the basic concepts underlying medical terminology, including examples of base or root elements, prefixes, suffixes, compounding and/or combining word elements, that are of use in the analysis of terms. It is important to emphasize that not all medical terms can be broken down exactly, or even consistently in this manner, and that there are many exceptions to the general "rules" of word formation. A medical terminology text is a guide to usage, and as such it must be combined with experience to achieve the ultimate goal of understanding.

Chapters 2 through 14 treat disorders of the major body systems. Within these chapters medical terms are divided into several pedagogic categories:

- *Origin of terms*, offering the student an orientation to key word elements that pertain to the body system or disorder under discussion.
- *Anatomic terms*, designating body system structure.
- *Diagnostic terms*, dealing with specific clinical disorders.
- *General terms*, relating closely to, although not exactly the same as, the body system or disorder. These terms may replace the anatomic classification wherever appropriate (e.g., see chapter 4 under Psychiatric Disorders). This classification of terms also may be used in addition to the anatomic terms (e.g., see chapter 11 under Obstetrical, Fetal, and Neonatal Conditions).
- *Operative terms*, relating to methods of surgical intervention employed to relieve or cure the impact of the clinical disorder, trauma, or other conditions on the system.
- *Symptomatic terms*, describing the presence of subjective evidence or symptoms experienced by the patient that characterize system disorders or conditions. In this text we also extend the meaning of "symptomatic term" to include any evidence of disturbed physiology perceived by either the patient or physician.
- *Abbreviations*, which are shortened forms of words or phrases used to represent the full form. Abbreviations are distributed throughout each chapter.
- *Verbalized terms*, (see Oral Reading Exercises). Pronunciation of medical terms may vary drastically, and some of the most widely accepted medical term pronunciations have little validity linguistically. We offer reading exercises that include brief

discussions of medical topics that provide the student with opportunities for verbal pronunciation of terms within a particular scientific-medical context, to help overcome inhibitions limiting the effective use of medical terminology.

- *Surgery-related terms,* detailed in tabular listings (see Conditions Amenable to Surgery) of organs affected by specific disorders, and of the title and type of surgical procedure employed to relieve or cure the impact of the disorder, trauma, or other condition on the body.
- *Special procedure terms,* relating to the type of method or mechanism employed for further investigation or utilized to cure or relieve impending disorders or conditions.
- *Illustrations,* (figures and tables) organize terminology primarily with regard to anatomic structures and/or significant procedures, to assist overall integration of material, and better general comprehension of the subject matter.

Chapter 15, "Multisystem Disorders," introduces the student to a threefold topical classification of these disorders: infectious diseases, immunologic diseases, and diseases of connective tissue. Each of these three topics has its own expository subcategories, the first of these always concerning the origin of terms. In outline form, the triad of disorder types, with subcategories, would read as follows:

Infectious Diseases
- Origin of terms
- General terms
- Terms related to specific infections of this type

Immunologic Diseases
- Origin of terms
- General terms
- Diagnostic terms

Diseases of Connective Tissue
- Origin of terms
- Anatomic terms
- Diagnostic terms

This chapter also contains abbreviations and oral reading practice.

Part Two. In the second section of the text, "Terms and Exercises," chapters 16 through 22 deal with medical terminology in a variety of subject settings, including anesthesiology, gerontology, oncology, clinical laboratory, radiology, diagnostic ultra-sound and magnetic resonance imaging, nuclear medicine, and physical therapy. Magnetic resonance imaging is a new and expanded addition to the radiology and diagnostic ultrasound chapter in the eighth edition. Revisions in the other chapters in this section reflect the proliferation of specialty terms.

Part Three. The third and concluding section of the text, "Review Guide," represents a distinctly important component of the eighth edition. This section provides the student with a review of the key concepts underlying the usage of medical terminology and also includes review guides for each chapter. These review guides permit the student to practice newly acquired spelling skills and offer resource material for midterm and final examinations. Some of the testing format is similar to that which the students may encounter when taking their registration and/or accreditation examinations.

Syllabus Structure

Ideally, the course in medical terminology should be taught in 48 50-minute hours (three semester credits) in order to ensure adequate coverage of the subject matter. This schedule also gives the learner the opportunity to digest and assimilate the material. The more common practice, however, is to cover this material in 32 50-minute hours (two semester credits). This type of course arrangement necessitates selective elimination of several key areas or chapters. Whatever time constraint is placed upon the instructor, it is recommended that chapters 1 through 15 be considered "core curriculum" chapters and that selection of material from other chapters be dependent upon the decision of the instructor, student needs, and the time that is available. The thorough student will make a point of reading all the material and would be well advised to keep the text at hand as a ready reference.

Conclusion

I wish to reaffirm my gratitude to all those who have offered assistance during the development of this eighth edition. A special debt of appreciation is warranted for those instructors at the collegiate and technical levels who took time to reflect on their experiences with previous editions of the text, enabling them to provide very valuable firsthand comments and criticisms. I am appreciative also for the feedback received from instructors in healthcare institutions and clinics in which the text has been used to teach medical terminology to staff personnel.

I am pleased to present this eighth edition of *Understanding Medical Terminology,* and I look forward to continued constructive response from teachers and students.

P
A
R
T

1

1 Orientation to Medical Terminology

2 Disorders of the Skin and Breast

3 Musculoskeletal Disorders

4 Neurologic and Psychiatric Disorders

5 Cardiovascular Disorders

6 Disorders of the Blood and Blood-Forming Organs

7 Respiratory Disorders

8 Digestive Disorders

9 Urogenital Disorders

10 Gynecologic Disorders

11 Obstetrical, Fetal, and Neonatal Conditions

12 Endocrine and Metabolic Disorders

13 Disorders Pertaining to the Sense Organ of Vision

14 Disorders Pertaining to the Sense Organ of Hearing

15 Multisystem Disorders

Orientation to Medical Terminology

CHAPTER 1

Objectives and Values

Medical terminology is the professional language of those who are directly or indirectly engaged in the art of healing. Its strangeness may seem bewildering at first to the student, and its complexity may tax his or her powers of concentration. These difficulties, however, gradually disappear as the student assimilates a working knowledge of the elements of medical terms, which enables the student to analyze words etymologically and according to their meaning. The drudgery of memorizing is somewhat annoying to the beginner, but memory work is only a stepping-stone to a keener understanding of the professional language. It is obvious that the intellect is constantly engaged in the study of medical terms in various types of mental processes: the analysis of words, their interpretation, and to a moderate degree, the transfer of knowledge by combining word roots synthetically with prefixes, suffixes, compound or combining word elements.

The primary goal of introducing the student to medical terminology is to help him or her develop the ability to read and understand the language of medicine. Efforts are directed to promote a knowledge of the elements of medical terms, and understanding of standard abbreviations, the ability to spell medical terms, and an appreciation of the logical method found in medical terminology.

Basic Concepts

The majority of medical terms claim Greek and Latin ancestry. Some have been adopted from modern languages, especially from the German and French. The study of medical terminology can enrich our understanding of history, language, and medicine. As time goes on, additional scientific advances occur that herald newer terms or evoke usage of previously coined medical terms.

The pronunciation of medical terms follows no rigid rules; flexibility appears to be one of its outstanding characteristics. Flexibility, however, may be a hindrance rather than a help, since it may lead to confusion or intimidation in the instance of a firm but strong pronunciation by an established medical person whose authority junior staff members prudently wish to avoid testing.

We emphasize that the student should not be intimidated when faced with common usage of an unfamiliar pronunciation. Remember the different traditions used in the teaching of these languages. For instance, in the German tradition of teaching, instruction emphasizes a pronunciation of Latin words that would have made little sense to ancient Romans or to their modern Italian counterparts. Nevertheless, the powerful influence of German scholarship in medicine and language helped to entrench these linguistically bizarre pronunciations of Latin and Greek terms; their ancient meaning, grammatical usage, and modern application all contributed to the medical terminology of today.

Many medical terms are combinations of components from these ancient languages. As our vocabulary grows, we begin to notice patterns of frequent usage that employ some of these components. Over time our growing familiarity with the more common components will enable us to recognize more quickly or recall more easily the modern meaning of the term. Sometimes this process of recognition is called *word-building*, which is a well-meaning but misleading term. Actually we are taking apart rather than building words to discover, remember, and use their meaning. As we break these words apart to arrive at their inner meaning, we begin to develop a knowledge of word form and usage that eventually will enable us to read modern medical terminology with intelligence. The student should not expect to develop this analytic perception overnight but only after extensive vocabulary study. One day he or she may use these building blocks to fashion new words for the medical vocabulary.

In this edition, as in previous editions, the text seeks to develop an analytic attitude in the student. Becoming aware of the structural design of words and developing the habit of analyzing terms leads to a better understanding of the definitions throughout the book. To assist the student in developing the ability to speak the language of medicine, we have included brief discussions of medical topics in the text for oral reading exercises. As the student moves through the various categories of disorders, he or she will note recurrent appearances of certain prefixes, suffixes, roots, compounding and/or combining form word elements. A review of key terms applicable to each chapter may be found in the section entitled *Origin of Terms*. It is through a well-ordered learning of these terms that the student begins to penetrate definitions of terms and articulate this new learning through the oral reading exercises.

A revised section entitled *Review Guide* reinforces concepts learned and provides the student with the opportunity to practice newly acquired spelling skills.

Newly updated references and bibliography appear at the end of each chapter; the student will find reference numbers in parentheses throughout the text.

In analyzing terms it is advisable for the student to understand the key concepts that will enable the beginner to *tear apart* terms. These concepts are:

1. Root or base word element — refers to the main body of the word. It may be accompanied by a prefix or suffix.
   Example: adenoma
   aden- (base or root) = gland
   -oma (suffix) = tumor
   adenoma = gland tumor
2. Prefix — refers to one or two syllables or word parts placed before a word to modify or alter its meaning.
   Example: hemigastrectomy
   hemi- (prefix) = half
   gastr- (base or root) = stomach
   -ectomy (suffix) = removal or excision of
   hemigastrectomy = removal of half of the stomach

3. Suffix — one or two syllables or word parts attached to the end of a word to modify or alter its meaning.
   Example: hysterectomy
   > hyster- (base or root) = uterus
   > -ectomy (suffix) = removal or excision of
   > hysterectomy = removal of uterus

4. "Pertaining to" suffix — selected suffixes meaning "pertaining to" include -ac, -al, -ic, -eal, -ary, and -ous.
   Example: hemic
   > hem- (base or root) = blood
   > -ic (suffix) = pertaining to
   > hemic = pertaining to blood

5. "One who" suffix — selected suffixes meaning "one who" include -er and -ist.
   Example: pathologist
   > path- (root) = disease or morbid condition
   > o (combining form element, vowel)
   > -logy (suffix) = science or study of
   > -ist (suffix) = one who
   > pathologist = one who studies disease or morbid conditions

6. Combining form element — results when a vowel, usually a, i, e, or o, is added to a word root or base. The vowels used most commonly as combining form elements are a, i, or o. The vowel is usually deleted from a combining form when the next letter that follows is also a vowel.
   Example: proctitis
   > procto- = combining form denoting relationship to the rectum
   > -itis (suffix) = inflammation of
   > proctitis = correct combination
   > proctoitis = incorrect combination (o should be dropped)
   > proctitis = inflammation of the rectum

7. Compound words — result when two or more root or base word elements are used to form a word. Usually adjectives or nouns are added to a root word to form compound words. Also compound words may include a combining form, a root or base word element, and a suffix or word ending.
   Example: myocardiopathy
   > myo- = combining form element denoting relationship to muscle
   > cardio- = combining form element denoting relationship to heart
   > -pathy (suffix) = disease or morbid condition
   > myocardiopathy = disease of the heart muscle

Tearing apart the term anemia, we have:
anemia
-emia (suffix) = blood
a- (prefix) = without, not

In the strict sense anemia might seem to mean no blood, absence or total lack of blood, rather than the attenuated quality of blood. This example reminds us that an exact correspondence does not usually exist between the meaning of a modern term and the ancient language roots from which the term derives. The important point here is an understanding of the meaning of each term and the overall relationship of terms; pronunciation must be flexible both out of courtesy and in the interest of better communication. Patience in the face of questioned pronunciation followed by willing accommodation is a reasonable approach.

When analyzing terms the student is advised for practical considerations to begin with the suffix and proceed to the root or root and prefix. Although logic in the analysis of word elements would normally dictate beginning with the base or root word element and then analyzing the suffix and prefix added to it, the best analysis strategy suggests beginning with the suffix, which generally gives a clue as to how the root is being used.

Medical terminology is an exciting language; it lives, grows, changes, and develops. Old words may die; new words may be born.

Elements of Medical Terms

Suffixes and Compounding Elements

To simplify learning, modifying endings have been classified according to their meanings into diagnostic, operative, and symptomatic suffixes.

Selected Diagnostic Suffixes*

Suffix	Term	Analysis	Definition
-cele (G) hernia, tumor, protrusion	cystocele	*kystis:* bladder *kele:* hernia	Hernia of the bladder
	gastrocele	*gaster:* stomach; —;	Hernia of the stomach
	hydrocele	*hydor:* water *kele:* tumor	Serous tumor, as of testis
	myelocele	*myelos:* marrow *kele:* protrusion	Protrusion of spinal cord through the vertebrae
-ectasis (G) expansion, dilatation	angiectasis	*angeion:* vessel *ektasis:* dilatation	Abnormal dilatation of a blood vessel
	atelectasis	*ateles:* imperfect; —;	Airless, functionless lung
	—; neonatorum	—; *neos:* new *natus:* birth, born	Imperfect expansion of lungs at birth
	bronchiectasis	*bronchos:* bronchus; —;	Abnormal dilatation of a bronchus or bronchi
-emia (G) blood	hyperglycemia hyperglycosemia	*hyper:* excessive *glykys:* sweet, sugar *haima:* blood	Abnormally high blood sugar
	polycythemia	*polys:* many, excessive *kytos:* cell, —; —;	Abnormal increase of red blood cells and hemoglobin in the blood
-iasis (G) condition, formation of, presence of	lithiasis	*lithos:* stone *iasis:* presence of	Formation of stones
	cholelithiasis	*chole:* bile; —; —;	Presence of calculi in the gallbladder
	nephrolithiasis	*nephros:* kidney; —; —;	Stones present in the kidney

*NOTE: (G) means that the suffix is a Greek derivative, (L) a Latin. The dash and semicolon refer to the suffix that has already been given. In the analysis, the Greek and Latin words are used to show the derivation, but the student needs only to learn the English version.

Suffix	Term	Analysis	Definition
-itis (G) inflammation	carditis	*kardia:* heart *itis:* inflammation	Inflammation of the heart
	iritis	*iris:* rainbow, iris; —;	Inflammation of the iris
	poliomyelitis	*polios:* gray *myelos:* marrow; —;	Inflammation of the gray matter of the spinal cord
-malacia (G) softening	encephalomalacia	*enkephalos:* brain *malakia:* softening	Softening of the brain
	osteomalacia	*osteon:* bone; —;	Softening of the bones
	splenomalacia	*splen:* spleen; —;	Softening of the spleen
-megaly (G) enlargement	acromegaly	*akros:* extreme *megas:* large	Disease marked by enlargement of the bones of head and the soft part of extremities and face
	hepatomegaly	*hepat:* liver; —;	Enlargement of the liver
	splenomegaly	*splen:* spleen; —;	Enlargement of the spleen
-oma (G) tumor	adenoma	*aden:* gland *oma:* tumor	Glandular tumor
	carcinoma	*karkinos:* cancer; —;	Malignant tumor of epithelial tissue
	sarcoma	*sark:* flesh; —;	Malignant tumor of connective tissue
-pathy (G) disease	adenopathy	*aden:* gland *pathos:* disease	Any glandular disease
	myelopathy	*myelos:* marrow; —;	Any pathologic disorder of the spinal cord
	myopathy	*mys:* muscle; —;	Any disease of a muscle
-ptosis (G) falling, downward displacement	blepharoptosis	*blepharon:* eyelid *ptosis:* a falling	Drooping of the eyelid
	gastroptosis	*gaster:* stomach; —;	Downward displacement of the stomach
	nephroptosis	*nephros:* kidney; —;	Downward displacement of the kidney
-rhexis (G) rupture	angiorrhexis	*angeion:* vessel *rhexis:* rupture	Rupture of a blood vessel or lymphatic
	cardiorrhexis	*kardia:* heart; —;	Rupture of the heart
	hysterorrhexis	*hystera:* uterus; —;	Rupture of the uterus

Selected Operative Suffixes

-centesis (G) puncture	paracentesis	*para:* beside *kentesis:* a puncture	Puncture of a cavity
	abdominal paracentesis	*abdomen:* belly; —;	Puncture and aspiration of the peritoneal cavity
	thoracentesis	*thorax:* chest; —;	Aspiration of the pleural cavity

Suffix	Term	Analysis	Definition
-desis (G) binding, fixation	arthrodesis	*arthron:* joint *desis:* fixation	Surgical fixation of a joint
	spondylosyndesis	*spondylos:* vertebra; —;	Surgical fixation of the vertebrae
	tenodesis	*tenon:* tendon; —;	Fixation of a tendon to a bone
-ectomy (G) excision	myomectomy	*mys:* muscle *oma:* tumor *ektome:* excision	Excision of a tumor of the[1] muscle
	oophorectomy	*oophor:* ovary; —;	Removal of an ovary
	tonsillectomy	*tonsilla:* tonsil; —;	Removal of tonsils
-lithotomy (G) incision for removal of stones	cholelithotomy	*chole:* bile, gall; —;	Incision into gallbladder for removal of stones
	nephrolithotomy	*nephros:* kidney; —;	Incision into kidney for removal of stones
	sialolithotomy	*sialon:* saliva; —;	Incision into salivary gland for removal of stones
-pexy (G) suspension, fixation	hysteropexy	*hystera:* uterus *pexis:* fixation	Abdominal fixation or suspension of the uterus
	mastopexy	*mastos:* breast; —;	Fixation of a pendulous breast
	orchiopexy	*orchis:* testis; —;	Fixation of an undescended testis
-plasty (G) surgical correction, plastic repair of	arthroplasty	*arthron:* joint *plassein:* to form	Reconstruction operation on joint
	hernioplasty	*hernos:* a young shoot; —;	Plastic repair of hernia
	proctoplasty	*proktos:* anus, rectum; —;	Surgical repair of rectum
-rhaphy (G) suture	perineorrhaphy	*perinaion:* perineum *rhaphe:* suture	Suture of a lacerated perineum
	staphylorrhaphy	*staphyle:* uvula; —;	Suture of a cleft palate
	trachelorrhaphy	*trachelos:* neck; —;	Suture of a torn cervix uteri
-scopy (G) inspection, examination	bronchoscopy	*bronchos:* windpipe *skopein:* to examine	Examination of the bronchi with an endoscope
	cystoscopy	*kystis:* bladder; —;	Inspection of the bladder with a cystoscope
-stomy (G) creation of an artificial opening	colostomy	*kolon:* colon *stoma:* opening	Creation of an opening into the colon through the abdominal wall
	cystostomy	*kystis:* bladder; —;	Creation of an opening into the urinary bladder through the abdomen
	gastroduodenostomy	*gaster:* stomach *duoden:* duodenum	Creation of an opening between the stomach and duodenum

Suffix	Term	Analysis	Definition
-tomy (G) incision into	antrotomy	*antron:* antrum *tome:* incision	Incision into an antrum to establish drainage
	neurotomy	*neuron:* nerve; —;	Dissection of a nerve
	thoracotomy	*thorax:* chest; —;	Opening of the chest
-tripsy (G) crushing, friction	lithotripsy	*lithos:* stone *tripsis:* crushing	Crushing of a stone
	phrenicotripsy	*phren:* diaphragm; —;	Crushing of the phrenic nerve

Selected Symptomatic Suffixes

Suffix	Term	Analysis	Definition
-algia (G) pain	gastralgia	*gaster:* stomach *algos:* pain	Epigastric pain
	nephralgia	*nephros:* kidney; —;	Renal pain
	neuralgia	*neuron:* nerve; —;	Lancinating nerve pain
-genic (G) origin	bronchogenic	*bronchos:* windpipe *gennan:* to originate	Originating in the bronchi
	neurogenic	*neuron:* nerve; —;	Originating in the nerves
	osteogenic	*osteon:* bone; —;	Originating in the bones
	pathogenic	*pathos:* disease; —;	Disease producing
-lysis (G) dissolution, breaking down	hemolysis	*haima:* blood *lysis:* breaking down	Breaking down of red blood cells
	myolysis	*mys:* muscle; —;	Destruction of muscular tissue
	neurolysis	*neuron:* nerve; —;	Disintegration of nerve tissue
-oid (G) like	fibroid	*fibra:* fiber *eidos:* resembling	Tumor of fibrous tissue, resembling fibers
	lipoid	*lipos:* fat; —;	Fatlike
	lymphoid	*lympha:* lymph; —;	Resembling lymph
-osis (G) increase, disease condition	anisocytosis	*anisos:* unequal *kytos:* cell *osis:* condition	Inequality of size of cells
	lymphocytosis	*lympha:* lymph; —; —;	Excess of lymph cells
-penia (G) deficiency, decrease	leukopenia	*leukos:* white *penia:* decrease	Abnormal decrease of leukocytes in the blood
	neutropenia	*neuter:* neutral; —;	Abnormal decrease of neutrophils in the blood
-spasm (G) involuntary contractions	chirospasm	*cheir:* hand *spasmos:* spasm or contraction of muscles	Spasm or contraction of the hand (writer's cramp)
	dactylospasm	*dactylos:* finger; —;	Spasm or cramp in fingers or toes
	enterospasm	*enteron:* intestine; —;	Painful intestinal contractions

Selected Roots*

Root	Term	Analysis	Definition
aden- (G) gland	adenectomy	*aden:* gland *ektome:* excision	Excision of a gland
	adenoma	—; *oma:* tumor	Glandular tumor
	adenocarcinoma	—; *karkinos:* cancer —;	Malignant tumor of glandular epithelium
aer- (G) air	aerated	*aer:* air	Filled with air
	aerobic	—; *bios:* life	Pertaining to an organism that lives only in the presence of air
	aeroneurosis	—; *neuron:* nerve *osis:* condition, disease, process	Functional nervous disorder affecting airplane pilots
arth- (G) joint	arthralgia	*arthron:* joint *algos:* pain	Pain in the joints
	arthritis	—; *itis:* inflammation	Inflammation of the joints
	arthrology	—; *logos:* study, science	The science of the joints
blephar- (G) eyelid	blepharedema	*blepharon:* eyelid *oidema:* swelling	Swelling of the eyelids
	blepharoplasty	—; *plassein:* to form	Plastic operation on the eyelid
	blepharoptosis	—; *ptosis:* a falling	Drooping of the upper eyelid
card- (G) heart	cardiac	*kardia:* heart	Pertaining to the heart or esophageal orifice of the stomach
	electrocardiogram	*elektron:* amber; —; *gramma:* mark	Graphic record of the heartbeat by an electrometer
	phonocardiography	*phono:* sound; —; *graphein:* to write	Graphic recording of heart sounds
cephal- (G) head	cephalad	*kephale:* head *ad:* toward	Toward the head
	cephalic	—; *ic:* pertaining to	Pertaining to the head
	cephalitis	—; *itis:* inflammation	Inflammation of the brain
cerv- (L) neck	cervical	*cervix:* neck *al:* pertaining to	Pertaining to the neck
	cervicectomy	—; *ektome:* excision	Excision of the neck of the uterus
	cervicovesical	—; *vesica:* bladder; —;	Relating to the cervix uteri and bladder
cheil-, chil- (G) lip	cheilitis	*cheilos:* lip *itis:* inflammation	Inflammation of the lip
	cheiloplasty	—; *plassein:* to form	Plastic operation of the lip
	cheilosis	—; *osis:* disease condition	Morbid condition of the lips caused by vitamin B deficiency

*NOTE: The dash and semicolon refer to the root that has already been given.

Root	Term	Analysis	Definition
*chir- (G) hand	chiromegaly	cheir: hand megas: large	Abnormal size of the hands.
	chiroplasty	—; plassein: to form	Plastic surgery on the hand
	chiropody	—; pous: foot	Treatment of conditions of the hands and feet
chol- (G) bile	cholangitis	chole: bile angeion: vessel itis: inflammation	Inflammation of the bile duct
	cholecyst	—; kystis: bladder, sac	Gallbladder
	cholecystogram	—; —; gramma: mark	Radiograph of the gallbladder
chrondr- (G) cartilage	chondrectomy	chondros: cartilage ektome: excision	Excision of a cartilage
	chondrofibroma	—; fibra: fiber oma: tumor	Mixed tumor composed of fibrous tissue and cartilage
	chondroma	—; —;	Cartilaginous tumor
cost- (L) rib	costochondral	costa: rib chrondros: cartilage al: pertaining to	Pertaining to a rib and its cartilage
	costophrenic angle	—; phren: diaphragm angle: corner	The angle formed by the ribs and diaphragm
	costosternal	—; sternon: breast	Referring to the ribs and sternum
cyst- (G) bladder, sac	cyst	kystis: bladder, sac	Bladder; any sac containing a liquid
	cystography	—; graphein: to write	Radiographic examination of the urinary bladder following the introduction of air or opaque solution
	cystoscope	—; skopein: to examine	Instrument for internal examination of the bladder
cyt- (G) cell	cytology	kytos: cell logos: study	The study of cell life
	erythrocyte	erythros: red; —;	Red blood cell
	lymphocyte	lympha: lymph; —;	Lymph cell, a nongranular leukocyte
dactyl- (G) finger, toe	dactylitis	dactylos: finger itis: inflammation	Inflammation of bones of fingers or toes
	dactylogram	—; gramma: mark	Fingerprint
	dactylomegaly	—; megas: large	Abnormal size of fingers or toes
derm- (G) skin	dermal	derma: skin al: relating to	Relating to the skin
	dermatitis	—; itis: inflammation	Inflammation of the skin
	dermopathy	—; pathos: disease	Any skin disease

*Chir may suggest of the hand as in chiromegaly, or by the hand as in the broad sense of "treatment" as in chiropody.

Root	Term	Analysis	Definition
encephal- (G) brain	encephalitis	*enkephalos:* brain *itis:* inflammation	Inflammation of the brain
	encephalography	—; *graphein:* to write	Radiographic examination of the head after withdrawing fluid and replacing it with air
	encephaloma	—; *oma:* tumor	Brain tumor
enter- (G) intestine	enteritis	*enteron:* intestine *itis:* inflammation	Inflammation of the intestines
	enterocele	—; *kele:* hernia	Hernia of the intestines
	enterocolitis	—; *kolon:* colon; —;	Inflammation of the intestines and colon
gastr- (G) stomach	gastrectasis	*gaster:* stomach *ectasis:* dilatation	Dilatation of the stomach
	gastroenterostomy	—; *enteron:* intestine *stoma:* opening	Formation of a passage between the stomach and intestine
	gastrointestinal	—; *intestinum:* intestine *al:* pertaining to	Pertaining to the stomach and intestines
hem-, hemat- (G) blood	hematemesis	*haima:* blood *emesis:* vomiting	Vomiting of blood
	hematoma	—; *oma:* tumor	Blood tumor
	hemophilia	—; *philein:* to love	Inability of the blood to coagulate
hepat- (G) liver	hepatic flexure	*hepat:* liver *flexura:* a curved part	Right bend of colon under the liver
	hepatitis	—; *itis:* inflammation	Inflammation of the liver
	hepatolysis	—; *lysis:* destruction	Destruction of liver cells
hyster- (G) uterus	hysterectomy	*hystera:* uterus *ektome:* excision	Excision of the uterus
	hysteria	—; *ia:* disease of	Psychoneurosis marked by emotional instability and somatic symptoms
	hysteropexy	—; *pexis:* fixation	Abdominal fixation of or suspension of the uterus
ile- (L) ileum	ileum	*ileum:* ileum	Distal part of the small intestine
	ileocecal valve	—; *caecus:* blind *valva:* one leaf of a double door	Two lips or folds at opening between the ileum and cecum
	ileostomy	—; *stoma:* opening	Creation of an opening through the abdomen into the ileum

Root	Term	Analysis	Definition
ili- (L) ilium	ilium	*ilium:* flank	The wide, upper part of the hipbone
	iliofemoral	—; *femoralis:* femur	Referring to the ilium and femur
	iliosacral	—; *sacralis:* sacrum	Pertaining to the ilium and sacrum
leuk- (G) white	leukemia	*leukos:* white *haima:* blood	Disease characterized by an extremely high leukocyte count
	leukocytosis	—; *osis:* condition, excess	Excessive increase in number of leukocytes
	leukopenia	—; *penia:* lack	Abnormal decrease in number of leukocytes
lip- (G) fat	lipectomy	*lipos:* fat *ektome:* excision	Excision of fatty tissues
	lipemia	—; *haima:* blood	Fat in the blood
lith- (G) stone	lithiasis	*lithos:* stone *iasis:* presence of	Presence of concretions or stones
	lithocystotomy	—; *kystis:* bladder *tome:* incision	Incision into the bladder to remove calculus or calculi
mening- (G) membrane	meningeal	*meninx:* membrane *al:* relating to	Related to the meninges
	meningioma	—; *oma:* tumor	Tumor of the meninges
	meningitis	—; *itis:* inflammation	Inflammation of the membranes of the spinal cord and brain
	meningococcus	—; *kokkos:* berry	Microorganism responsible for meningitis
metr- (G) uterus	metritis	*metra:* uterus *itis:* inflammation	Inflammation of the uterine musculature
	metrorrhagia	—; *regnunai:* to burst forth	Bleeding from the uterus
	metrorrhexis	—; *rhexis:* a rupture	Rupture of the uterus
my- (G) muscle	myitis or myositis	*mys:* muscle *itis:* inflammation	Inflammation of a muscle
	myocardium	—; *kardia:* heart	Heart muscle
myel- (G) marrow	myelitis	*myelos:* marrow *itis:* inflammation	Inflammation of the spinal cord or of bone marrow
	myelogenous	—; *gennan:* to produce	Originating in the marrow
	myelosarcoma	—; *sark:* flesh	Malignant tumor of the bone marrow

Root	Term	Analysis	Definition
nephr- (G) kidney	nephropexy	*nephros:* kidney *pexis:* fixation	Surgical attachment of a floating kidney
	nephrosclerosis	—; *sklerosis:* hardening	Hardening of the kidney
	nephrosis	—; *osis:* condition	Condition marked by degeneration of renal substance
ophthalm- (G) eye	ophthalmia	*ophthalmos:* eye *ia:* disease of	Severe inflammation of the eye, including the conjunctiva
	—; neonatorum	—; *neos:* new *natus:* born, birth	Purulent conjunctivitis in the newborn
	ophthalmology	—; *logos:* study	Science of the eye and its diseases
pneum- (G) lung, air	pneumococcus	*pneumon:* lung *kokkos:* berry	Microorganism causing pneumonia and other diseases
	pneumonia	—; *ia:* disease of	Inflammation of the lungs with consolidation and exudation
	pneumoperitoneum	—; *peritonaion:* peritoneum	Introduction of air into the peritoneal cavity
	pneumothorax	*pneumon:* lung *thorax:* chest	Introduction of air into the pleural cavity
proct- (G) rectum, anus	proctology	*proktos:* rectum *logos:* science	Medical specialty dealing with diseases of the rectum
	proctopexy	—; *pexis:* fixation	Suture of the rectum to some other part
	proctoscopy	—; *skopein:* examine	Instrumental examination of the rectum
psych- (G) soul, mind	psychiatry	*psyche:* mind *iatreia:* healing	Medical specialty treating mental and neurotic disorders
	psychoneurosis	—; *neuron:* nerve *osis:* disease or condition	Functional disorder of mental origin without demonstrable lesion
	psychopathy	—; *pathos:* disease	Any mental disease, usually related to defective character and personality
pyel- (G) pelvis	pyelitis	*pyelos:* pelvis *itis:* inflammation	Inflammation of the pelvis of the kidney
	pyelogram	—; *gramma:* mark	Radiograph of the ureter and renal pelvis
	pyelography	—; *graphein:* to write	Radiography of a renal pelvis and ureter

Root	Term	Analysis	Definition
pylor- (G) pylorus, gatekeeper	pylorus	*pyloros:* gatekeeper	Orifice between stomach and duodenum
	pyloromyotomy	—; *mys:* muscle *tome:* a cutting	Incision of the pyloric sphincter to relieve pyloric stenosis
	pylorostenosis	—; *stenosis:* narrowing	Constriction of pylorus
radi- (L) ray	radioactivity	*radius:* ray *activus:* acting	The ability to emit rays that can penetrate various substances
	radiosensitive	—; *sensitivus:* feeling	Capable of being destroyed by radioactive substances
	radiotherapy	—; *therapeia:* treatment	The use of radiation of any type in treating diseases
spondyl- (G) vertebra	spondylitis	*spondylos:* vertebra *itis:* inflammation	Inflammation of vertebrae
	spondylolisthesis	—; *olisthesis:* a slipping	Forward dislocation of lumbar vertebrae with pelvic deformity
	spondylosyndesis	—; *syndesis:* a binding together	Surgical formation of an ankylosis between vertebrae
trachel- (G) neck	trachelitis	*trachelos:* neck *itis:* inflammation	Inflammation of the cervix uteri
	tracheloplasty	—; *plassein:* to form	Plastic operation of the cervix uteri
	trachelorrhaphy	—; *rhaphe:* suture	Suturing of a torn cervix uteri
tubercul- (L) tubercle	tubercle	*tuberculum:* a little swelling	The lesion of tuberculosis; also, a nodular bony prominence
	tubercle bacillus	—; *bacillus:* rod	Microorganism causing tuberculosis
	tubercular	—; *aris:* akin to	Relating to a bony prominence
	tuberculoma	—; *oma:* tumor	Tuberculous tumor
	tuberculosis	—; *osis:* process	Infectious condition marked by the formation of tubercles in any tissue
	tuberculous	—; *ous:* full of	Affected with tuberculosis
viscer- (L) organ	visceral	*viscus:* organ *al:* pertaining to	Pertaining to the internal organs
	viscus	—;	Organ
	viscera	—;	Organs
	visceroptosis	—; *ptosis:* a dropping	Prolapse of the viscera; splanchnoptosis

Selected Prefixes*

Prefix	Term	Analysis	Definition
a, an- (G) without, not	anesthesia	*an:* without *aesthesis:* sensation	Loss of sensation
	apnea	*a:* without *pnoe:* breath	Temporary absence of respiration
	asthenia	—; *sthenos:* strength	Debility; loss of strength
	atresia	—; *tresis:* a perforation	Absence or closure of a normal opening or passage
ab- (L) from, away from	abductor	*ab:* away from *ductor:* that which draws	That which draws away from a common center, as a muscle
	abnormal	—; *norma:* rule	Away from or not corresponding to rule
	abruptio placentae	—; *ruptere:* break *placenta:* a flat cake	Tearing away from or premature detachment of a normally situated placenta
ad- (L) adherence, increase, near, toward	adductor	*ad:* toward *ductor:* that which draws	That which draws toward a common center
	adhesion	*ad:* to *haerere:* to stick	Abnormal joining of surfaces to each other
	adrenal	*ad:* near *ren:* kidney	Ductless gland above the kidney
ante- (L) before	anteflexion	*ante:* forward *flectere:* to bend	Forward displacement of an organ; for example, the uterus
	antenatal	—; *natus:* birth	Before birth
	antepartum	—; *partum:* labor	Before the onset of labor
anti- (G) against	antipyretic	*anti-:* against —; *pyretos:* fever	Drug that reduces fever
	antisepsis	—; *sepsis:* putrefaction	The exclusion of putrefactive germs
	antitoxin	—; *toxikon:* poison	Protein that defends the body against a toxin
bi- (L) two, both, double	biceps	*bis:* two *caput:* head	Two-headed
	—; brachii	—; *brachii:* arm	Muscle of the upper arm having two heads
	—; femoris biconvex	—; *femoris:* thigh —; *convexus:* rounded surface	Muscle of the thigh Having two convex surfaces, as in a lens
co-, con- (L) together, with	congenital defect	*con:* with *genitus:* born *defectus:* imperfection	Born with a defect; hereditary
	conjunctiva	—; *jungere:* to join	Mucous membrane that lines eyelids
	connective tissue	*con:* together *nectere:* to bind	Tissue that connects or binds together

*NOTE: The dash and semicolon refer to the prefix that has already been given.

Prefix	Term	Analysis	Definition
contra- (L) against, opposite	contraception	*contra:* against, *concipere:* to conceive	The prevention of conception
	contraindication	—; *indicare:* to point out	Condition antagonistic to a type of treatment
	contralateral	*contra:* opposite *latus:* side	Affecting the opposite side of the body
ec- (G) out	ectropion of eyelid, cervix uteri	*ek:* out *trepein:* to turn *cervix:* neck *uteri:* of womb	Eversion, as of the edge of the eyelid, or the turning out of the cervical canal of the uterus
ecto- (G) outside	ectopic pregnancy	*ecto:* outside *topos:* place *prae:* before *natus:* birth	Gestation outside the uterine cavity
em-, en- (G) in	empyema	*em:* in *pyon:* pus	Pus in a body cavity, especially in the pleural cavity
	encephalopathy	*en:* in *kephale:* head *pathos:* disease	Any disease of the brain
endo- (G) within	endocardium	*endon:* within *kardia:* heart	Membrane lining the inner surface of the heart
	endocrine gland	—; *krinein:* to secrete *glans:* gland	Ductless gland in which forms an internal secretion
epi- (G) upon, at, in addition to	epidermis	*epi:* upon *derma:* skin	Cuticle or outer layer of the skin
	epigastrium	—; *gaster:* stomach	Region over the pit of the stomach
	epiphysis	*epi:* at *physis:* a growing upon	Center of ossification at both extremities of long bones
ex- (L, G) out, away from, over	exacerbation	*ex:* over *acerbus:* harsh	Aggravation of symptoms
	exeresis	*ex:* out *eiresis:* taking	Excision of any part
hemi- (G) half	hemigastrectomy	*hemi:* half —; *gaster:* stomach *ektome:* excision	Removal of half of the stomach
	hemiglossectomy	—; *glossa:* tongue —;	Removal of half of the tongue
hyper- (G) above, excessive, beyond	hyperacidity	*hyper:* excessive *acidus:* sour	Excess of acid in the stomach
	hyperadrenalism	—; *ad:* near *ren:* kidney *ismos:* state of	Excess of adrenal secretion

Prefix	Term	Analysis	Definition
hypo- (G) beneath, below, deficient	hypochondriac region	hypo: beneath chondros: cartilage regio: area	Part of abdomen beneath the ribs
	hypoglycemia	hypo: deficient glykys: sugar haima: blood	Low blood sugar
infra- (L) beneath, below	infracostal	infra: below costa: ribs	Below the ribs
	infrasternal	infra: below sternon: sternum	Below the sternum
inter- (L) between	interannular	inter: between annulus: ring	Situated between two rings or constrictions
	interarticular	inter: between articulus: joint	Situated between articular surfaces
intra- (L) within	intracordal	intra: within cor: heart	Within the heart
	intrapyretic	intra: within pyrexia: fever	During the stages of fever
iso- (G) equal, alike, same	isocellular	isos: same cellula: cell	Composed of same kinds of cells
	isocytosis	isos: equal kytos: cell osis: condition	Equality of the size of cells
meso- (G) middle, intermediate	mesoderm	meso: middle derma: skin	Middle layer of skin
	mesotarsal	meso: middle tarsalis: tarsal	Midtarsal
pan- (G) all	panarthritis	pan: all arthron: joint itis: inflammation of	Inflammation of all joints
	pancolectomy	pan: all kolon: colon ektome: removal	Removal of entire colon with creation of an ileostomy
para, par- (G) beside, around, near, abnormal	paracentesis	para: beside kentesis: a puncture	Puncture of a cavity with tapping
	parametrium	para: around metra: uterus	Fat and connective tissue around the uterus
peri (G) around, about	pericardium	peri: around kardia: heart	The double membranous sac enclosing the heart
	pericarditis	—; —; itis: inflammation	Inflammation of the pericardium
	perimetrium	—; metra: womb	Peritoneum covering the uterus
	perimetritis	—; —; itis: inflammation	Inflammation of the peritoneum covering of the uterus

Prefix	Term	Analysis	Definition
post- (L) after, behind	postembryonic	*post:* after *embryon:* embryo	Occurring after the embryonic stage
	postprandial	*post:* after *prandium:* breakfast	Occurring after a meal
pre- (L) before, in front of	precancerous	*prae:* before *cancer:* crab	Before the development of carcinoma
	precordium	—; *cor:* heart	Region over the heart
	preeclampsia	—; *ek:* out *lampein:* to flash	Eclampsia before delivery (Eclampsia is a major toxemia during pregnancy)
	prepatellar bursitis	*prae:* in front of *patella:* kneecap *bursa:* sac *itis:* inflammation	Inflammation of the bursa in front of the patella (housemaid's knee)
	presentation	*praesentatio:* a placing before	Manner in which fetus is presented at the cervix
pro- (L, G) in front of, before, forward	procidentia	*procidentia:* a falling forward	Complete prolapse, especially of the uterus
	prognosis	*pro:* before *gnosis:* a knowing	Prediction of the probable outcome of a disease
	prolapse	*pro:* forward *lapsus:* slide	A downward displacement of an organ, as the rectum or the uterus
retro- (L) backward, behind, back of	retroflexion	*retro:* backward *flexio:* a bending	Bending or flexing backward; as of the uterus
	retrogasserian neurotomy	*retro:* back of *gasserian:* pertaining to a ganglion *neuron:* nerve *tome:* incision into	Transection of the posterior root of the retrogasserian ganglion
	retroperitoneal	*retro:* behind *peritonaion:* peritoneum	Located behind the peritoneum
	retroversion	*retro:* backward *versio:* a turning	State of being turned back; as of the uterus
semi- (L) half	semicircular canal	*semi:* half *circulus:* a ring *canal:* a channel	One of the three canals in the labyrinth of the ear
	semicoma	—; *koma:* lethargy	Mild degree of coma
	semilunar valves	—; *luna:* moon *valva:* one leaf of a double door	Half-moon–shaped valves of the aorta and pulmonary arteries
sub- (L) under, beneath, below	subclavicular	*sub:* beneath *clavicular:* a little key	Beneath the clavicle (collarbone)
	subcostal	—; *costa:* rib	Beneath the ribs
	subcutaneous	—; *cutis:* skin	Beneath the skin
	subinvolution	—; *involutio:* a turning into	Failure of the uterus to reduce to normal size after childbirth

Prefix	Term	Analysis	Definition
super-, *supra-* (L) above, beyond, superior	supernatant	*super:* above *natare:* to float	Floating on the surface
	supraoccipital	—; *occiput:* back part of the skull	Situated above the occiput
	suprapubic cystotomy	—; *pubis:* bone of pelvis *kystis:* bladder *tome:* incision	Surgical opening into the bladder from above the symphysis pubis
	suprarenal	—; *ren:* kidney *al:* pertaining to	Adrenal gland above the kidney
sym-, *syn-* (G) with, along, together, beside	symphysis pubis	*sym:* together *physis:* a growing	Fusion of pubic bones on midline anteriorly
	synarthrosis	*syn:* together *arthron:* joint *osis:* condition	Immovable joint
	syndactylism	*daktylos:* digit, finger *ismos:* condition	Fusion of two or more fingers or toes; webbing
trans- (L) across, over	transection	*trans:* across *sectio:* cutting	Incision across the long axis; cross section
	transfusion	—; *fusio:* a pouring	Injection of the blood of one person into the blood vessels of another
	transurethral prostatectomy	—; *ourethra:* urethra *prostates:* prostate *ektome:* excision	Excision of the prostate gland through the urethra
tri- (G) three	tricuspid	*tres, tria:* three *cuspis:* a point	Having three cusps or points; tricuspid valve
	trifacial	—; *facialis:* facial	Fifth cranial nerve
	trigone	*trigonon:* a three-cornered figure	A triangular space, especially that of the lower part of the urinary bladder
uni- (L) one	uniarticular	*unus:* one *articulus:* joint	Pertaining to a single joint
	unicellular	—; *cellula:* cell	Made up of a single cell

Combining Form Word Elements

Combining form word elements results when a vowel, usually a, i, e, or o, is added to the word root or base. The vowels most commonly used as combining forms are a, i, or o. Listed below are examples of selected combining form word elements.

Selected Combining Form Word Elements and Definitions

angi(o)- (G) vessel	anthrop(o)- (G) human being, man	blenn(o)- (G) mucus	celi(o)- (G) belly, abdomen
anis(o)- (G) unequal, uneven, dissimilar	arthr(o)- (G) joint(s)	carcin(o)- (G) cancer	cephal(o)- (G) head

Selected Combining Form Word Elements and Definitions

chlor(o)-
(G)
green

chrom(o)-
(G)
color

colp(o)-
(G)
vagina

duoden(o)-
(L)
duodenum

enter(o)-
(G)
intestine(s)

fibr(o)-
(L)
fiber(s)

galact(o)-
(G)
milk

gam(o)-
(G)
marriage,
sexual union

gangli(o)-
(G)
ganglion

gastr(o)-
(G)
stomach

geni(o)-
(G)
chin

ger(o)-
(G)
old age,
aged

glyc(o)-
(G)
sweet,
sugar,
glucose

gon(o)-
(G)
semen,
seed

gynec(o)-
(G)
woman,
female
reproductive
organ(s)

gyr(o)-
(G)
circle,
gyrus

hal(o)-
(G)
salt

hamart(o)-
(G)
defect

hemat(o)-
(G)
blood

heter(o)-
(G)
different,
other,
abnormal

hist(o)-
(G)
tissue, web

hydr(o)-
(G)
water

kary(o)-
(G)
nucleus,
kernel,
nut

kerat(o)-
(G)
cornea,
horn

kinesi(o)-
(G)
movement

mening(o)-
(G)
membrane

micr(o)-
(G)
small

mon(o)-
(G)
one,
single

neur(o)-
(G)
nerve(s)

olig(o)-
(G)
little,
scanty

onc(o)-
(G)
tumor,
swelling,
mass

oophor(o)-
(G)
ovary,
bearing eggs

oste(o)-
(G)
bone(s)

ov(o)-
(L)
egg(s)

pulmon(o)-
(L)
lung

py(o)-
(G)
pus

pyel(o)-
(G)
pelvis
of the
kidney

pyret(o)-
(G)
fever

rachi(o)-
(G)
spine

rect(o)-
(L)
rectum

ren(o)-
(L)
kidney

rhin(o)-
(G)
nose

sapr(o)-
(G)
rotten,
decay

sarc(o)-
(G)
flesh

schiz(o)-
(G)
division

scot(o)-
(G)
darkness

strept(o)-
(G)
twisted

PLEASE NOTE: The parentheses surrounding the vowel in the above examples have been deleted from the combining form word elements that appear in the "Origin of Terms" sections throughout the book, as well as in the "Review Guide" sections of the text.

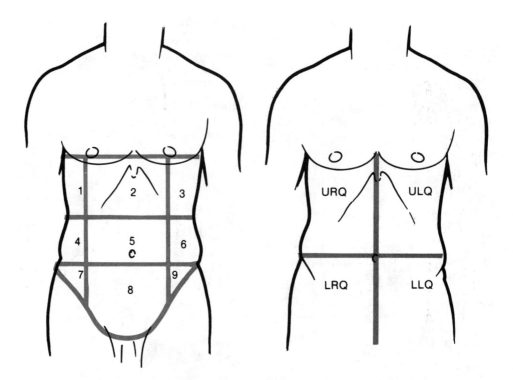

Figure 1 Abdomen divided into nine regions by two horizontal planes (subcostal and transtubercular or intertubercular) and two sagittal planes (left and right lateral, through the midinguinal points).

Figure 2 Abdomen divided into four quadrants by one horizontal and one vertical (median plane).

Terms Pertaining to the Body as a Whole
Anatomic Division of the Abdomen (Fig. 1)
hypochondriac regions (upper lateral regions beneath the ribs) .... 1 and 3
epigastric region (region of the pit of the stomach) 2
lumbar regions (middle lateral regions) .... 4 and 6
umbilical region (region of the navel) 5
inguinal regions (lower lateral regions) .... 7 and 9
hypogastric region (region below the umbilicus) 8

Clinical Division of the Abdomen (Fig. 2)
upper right quadrant .... URQ
upper left quadrant .... ULQ
lower right quadrant .... LRQ
lower left quadrant .... LLQ

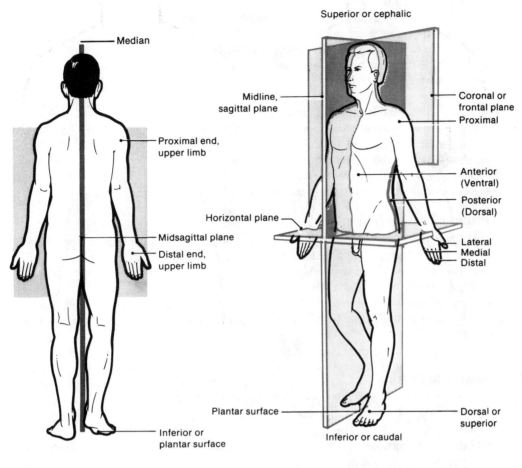

Figure 3 Posterior view of body   **Figure 4** Directional planes of body

Anatomic Division of the Back

cervical region .... neck
thoracic region .... chest
lumbar region .... loin
sacral region .... sacrum

Position and Direction

afferent — conducting toward a structure.
anterior or ventral — front of the body (not synonymous in lower limb).
central — toward the center.

deep — away from the surface.

distal or peripheral — away from the beginning of a structure; away from the center.

efferent — conducting away from a structure.

inferior or caudal — away from the head; situated below another structure.*

intermediate — between median and lateral.

lateral — toward the side.*

medial — toward the median plane.*

median — in the middle of a structure.

posterior or dorsal — back of the body (not synonymous in lower limb). (See Fig. 3 for posterior view of body.)

proximal — toward the beginning of a structure.

superficial — near the surface.

superior or cephalic — toward the head; situated above another structure.*

Planes of the Body (Fig. 4)

frontal or coronal — vertical plane parallel to the coronal suture of the skull. It divides the body or structure into anterior and posterior portions.

horizontal — plane parallel to the horizon.

longitudinal — plane parallel to the long axis of the structure.

median — lengthwise plane that divides the body or structure into right and left halves.

sagittal — any vertical plane parallel to the sagittal suture of the skull and the median plane.

transverse — plane at a right angle to the long axis of a structure.

Anatomic Position

Anatomists all over the world apply anatomic terms to the body as though it were in what is known as the anatomic position. In this position, the body is erect, the eyes look straight to the front, the upper limbs hang at the sides with palms facing forward, and the lower limbs are parallel with the toes pointing forward. Whether the body lies face upward or downward, or in any other position, the positions and relationships of structure are always described as if the body were in the anatomic position.

---

*Refer to section on "Anatomic Positions."

References and Bibliography

1. Dorland's *Illustrated Medical Dictionary,* 27th ed. Philadelphia: W.B. Saunders Co., 1988.
2. Logan, Carolynn M., and Rice, M. Katherine *Logan's Medical and Scientific Abbreviations,* Philadelphia: J.B. Lippincott Co., 1987.
3. Stedman's *Medical Dictionary Illustrated,* 24th ed. Baltimore: Williams & Wilkins, 1982.
4. Taber's *Cyclopedia Medical Dictionary,* 15th ed. Philadelphia: F.A. Davis Co., 1985.

CHAPTER 2

Disorders of the Skin and Breast

Skin

Origin of Terms

cutis (L)—skin
cryo- (G)—cold
cyan-, cyano- (G)—blue
derma-, dermat-, dermato-, dermo-, (G)—skin
erythema (G)—flush
hidro- (G)—sweat
kerato- (G)—horny, tissue, cornea
leuko- (F)—white
macula (L)—spot, stain
melano- (G)—black, melanin

onych-, onycho- (G)—nail
papula- (L)—pimple
phyto- (G)—plant
pilo- (L)—hair
pruritus (L)—itching
pyo- (G)—pus
sclero- (G)—hard
squama (L)—scale
sudor (L)—sweat
tinea (L)—worm
vesico- (L)—blister, bladder

Anatomic Terms (Refs. 5, 14, 31, 34)

- *corium*—the true skin or deeper layer containing blood vessels, lymphatics, hair follicles, nerve endings, connective tissue fibers, and sweat and sebaceous glands.
- *derma, dermis*—synonymous with corium.
- *epidermis*—cuticle or outer layer of the skin.
- *epithelium*—the layers of cells covering the surface of the body, external as well as internal.
- *integument*—the skin, composed of the corium and epidermis.
- *pigment*—a coloring substance. (See Fig. 5.)
- *pilosebaceous*—pertaining to hair and oil glands.
- *sebaceous glands*—oil glands of the skin.
- *sebum*—oily substance secreted by sebaceous glands.
- *subcutaneous tissue*—layer of loose, connective tissue containing fat.
- *sudoriferous glands*—sweat glands.

Diagnostic Terms

- *acne*—any inflammatory condition of the sebaceous glands. The more common forms are:
    - *acne conglobata*—severe cystic process of acne with the appearance of multiple deep cysts, sinus tracts, and erythematous papules.
    - *acne pomade*—seen mostly in the black population. The pomade lesions are of the blackhead type and are usually found packed together around the hairline, scalp, and forehead.
    - *acne rosacea, simple rosacea*—condition characterized by thickened skin, especially on the nose, due to hypertrophy of sebaceous glands.
    - *acne vulgaris*—a common form of acne, marked by papules, pustules, and comedones. (35, 37, 39)

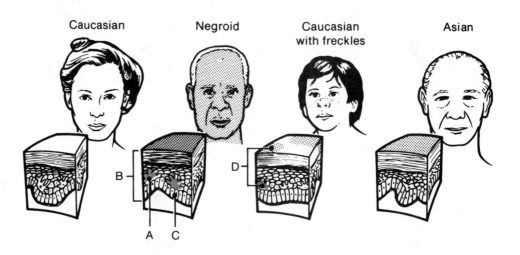

Figure 5 Skin-coloring process. Skin coloring is caused by production of the pigment melanin from melanocyte cells (A) in the epidermis layer of the skin (B). Although people of all races have equal melanocyte numbers, their genetic variations control the amount of melanin introduced into the cells. These cells are manufactured in the germinative layer (C). Ultraviolet rays of the sun play a key role in melanin production. The melanin absorbs these rays, and as a result, the skin becomes tanned or sunburned. Freckles result when only some of the melanocyte cells (D) manufacture melanin.

- *albinism*—congenital lack of normal skin pigment. (14)
- *alopecia*—loss of hair; baldness. (2, 37)
- *angioedema, angioneurotic edema, Quincke's edema*—diffuse swelling of the loose tissues of the face, eyelids, lips, tongue, larynx, gastrointestinal tract, and other areas. (28)
- *atopic skin disorders*—allergic skin conditions such as angioedema, urticaria, atopic drug reactions, and food allergy in atopic dermatitis. Atopy or allergy tends to be of the familial type. (17, 34, 37)
- *burn*—the effect of exposure to heat, chemicals, electricity, or sunshine.
    - *first degree*—redness or hyperemia involving superficial layers of skin.
    - *second degree*—blisters or vesication involving deeper layers of skin.
    - *third degree*—destruction involving any tissue below the skin. (2, 10)
- *callositas, keratosis*—a circumscribed thickening and hypertrophy of the horny cells of the epidermis. (37)

- *carbuncle*—a circumscribed inflammation of the skin and deeper tissue causing necrosis and suppuration. (14, 15)
- *cellulitis*—inflammation of skin and subcutaneous tissue with or without formation of pus. (11, 37)
- *decubitus ulcer, bedsore, pressure sore*—an ulcer that develops in an area where the skin covers a bony prominence and is damaged by continuous pressure, impoverished circulation, and nutrition. (5)
- *dermatitis*—inflammation of the skin. Some common forms are:
    - —*contact dermatitis, dermatitis venenata*—inflammatory reaction to an irritant or a sensitizer; for example, poison ivy, ragweed, metal, chemical, rubber, and others. (13, 37)
    - —*exfoliative dermatitis*—exfoliation or scaling off of dead skin, associated with crust formation, generalized redness, and edema. (37)
    - —*stasis dermatitis*—brown, mottled hyperpigmentation. There may be evidence of scaling, thinning of the epidermis, pitting edema, varicosities, venous insufficiency, and ulceration. It is found most frequently on the skin over the medial malleolus. Stasis dermatitis may appear bilaterally. (11, 40)
- *dermatophytosis*—superficial fungus infection (mycosis) that is readily transmitted from person to person; attacks the skin, nails, and hair; thrives in moisture; and is caused by dermatophytes. (9)
    - —*Epidermophyton*—fungus that infects the skin.
    - —*Microsporum*—fungus that is found in the skin and hair.
    - —*Trichophyton*—fungus that attacks the skin, nails, and hair.
- *dermatophytosis of foot, epidermophytosis, tinea pedis, athlete's foot*—parasitic or fungal infection, chiefly affecting the skin between the toes and associated with intense itching, sogginess, fissures, small blisters, and scaling of skin. (9, 34)
- *eczema*—cutaneous inflammatory condition producing red papular and vesicular lesions, crusts, and scales. (37)
- *epidermolysis bullosa, acantholysis bullosa, Goldschneider's disease*—hereditary condition characterized by dissolution of the layers of the skin and blister formation in response to slight irritation. (27, 34, 37)
- *erysipelas, St. Anthony's fire*—a tender, erythematous area with sharp margin, with or without vesicle or bulla formation. The face and lower limbs are the most involved areas of the skin. (6, 37)
- *gangrene*—a form of necrosis or putrefaction of tissue.
    - —*diabetic gangrene*—associated with diabetes mellitus.
    - —*embolic gangrene*—caused by circulatory obstruction caused by embolus.
    - —*gas gangrene*—resulting from infection with bacillus *Clostridium perfringens*, an anaerobic microorganism. (27)
- *leukoderma*—white patches of skin due to local absence of pigment.
- *lichen planus*—inflammatory condition of skin and mucous membrane characterized by small, flat papules that appear shiny, dry, and violet in color. Linear, annular, and irregular patches are found on neck, wrists, and thighs. (24, 37)
- *lupus vulgaris*—a type of cutaneous tuberculosis, marked by reddish brown patches in which tiny nodules are embedded.
- *melanoderma*—abnormal brown or black pigmentation of the skin.
- *onychia*—inflammation of the nail bed.
- *paronychia*—infected skin around the nail. (22, 37)
- *pediculosis*—infestation with lice. (33)
- *pemphigus*—skin disease characterized by the appearance of crops of bullae of various sizes. (20, 21, 27, 37)

- *psoriasis*—eruption appearing in circular patches of various sizes and showing a definite line of demarcation. Remissions and exacerbations are common. (22, 24, 34, 37)
- *pyoderma*—bacterial infection affecting:
    - *the skin (22)*
        - *impetigo contagiosa*—infectious skin disease characterized by discrete vesicles that change to pustules and crusts; appear in crops, usually on the face; and are caused by staphylococci and streptococci. (15, 37)
        - *pyoderma faciale*—cyanotic or reddish erythema associated with deep or superficial cystic lesions or abscesses. (22, 43)
    - *pilosebaceous apparatus (hair and oil glands), causing:*
        - *furunculosis*—purulent infection of hair follicles usually by *Staphylococcus aureus*, which may result in necrosis of hair follicles and formation of furunculoid abscesses.
        - *staphylococcic folliculitis*—intradermal pustules surrounding hair follicles, usually due to *Staphylococcus aureus*. (15, 37)
- *rhinophyma*—red, large, nodular hypertrophic masses around the tip and wings of the nose; seen in men past 40 years of age.
- *scabies*—contagious skin condition caused by the mite *Sarcoptes scabiei*, which lays her eggs in burrows under the skin, causing an intensely pruritic, vesicular eruption between the fingers, folds of axillae, buttocks, under the breasts, and in other areas. (33, 37)
- *steatoma*—sebaceous cyst.
- *tinea*—any fungal skin disease, frequently caused by ringworms.
    - *tinea barbae, tinea sycosis*—ringworm of the beard.
    - *tinea capitis, tinea tonsurans*—ringworm of the scalp, forming bold circular patches.
    - *tinea corporis, tinea circinata*—ringworm of the body, usually noted by ring-shaped eruptions, scaling, vesiculation, and itching. It is transmitted by animal contact.
    - *tinea pedis*—athlete's foot. (37)
    - *tinea unguium, onychomycosis*—ringworm of the nails, especially toe nails, causing thickening and scaling under the nail plate. (37)
- *tumors of the skin*—new growths of skin.
    - *angiosarcoma*—extremely aggressive malignant tumor arising from the vascular structures within the skin. The lesions have a highly metastatic potential. (6, 37)
    - *basal cell carcinoma of the skin*—present on sun-exposed skin as a small papule area, which in time forms a pearly, translucent surface. Lesions grow slowly. The large lesions may have a telangiectasia, which is a rolled, raised border with a depressed center. (34, 37)
    - *keloid*—new growth of scar tissue. (23)
    - *keratoacanthoma*—rapidly growing nodule arising from the epidermis and containing a horn-filled crater; usually a benign lesion. (6, 19)
    - *nevus, mole, birthmark*—congenital pigmentation of a circumscribed area of the skin. (8, 9, 30)
    - *seborrheic keratosis, basal cell papilloma*—a benign superficial, epithelial tumor; few or many in number; light tan to black in color (depending on melanin content); characterized by horny overgrowth (hyperkeratosis); primarily occurring in middle-aged and elderly persons. (6, 19)

- *ulcer*—break in the skin or mucous membrane resulting from varicose veins or other causes. (37)
- *urticaria, hives, nettle rash*—skin eruption of pale or reddish wheals, usually associated with intense itching. May occur as an acute self-limited episode caused by food allergy, drug reaction, or emotional stress or in chronic form as a characteristic feature of rheumatic and connective tissue disorders. (28, 37, 42)

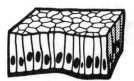
A. Simple columnar

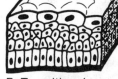
B. Transitional

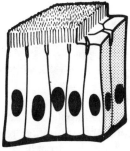
C. Ciliated columnar

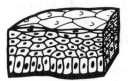
D. Stratified squamous

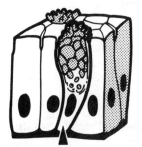
E. Goblet cell
Located in
simple columnar
epithelium

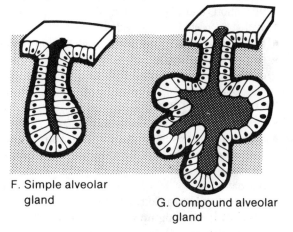
F. Simple alveolar
gland

G. Compound alveolar
gland

Figure 6 Various types of simple epithelium (A, B, C, D) and glands (E, F, G).

Operative Terms

- *cryosurgery of skin*—freezing the skin with liquid nitrogen or solid carbon dioxide to destroy a lesion. (6)
- *curettage of skin*—removal of superficial lesions with a skin curette. (6)
- *dermabrasion*—surgical removal of nevi or scars using sandpaper or other abrasives. (37)

- *electrodesiccation*—the use of short, high-frequency electric sparks for drying cells and tissues. (6)
- *electrosurgical excision of burn*—excision of full-thickness burn using the electrosurgical unit at the level of the fascia. The procedure leaves a dry fascial bed for immediate grafting.
- *fulguration of skin*—the use of long, high-frequency electric sparks for destroying tissue.
- *incision and drainage of infected skin lesion.* (11)
- *laser surgery*—devices that generate light amplification by stimulated emission radiation. Laser light lies in the infrared and visible light portions of the electromagnetic spectrum. Two lasers that have broad application in dermatology are the argon laser and the carbon dioxide laser. The argon laser penetrates 1 to 2 mm in tissue depth and produces considerable scatter to the tissue. The carbon dioxide laser penetrates 0.1 to 0.2 mm in tissue depth and produces minimal scatter to the tissue.
  - —Argon laser is used for:
    - –treatment of port wine hemangiomas
    - –destruction of blood vessel lesions, hemangiomas, senile angiomas, pyogenic granulomas, telangiectasia, melanin-containing lesions, nevi, café-au-lait spots, and seborrheic keratoses.
  - —Carbon dioxide laser is used for:
    - –removal of benign and malignant tumors
    - –debridement of burns and decubitus ulcers
    - –removal of viral verrucae, actinic keratosis, and leukoplakia. (32)
- *Linton flap procedure*—operation for stasis dermatitis and ulceration refractory. All incompetent communicating veins are ligated and divided to relieve ambulatory venous hypertension in superficial veins. This prevents progression of dermatitis, ulceration, and pigmentation of overlying skin in the lower limb.
- *local excision of skin lesion.* (1)
- *plastic operation on skin*—surgical correction of defect.
- *skin grafting*—transfer of skin from a normal area to cover denuded areas. A dermatome may be used to obtain these skin transplants. (11)

Symptomatic Terms

- *anular (annular)*—ring-shaped. (14, 34)
- *café-au-lait spots*—light brown, flat spots, variable in shape and size, seen in neurofibromatosis (von Recklinghausen's disease). (1, 34)
- *chloasma*—patches of brown or yellowish pigmentation on skin that is otherwise normal. (34)
- *cicatrix of skin*—scar left by a healed wound.
- *cicatrization*—healing by scar formation.
- *comedo (pl. comedones), blackhead*—excretory duct of skin plugged by discolored sebum. (39)
- *confluent*—lesions joined or run together.
- *depigmentation*—partial or complete loss of pigment; occurs in albinism, atrophic skin, and scars.
- *dermatographism, dermographia*—skin writing. Urticarial wheals appear where skin was marked by pencil or blunt instrument. (14, 28)
- *discoid*—shaped like a disk. (14)
- *discrete*—lesions that are disconnected and separate from one another.
- *ecchymosis (pl. ecchymoses)*—purple spot or bruise caused by seepage of blood into the skin. (14, 26)

- *eczematoid, eczematous*—eczema-like inflammatory lesion that tends to thicken and become scaly, vesicular, crusty, or weeping. (34, 37)
- *eruption*—rash or skin lesion.
- *erythema*—diffuse redness of skin. (4, 14, 34, 43)
- *excoriation*—linear break of skin or scratch mark resulting from surface trauma.
- *granulation*—method of repair or healing following loss of tissue or pyogenic infection.
- *guttate*—droplike. (14)
- *keratotic*—pertaining to a horny thickening. (14)
- *hyperpigmentation*—the presence of an abnormal amount of pigment in the skin; seen in a number of systemic diseases, such as adrenal insufficiency, acromegaly, and others. In the familial progressive type of hyperpigmentation, patches of excessive pigmentation enlarge in size with increasing age. (14)
- *intertriginous*—between two folds of skin. (37)
- *macule*—discolored patch or spot on the skin. (14)
- *milia (sing. milium)*—tiny white nodules appearing on the skin, frequently below the eyes.
- *moniliform*—beaded.
- *multiform*—several forms of a skin lesion.
- *papule*—pimple. (14)
- *petechiae*—pin-sized hemorrhagic spots in the skin. (14, 26)
- *proliferation*—process of rapid reproduction of similar cells.
- *pustule*—small elevation of the skin containing pus or lymph. (14, 34)
- *seborrheal, seborrheic*—pertaining to seborrhea, an oversecretion of sebaceous glands. (34)

Breasts

Origin of Terms

areola (L)—a small area or space
-gram (G)—a writing, a mark
grapho- (G)—writing, record
-graphy (G)—to write or record
hyper- (G)—above, excessive; beyond
hypo- (G)—beneath, below; deficient
lacto- (L)—milk

mamma- (L)—breast
mammo- (G)—breast
mast-, masto, (G)—breast
-pexy (G)—suspension, fixation
-plasty (G)—surgical correction or formation
thele- (G)—nipple

Anatomic Terms (4, 7, 41)

- *areola*—area of pigmented skin surrounding the nipple. It becomes dark during pregnancy and remains so thereafter.
- *mammary gland*—glandular tissue of the breast composed of 15 to 20 compound alveolar lobes, each connected with the nipple by a lactiferous duct.
- *papilla mammae*—the nipple.

Diagnostic Terms

- *abscess of breast, mammary abscess*—localized collection of pus in mammary tissue.
- *amastia*—absence of a breast. (16)
- *athelia*—absence of a breast nipple.
- *breast cancer*—malignant mammary tumor, a painless or painful mass that may be associated with skin and muscle attachment, discharge, crusting, and retraction of

nipple, changes in contour of affected breast; and metastasis to regional lymph nodes. (Contrary to past belief that the breast cancer spreads from the primary tumor to the lymph nodes and then to other distant sites, the malignant tumor may bypass lymph nodes and spread directly to the bloodstream. Thus the malignant tumor may appear as a metastasis without evidence of a primary tumor, giving rise to the consideration of breast cancer as a systemic disease.) (1, 2, 3, 7)

- *chronic cystic mastitis*—describes a family of lesions found in the breast. These include papillomatosis, blunt duct adenosis, periductal mastitis, fat necrosis, hyperplasia of duct epithelium, and fibroadenoma. Mastitis first appears in the late twenties age range, with increased evidence in the thirties and forties. Cysts may vary in size. (16, 37)
- *fissure of nipple*—a deep furrow in the nipple.
- *hyperplasia of breast, hypermastia*—abnormally large breast, usually pendulous and sagging.
- *hypoplasia of breast, hypomastia*—abnormally small breast.
    —*unilateral hypomastia*—one breast underdeveloped, with the other normal or overdeveloped. This results in mammary asymmetry and disfigurement.
    —*bilateral hypomastia*—both breasts are abnormally small.
- *occlusion of lactiferous ducts*—blockage of lumen of milk-conveying ducts.
- *Paget's disease of nipple*—cancer directly beneath the nipple, seen in elderly women. Areola, nipple, and surrounding skin may be weeping and eczematoid. (16, 19)
- *thelitis*—inflammation of the nipple.
- *tuberculosis of breast*—the breast is rarely infected by tubercle bacilli. The presenting lump may be mistaken for cancer or as sinuses discharging purulent material. Breast tuberculosis appears to be secondary to tuberculosis of the internal mammary lymph nodes. (37)

Operative Terms

- *biopsy of breast*—excision of small piece of mammary tissue for diagnostic evaluation. (16)
- *frozen section*—microscopic study of slides prepared with fresh tissue of a lesion. It is valuable for rapid diagnosis while the patient awaits surgery to determine the need for a conservative approach, if the tissue section shows a benign lesion; or a radical approach, if a malignant lesion is found. (16)
- *incisional biopsy*—tissue of lesion obtained for pathologic verification. This procedure is indicated when the tumor mass is very large. Otherwise excisional biopsy is the method of choice.
- *mammaplasty, mammoplasty, mastoplasty*—surgical reconstruction of a breast. (16)
    —*augmentation mammaplasty*—implantation of a retromammary prosthesis for an underdeveloped breast.
    —*reduction mammaplasty*—repair of an overdeveloped, pendulous breast by partial removal of the mammary gland and fixation of the breast to its normal position. (3, 16, 18, 25)
- *mastectomy, mammectomy*—removal of a breast.
    —*modified radical mastectomy*—consists of an en bloc removal of the breast with the underlying pectoralis major fascia (but not muscle) and axillary lymph nodes. Modified radical mastectomy provides much better cosmetic and functional outcome compared to the standard radical mastectomy.
    —*radical mastectomy*—removal of an entire breast, including axillary dissection and surgical division of pectoralis major and minor muscles.
    —*segmental mastectomy*—quadrant excision, partial mastectomy, or lumpectomy may be another option available for consideration. An additional option may be

to use radiation therapy with segmental mastectomy.

—*simple mastectomy*—removal of a breast without dissection of axillary lymph nodes. (7, 16, 25)

- *mastopexy*—surgical fixation of a pendulous breast.
- *mastotomy*—incision and drainage of a breast abscess.

Symptomatic Terms

- *mastalgia, mastodynia*—breast pain occurring in premenstrual period, mastitis, breast cancer, and other disorders.
- *peau d'orange*—skin simulating orange peel; seen in inflammatory breast cancer. (14)
- *skin retraction*—dimpling and puckering of skin caused by benign or malignant lesions underneath. (3)

Abbreviations

General

BP—blood pressure
CC—chief complaint
Dx—diagnosis
FH—family history
FS—frozen section

MH—marital history
PH—past history
PI—present illness
TPR—temperature, pulse, and respiration

Coding Systems and Nomenclatures

CPHA—Commission on Professional Hospital Activities
CPT—Common Procedural Terminology
ICD-9-CM—International Classification of Diseases, 9th Revision, Clinical Modification
SNDO—Standard Nomenclature of Diseases and Operations

Paramedical Organizations

AAPA—American Academy of Physicians' Assistants
AART—American Association for Respiratory Therapy
ADA—American Dietetic Association
AMRA—American Medical Record Association
APAP—Association of Physician Assistant Programs
APTA—American Physical Therapy Association
ASHP—American Society of Hospital Pharmacists
ASRT—American Society of Radiologic Technologists

Oral Reading Practice

Pemphigus

There are several forms of **dermatitis** in which a **bullous eruption** develops, but they are distinguished from true bullous diseases by a short duration and good prognosis.

The term **pemphigus,** derived from the Greek **pemphix,** "blister," points up the chief characteristic of **pemphigus vulgaris,** namely, the formation of blisters. These **blebs** arise suddenly on apparently normal or slightly **erythematous** skin and form oval-shaped or round blisters containing clear **serum.** The blisters tend to be **flaccid** and break easily. The **epidermis** becomes detached, leaving increasingly larger areas of

denudation. The **Nikolsky sign** is always positive. It is obtained by pressing on the skin with the fingertip. The epidermis then slides off, and a raw surface remains. The **denuded** areas are slow in healing and constitute a continuous threat of infection.

Pemphigus has been compared to a serious burn, but the trauma of a burn is a single occasion and the lesion is frequently localized. On the other hand, the injury inflicted on the skin by numerous crops of **bullae** followed by widespread denudation presents a still more serious problem than that of many burns. The blisters vary in size from a few **millimeters** in diameter to 10 **centimeters.** New lesions develop as old ones disappear. Since the crops arise rapidly, often overnight, and old lesions heal slowly, the areas of denudation are extensive. Eventually, crusts form over the raw surface. If **pyogenic bacteria** get beneath these crusts, foul-smelling pus collects and increases the patient's physical distress. There is no scarring; only a **hyperpigmented** lesion remains after healing. The formation of bullae in the **oral cavity** is particularly painful. Blebs about five millimeters in diameter are scattered over the **buccal mucosa.** They appear spontaneously, rupture, and leave new, painful ulcers. Blebs may also occur on other orificial mucous membranes.

The etiology of pemphigus is still unknown. Some authorities believe that it is metabolic in nature or caused by **bacterial** or **viral** infections; however, no theory has yielded convincing evidence.

The common type of pemphigus is a chronic, recurrent disease, afflicting only adults. Acute **exacerbations** may be followed by brief or prolonged periods of remission. As a rule pemphigus vulgaris lasts from several months to years. Untreated, it is a fatal disease, but with the judicious use of **cortisone** the **prognosis** is favorable. (20, 21, 27, 29, 34, 37)

Table 1
Some Conditions of the Skin and Breast Amenable to Surgery

Organs Involved	Diagnosis	Type of Surgery	Operative Procedures
Skin	Seborrheic keratoses	Epidermal curettage	Lesions frozen with ethyl chloride and curetted
	Basal cell carcinoma— small lesion	Curettage	Lesion and all extensions removed with skin curette
		Electrodesiccation	Remaining cells destroyed by surgical diathermy
Skin	Basal cell carcinoma— small lesion	Cryosurgery of skin lesion	Freezing with cryosurgical spray or by insertion of microthermocouple
Skin Sebaceous glands Hair follicles Nail bed Nail fold	Infected steatoma Furuncle or carbuncle of hair follicles Onychia, paronychia Infected ingrowing toenail	Incision and drainage of glands of skin; of hair follicles; of nail bed or fold	Surgical opening of infected sebaceous glands, etc., to induce drainage

Organs Involved	Diagnosis	Type of Surgery	Operative Procedures
Subcutaneous areolar tissue	Cellulitis of forearm	Incision and drainage of subcutaneous areolar tissue	Surgical opening of infected area and insertion of drain
Skin, subcutaneous tissue	Dermoid of skin Lipoma of subcutaneous tissue	Local excision of dermoid or lipoma	Removal of benign neoplasm
Skin	Cicatrix of skin caused by burn (structures beneath skin undamaged)	Excision of cicatricial skin lesion Use of split-thickness or full-thickness skin graft	Removal of excess scar tissue and replacement by covering area with either half or full thickness of skin removed by knife or dermatome
Skin, subcutaneous tissue	Thermal burn injury	Electrosurgical excision of full-thickness burn	Burned skin and subcutaneous tissue removed by electrosurgery at level of fascia Immediate skin grafting of dry fascial bed
Skin of neck, chin, or cheek	Contracture from scar of old burns or injuries	Reconstruction operation *First stage:* Preparation of pedicle or Gillies' tube flap *Second stage:* Excision of scar Coverage of denuded area with pedicle *Third stage:* Removal of pedicle	Skin and subcutaneous tissue from donor area raised and pedicle tubed Removal of deep scar; distal end of pedicle severed and sutured into defect with pedicle still attached Pedicle opened and returned to donor area
Skin of axilla	Cicatricial contracture of axilla	Z-plasty	Defect corrected by using sliding flaps of skin
Breast	Abscess of breast caused by *Staphylococcus aureus* or other infectious agents	Mastotomy with drainage	Surgical opening and evacuation of abscess Insertion of drain
Breast	Carcinoma of breast	Radical mastectomy	Removal of breast, pectoral muscles, and lymph nodes
Breast	Overdevelopment of breast (pendulous breast)	Mastopexy	Fixation of pendulous breast

Root	Term	Analysis	Definition
Breast	Unilateral hypomastia	Augmentation mammaplasty of underdeveloped breast	Implantation of Cronin silicone prosthesis in retromammary pocket
	Hypermastia of contralateral breast	Reduction mammaplasty of overdeveloped breast	Partial excision of mammary tissue
Breast	Cystic disease of breast—benign lesions	Subcutaneous mastectomy	Excision of cystic mammary gland below the skin Subcutaneous reconstruction by implanting prosthesis

References and Bibliography

1. Aminoff, Michael J. Nervous system. In Schroeder, Steven A., Krupp, Marcus A., and Tierney, Lawrence M., Jr., eds. *Current Medical Diagnosis & Treatment—1988*, Norwalk, CT: Appleton & Lange, 1988, pp. 571-602.

2. Bergfeld, Wilma F. Hair disorders. In Rakel, Robert E., ed. *Conn's Current Therapy—1988*, Philadelphia: W.B. Saunders Co., 1988, pp. 659-662.

3. Berrino, Pietro, et al. Unilateral mammoplasty: Sculpturing the breast from the undersurface. *Plastic and Reconstructive Surgery* 82:88-98, July 1988.

4. Copeland, Edward M., and Bland, Kirby I. The breast. In Sabiston, David C., Jr., ed. *Essentials of Surgery*, Philadelphia: W.B. Saunders Co., 1987, pp. 288-326.

5. Cruz, A.B., Jr., and Aust, J. Bradley. Lesions of the skin and subcutaneous tissue. In Hardy, James D., ed. *Hardy's Textbook of Surgery*, 2nd ed. New York: J.B. Lippincott Co., 1988, pp. 320-338.

6. d'Aubermont, Peter C. Cancer of the skin. In Rakel, Robert E., ed. *Conn's Current Therapy—1988*, Philadelphia: W.B. Saunders Co., 1988, pp. 663-668.

7. Donovan, Arthur. Breast. In Hardy, James D., ed. *Hardy's Textbook of Surgery*, 2nd ed. New York: J.B. Lippincott Co., 1988, pp. 339-364.

8. Dunagin, William G. Verruca vulgaris (warts). In Rakel, Robert E., ed. *Conn's Current Therapy—1988*, Philadelphia: W.B. Saunders Co., 1988, pp. 689-690.

9. Elgart, Mervyn L. Fungal diseases. In Rakel, Robert E., ed. *Conn's Current Therapy—1988*, Philadelphia: W.B. Saunders Co., 1988, pp. 706-711.

10. Epstein, John H. Sunburn and photosensitivity. In Rakel, Robert E., ed. *Conn's Current Therapy—1988*, Philadelphia: W.B. Saunders Co., 1988, pp. 739-741.

11. Falanga, Vincent. Venous ulcers and other cutaneous ulcerations. In Rakel, Robert E., ed. *Conn's Current Therapy—1988*, Philadelphia: W.B. Saunders Co., 1988, pp. 719-722.

12. Fischl, Margaret A., and Dickerson, Gordon M. Acquired immunodeficiency syndrome (AIDS). In Rakel, Robert E., ed. *Conn's Current Therapy—1988*, Philadelphia: W.B. Saunders Co., 1988, pp. 31-40.

13. Fisher, Alexander A. Occupational dermatitis. In Rakel, Robert E., ed. *Conn's Current Therapy—1988*, Philadelphia: W.B. Saunders Co., 1988, pp. 738-739.

14. Fitzpatrick, Thomas B., and Bernhard, Jeffrey D. The structure of the skin and fundamentals of diagnosis. In Fitzpatrick, Thomas B., et al., eds. *Dermatology in General Medicine*, 3rd ed. New York: McGraw-Hill Book Co., 1987, pp. 20-49.

15. Goldfarb, Michael T., and Anderson, Thomas F. Bacterial diseases of the skin. In Rakel, Robert E., ed. *Conn's Current Therapy—1988*, Philadelphia: W.B. Saunders Co., 1988, pp. 697-700.

16. Giuliano, Armando. Breast. In Schroeder, Steven A., Krupp, Marcus A., and Tierney, Lawrence M., Jr., eds. *Current Medical Diagnosis & Treatment—1988*, Norwalk, CT: Appleton & Lange, 1988, pp. 429-446.

17. Hanifin, Jon M. Atopic dermatitis. In Rakel, Robert E., ed. *Conn's Current Therapy—1988*, Philadelphia: W.B. Saunders Co., 1988, pp. 722-725.

18. Hayes, Harry, Jr., et al. Mammography and

breast implants. *Plastic and Reconstructive Surgery* 82:1-6, July 1988.

19. Hill, Thomas G. Premalignant lesions. In Rakel, Robert E., ed. *Conn's Current Therapy—1988*, Philadelphia: W.B. Saunders Co., 1988, pp. 693-697.

20. Jordan, Robert. Pemphigus. In Fitzpatrick, Thomas B., et al., eds. *Dermatology in General Medicine*, 3rd ed. New York: McGraw-Hill Book Co., 1987, pp. 571-579.

21. ———. Bullous pemphigoid, ciatricial pemphoid, and chronic bullous dermatosis of childbed. Ibid., pp. 580-586.

22. Kechijian, Paul. Diseases of the nails. In Rakel, Robert E., ed. *Conn's Current Therapy—1988*, Philadelphia: W.B. Saunders Co., 1988, pp. 6811-687.

23. Kelly, A. Paul. Keloids. In Rakel, Robert E., ed. *Conn's Current Therapy—1988*, Philadelphia: W.B. Saunders Co., 1988, pp. 687-689.

24. Lamkin, Barry C. Papulosquamous eruptions. In Rakel, Robert E., ed. *Conn's Current Therapy—1988*, Philadelphia: W.B. Saunders Co., 1988, pp. 668-675.

25. Lewis, Bian J. Breast cancer. In Wyngaarden, James B., and Smith, Lloyd H., Jr., eds. *Cecil's Textbook of Medicine*, 18th ed. Philadelphia: W.B. Saunders Co., 1988, pp. 1452-1458.

26. Linker, Charles. Blood. In Schroeder, Steven A., Krupp, Marcus A., and Tierney, Lawrence M., Jr., eds. *Current Medical Diagnosis & Treatment—1988*, Norwalk, CT: Appleton & Lange, 1988, pp. 294-338.

27. Marshall, John C., and Meakins, Jonathan L. Anaerobic and necrotizing infections including gas gangrene. In Rakel, Robert E., ed. *Conn's Current Therapy—1988*, Philadelphia: W.B. Saunders Co., 1988, pp. 60-63.

28. Monroe, Eugene W. Urticaria and angioedema. In Rakel, Robert E., ed. *Conn's Current Therapy—1988*, Philadelphia: W.B. Saunders Co., 1988, pp. 732-734.

29. Morrison, Lynne H., and Diaz, Luis A. Bullous diseases. In Rakel, Robert E., ed. *Conn's Current Therapy—1988*, Philadelphia: W.B. Saunders Co., 1988, pp. 727-729.

30. Newcomer, Victor D. Nevi and malignant melanoma. In Rakel, Robert E., ed. *Conn's Current Therapy—1988*, Philadelphia: W.B. Saunders Co., 1988, pp. 690-693.

31. Olmstead, P. Michael, and Graham, William P., III. Surgical disorders of the skin. In Sabiston, David C., Jr., ed. *Essentials of Surgery*, Philadelphia: W.B. Saunders Co., 1987, pp. 791-801.

32. Parish, John A., and Tan, O.T. Laser photomedicine. In Fitzpatrick, Thomas B., et al., eds. *Dermatology in General Medicine*, 3rd ed. New York: McGraw-Hill Book Co., 1987, pp. 1558-1566.

33. Parish, Laurence C., and Witkowski, Joseph A. Parasitic diseases. In Rakel, Robert E., ed. *Conn's Current Therapy—1988*, Philadelphia: W.B. Saunders Co., 1988, pp. 703-706.

34. Parker, Frank. Skin diseases. In Wyngaarden, James B., and Smith, Lloyd H., Jr., eds. *Cecil's Textbook of Medicine*, 18th ed. Philadelphia: W.B. Saunders Co., 1988, pp. 2300-2353.

35. Pochi, Peter E. Acne vulgaris and roseacea. In Rakel, Robert E., ed. *Conn's Current Therapy—1988*, Philadelphia: W.B. Saunders Co., 1988, pp. 655-659.

36. Rapaport, Marvin. Pigmentary disorders. In Rakel, Robert E., ed. *Conn's Current Therapy—1988*, Philadelphia: W.B. Saunders Co., 1988, pp. 734-737.

37. Rees B., Jr., and Odom, Richard B. Skin and appendages. In Schroeder, Steven A., Krupp, Marcus A., and Tierney, Lawrence M., Jr., eds. *Current Medical Diagnosis & Treatment—1988*, Norwalk, CT: Appleton & Lange, 1988, pp. 47-93.

38. Sparling, P. Frederick. Sexually transmitted diseases. In Wyngaarden, James B., and Smith, Lloyd H., Jr., eds. *Cecil's Textbook of Medicine*, 18th ed. Philadelphia: W.B. Saunders Co., 1988, pp. 1701-1723.

39. Straus, John S. Sebaceous glands. In Fitzpatrick, Thomas B., et al., eds. *Dermatology in General Medicine*, 3rd ed. New York: McGraw-Hill Book Co., 1987, pp. 666-685.

40. Tierney, Lawrence M., Jr., and Erskine, John M. Blood vessels & lymphatics. In Schroeder, Steven A., Krupp, Marcus A., and Tierney, Lawrence M., Jr., eds. *Current Medical Diagnosis & Treatment—1988*, Norwalk, CT: Appleton & Lange, 1988, pp. 266-293.

41. Tolis, George. Nonmalignant diseases of the breast. In Wyngaarden, James B., and Smith, Lloyd H., Jr., eds. *Cecil's Textbook of Medicine*, 18th ed. Philadelphia: W.B. Saunders Co., 1988, pp. 1449-1452.

42. Wallerstein, Ralph O. Blood transfusions. In Schroeder, Steven A., Krupp, Marcus A., and Tierney, Lawrence M., Jr., eds. *Current Medical Diagnosis & Treatment—1988*, Norwalk, CT: Appleton & Lange, 1988, pp. 338-341.

43. Zugerman, Charles. Erythemas. In Rakel, Robert E., ed. *Conn's Current Therapy—1988*, Philadelphia: W.B. Saunders Co., 1988, pp. 725-727.

Musculoskeletal Disorders

Bones

Origin of Terms

calcaneus (L)—heel bone
cancellus (L)—lattice
coxa (L)—hipbone
di- (G)—twice, double
dia- (G)—through, between
diploë (G)—fold
femur (L)—thigh
genu (L)—knee

ischio- (G)—hip
lacuna (L)—lake
medulla (L)—marrow
myel-, myelo- (G)—marrow
os (pl. ossa) (L)—bone
osteo- (G)—bone
pelvis (L)—basin
physis (G)—growth

Anatomic Terms (Ref. 11)

- *bone, osseous tissue*—the hardest type of connective tissue, which provides a supporting framework for the body.
- *bone marrow, medulla*—soft, central part of bone.
    - *red marrow*—fills cancellous bone and manufactures red blood cells and hemoglobin.
    - *yellow marrow*—fills the medullary cavity and contains fat cells.
- *cancellous bone*—spongy bone composed of a loose latticework of bony trabeculae and bone marrow within the interspace.
- *compact bone, cortex of bone*—solid bone rich in calcium.
- *diaphysis*—shaft of long bone.
- *diploë*—spongy bone between the two tables of the skull.
- *endosteum*—membrane lining the walls of the medullary cavity.
- *epiphysis (pl. epiphyses)*—extremity of long bones and center of ossification for growing bone.
- *matrix of bone*—collagenous fibers and a ground substance in which calcium is deposited.
- *medullary cavity*—marrow-filled cavity within the shaft of long bones.
- *metaphysis*—enlarged part of the shaft near the epiphysis of a long bone.
- *ossification*—bone formation.

Figure 7 Skeleton, anterior view.

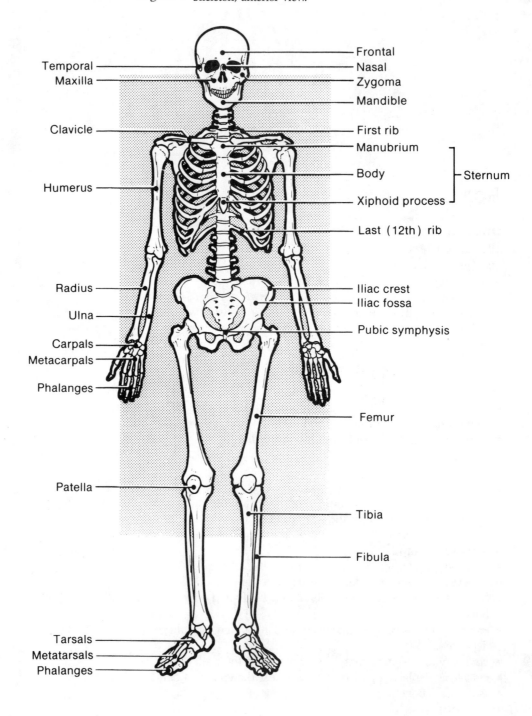

Temporal

Maxilla

Clavicle

Humerus

Radius

Ulna

Carpals

Metacarpals

Phalanges

Patella

Tarsals

Metatarsals

Phalanges

Frontal

Nasal

Zygoma

Mandible

First rib

Manubrium

Body

Xiphoid process

Sternum

Last (12th) rib

Iliac crest

Iliac fossa

Pubic symphysis

Femur

Tibia

Fibula

Figure 8 Skeleton, posterior view.

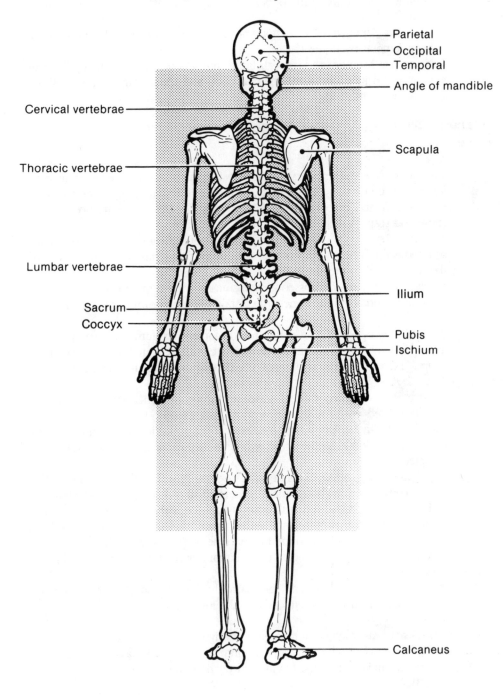

Parietal

Occipital

Temporal

Angle of mandible

Cervical vertebrae

Scapula

Thoracic vertebrae

Lumbar vertebrae

Ilium

Sacrum

Coccyx

Pubis

Ischium

Calcaneus

- *osteoblasts*—bone-forming cells.
- *osteoclasts*—bone-absorbing cells.
- *osteocytes*—bone cells lying in lacunae within intercellular substance.
- *osteoid*—calcifiable osseous tissue, yet uncalcified.
- *periosteum*—outer covering of bone.
- *trabeculae*—slender spicules or anastomosing bars of spongy bone.
- *trochanter*—bony prominence of the upper extremity of the femur below the femoral neck.
    —*major or greater trochanter*—large bony projection located externally and laterally between femoral neck and shaft.
    —*minor or lesser trochanter*—conical bony prominence located medially and laterally at the junction of the femoral neck and shaft. (Figs. 7 and 8 show major bones of the body.)

Diagnostic Terms

- *bone neoplasms:*
    —*benign:*
    —*aneursymal bone cyst*—solitary vascular lesion that usually arises from medullary or cancellous structures; affects the ends of the shaft and pushes outward, eroding soft and osseous tissue. Other possible sites of occurrence are the spine and scapula. (7)
    —*epidermoid cyst*—cyst filled with keratinaceous material and lined with squamous epithelium. Epidermoid cysts occur frequently in the phalanges of the fingers and in the skull. (7)
    —*ganglion cyst of bone*—intraosseous extensions of ganglia of local soft tissues that occur at the ends of long bones; the distal tibia is a common site for this cyst. (7)
    —*giant cell tumor, benign*—osteolytic tumor containing numerous giant cells. It arises at the epiphysis and does not interfere with joint motion until late in its course. It may undergo malignant transformation or recur after removal. (8, 43)
    —*hemangioma*—common benign vascular tumor of bone. These lesions are usually located in the vertebral body or skull. (7)
    —*osteoblastoma*—a benign lesion consisting of a collection of reparative bone reactions. It is found in the spine, where it may cause cord compression and paraplegia. (8)
    —*osteochondromas*—cartilaginous nodules originating within the periosteum. The lesion consists of a bony mass generated by progressive endochondral ossification of a growing cartilaginous cap. Growth of the lesion usually parallels that of a person and ceases when skeletal maturity is reached. Osteochondromas may be found in any bone preformed in cartilage; however, they usually occur on the metaphysis of a long bone near the epiphyseal plate. (7)
    —*osteoid osteoma*—benign, small, very painful tumor, found in almost any bone of the skeleton but most frequently in the lower extremities. (7)
    —*malignant:*
    —*Ewing's sarcoma*—malignant new growth originating in the shaft of long bones and spreading through the periosteum into soft tissues. Metastases occur early. The femur, tibia, humerus, fibula, and pelvic bones are frequently involved. (8, 33)

—*fibrosarcoma of the bone*—malignant tumor derived from bone marrow, metaphysis, or periosteum and found on the femur, humerus, and jawbone. (8, 43)

—*myeloma, plasmacytoma*—malignant neoplasm derived from plasma cells and usually associated with abnormal protein metabolism. It may occur as:

—*multiple myeloma*—a malignant type of widespread bone destruction with gradual replacement of cancellous bone by neoplasm; usually seen in persons over 50 years old. (8, 33)

—*solitary myeloma*—single lesion found in any location but most frequently in vertebral column. Back pain is severe. (8, 33)

—*osteogenic sarcoma*—highly malignant, vascular tumor usually involving the upper shaft of long bones, the pelvis, or knee. Metastases are common and life threatening. (8, 33)

- *cervical rib*—a supernumerary rib attached to cervical vertebra. (2)
- *coxa plana*—flattening of the head of the femur. (29)
- *coxa valga*—widening of angle between the shaft and neck of the femur. (29, 47)
- *coxa vara*—diminishing of angle between the shaft and neck of the femur. (29, 47)
- *epiphysitis, acute*—inflammatory process of the epiphyseal region of a long bone, marked by tenderness and pain of the joint. (5)
- *fracture*—a broken bone. Long bone fractures are frequently associated with nerve injury. (Figs. 9 to 16 show mature and immature femur, various fractures, and surgical fixation of fractures.)

—*nonpenetrating or closed fracture*—no external wound present.

—*penetrating or open fracture*—an external wound communicating with the fracture.

Fractures may be:

—*capillary*—hairlike line of break.

—*comminuted*—bone splintered into small fragments (Fig. 12).

—*complicated*—broken bone injuring adjacent structure; for example, fractured rib piercing the lung.

—*compound*—an open wound leading down to the fracture.

—*depressed*—bone broken inward, as in certain skull fractures.

—*greenstick*—incomplete break that may be associated with bowing of shaft (Fig. 11).

—*impacted*—broken fragment wedged into another bony fragment.

—*pathologic*—spontaneous fracture caused by bone destruction in certain diseases: cancer, syphilis, osteomalacia, osteoporosis, and others.

—*simple*—uncomplicated fracture with no open wound.

—*transverse*—break across the bone (Fig. 10). For example, Colles' fracture—transverse fracture of the radius above the wrist with displacement of the hand. (51, 53)

- *fracture of hip*—a break in the upper end of the femur. The two main types are:

—*femoral neck fracture*—bone broken through the neck of the femur.

—*trochanteric fracture*—bone broken below, around, or between the greater or lesser trochanters. (53)

- *genu valgum*—knock-knee. (29)
- *genu varum*—bowleg; deformity involving either tibia alone or femur, tibia, and fibula; seen in rickets and corrected by high doses of vitamin D. (29)
- *osteitis deformans,*—*Paget's disease of bone*—slowly progressive disease occurring in advanced age; characterized by extensive bone destruction and followed almost

immediately by abnormal bone repair of the weakened, deossified skeleton, which yields deformities and pathologic features. (31)

- *osteochondritis deformans juvenile, coxa plana, Legg-Calvé-Perthes disease*—self-limited disease in children aged four to nine; characterized by flattening of the femoral head and resulting in limping and restricted motion. (5)
- *osteoclasia, osteolysis*—resorption and destruction of osseous tissue. (3)
- *osteomalacia*—softening of bone caused by deficiency in calcium or phosphorus or both, needed for ossification of mature bone in adults. In children the primary cause is lack of Vitamin D and sunlight necessary for the normal absorption of the vitamin. (32, 47)
- *osteomyelitis*—inflammation of the bone and bone marrow. Infective agents may be pyogenic bacteria, *Brucella*, *Salmonella*, or other organisms. (26)
- *osteoporosis, porous bone*—disorder of protein metabolism characterized by diffuse decrease of bone density and marked increase in porosity, which are most pronounced in the spine and pelvis. (32)
- *renal (azotemic) osteodystrophy*—bone disorder caused by defective mineralization complicating chronic renal failure. (47)
- *rickets, rachitis*—calcium and vitamin D deficiency of early childhood that leads to demineralization of bones and deformities. (32, 47)
- *sequestrum*—dead bone separated from surrounding tissue. (6)
- *supernumerary bone*—extra bone. (40)
- *vitamin D refractory rickets, familial hypophosphatemia*—a relatively common type of rickets in which abnormal phosphate loss and deficient mineralization are associated with renal tubule insufficiency. (32, 47)
- *whiplash injury of neck*—compression of cervical spine involving the bones, joints, and intervertebral disks. It results from a sudden throwing forward and then backward of the head, usually caused by a car accident when the collision is from the rear. (2)

Operative Terms

- *amputation*—partial or complete removal of limb necessitated by crushing injury, intractable pain, gangrene, vascular obstruction, or uncontrollable infection. (59, 60)
- *bone grafting, transplantation of bone*—insertion of a bone graft.
    - *autografting or autotransplantation of bone*—removal of bone from one site and implanting it at another site to promote bone union, to replace destroyed bone, or to immobilize joint in surgical fusion.
    - *homografting or homotransplantation of bone*—surgical use of bone from bone bank obtained from amputations, ostectomies, or rib resections of nonmalignant, noninfectious cases. (4, 14)
- *epiphyseal arrest*—surgical procedure for retarding growth at the epiphysis by equalizing length of lower extremities. (1)
- *epiphyseal stapling*—temporary arrest of epiphyseal growth by stapling the epiphysis to control leg length discrepancy. (1)
- *epiphysiodesis*—implanting bone grafts across the epiphyseal plate to secure immobilization of epiphysis. Operation is done for slipped femoral epiphysis following insertion of metal pins. (1)
- *exostectomy*—removal of a benign bone tumor (exostosis), such as a bunion (hallux valgus).
- *ostectomy*—excision of a bone. (1)
- *osteoclasis*—surgical refracture of a bone in case of malunion of broken parts. (27)
- *osteoplasty*—reconstruction or repair of a bone.

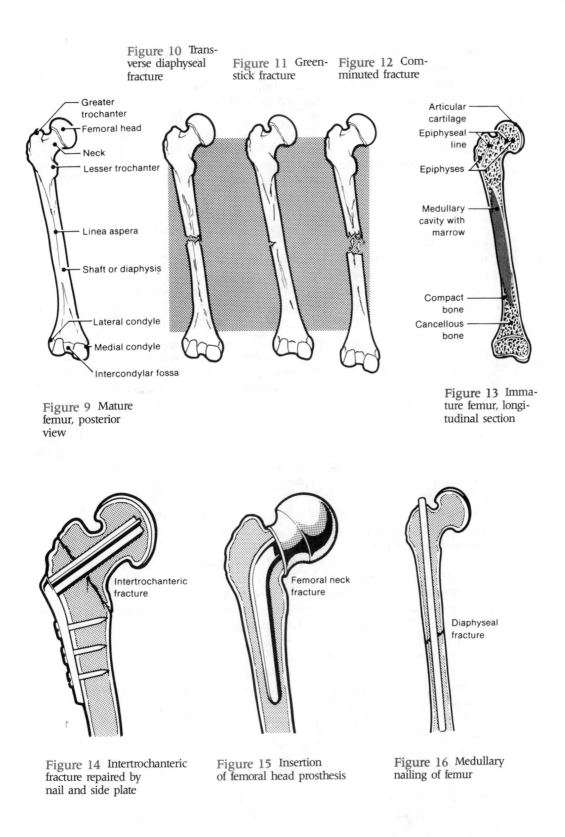

Figure 10 Transverse diaphyseal fracture

Figure 11 Greenstick fracture

Figure 12 Comminuted fracture

Figure 9 Mature femur, posterior view

Greater trochanter
Femoral head
Neck
Lesser trochanter
Linea aspera
Shaft or diaphysis
Lateral condyle
Medial condyle
Intercondylar fossa

Articular cartilage
Epiphyseal line
Epiphyses
Medullary cavity with marrow
Compact bone
Cancellous bone

Figure 13 Immature femur, longitudinal section

Intertrochanteric fracture

Femoral neck fracture

Diaphyseal fracture

Figure 14 Intertrochanteric fracture repaired by nail and side plate

Figure 15 Insertion of femoral head prosthesis

Figure 16 Medullary nailing of femur

- *osteotomy*—surgical division or section of a bone.
- *replantation of an extremity*—restorative surgery of an accidentally amputated limb to its functional capacity, including:
    —restoration of circulation by anastomoses of blood vessels.
    —internal fixation of diaphyseal fracture of bone by intramedullary nail.
    —repair of nerves and tendons.
    —debridement of devitalized tissue.
    —closure by suturing undamaged soft tissue of dismembered limb to stump.
    —split-thickness grafts for denuded skin areas. (64)
- *sequestrectomy*—surgical removal of a piece of dead bone. (6)
- *surgical correction of fracture*—this may be achieved by:
    —*closed reduction*—manipulation and application of cast or application of splint or traction apparatus in selected cases when the fractured ends are not in alignment. (51)
    —*open reduction and internal fixation*—manipulation and:
        —insertion of plate and screws.
        —insertion of medullary nail for diaphyseal fractures (shaft of long bones); extraction of nail after bone union.
        —insertion of a nail with a side plate, such as a Jewett nail, for trochanteric or femoral neck fractures.
        —insertion of a hip prosthesis, Fred Thompson or Austin Moore type, in selected femoral neck fractures. Occasionally prostheses are used for severe fractures of the upper or lower end of the humerus. (51, 52, 53)
    —*simple immobilization*—application of a cast or splint when the fractured ends are in apposition. (54)

Symptomatic Terms

- *callus*—substance growing between ends of fractured bone and converted into osseous tissue in the process of repair.
- *crepitation*—grating sound made by movement of fractured bones. (15, 20)
- *decalcification*—the removal of lime salts, especially from the bone.
- *demineralization*—deficiency or loss of bone minerals that occurs in osteoporosis, osteomalacia, cancer, or other disorders.
- *necrosis of bone*—devitalization of osseous tissue; formation of dead bone.
    —*aseptic*—without infection.
    —*avascular*—from deprivation of blood supply caused by fracture, loss of periosteum, exposure to radioactive substances, or other causes.
    —*ischemic*—same as avascular necrosis of bone. (47)
- *nidus*—focal point from which a pathologic lesion develops.
- *ostealgia, osteodynia*—bone pain. (31)
- *osteophyte*—bony outgrowth (osseous excrescence). (20)
- *phantom limb pain*—painful sensation felt by amputee as if the limb were still intact. (59)
- *sequestration*—process of bone necrosis resulting in dead bone. (6)

Joints, Bursae, Cartilages, Ligaments

Origin of Terms

arthr-, arthro- (G)—joint
bursa (L)—saclike cavity, sac

chondr-, chondro- (G)—cartilage, gristle
condyle (G)—rounded bone projection, knuckle
ligamentum (pl. ligamenta) (L)—that which ties, tissue that binds
scolio- (G)—twisted, crooked
spondyl-, spondylo- (G)—vertebra, spinal column

Anatomic Terms (12)

- *acetabulum*—cup-shaped socket on the external surface of the innominate bone in which the head of the femur lies.
- *articulation*—joint
  —*cartilaginous joint*—bones united by fibrocartilage or hyaline cartilage.
  —*fibrous joint*—bones united by fibrous tissue.
  —*synovial joint, diarthrodial joint*—bones united by a joint capsule and ligaments. Cartilage covers the articular surface of the bones. The joint capsule is composed of a fibrous layer lined by synovial membrane.
- *bursa (pl. bursae)*—connective tissue sac containing lubricating fluid, sometimes synovia.
- *intervertebral disc*—fibrocartilage between the bodies of the vertebrae composed of:
  —*anulus fibrosus*—outer fibrous ring encircling the nucleus pulposus.
  —*nucleus pulposus*—inner gelatinous mass.
- *ligaments*—fibrous, connective tissue bands uniting articular ends of bones.
- *meniscus*—fibrocartilage found in certain joints.
- *synovial membrane*—inner lining of a joint capsule secreting synovia.
- *volar*—pertaining to the palm of the hand or sole of the foot.

Diagnostic Terms

- *ankylosis*—stiff joint. (20)
- *arthritis*—inflammation of joints.
  —*atrophic or rheumatoid arthritis*—produces constitutional symptoms in addition to painful, inflammatory, multiple joint involvement. (34, 50)
  —*gouty arthritis*—metabolic disorder, usually involving one joint (monarticular). Urate crystals are highly increased and found in various tissues. Pain is relieved by colchicine. (30)
  —*infectious arthritis, pyogenic arthritis, septic arthritis:*
  —*acute infectious arthritis*—acute inflammatory process affecting synovial and subchondrial tissues and causing articular destruction. It is usually caused by pyogenic cocci such as gonococci, meningococci, pneumococci, staphylococci, and streptococci. (24, 50)
  —*chronic infectious arthritis*—persistent infection of joint causing pain, swelling, restricted joint motion, and deformity. (24, 50)
  —*hypertrophic arthritis, osteoarthritis*—a degenerative condition of cartilage and enlargement of bone at the joint margins, occurring particularly in older persons. It often affects the terminal phalanges, knees, hips, and spine and results in contractures, deformities, and stiffness of affected joints. (20, 50)
  —*Marie-Strümpell arthritis, ankylosing spondylitis*—painful inflammatory joint disease characterized by progressive stiffening of the spine caused by fusion of vertebral bodies. (19, 35)
  —*traumatic arthritis*—a group of disorders resulting from single or repetitive trauma to joints:
  —*acute synovitis, traumatic synovitis*—this may result from a single episode of articular trauma to the synovial membrane of a joint and may be associated

with hemarthrosis and sprains. The articular cartilage is intact. (20)

    —disruptive trauma of joint—the major supporting structures have ruptured and the articular cartilage is damaged. Meniscal tears, intra-articular fractures, and severe sprains may be present.

    —post-traumatic osteoarthritis—residual damage from disruptive trauma may lead to restricted mobility, deformity, and articular instability. (20, 24)

    —repetitive articular trauma—chronic arthritis of the affected joints may develop due to occupational hazards or sports.

    —other types of trauma—arthropathy may develop following decompression, radiation, frostbite, or the like. (20, 24)

- *arthropathy*—any disease of the joints. (20, 24)
- *Baker's cyst*—synovial fluid-filled popliteal lesion found in muscles, other tissues, or near a joint in advanced osteoarthritis.
- *bursitis*—inflammation of a bursa. (23)
- *chondritis*—inflammation of a cartilage. (20)
- *chondrocalcinosis, pseudogout*—acute, recurrent joint disease affecting the cartilaginous structures of large joints, especially the knee. Synovial fluid contains calcium pyrophosphates. (21)
- *destructive coxarthropathy*—painful inflammatory disability of hip joint. Joint motion is moderately impaired.
- *dislocation*—displacement of a bone from its natural position in a joint. (2)
- *hallux malleus*—hammer toe. (46)
- *hallux valgus*—deflection of great toe to outer side of foot and subsequent development of bony prominence. (46)
- *hallux varus*—deflection of great toe to inner side of foot. (46)
- *hemarthrosis*—bloody effusion in a joint cavity. It is prone to occur in hemophiliacs. (50)
- *internal derangement of knee joint*—refers to various joint lesions that interfere with motion (locking, snapping, buckling) due to atrophy of thigh muscles, tenderness or pain, and joint swelling. Some leading causes are tears of menisci, ligaments, patellar or quadriceps tendons, loose bodies, fracture, or chondromalacia of patellae. (20)
- *kyphosis*—hunchback; abnormal posterior curvature of thoracic spine. (17)
- *lordosis*—hollow-back; anterior convexity of lower spine. (32)
- *neoplasms:*
    - *—benign:*
    - *—chondroblastoma*—benign, vascular, cartilaginous tumor arising from the epiphysis of a long bone. (8)
    - *—chondroma*—benign neoplasm arising from cartilage. (50)
    - *—hemartoma, benign mesenchymoma*—tumor containing multiple mesenchymal tissues. They have bizarre roentgenographic and histologic features and may be mistaken for malignant connective tissue tumors. This type of tumor usually tends to regress after puberty. These tumors appear most often in bones and are hard to distinguish from other connective tissue tumors. (7)
    - *—malignant:*
    - *—chondrosarcoma*—malignant tumor derived from cartilage. These tumors usually affect the femur, pelvis, tibia, humerus, scapula, and ribs. (9, 33)
    - *—chordoma*—originates from embryonic notochordal remnants. Ninety percent of tumors occur in the upper and lower ends of the vertebral column. Benign and malignant distinction is clinically and histologically difficult. Cellular differentiation, anaplasia, and mitotic activity do not relate to the usual indolent and progressive course, with presence for years without metastasis. When metastases do occur, it is usually late in the growth process. (9)

—*synovioma, synovial sarcoma*—a highly malignant fibroblastic sarcoma, originating in periarticular structures and occurring in older children and young adults. The tumor presents as a slow-growing mass near a joint and spreads along tissue planes. The most common site of visceral metastases is the lung. (10, 33)

■ *painful shoulder, cervicobrachial pain syndromes*—articular or extra-articular disorders characterized by tenderness, moderate to agonizing pain, and limitation of motion in the shoulder girdle, neck, and arm. All or some of these symptoms are present in:

—*adhesive capsulitis, adhesive bursitis, frozen shoulder, periarthritis of the shoulder joint*—adhesions within the bursa, articular tendosynovitis, and calcareous deposits causing stiffness and atrophic changes. (23)

—*carpal tunnel syndrome*—painful condition resulting from a compression of the median nerve within the carpal tunnel, as evidenced by a flattening or circular constriction of the nerve. Tingling, aching, or burning pain in fingers, radiating to forearm and shoulder; may be constant or episodic and aggravated by strenuous manual activity. (23, 42)

—*cervical spondylosis, cervical disk disease*—degenerative disorder of cervical disk, characterized by progressive thinning of the joint cartilage; spinal cord and nerve root compression, resulting from extrusion of the nucleus pulposus; and subsequent pain radiating to the back of the neck and head, shoulder, and arm. (35, 62)

—*epicondylalgia, epicondylitis, tennis elbow*—pain syndrome primarily affecting the lateral and median regions of the elbow and radiating to the upper arm and forearm. It is accentuated by repetitive grasping. (64)

—*hand-shoulder syndrome*—peculiar clinical entity in which pain radiates from shoulder to fingertips. The patient spontaneously immobilizes the affected extremity, which leads to atrophy and edema of the hand. Later overactivity of sympathetic nerves results in a sweaty, cold, painful hand followed by stiffness and fibrosis of joints. Syndrome may occur in myocardial ischemia, following myocardial infarction, and infrequently in bronchogenic carcinoma. (35)

—*supraclavicular nerve entrapment syndrome*—compression of middle branch of supraclavicular nerve at its passage through the bone canal in the clavicle, causing pain and numbness. Neuralgia can be relieved by decompression of the nerve. (35)

—*supraspinatus syndrome*—disorder caused by adhesions, calcium deposits, or tears in rotator cuff, resulting in a painful shoulder, limited motion, muscle atrophy, and spasm. (64)

■ *Reiter's syndrome*—a triad of inflammatory states: urethritis (nongonococcal), conjunctivitis, and arthritis, probably due to chlamydial or mycoplasmal infection. (22, 44)

■ *scoliosis*—lateral spinal curvature. (16, 50)

■ *skeletal dysplasias*—disturbances of bony growth, congenital or inherited; most severe if present in early infancy; less harmful if developing in adult life, causing progressive destruction of osseous tissue as a result of chondroid and osteoid abnormalities. Examples are:

—*dysplasias caused by impaired chondroid production*—probably a metabolic defect of the maturation of chondroblasts (immature cartilage cells).

—*achondroplasia*—congenital, hereditary abnormality of chondroblastic cell growth at the epiphyses; subsequent development of a peculiar dwarfism. (33)

—*enchondromatosis, dyschondroplasia, Ollier's disease*—a disorder affecting the growth plate in which hypertrophic cartilage is not resorbed and ossified in a normal manner. Masses of cartilage are present in the metaphyses in close association with the growth plate in very young children, but diaphyseal in teenagers and adults. The usual sites of involvement are ends of long bones and the pelvis. (33)

　　*—osteochondromatosis, hereditary multiple exostoses—*osteochondromas or bony outgrowths from the ends of cortical bone that may be associated with deformities of the knee, wrist, elbow, and long bones, or other defects. (33)

　*—dysplasias caused by impaired osteoid production—*a group of developmental abnormalities characterized by the presence of insufficient, excessive, or immature osteoid. Examples are:

　*—fibrous dysplasia of bone, Albright's syndrome—*metabolic bone disease characterized by rapid resorption of bone and fibrous replacement of marrow, distortion of one or several bones, brownish pigmentation of skin, and precocious puberty in girls. (33)

　*—osteogenesis imperfecta, brittle bones—*an inherited connective tissue disorder affecting the skeleton and occurring as:

　　*—osteogenesis imperfecta congenita—*a severe form that develops prenatally and may be fatal in infancy.

　　*—osteogenesis imperfecta tarda—*a moderately severe form that develops in childhood. Clinical features include fragility of bones; fracture proneness at an early age; multiple pathologic fractures; deformities of long bones; excessive digital laxity; white or blue sclerae; deafness; a peculiar squeaky voice; and a crackling laugh. (45)

　*—osteopetrosis, marble bones, Albers-Schönberg disease—*rare congenital bone disorder thought to be caused by a persistence of primitive chondro-osteoid that interferes with its replacement by mature bone. Since osteoid formation is insufficient, the bones are fracture prone, marblelike, and chalklike. (33)

　*—spondyloepiphyseal dysplasia—*disorder in which growth abnormalities occur in various bones, including vertebrae, pelvis, carpal and tarsal bones, and the epiphyses of tubular bones. (33)

- *spondylolisthesis—*forward slipping of a lumbar vertebra on the adjacent vertebra below, usually associated with pelvic deformity. (17, 50)
- *spondylosis—*ankylosis of vertebrae; also any degenerative lesion of the spine. (20)
- *sprain—*injury to joint with tearing of tendons and ligaments.
- *Still's disease—*painful rheumatoid arthritis in children associated with retarded growth and glandular and splenic enlargement. (4, 50)
- *subluxation—*incomplete dislocation.
- *talipes—*clubfoot:
　*—equinus—*forefoot touches ground; walking on toes.
　*—planus—*arch broken; entire sole rests on ground.
　*—valgus—*foot everted; inner side of sole touches ground.
　*—varus—*foot inverted; outer side of sole rests on ground. (27)
- *vertebral injuries—*trauma to the spine resulting in compression fractures of the vertebrae and fractures and dislocations or flexion fractures of the spine associated with minimal spinal cord damage. (20, 63)

Operative Terms

- *arthroclasia—*surgical breaking of a stiff joint.
- *arthrodesis, artificial ankylosis—*surgical fixation of a joint to immobilize the joint. (27, 48)
- *arthrolysis—*freeing the joint from fibrous bands or excess cartilage to restore its mobility.

Figure 17 Acetabular component with socket for prosthetic head of femoral component

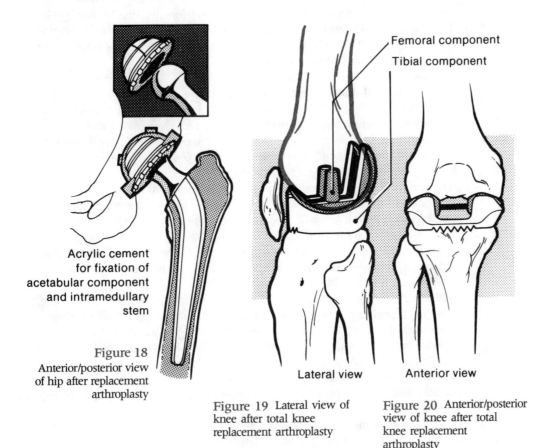

Femoral component

Tibial component

Acrylic cement for fixation of acetabular component and intramedullary stem

Figure 18
Anterior/posterior view of hip after replacement arthroplasty

Lateral view

Anterior view

Figure 19 Lateral view of knee after total knee replacement arthroplasty

Figure 20 Anterior/posterior view of knee after total knee replacement arthroplasty

- *arthroplasty*—surgical repair of a joint. The hip, knee, elbow, and temporomandibular joints are best suited for reconstruction.

  —*arthroplasties of the hip joint* (see Figs. 17 and 18):

    –*Charnley low-friction arthroplasty*—a total hip arthroplasty or total hip replacement for rheumatoid arthritis or any type of destructive hip disease. The prosthesis has two components: (1) an acetabular cup or socket of high-density polyethylene and (2) a femoral component of vitallium or stainless steel, consisting of a small femoral head for low friction that lodges in the socket and a prosthetic stem embedded in the intramedullary canal of the femur. Acrylic cement is used to seat the acetabular cup and prosthetic stem. The cement provides rigid fixation and stability. Modifications of Charnley total hip replacement are those of McKee and Watson-Farrar. (4)

    –*Colonna capsular arthroplasty*—surgery for congenital dislocation of the hip. This procedure retains the gliding mechanisms between the displaced head of the femur and its capsule. The acetabulum is usually deepened and enlarged. (4)

—*Moore or Thompson prosthetic arthroplasty*—surgical repair of arthritic hip including amputation of head and neck of femur, acetabular remodeling and reconstruction, and seating of prosthesis in femoral shaft and acetabulum. (4)

—*vitallium mold arthroplasty*—molding a joint and interposing a nonirritating substance between bony surfaces to improve joint function and lessen pain in rheumatoid arthritis and bony or fibrous ankylosis. Interposition of material between joint surfaces, such as autogenous fascia or inert metal (vitallium), also prevents recurrence of ankylosis. (4)

—*arthroplasties of the knee:*

—*compartmental total knee arthroplasty*—reconstruction of the articulating surfaces limited to the affected compartment of the knee joint and correction of deformities in the presence of intact ligaments, providing joint stability.

—*geomedic (or geometric) total knee arthroplasty*—removal of sufficient bone and insertion of femoral and tibial components of the geomedic prosthesis for total knee replacement. (See Figs. 19 to 20.) (61)

—*patellofemoral joint replacement*—conservative surgical procedure in which a minimum of diseased bone is removed, a knee implant for resurfacing the patellofemoral joint is inserted, and any interference with patellar ligaments is avoided to safeguard joint stability.

—*polycentric total knee arthroplasty*—replacement of the involved articulating surfaces of the tibial plateaus and femoral condyles to relieve pain and restore joint motion and stability. (61)

—*Walldius arthroplasty*—salvage operation for severe pain and instability of the knee joint in rheumatoid arthritis using a vitallium hinge prosthesis (Walldius) with 10-centimeter stems. Insertion of the prosthesis is done by the anterior transverse approach with retention of the patella and usually without acrylic cement, since it fails to achieve joint stabilization. (61)

—*arthroplasties of the shoulder:*

—*partial shoulder arthroplasty, hemireplacement of shoulder*—replacement of the articular surface of the humeral head by a Neer prosthesis in the presence of an intact rotator cuff and glenoid cavity.

—*total shoulder arthroplasty, total glenohumeral joint replacement*—replacement of both the head of the humerus and the glenoid fossa in the presence of a massive tear or other defect in the rotator cuff.

Indications for surgical intervention are disabling rheumatoid arthritis or osteoarthritis, with a painful shoulder and limited joint motion that remain uncontrolled by conservative treatment. (58)

—*arthroplasty of temporomandibular joint*—surgical breaking of a stiff joint to relieve disabling ankylosis caused by rheumatic, degenerative, infectious, or traumatic arthritis. The mandibular condyle is resected and remodeled.

- *arthroscopy*—endoscopic examination of the magnified joint, enhanced by fiberoptic light transmission, and provision for joint irrigation to relieve pain from injury or arthritis. The procedure is primarily indicated in the detection of articular and meniscal lesions or other internal derangements of the knee. Its usefulness in evaluating the hip, ankle, shoulder, and elbow joints needs to be established. (55, 56, 57)

- *arthrotomy*—surgical opening of a joint.

- *bunionectomy, surgical correction of valgus deformity*—removal of bony prominence (bunion) from medial aspect of first metatarsal head. (46)

- *chondrectomy*—removal of a cartilage.

- *chondroplasty*—plastic repair of a cartilage.

- *Harrington instrumentation and fusion*—surgery for correcting scoliosis and spondylolisthesis. Metal rods and hooks are directly implanted on the spine. Articular fusion is achieved by inserting bone grafts from the ilium. (16)
- *synovectomy*—partial or total removal of a synovial membrane lining of a joint capsule. (47)

Symptomatic Terms

- *arthralgia, arthrodynia*—joint pain.
- *capsular laceration*—tear of a joint capsule.
- *crepitus, articular*—the grating of joints. (20)
- *detachment of cartilage*—separation of cartilaginous material from a joint. Loose bodies limit motion.
- *effusion, hemorrhagic*—bleeding into synovial sac.
- *effusion, synovial*—an overproduction of joint fluid. (20)
- *Heberden's nodes*—hard nodules at the distal phalangeal joints of the fingers in osteoarthritis. (20)
- *lipping*—liplike bony growths at the joints in osteoarthritis; for example, the marginal lipping of the acetabular rim and head of the femur in degenerative hip disease. (31)
- *lumbago*—dull, aching pain in the lumbar region of the back.
- *rheumatoid nodules*—subcutaneous nodules located over bony prominences, such as the elbow or back of the heel. They exert pressure and are present in advanced rheumatoid arthritis.
- *spur*—projection from a bone. (20, 34)
- *tophus (pl. tophi)*—deposit of urate crystals in subcutaneous tissue near a joint. (30)

Diaphragm, Muscles, Tendons

Origin of Terms

fascia (L)—band
leio- (G)—smooth
my-, myo- (G)—muscle

rhabdo- (G)—rod, striated
teno-, tenonto- (G)—tendon
tendo- (L)—tendon

Anatomic Terms (13)

- *aponeurosis*—flat sheet of fibrous tissue that usually serves as an attachment for a muscle.
- *diaphragm*—the muscular, dome-shaped septum between the thoracic and abdominal cavities.
- *fascia*—sheet of connective tissue that covers, supports, and separates muscles.
- *insertion of muscle*—end attached to the bone or cartilage that moves when the muscle contracts (or shortens).
- *muscle*—contractile tissue composed of units that have the power to contract when stimulated by a nerve impulse.
- *origin of muscle*—end attached to the bone or cartilage that does not move when the muscle contracts (or shortens).
- *tendons*—bands of fibrous tissue that attach muscles to bones.

Diagnostic Terms

- *carpoptosia*—wristdrop.
- *claudication*—limping, intermittent type caused by ischemia of leg muscles. (28)

Figure 21 Muscles, anterior view.

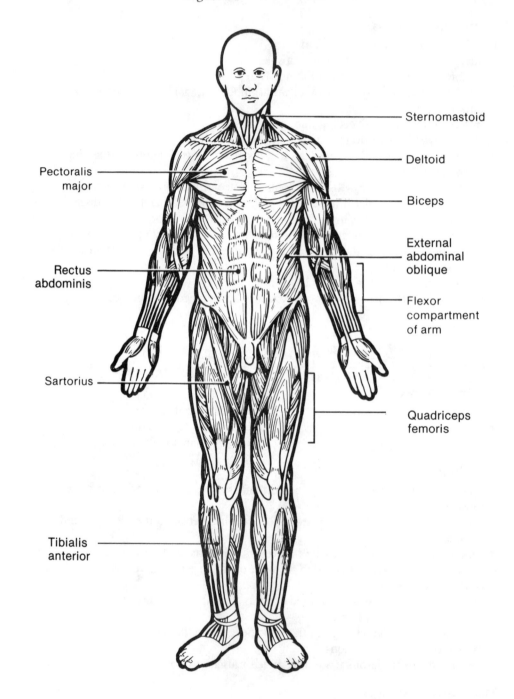

Sternomastoid

Deltoid

Pectoralis major

Biceps

External abdominal oblique

Flexor compartment of arm

Rectus abdominis

Sartorius

Quadriceps femoris

Tibialis anterior

Figure 22 Muscles, posterior view.

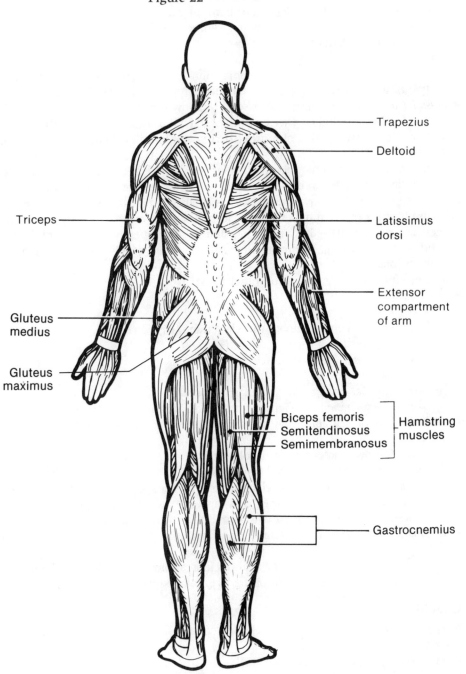

Trapezius

Deltoid

Triceps

Latissimus dorsi

Extensor compartment of arm

Gluteus medius

Gluteus maximus

Biceps femoris
Semitendinosus
Semimembranosus

Hamstring muscles

Gastrocnemius

- *contracture*—permanent shortening of one or more muscles caused by paralysis, spasm, or scar formation.
  - *Dupuytren's contracture*—shrinkage of palmar fascia, resulting in flexion deformity of one or more fingers. (41)
  - *Volkmann's contracture*—flexion deformity of wrist and fingers that may be caused by circulatory interference from a tight cast. (39)
- *disuse atrophy*—muscle wasting caused by immobilization. (31)
- *fascitis, fasciitis*—inflammation of the fascia.
- *graphospasm*—writer's cramp.
- *hiatus hernia, diaphragmatic hernia*—protrusion of an abdominal organ, usually a portion of the stomach, through the esophageal opening of the diaphragm. (25)
- *muscular dystrophy*—progressive disease of unknown etiology, marked in infants by enlarged calves, waddling gait, swayback, and winged shoulders. As the disease advances, extensive wasting of muscles occurs and bizarre deformities develop. (36, 49)
- *myasthenia gravis*—chronic neuromuscular disorder characterized by weakness, usually first manifested in ocular muscles, resulting in bilateral ptosis of eyelids and sleepy appearance. The myasthenic facies is apathetic and expressionless. There may be involvement of the muscles of speech, mastication, and swallowing. When the chest muscles are affected, dyspnea may develop. Infrequently, weakness of the legs interferes with walking. Symptoms fluctuate in severity, ranging from exacerbations to remissions. (18)
- *myositis*—inflammatory process of muscles. (3)
- *neoplasms:*
  - *benign:*
    - *leiomyoma*—benign smooth muscle tumor. (10)
    - *myoma*—benign muscular tumor. (10)
    - *rhabdomyoma*—striated muscle tumor. (10)
  - *malignant:*
    - *myosarcoma*—malignant muscular tumor. (10)
    - *rhabdomyosarcoma*—malignant tumor of striated muscle. (10, 13)
- *paralysis*—loss of sensation and voluntary movements, either temporary or permanent.
  - *flaccid*—lower motor neuron involvement.
  - *spastic*—upper motor neuron involvement. (38)
- *polymyositis*—primary myopathy characterized by muscle weakness in pelvic and shoulder girdles and distal lower and upper extremities and muscle pain or tenderness. It may be associated with connective tissue disease. (3)
- *tenosynovitis, tendosynovitis*—inflammation of a tendon and its synovial sheath. (23, 42)
- *torticollis, wryneck*—contraction of a sternocleidomastoid muscle, drawing the head to one side and causing asymmetry of the face; may be congenital or acquired. (2)

Operative Terms

- *myoplasty*—surgical repair of a muscle; for example, by free muscle graft or pedicle graft.
- *myorrhaphy*—suture of a muscle.
- *myotasis*—stretching of a muscle.
- *tenodesis*—suture of end of tendon to skeletal attachment (tendon torn at point of insertion). (37)
- *tenoplasty, tendoplasty*—surgical repair of a tendon. (27)
- *tenosynovectomy*—resection or removal of a tendon sheath. (42)

Symptomatic Terms

- *clonic spasm*—rapid, repeated muscular contractions.
- *cramp*—prolonged, intense spasm of one muscle.
- *hyperkinesia*—purposeless, excessive involuntary movements.
- *hypotonia*—reduced muscle tension associated with muscular atrophy.
- *rigidity, rigor*—stiffness, muscular hardness.
- *tonic spasm*—excessive, prolonged muscular contractions.
- *tremors*—oscillating, rhythmic movements of muscle groups.

Abbreviations

General

AP—anteroposterior
ASS—anterior superior spine
C_1—first cervical vertebra
C_2—second cervical vertebra
Ca—calcium, cancer
CDH—congenital dislocation of the hip
DIP—distal interphalangeal (joint)
EMG—electromyogram
Fx—fracture
IDK—internal derangement of the knee
IM—intramuscular
IS—intercostal space
L_1—first lumbar vertebra
L_2—second lumbar vertebra
LCP—Legg-Calvé-Perthes (disease)

LIF—left iliac fossa
LLE—left lower extremity
LOM—limitation of motion
LUE—left upper extremity
MP—metacarpal-phalangeal
MSL—midsternal line
Ortho—orthopedics
PIP—proximal interphalangeal (joint)
RIF—right iliac fossa
RLE—right lower extremity
ROM—range of motion
RUE—right upper extremity
T_1—first thoracic vertebra
T_2—second thoracic vertebra

Amputations and Prostheses

AE—above the elbow
AK—above the knee
BE—below the elbow
BK—below the knee
HD—hip disarticulation
HP—hemipelvectomy
KB—knee bearing

KD—knee disarticulation
PTB—patellar tendon bearing (prosthesis)
SACH—solid ankle cushion heel (foot prosthesis)
SD—shoulder disarticulation
THR—total hip replacement
TKR—total knee replacement

Organizations

MDAA—Muscular Dystrophy Association of America, Inc.
NSCCA—National Society for Crippled Children and Adults

Oral Reading Practice

Paget's Disease of Bone

Paget's disease of bone **(osteitis deformans)** is a peculiar bone disorder with an insidious onset, an **asymptomatic** early phase, a plateau of apparent stationary involvement, perhaps lasting years, followed by progressive disease and complications that may terminate life. The **etiology** of Paget's disease is unknown. It is not a metabolic disturbance, since it primarily attacks bones under pressure of weight bearing, leaving those of the upper body relatively untouched. An exception is the skull, which shows

roentgenographic evidence of **osteoporosis circumscripta,** so termed because **osteoporotic** changes are limited to a circumscribed area. A lesion of **decalcification** forms, particularly in the outer **cranial** table. Gradually, dense areas resembling tufts of cotton appear in the **rarefied** lesion, and the **demarcation** between **diploë,** the two cranial tables, becomes indistinct. Another serious neurologic complication that may result from overgrowth of pagetic bone at the base of the skull **(platybasia)** is due to compression of the **brain stem.**

The incidence of Paget's disease of bone is highest in advancing years and greater in males than females. It is a rather common affliction, affecting 3 percent in the age-group past 40.

The pathologic characteristics comprise concurrent processes of **osteoclastic** and **osteoblastic** activity, resulting in marked bone destruction and rapid bone repair, architectural abnormality of new bone, and increased **vascularity** and **fibrosis.** Instead of normal resorption and replacement of bone, metabolic processes are disorganized and irregular. New bone may undergo **osteolysis** as soon as it is formed. Osteoblasts produce coarse, distorted **trabeculae** that **anastomose** in a peculiar fashion, exhibiting a mosaic design.

In advanced Paget's disease the patient's **contour** portrays the influence of pathologic skeletal changes. The spine is **kyphotic,** stature shortened, position crouched, and abdomen pendulous. Pain develops with progressive bone involvement and varies from dull ache to intermittent or persistent **ostealgia.** Also, pain may be caused by involvement of the hip joint resembling **degenerative joint disease,** with varying degrees of **intrapelvic** protrusion of the **acetabulum, varus deformity** of the **femur,** and anterolateral bowing of the shaft. The **anterolateral** bowing of the legs results in a waddling, slow gait. The face appears small compared to the protruding skull, which characteristically shows **bitemporal** enlargement. Paget's disease produces one type of spinal stenosis that appears to respond well to treatment with **calcitonin. Hearing loss deficits** can occur because of pagetic bone involvement of the **ossicles** of the inner ear or of the **cochlear** bone; they can also result from impingement of the eighth **cranial nerve** by pagetic bone narrowing the **auditory foramen.**

Fractures occur frequently, heal rapidly, and are the most common complication of Paget's bone disease. They may be caused by trivial incidents such as tripping on stairs or turning in bed. Two most common sites of fracture are the **subtrochanteric** area and the upper shaft area of the femur. Total hip **arthroplasty** is usually the procedure of choice. **Heterotopic** bone formation may occur as a postoperative complication; however, the administration of calcitonin before and after surgery tends to decrease the **osteoclastic** activity and thereby hopefully reduce the risk of loosening secondary to inadequate support by osteoporotic bone.

The patient with Paget's disease, immobilized because of fracture or intercurrent disease, is likely to develop **hypercalciuria, renal calculi,** and **hypercalcemia.** Since bone repair is markedly dec   ƒed during immobilization, **osteoporosis** resulting from disuse becomes problematic. Bone destruction persists unabated, thus liberating an excessive amount of calcium, which is spilled into urine instead of being deposited in bone. This may lead to **nephrolithiasis** and serious **sequelae.** If the kidneys are unable to handle the high surplus of calcium, hypercalcemia is prone to develop. It is signaled by dryness of mouth and nose, nausea, and vomiting. Untreated, the **prognosis** may be fatal. Techniques of measuring disappearance rates of injected **radioisotopes** of calcium or strontium have shown that rates of bone turnover may be increased enormously in patients with active Paget's disease, occasionally more than 20 times normal. The magnitude of the increase varies with the extent and activity of the disease.

Malignant degeneration of diseased bone is a constant threat. Whenever **osteogenic sarcoma, chondrosarcoma,** malignant **fibrous histiocytoma, fibrosarcoma** or malignant **osteoclastoma** develop, the patient has probably reached the terminal phase of life. **Palliative** measures must be instituted to bring relief of ostealgia and other distressing symptoms. (4, 10, 31, 52, 63)

Table 2
Some Orthopedic Conditions Amenable to Surgery

Organs Involved	Diagnosis	Type of Surgery	Operative Procedures
Shoulder	Calcified deposits in rotator cuff	Curettement of rotator cuff	Split deltoid approach and scraping of cuff to remove deposits
Knee	Recurrent dislocation of patella	Hauser operation	Medial and distal transplantation of tibial tubercle and its patellar tendon
Knee	Chondromalacia of patella	Patellaplasty	Partial resection and plastic repair of patella
		Complete patellectomy	Removal of patella
Ulna Radius	Crushing injury with loss of blood supply to hand and wrist	Amputation of forearm	Removal of forearm below elbow
		Biceps cineplasty for operating prosthetic device	Construction of skin tunnel through biceps muscle; tunneled muscle to move artificial hand
Hand Wrist joint	Traumatic severance of hand	Replantation of hand	First wire passed through carpus and up medullary cavity of radius
	Disarticulation at wrist joint	Internal fixation with Kirschner wires	Second wire crossed from base of 5th metacarpal through cortex of radius. Repair of vessels and tendons
Carpal tunnel Transverse carpal ligament Median nerve	Carpal tunnel syndrome	Surgical division and partial excision of transverse carpal ligament	Complete section and partial removal of carpal ligament
		Synovectomy of flexor synovialis	Removal of thickened synovial membrane to decompress the median nerve

Organs Involved	Diagnosis	Type of Surgery	Operative Procedures
Spine	Scoliosis	Harrington's operation: instrumentation and fusion for correction of scoliosis	Implantation of metal rods and hooks directly on the spine, followed by fusion to provide distractive and compressive forces of spinal curve
Spine	Spondylolisthesis	Modified Hibbs arthrodesis of spine	Excision of cartilage from articular facets, packing bone chips into joint spaces; iliac bone grafting
Hip joint	Early degenerative arthritis	High femoral osteotomy	Incision through upper end of femur, usually in subtrochanteric region Medial displacement of distal femur resulting in change in weight-bearing position of femoral head
Hip joint	Degenerative arthritis	Vitallium mold arthroplasty	Reconstruction of femoral head and placement of deep cup over femoral head
		Austin Moore or Fred Thompson arthroplasty	Replacement of femoral head with hip prosthesis
Hip joint	Advanced rheumatoid arthritis and ankylosing spondylitis of hip—or Advanced osteoarthritis	Charnley low-friction arthroplasty for total hip replacement	Lateral oblique incision to expose upper end of femoral shaft Dislocation of hip and removal of femoral head and neck and of destructive joint lesions Insertion of small femoral head and stem in shaft Cement used for seating the acetabular cup and prosthetic stem to provide rigid fixation
Hip joint	Congenital dislocation of hip	Colonna capsular arthroplasty	*First stage:* Hamstring stretching and surgical division of adductor tendon *Second stage:* Reconstruction of acetabulum Placement of capsule-covered femoral head into reconstructed acetabulum

Organs Involved	Diagnosis	Type of Surgery	Operative Procedures
Femur	Fracture of femoral neck	Excision of femoral head and insertion of hip prosthesis (Fred Thompson or Austin Moore type)	Removal of femoral head and most of neck; replacement by metal prosthesis
		Internal fixation by insertion of Smith-Petersen nail	Three-flanged nail driven over guide wire through femoral neck and head; then guide wire removed
Femur	Intertrochanteric fracture of femur	Internal fixation by insertion of hip nail (Jewett, Neufeld, Holt, or Key type)	Nail driven over guide wire through femoral neck and into head of femur; side plate fixed to shaft with screws
Femur	Transverse diaphyseal fracture of femur	Internal fixation by insertion of intramedullary nail (Kuntscher type or Lottes type)	Medullary nail driven over guide wire into medullary cavity, occupying the entire canal
Tibia Fibula Foot	Crushing injury; uncontrollable infection of distal portion of lower extremity	Below-knee amputation	Incision of skin flaps Division of anterolateral muscles Ligation of blood vessels Removal of leg and stump closure Application of rigid elastic plaster dressing and prosthetic unit
Foot	Hallus valgus deformity	Keller operation	Resection of proximal half of first phalanx of great toe Excision of bony prominence
Anterior cruciate ligament	Tear of anterior cruciate ligament; separation of anterior attachment	Reconstruction of torn anterior cruciate ligament	Repair of ligament by restoring the anterior attachment
Achilles tendon or Tendon calcaneus	Abnormal shortening of tendon calcaneus	Tenoplasty with lengthening of tendon calcaneus	Surgical repair of tendon
Sternoclei-domastoid muscle	Torticollis, congenital	Brown and McDowell excision of sternocleidomastoid muscle	Abnormal muscle freed from underlying structures and excised
		Tenotomy of upper and lower end of sternocleidomastoid muscle or both ends	Muscle lengthened by division of one or both ends, allowing shortened muscle to retract

References and Bibliography

1. Beaty, James H. Congenital anomalies of lower extremity. In Crenshaw, A.H., ed., *Campbell's Operative Orthopaedics,* 7th ed., vol. 4. St. Louis: The C.V. Mosby Co., 1987, pp. 2623-2712.

2. ———. Congenital anomalies of trunk and upper extremity. Ibid., pp. 2759-2780.

3. Bradley, Walter G. Dermatomyositis and polymyositis. In Braunwald, Eugene, et al., eds., *Harrison's Principles of Internal Medicine,* 11th ed. New York: McGraw-Hill Book Co., 1987, pp. 2069-2072.

4. Calandruccio, Rocco A. Arthroplasty of hip. In Crenshaw, A.H., ed., *Campbell's Operative Orthopaedics,* 7th ed. vol. 2. St. Louis: The C.V. Mosby Co., 1987, pp. 1213-1501.

5. Canale, S. Terry. Osteochondrosis. In Crenshaw, A.H., ed., *Campbell's Operative Orthopaedics,* 7th ed., vol. 2. St. Louis: The C.V. Mosby Co., 1987, pp. 989-1003.

6. Carnesale, Peter G. Osteomyelitis. In Crenshaw, A.H., ed., *Campbell's Operative Orthopaedics,* 7th ed., vol. 2. St. Louis: The C.V. Mosby Co., 1987, pp. 651-675.

7. ———. Benign tumors of bone. Ibid., pp. 747-764.

8. ———. Sometimes malignant tumors of bone. Ibid., pp. 765-775.

9. ———. Malignant tumors of the bone. Ibid., pp. 777-805.

10. ———. Soft tissue tumors. Ibid., pp. 807-826.

11. Clemente, Carmine D., ed. Osteology. In *Gray's Anatomy of the Human Body,* 30th ed. Philadelphia: Lea & Febiger, 1985, pp. 114-328.

12. ———. The joints. Ibid., pp. 329-428.

13. ———. Muscles and fasciae. Ibid., pp. 429-605.

14. Crenshaw, A.H. Delayed union and nonunion of fractures. In Crenshaw, A.H., ed., *Campbell's Operative Orthopaedics,* 7th ed., vol. 3. St. Louis: The C.V. Mosby Co., 1987, pp. 2053-2118.

15. Cush, John J., and Lipsky, Peter E. Approach to disorders of the joints and musculoskeletal disorders. In Braunwald, Eugene, et al., eds., *Harrison's Principles of Internal Medicine,* 11th ed. New York: McGraw-Hill Book Co., 1987, pp. 1454-1456.

16. Edmonson, Allen S. Scoliosis. In Crenshaw, A.H., ed., *Campbell's Operative Orthopaedics,* 7th ed., vol. 4. St. Louis: The C.V. Mosby Co., 1987, pp. 3167-3236.

17. ———. Kyphosis and spondylolisthesis. Ibid., pp. 3237-3253.

18. Engle, Andrew G. Myasthenia gravis and other disorders of neuromuscular transmission. In Braunwald, Eugene, et al., eds., *Harrison's Principles of Internal Medicine,* 11th ed. New York: McGraw-Hill Book Co., 1987, pp. 2079-2082.

19. Gilliland, Bruce C. Ankylosing spondylitis. In Braunwald, Eugene, et al., eds., *Harrison's Principles of Internal Medicine,* 11th ed. New York: McGraw-Hill Book Co., 1987, pp. 1434-1436.

20. ———. Degenerative joint disease. Ibid., pp. 1456-1458.

21. ———. Calcium pyrophosphate (pseudogout) and calcium hydroxyapatite deposition diseases. Ibid., pp. 1458-1460.

22. ———. Psoriatic arthritis and arthritis associated with gastrointestinal diseases. Ibid., pp. 1460-1461.

23. ———. Miscellaneous arthritides and extraarticular rheumatism. Ibid., pp. 1465-1469.

24. Gilliland, Bruce C., and Petersdorf, Robert G. Infectious arthritis. In Braunwald, Eugene, et al., eds., *Harrison's Principles of Internal Medicine,* 11th ed. New York: McGraw-Hill Book Co., 1987, pp. 1462-1465.

25. Goyal, Raj K. Diseases of the esophagus. In Braunwald, Eugene, et al., eds., *Harrison's Principles of Internal Medicine,* 11th ed. New York: McGraw-Hill Book Co., 1987, pp. 1231-1239.

26. Hirschmann, Jan V. Osteomyelitis. In Braunwald, Eugene, et al., eds., *Harrison's Principles of Internal Medicine,* 11th ed. New York: McGraw-Hill Book Co., 1987, pp. 1910-1912.

27. Ingram, Alvin J. Paralytic disorders. In Crenshaw, A.H., ed., *Campbell's Operative Orthopaedics,* 7th ed., vol. 4. St. Louis: The C.V. Mosby Co., 1987, pp. 2925-3068.

28. Justis, E. Jeff, Jr. Traumatic disorders. In Crenshaw, A.H., ed., *Campbell's Operative Orthopaedics,* 7th ed., vol. 3. St. Louis: The C.V. Mosby Co., 1987, pp. 2221-2246.

29. ———. Nontraumatic disorders. Ibid., pp. 2247-2261.

30. Kelley, William N., and Palella, Thomas D. Gout and other disorders of purine metabolism. In Braunwald, Eugene, et al., eds., *Harrison's Principles of Internal Medicine,* 11th ed. New York: McGraw-Hill Book Co., 1987, pp. 1623-1632.

31. Krane, Stephen M. Paget's disease of bone. In Braunwald, Eugene, et al., eds., *Harrison's Principles of Internal Medicine,* 11th ed. New York: McGraw-Hill Book Co., 1987, pp. 1900-1902.

32. Krane, Stephen M., and Holick, Michael F. Metabolic bone disease. In Braunwald, Eugene, et al., eds., *Harrison's Principles of Internal Medicine,* 11th ed. New York: McGraw-Hill Book Co., 1987, pp. 1889-1900.

33. Krane, Stephen M., and Schiller, Alan L. Hyperostosis, neoplasms, and other disorders of bone and cartilage. In Braunwald, Eugene, et al., eds., *Harrison's Principles of Internal Medicine,* 11th ed. New York: McGraw-Hill Book Co., 1987, pp. 1902-1910.

34. Lipsky, Peter E. Rheumatoid arthritis. In Braunwald, Eugene, et al., eds., *Harrison's Principles of Internal Medicine,* 11th ed. New York: McGraw-Hill Book Co., 1987, pp. 1423-1428.

35. Mankin, Henry J., and Adams, Raymond D. Pain in back and neck. In Braunwald, Eugene, et al., eds., *Harrison's Principles of Internal Medicine,* 11th ed. New York: McGraw-Hill Book Co., 1987, pp. 34-42.

36. Mendell, Jerry R., and Griggs, Robert C. Muscular dystrophy and other chronic myopathies. In Braunwald, Eugene, et al., eds., *Harrison's Principles of Internal Medicine,* 11th ed. New York: McGraw-Hill Book Co., 1987, pp. 2072-2078.

37. Milford, Lee. Paralytic hand. In Crenshaw, A.H., ed., *Campbell's Operative Orthopaedics,* 7th ed., vol. 2. St. Louis: The C.V. Mosby Co., 1987, pp. 325-362.

38. ———. Cerebral palsied hand. Ibid., pp. 363-375.

39. ———. Volkmann's contracture and compartment syndromes. Ibid., pp. 409-418.

40. ———. Congenital abnormalities. Ibid., pp. 419-449.

41. ———. Dupuytren's contracture. Ibid., pp. 451-457.

42. ———. Carpal tunnel syndrome and ulnar tunnel syndrome and stenosing tenosynovitis. Ibid., pp. 459-468.

43. ———. Tumors and tumorous conditions of the hand. Ibid., pp. 469-494.

44. Moutsopoulos, Haralampos M. Reiter's syndrome and Behcet's syndrome. In Braunwald, Eugene, et al., eds., *Harrison's Principles of Internal Medicine,* 11th ed. New York: McGraw-Hill Book Co., 1987, pp. 1436-1438.

45. Prockop, Darwin J. Heritable disorders of connective tissue. In Braunwald, Eugene, et al., eds., *Harrison's Principles of Internal Medicine,* 11th ed. New York: McGraw-Hill Book Co., 1987, pp. 1680-1688.

46. Richardson, E. Greer. The foot in adolescents and adults. In Crenshaw, A.H., ed., *Campbell's Operative Orthopaedics,* 7th ed., vol. 2. St. Louis: The C.V. Mosby Co., 1987, pp. 829-988.

47. ———. Miscellaneous nontraumatic disorders. Ibid., pp. 1005-1088.

48. Russell, Thomas A. Arthrodesis of lower extremity. In Crenshaw, A.H., ed., *Campbell's Operative Orthopaedics,* 7th ed., vol. 2. St. Louis: The C.V. Mosby Co., 1987, pp. 1091-1130.

49. Sage, Fred P. Inheritable progressive neuromuscular diseases. In Crenshaw, A.H., ed., *Campbell's Operative Orthopaedics,* 7th ed., vol. 4. St. Louis: The C.V. Mosby Co., 1987, pp. 3061-3088.

50. Shearn, Martin A. Arthritis and musculoskeletal disorders. In Schroeder, Steven A., Krupp, Marcus A., and Tierney, Lawrence M., Jr., eds., *Current Medical Diagnosis and Treatment—1988,* Norwalk, CT: Appleton & Lange, 1988, pp. 496-532.

51. Sisk, T. David. General principles of fracture treatment. In Crenshaw, A.H., ed., *Campbell's Operative Orthopaedics,* 7th ed., vol. 3. St. Louis: The C.V. Mosby Co., 1987, pp. 1557-1606.

52. ———. Fractures of lower extremity. Ibid., pp. 1607-1718.

53. ———. Fractures of the hip and pelvis. Ibid., pp. 1719-1791.

54. ———. Fractures of shoulder girdle and upper extremity. Ibid., pp. 1783-1831.

55. ———. General principles of arthroscopy. Ibid., vol. 4, pp. 2527-2546.

56. ———. Arthroscopy of knee and ankle. Ibid., vol. 4, pp. 2547-2608.

57. ———. Arthroscopy of shoulder and elbow. Ibid., vol. 4, pp. 2609-2620.

58. Sisk, T. David, and Wright, Phillip E. Arthroplasty of shoulder and elbow. In Crenshaw, A.H., ed., *Campbell's Operative Orthopaedics,* 7th ed., vol. 2. St. Louis: The C.V. Mosby Co., 1987, pp. 1503-1554.

59. Tooms, Robert E. General principles of amputation. In Crenshaw, A.H., ed., *Campbell's Operative Orthopaedics,* 7th ed., vol. 1. St. Louis: The C.V. Mosby Co., 1987, pp. 597-606.

60. ———. Amputations of lower extremity. Ibid., pp. 607-627.

61. ———. Arthroplasty of ankle and knee. Ibid., vol. 2, pp. 1145-1211.

62. Wood, George W. Lower back pain and disorders of intervertebral disc. In Crenshaw, A.H., ed., *Campbell's Operative Orthopaedics,* 7th ed., vol. 4. St. Louis: The C.V. Mosby Co., 1987, pp. 3255-3321.

63. ———. Other disorders of spine. Ibid., pp. 3347-3374.

64. Wright, Phillip E. Shoulder and elbow injuries. In Crenshaw, A.H., ed., *Campbell's Operative Orthopaedics,* 7th ed., vol. 3. St. Louis: The C.V. Mosby Co., 1987, pp. 2497-2524.

Neurologic and Psychiatric Disorders

Nerves

Origin of Terms

axon (G)—axis
gangli-, ganglio- (G)—knot, ganglion
neur-, neuro- (G)—nerve(s)
nucleus (pl. nuclei) (L)—little kernel

plexus (L)—braid, network
radicle (L)—root, small branches
synapse (G)—clasp, connection

Anatomic Terms (Ref. 84)

- *nerve*—a collection of many nerve fibers.
  - —*cranial nerves*—12 pairs of nerves made up of either motor or sensory fibers or both.
  - —*spinal nerves*—31 pairs of mixed nerves.
- *nerve cell, neuron*—basic component of nerve tissue consisting of a cell body or neuron body and one or more processes. The neuron is the anatomic unit of the central nervous system.
  - —*structure of neurons:*
    - —*axon, axone*—slender process of a neuron body arising from specialized protoplasm known as an axon hill. It contains many neurofibrils but no Nissl bodies.
    - —*cell body*—neuron body composed of a nucleus embedded in cytoplasm, which contains neurofibrils, Nissl bodies, mitochondria, and others. The cell body maintains the nutrition of the whole neuron.
    - —*dendrite, dendron*—a protoplasmic extension from the cell body forming an irregular knobby process, which is wide at the base and narrows down rapidly. Dendrites greatly increase the cell body's receptive surface.
    - —*effector*—organ of response that reacts to the impulse, for example, a muscle or a gland.
    - —*ganglion (pl. ganglia)*—a collection of neural cell bodies lying outside the central nervous system.
    - —*myelin sheath*—protective covering of axons, composed of lipids and protein and interrupted by constrictions, the nodes of Ranvier.
    - —*neurilemma, neurolemma, sheath of Schwann*—a thin, cellular membrane covering the axis cylinder of a nonmedullated nerve fiber or enclosing the

myelin sheath of a medullated nerve fiber of peripheral nerves.

  —*neurofibrils*—delicate threads found in the cell bodies and processes of neurons.

  —*Nissl bodies*—RNA (ribonucleic acid) granules present in the cell bodies of neurons.

  —*receptor*—end organ that responds to various stimuli (pain, touch, and others) and converts them into nervous impulses.

  —*classification according to function:*

  —*afferent neurons*—conduct impulses from receptor to central nervous system.

  —*association, intercalated, or internuncial neurons*—located within the central nervous system; these transmit impulses between neurons.

  —*efferent neurons*—conduct impulses away from the central nervous system to the effector organ.

- *nerve fiber*—the axon with its sheaths.
- *plexus (pl. plexuses) of spinal nerves*—a network of nerve fibers. For example:

  —*brachial plexus*—an intermingling of the fifth to the eighth cervical nerves and the first thoracic nerve, which supply the upper limb.

  —*sacral plexus*—an intermingling of the fourth and fifth lumbar and first four sacral nerves, which help to supply the lower limb.

- *roots of spinal nerves*—these attach the nerves to the spinal cord.

  —*ventral (anterior) root*—composed of efferent fibers, with no ganglion.

  —*dorsal (posterior) root*—composed of afferent fibers, with a small ganglion.

- *synapse*—the point of contact between the axon of one neuron and a dendrite or cell body of another neuron.

(See Figs. 23 to 26 for structure of nerves and neurons.)

Diagnostic Terms

- *Bell's palsy*—functional disorder of the seventh cranial nerve that may result in a unilateral paralysis of facial muscles and distortion of taste perception. Etiology is unknown. (13, 40)
- *causalgia*—posttraumatic paroxysms of unbearable peripheral nerve pain of a burning quality aggravated by heat, slight friction, anxiety, and emotion. It appears to be stimulated by efferent sympathetic nerve impulses. (51)
- *Guillain-Barré syndrome, acute idiopathic polyneuropathy*—widespread disorder of the peripheral motor nerves, characterized by progressive flaccid paralysis of an ascending type associated with sensory disturbances. When the chest muscles and diaphragm become affected, respiratory difficulties arise. Cranial nerve involvement, particularly that of the facial nerve, may develop last in the course of the disease, or it may be the initial pathology followed by motor impairment of a descending type. (13, 40)
- *herniated nucleus pulposus, herniated intervertebral disk*—tear in posterior joint capsule and bulging of portions of intervertebral disk, resulting in nerve root irritation and compression followed by sciatic pain and paresthesias and occasionally by paresis or paralysis. (52)
- *neurilemoma, neurilemmoma (also neurolemoma, neurolemmoma)*—usually a benign, encapsulated, solitary tumor, produced by the proliferation of Schwann cells. It may originate from a sympathetic, peripheral, or cranial nerve. (24)
- *neuroma*—a tumor of tissue found in the nervous system. Neuroma is an obsolete term and a more specific designation is preferable, for example:

  —*ganglioneuroma*—true neuroma.

  —*pseudoneuroma, amputation neuroma*—false neuroma or traumatic neuroma. (71, 75)

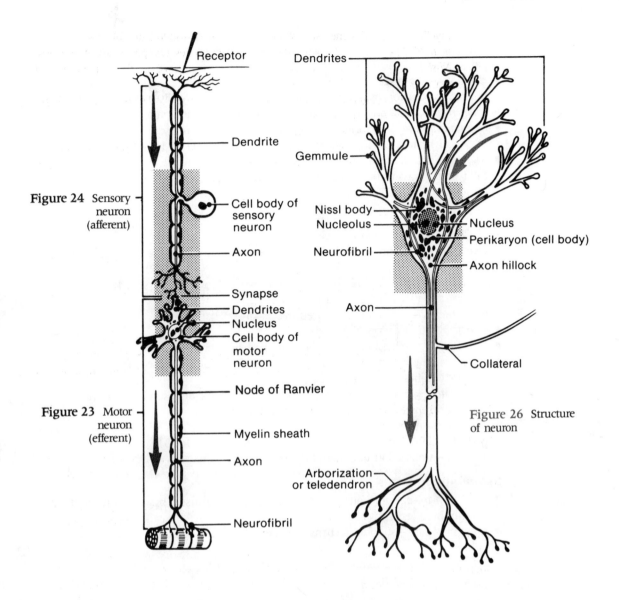

Figure 24 Sensory neuron (afferent)

Receptor

Dendrite

Cell body of sensory neuron

Axon

Synapse
Dendrites
Nucleus
Cell body of motor neuron

Node of Ranvier

Figure 23 Motor neuron (efferent)

Myelin sheath

Axon

Neurofibril

Dendrites

Gemmule

Nissl body
Nucleolus

Neurofibril

Nucleus
Perikaryon (cell body)

Axon hillock

Axon

Collateral

Figure 26 Structure of neuron

Arborization or teledendron

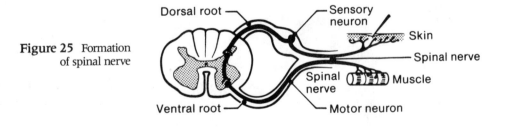

Figure 25 Formation of spinal nerve

Dorsal root

Sensory neuron

Skin

Spinal nerve

Spinal nerve

Muscle

Ventral root

Motor neuron

- *polyneuritis, polyneuropathy*—widespread neural lesions caused by nutritional deficiencies, especially of vitamin B complex. The chief symptoms are pain and paresthesia. (13, 40)
- *radiculitis*—any involvement of the spinal nerve roots due to either infection, toxins, trauma, protrusion of intervertebral disk, or degenerative diseases. (52)
- *sciatic neuritis, sciatica*—a very painful involvement of the sciatic nerve. (13)
- *trigeminal neuralgia, trifacial neuralgia, tic douloureux*—paroxysms of lancinating pain of one or more areas innervated by the fifth cranial nerve. (46, 81)
- *trigeminal neurinoma*—rare, benign tumor of the trigeminal nerve characterized by mild pain or paresthesia, diminished corneal reflex, and weakness of muscles of mastication. (27, 77)

Operative Terms

- *ganglionectomy*—excision of a ganglion.
- *neurectomy*—excision of a nerve or lesion of a nerve, for example, a solitary neuroma. (23)
- *neuroanastomosis*—surgical communication between nerve fibers. (54)
- *neuroplasty*—plastic repair of a nerve.
- *neurorrhaphy*—suture of an injured nerve. (54)
- *neurotomy*—transection of a nerve.
- *sympathectomy*—excision of part of a sympathetic nerve.
    - *thoracic ganglionectomy*—for causalgia or Raynaud's disease affecting the upper extremities.
    - *lumbar ganglionectomy*—for causalgia, Raynaud's disease, and thromboangiitis obliterans affecting the lower extremities. (15)
- *trigeminal decompression*—compression of ganglion and root of trigeminal complex with dry cottonoid to relieve pain in tic douloureux. (46, 81)
- *vagotomy*—transection of a vagus nerve.

Symptomatic Terms

- *aural vertigo*—episodic attacks of severe dizziness caused by a lesion in the ear (labyrinthine lesion). (71)
- *paroxysmal pain*—sudden, recurrent, or periodic attack of pain, as in tic douloureux. (46, 81)
- *tactile stimulation*—evoking a response by touch. (12)
- *trigger area*—point from which the pain starts, as in trigeminal neuralgia. (77)

Brain and Spinal Cord

Origin of Terms

cerebro- (G)—brain
chordo- (G)—cord, string
cingulum (L)—girdle
cord (L)—string
encephalo- (G)—brain
hemi- (G)—one half
gyrus (L)—convolution
lamina (L)—thin plate
medulla (L)—marrow
meninges (G)—membrane
meningo- (G)—membrane

myel-, myelo- (G)—marrow
neur-, neuro- (G)—nerve
-oma (G)—tumor
paresis (G)—relaxation
peri- (G)—around
plexus (L)—braid, network
pons (L)—bridge
spina (L)—thornlike projection or process, spine
thalmo- (G)—chamber
ventricle (L)—small cavity

Anatomic Terms (84)

- *brain, encephalon*—major part of central nervous system. It is divided into the forebrain or prosencephalon, midbrain or mesencephalon, and hindbrain or rhombencephalon and comprises the following structural and functional components:
  - *cerebellum*—second largest part of the brain, which serves as a reflex center for the coordination of muscular movements. It is divided into two hemispheres and a median portion, the vermis.
  - *cerebrum*—the largest part of the brain, which is divided into two hemispheres by a deep groove, the longitudinal fissure.
  - *cerebral cortex*—the surface of the cerebrum, composed of gray matter and arranged in folds known as convolutions or gyri.
  - *cerebral localization*—definite regions of the cerebral cortex performing special functions:
    - the motor areas, which influence voluntary muscular activity.
    - the sensory areas, where sensations reach the conscious level.
    - *corpus callosum*—a bridgelike structure of white fibers that joins the two hemispheres.
- *brain stem*—upward continuation of cervical cord that consists of numerous bundles of nerve fibers and nuclei. Its structural components include the following:
  - *diencephalon, interbrain*—small but important part of forebrain comprising:
    - *epithalamus*—area including several nuclei and the pineal body or epiphysis.
    - *hypothalamus*—small mass below the thalamus containing nuclei and fibers. It is an integrating center for the autonomic nervous system and through its relation to the hypophysis for the endocrine system.
    - *metathalamus*—area of the lateral and medial geniculate bodies.
    - *subthalamus*—a mass of nuclei and fibers important in regulating muscular activities.
    - *thalamus*—a mass of nuclei situated on either side of the third ventricle. It is the great sensory relay station.
  - *medulla oblongata, myelencephalon, marrow brain*—extends from upper cervical cord to pons; contains vital centers regulating heart action, vasomotor activity, respiration, deglutition, and vomiting.
  - *mesencephalon, midbrain*—extends from pons below to forebrain above and is composed of nuclei and bundles of fibers.
  - *pons*—part of metencephalon (afterbrain) composed of bundles of fibers and nuclei that are located between the medulla and midbrain.
- *meninges*—covering membranes of the brain and the spinal cord.
  - *dura mater*—serves as outer protective coat and is composed of strong fibrous tissue.
  - *arachnoid*—middle layer consisting of thin meshwork. The subarachnoid space contains cerebrospinal fluid.
  - *pia mater*—dips down between the convolutions and adheres closely to the brain.
- *nucleus (pl. nuclei)*—group of nerve cells within the central nervous system.
  - *basal nuclei, formerly basal ganglia*—masses of nerve cells deeply embedded in the white matter of the forebrain, for example, the lentiform nucleus.
- *ventricles and aqueduct:*
  - *lateral ventricles*—fluid-filled spaces, one in each cerebral hemisphere.
  - *third ventricle*—fluid-filled space beneath the corpus callosum.
  - *cerebral aqueduct*—a narrow canal that connects the third and fourth ventricles.
  - *fourth ventricle*—an expansion of the central canal of the medulla oblongata.

The ventricles contain cerebrospinal fluid, which is formed by the capillaries of the choroid plexuses. The fluid seeps from the third ventricle into the cerebral aqueduct and fourth ventricle and from there into the central canal. It reaches the subarachnoid space through openings in the roof of the fourth ventricle and circulates around the cord and brain in this space, thus providing a water-cushion and shock absorber for the delicate nerve tissue.

- *spinal cord*—portion of central nervous system located in the vertebral canal and giving rise to 31 pairs of spinal nerves. It extends from the foramen magnum to the second lumbar vertebra and is composed of white substance, which surrounds the inner gray matter of the cord. Several lengthwise grooves demarcate the white matter into long columns. The deepest groove is the anterior median fissure, which, together with the posterior median septum, almost separates the cord into two equal halves. The **white matter** consists of myelinated fibers arranged in longitudinal bundles and grouped into three columns: the anterior, lateral, and posterior funiculi. Afferent white fibers arise from the ascending nerve tracts, which carry impulses from the cord to the brain. Efferent white fibers represent descending nerve tracts, which bring messages from the brain to the cord. The **gray matter** is H-shaped in cross-section and consists mainly of cell bodies. The anterior horn contains motor cells from which the motor fibers of the peripheral neurons arise. Sensory relay neurons are located in the posterior horn.

(See Figs. 27 and 28 for median section of brain and spinal cord and transverse section of cord.)

Diagnostic Terms

- *amyotrophic lateral sclerosis*—degenerative disease of the lateral motor tracts of the spinal cord causing widespread muscle wasting, weakness, fasciculations, and usually a mild degree of spastic paralysis of lower extremities. (32, 62)
- *anencephalia, anencephalus*—absence of brain.
- *brain abscess*—localized lesion of suppuration within the brain, generally secondary to ear infection, sinusitis, or other infections.
- *brain tumor, intracranial tumor*—benign or malignant space-occupying brain lesion. (35)
  - *adnexal tumor*—derived from pineal body or choroid plexus. It may compress the aqueduct and cause obstructive hydrocephalus or exert pressure on the hypothalamus and may be associated with diabetes insipidus or precocious puberty. (59)
  - *congenital tumor*—a slowly growing, highly invasive tumor, for example, a dermoid or teratoma.
  - *medulloblastoma*—a highly malignant cerebellar tumor that metastasizes freely to the subarachnoid space, cerebrum, and cord. (44, 59)
  - *meningeal tumor*—neoplasm arising from the covering membranes of the brain or cord.
    The meningioma may cause compression and distortion of the brain. (59)
  - *metastatic tumor*—most primary tumors may metastasize to the brain, especially breast and lung tumors. (44, 60)
  - *pituitary tumor*—arises from anterior pituitary (adenohypophysis) and may compress the normal portion of the pituitary, the hypothalamus, and optic chiasm.
  - *primary brain tumors*—comprise a large number of intracranial tumors, especially the gliomas, which contain malignant glial cells. Some neoplasms of the glioma group are presented:

—*astrocytoma*—a slowly growing tumor containing astrocytes that infiltrate widely into neighboring brain tissue and may undergo cystic degeneration. (44, 59)

—*ependymoma*—tumor that arises from the lining of the ventricular wall and is highly malignant and invasive. (59)

—*glioblastoma multiforme*—the most malignant glioma, rapidly growing, causing edema and necrosis of brain tissue. (1, 44, 59)

—*oligodendroglioma*—similar to astrocytoma in behavior, different in histologic structure. (44)

- *cerebral concussion*—transient state of unconsciousness following head injury that is an immediate result of damage to the brain stem. (31, 72)

- *cerebral palsy*—condition characterized by paralysis, incoordination, and other aberrations of motor or sensory functions caused by damage to the brain. (27)

- *cerebrovascular disease*—any disorder in which one or more of the cerebral blood vessels have undergone pathologic changes (see Fig. 29).

—*cerebral aneurysm, intracranial aneurysm*—dilation of an artery of the brain, resulting in a thinning and weakening of the arterial wall. Common locations are the internal carotid and middle cerebral arteries. Rupture and hemorrhage may occur and cause serious brain damage.

—*cerebral arteriovenous malformation*—structural vascular defect, generally found in young patients with recurrent subarachnoid hemorrhage and epilepsy. (30)

—*cerebral atherosclerosis*—a primary degeneration of the intima by atheromatous plaques (lipid deposits) usually located in the basilar artery, the middle and posterior cerebral arteries, and at the branching of the internal carotids. The subsequent narrowing of the vessels may lead to inadequate oxygenation and nutrition of the brain by the reduced cerebral circulation. Brain softening, neural atrophy, and senile plaques add further damage and predispose to physical and mental deterioration. (30, 50)

—*cerebral embolism*—sudden occlusion of a cerebral blood vessel by a circulatory embolus composed of air bubble, blood clot, fat cells, or bacteria. (30)

—*cerebral infarction*—local necrosis of brain tissue resulting from loss of blood supply in vascular obstruction. (30, 50)

—*cerebral ischemia*—anemia of the brain resulting from diminished cerebral blood flow. Some important causes are circulatory obstruction of the intracranial or extracranial arteries by atheroma, thrombus or embolus, severe hypotension, arteritis, or stenosis of an artery. Recurrent ischemic episodes are thought to signal impending stroke. (30)

—*cerebral thrombosis*—formation of a thrombus within an intracranial artery, leading to its occlusion and subsequent necrosis of the area supplied by the thrombosed vessel. (30, 50)

—*cerebrovascular accident, stroke, apoplexy*—neurologic disorder caused by pathologic changes in the extracranial or intracranial blood vessels, primarily by atherosclerosis, thrombosis, embolic episodes, hemorrhage, or arterial hypertension. Cerebral infarction or necrosis of brain tissue may occur in the affected lesion. The completed stroke, usually recognized by a rather sudden loss of consciousness and other marked neurologic insult, is preceded by: (31, 48, 50)

—*transient ischemic attacks*—symptoms of minor brain damage evidenced by numbness, unilateral weakness, visual deficits, and motor disability, and similar symptoms. They last from minutes to hours. A complete return to the preattack status may occur, or there may be residual damage.

—*progressive stroke*—neurologic manifestations are persistent and become more serious, signaling impending stroke.

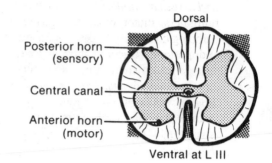

Figure 27 Transverse section of spinal cord at level of origin of third lumbar nerve.

Figure 28 Median section of brain and spinal cord, showing communication of ventricles with subarachnoid space and central canal. Choroid plexuses, generally thought to form cerebrospinal fluid, are tufts of capillaries located in ventricles.

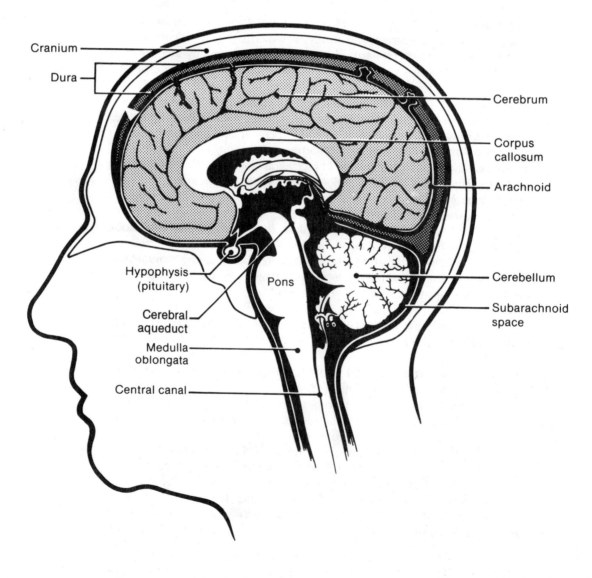

—*cerebrovascular insufficiency syndrome*—clinical evidence of minor brain damage: numbness, motor weakness, slurred speech, and others; may develop from pathologic changes of the intracranial vessels, especially the anterior, middle, and posterior cerebral arteries. More frequently it is caused by extracranial vascular obstruction leading to cerebral ischemia, as seen in the following: (50)

—*internal carotid syndrome, internal carotid stenosis, internal carotid ischemia*—stenotic lesion usually resulting from atheromatous process near the bifurcation of the common carotid artery. It may cause contralateral hemiparesis or hemiplegia, speech difficulties, visual defects, and other changes (Fig. 30).

—*subclavian steal syndrome, proximal subclavian stenosis, skeletal muscle ischemia of arm*—syndrome caused by impaired blood flow to the basilar artery or brachiocephalic trunk near the origin of the vertebral artery. The decreased vascular pressure beyond the occluded segment initiates retrograde flow in the vertebral artery and siphons the blood away from the brain. This stealing of blood, which reduces the cerebral circulation, thus causing neurologic deficit, is demanded by the muscles for exercise of the affected arm. The low or absent blood pressure and pulse on the site of the subclavian occlusion, in contrast to those markedly higher on the unaffected arm, are diagnostic evidence (Fig. 31).

—*vertebrobasilar syndrome, vertebral artery stenosis or basilar artery stenosis, vertebrobasilar ischemia*—syndrome manifests cerebellar involvement: vertigo, disequilibrium, ataxia and cranial nerve damage, facial paralysis, motor and sensory disturbances, and others.

—*intracranial hematoma*—local mass of extravasated blood formed as a result of intracranial hemorrhage. Chronic lesions may become encapsulated. Epidural and subdural hematomas, located above or below the dura mater, are usually caused by head injury. (63)

—*intracranial hemorrhage*—rupture of a vessel beneath the skull with seepage of blood into the brain coverings or substance. It may be caused by head injury, stroke, or ruptured aneurysm. Brain damage depends on the location and extent of the lesion involved. (30, 31)

—*subarachnoid hemorrhage*—bleeding into the subarachnoid space, which in some cases is associated with excruciating headache, convulsions, and coma. It is due to head injury or ruptured intracranial aneurysm. (31)

- *chorea*—nervous disorder characterized by bizarre, abrupt, involuntary movements.

   —*Huntington's chorea, adult chorea*—hereditary form with onset in adult life, involvement of basal ganglia and cortex, choreiform movements, and mental decline.

   —*Sydenham's chorea, juvenile chorea*—disorder of childhood and adolescence with insidious onset of jerky movements, usually occurring during rheumatic fever. (32, 62)

- *encephalitis lethargica*—inflammation of the brain marked by somnolence and ocular paralysis. It is caused by a filtrable virus. (38, 42)

- *encephalocele*—protrusion of some brain substance through a fissure of the skull.

- *epilepsy*—convulsive disorder consisting of recurrent seizures and impaired consciousness. (26, 28)

- *Friedreich's ataxia*—familial disease seen in young persons. Involvement of cerebellum, pyramidal tracts, and peripheral nerves results in sensory impairment, unsteady gait, contractures, and deformities such as lordosis and high-arching feet with toes cocking up. Optic atrophy and myocardial disease may occur. (62, 65)

- *head injury, craniocerebral trauma*—injury to the head, usually associated with a fractured skull and directly or indirectly affecting at varying degrees one or more

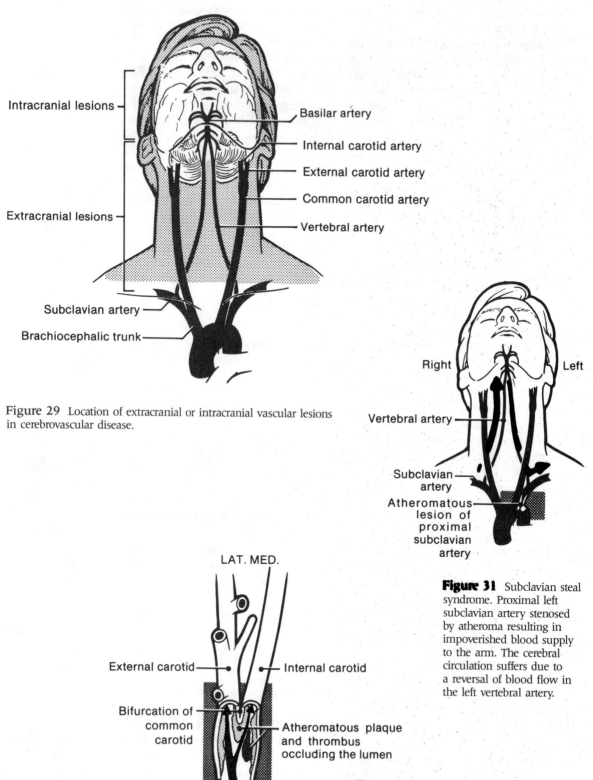

Intracranial lesions

Basilar artery

Internal carotid artery

External carotid artery

Common carotid artery

Vertebral artery

Extracranial lesions

Subclavian artery

Brachiocephalic trunk

Figure 29 Location of extracranial or intracranial vascular lesions in cerebrovascular disease.

Right   Left

Vertebral artery

Subclavian artery

Atheromatous lesion of proximal subclavian artery

Figure 31 Subclavian steal syndrome. Proximal left subclavian artery stenosed by atheroma resulting in impoverished blood supply to the arm. The cerebral circulation suffers due to a reversal of blood flow in the left vertebral artery.

LAT. MED.

External carotid

Internal carotid

Bifurcation of common carotid

Atheromatous plaque and thrombus occluding the lumen

Figure 30 Occlusive lesion of the bifurcation of the common carotid artery extending into the internal carotid artery.

cerebral centers. The severity and extent of brain damage is usually but not exclusively indicated by:
—state of consciousness
—intracranial pressure
—respiratory exchange
—circulatory ability to supply the brain with oxygen and nutrients
—prevention or control of cerebral hemorrhage, edema, and infection (31, 63, 72)

■ *hydrocephalus*—a pathologic condition characterized by a dilatation of the ventricles of the brain and an abnormal accumulation of intraventricular cerebrospinal fluid. It may be:
—obstructive or noncommunicating due to an interference with the circulation of the cerebrospinal fluid through the ventricular system.
—nonobstructive or communicating due to an interference in absorption of cerebrospinal fluid.
Other distinctions include the following: (27, 37, 62)
—*adult hydrocephalus, hydrocephalus ex vacuo*—a rare type in which the increased volume of cerebrospinal fluid develops as a compensatory response to brain atrophy in degenerative cerebral disease.
—*infantile hydrocephalus*—relatively common form that occurs before closure of fontanelles and is characterized by increasing cranial enlargement and prominent forehead. Occasionally the process is arrested.
—*post-traumatic hydrocephalus*—type caused by head injury that may result in ventricular hemorrhage or subarachnoid bleeding and blockage of the aqueduct and fourth ventricle by blood clot.

■ *hypertensive encephalopathy*—cerebral vasoconstriction and edema. The cerebral arteries are greatly constricted. The swollen, pale, and anemic brain is compressed against the skull and ventricles, causing increased intracranial pressure. (50, 82)

■ *meningitis*—inflammation of the meninges resulting from infectious agents such as bacteria, fungi, viruses, or other causes. (29)

■ *meningocele*—protrusion of the meninges through a cranial fissure.

■ *microcephalus*—abnormally small head sometimes associated with idiocy. (27)

■ *multiple sclerosis, disseminated sclerosis*—slowly progressive disease, striking the 20-to-40 age group. Areas of demyelination and scar tissue plaques are scattered throughout the nervous system, disrupting nerve transmission. Numbness, fatigability, clumsiness, difficulty in walking, and blurring vision may be followed by severe incoordination, spasticity, paralysis, incontinence, scanning speech, intention tremor, nystagmus, and blindness. (11, 41)

■ *myelitis*—inflammation of the spinal cord. (32)

■ *neurofibromatosis, von Recklinghausen's disease*—hereditary disorder of the nervous system in which multiple neurofibromas and café au lait spots are found on the skin. The tumors are usually asymptomatic and rarely cause compression of the spinal cord or sensory nerve damage. (27)

■ *paralysis agitans, Parkinson's disease*—slowly progressive neurologic disorder of middle life, primarily affecting the nuclei of the brain stem. Rigidity, slow movements, tremors, masklike facies, and a monotonous voice are clinical findings. Characteristically festination is present. The patient's body is stooped forward, the steps are short, and shuffling occurs with increasing pace once locomotion has started. The gait is propulsive or retropulsive. (62)

■ *poliomyelitis*—viral disease with lesions in the central nervous system and varying symptomatology. Forms include the following: (29)
—*asymptomatic, nonparalytic poliomyelitis*—abortive type, devoid of symptoms, referable to the central nervous system.

—*paralytic poliomyelitis:*
  –*bulbar poliomyelitis*—involvement of cranial nerve nuclei, particularly the respiratory center in the medulla. It is the most serious type of poliomyelitis, causing respiratory paralysis.
  –*spinal paralytic poliomyelitis*—usually an involvement of anterior horn cells of the spinal cord resulting in characteristic stiffness of the neck and spine and tightness of the hamstring muscles followed by paralysis of lower extremities. It presents as the classic form of poliomyelitis.

- *spina bifida*—congenital defect resulting from the absence of a vertebral arch of the spinal column. It may cause a:
  —*meningocele*—protrusion of the meninges through the defect in the spinal column.
  —*meningomyelocele*—herniation of the cord and meninges through the defect of the vertebral column.
  —*syringomyelocele*—protrusion of cord and meninges through the defect in the spine. Cord tissue is a thin-walled sac filled with fluid from the central canal. (27, 64)

- *spinal cord injury*—trauma to cord produced by fracture or dislocation of spine may cause irreversible damage and disability.
  —*compression of cervical cord*—complete transverse compression of cervical cord may cause lifelong quadriplegia (paralysis of arms and legs) and loss of sphincter control or be fatal due to phrenic nerve injury and subsequent respiratory paralysis.
  —*compression of thoracic or lumbar cord*—pressure on this area may cause paraplegia (paralysis below the waist) and sphincter disturbances.
  Compression of spinal cord may also be caused by a cord tumor and a herniated intervertebral disk affecting the spinal nerve root of the lesion. (31, 64)

- *subacute sclerosing panencephalitis (SSPE), Dawson's encephalitis*—uncommon form of inflammation of the brain occurring between 4 and 20 years of age. Three stages are recognized:
  —behavioral disorders at the onset
  —mental deterioration, myoclonic jerkings, and convulsive seizures as the disease progresses
  —stupor, dementia, rigidity, blindness, and coma in the terminal phase. (42)

- *tabes dorsalis, locomotor ataxia*—syphilis of the central nervous system clinically recognized by peculiar gait. (37)

Operative Terms

- *carotid artery ligation*—tying a carotid artery in its cervical portion (neck) or using a Selverstone or Crutchfield clamp to gradually occlude the blood flow in the extracranial portions of the common or internal carotid artery. (65)
- *carotid endarterectomy*—removal of plaques on the intimal lining of a carotid artery in occlusive cerebrovascular disease. This removal may be carried out at the carotid bifurcation and followed by a reconstruction of an internal carotid artery with a Dacron graft. (58, 65)
- *cingulumotomy*—cingulum destruction by stereotaxic surgery with positioning of electrodes in target area. Operation is done under roentgenographic 'guidance for relief of psychogenic pain, manic depressive reactions, and other disorders. (14)
- *cordectomy*—removal of a portion of the spinal cord to convert a spastic paraplegia to a flaccid paraplegia. This enhances rehabilitation.
- *cordotomy, chordotomy*—removal of a section of a nerve fiber tract (usually the spinothalamic tract) within the cord for relief of pain. (36, 66)

—*percutaneous cordotomy*—surgical interruption of the pain fibers in the high cervical cord by means of percutaneous electric needle. This is done under biplane roentgenographic control.

—*selective cordotomy*—palliative surgery for obtaining sensory loss in local pain region, as in arm, leg, or trunk.

- *craniectomy*—removal of part of the skull; a method of approach to the brain. (77)
- *craniotomy*—opening of the skull. Burr or trephine openings into the skull are made to prepare a bone flap. This osteoplastic flap is separated from the skull during brain surgery and replaced when the skull is closed. Osteoplastic craniotomy is a common method of approach to the brain. (68)
- *cryoneurosurgery*—the operative use of cold in the destruction of neurosurgical lesions. (23)
- *decompression of*

  —*brain*—removal of a piece of skull, usually in the subtemporal region, with opening of the dura mater to relieve intracranial pressure.

  —*spinal cord*—removal of bone fragments, hematoma, or lesion to relieve pressure on cord. (23)

- *drainage of meninges for abscess or hematoma*—evacuation of subarachnoid or subdural space.
- *excision of brain lesion*—complete removal if lesion does not encroach on vital centers.
- *laminectomy*—excision of one or more laminae of vertebrae; methods of approach to spinal cord.
- *microneurosurgery*—use of the surgical binocular microscope that provides a powerful light source, up to 25 times magnification, and a clear stereoscopic view of the brain. Microsurgical techniques and dissection are employed for:

  —*acoustic tumors*

  —*cerebral aneurysms*

  —*pituitary tumors*

  —*spinal cord tumors and other neurosurgical procedures* (54, 68)

- *operations for parkinsonism*—surgical procedures directed toward the destruction of areas of basal nuclei presumably affected by the disease.

  —*pallidotomy (formerly pallidectomy)*—surgical interruption of nerve pathways coming from the globus pallidus to relieve intractable tremor and rigidity. Division of nerve fibers is usually achieved by use of electrocautery or chemical solution. Cryogenic agents, ultrasonic waves, and stereotaxic techniques may be employed.

  —*thalamotomy (formerly thalamectomy)*—partial destruction of thalamus for relief of tremors and rigidity. The stereotaxic instrument is applied to the skull. By means of roentgenographic visualization the target area is located and lesions are created by electrolytic, chemical, ultrasonic, or cryogenic methods. (14)

- *stereotaxic neurosurgery*—operative procedure that uses three-dimensional measurement for precisely locating the neurosurgical target area in:

  —*acromegaly*

  —*cerebral aneurysm*

  —*diabetic retinopathy*

  —*manic depressive reactions*

  —*Parkinson's disease*

  —*psychogenic pain*

  —*temporal lobe epilepsy.* (74)

- *stereotaxy*—the use of a stereotaxic instrument fixed onto the skull with screws, as in a scaffold. From this a probe, containing either a chemical, electric, or cryogenic agent, is introduced through a burr opening into the target area of the brain. (74)

- *surgical shunts for hydrocephalus*—detour channels, surgically created to relieve an accumulation of cerebrospinal fluid in the brain.
    - *ventriculoatrial or ventriculocaval shunt*—insertion of a Holter, Pudenz, or Hakim valve to channel the cerebrospinal fluid from the lateral ventricle to either an atrium or the superior vena cava via the jugular vein. This operation is performed for communicating hydrocephalus.
    - *ventriculocisternostomy, Torkildsen's operation*—surgical procedure for obstructive hydrocephalus. A catheter is used to shunt the fluid from a ventricle to the cisterna magna.
    - *ventriculoperitoneal shunt*—detour channel shunting the cerebrospinal fluid from the enlarged ventricular system into the peritoneal cavity. (53)
- *tractotomy*—section of a nerve fiber tract within the brain stem for relief of intractable pain. (49)
- *trephination*—cutting a circular opening or boring a hole into the skull; a method of approach to the brain.

Symptomatic Terms

- *analgesia*—loss of normal sense of pain. (83)
- *anesthesia*—loss of sensation; may be associated with unconsciousness.
- *aphasia*—difficulty with the use or understanding of words due to lesions in association areas.
    - *motor aphasia*—verbal comprehension intact, but patient is unable to use the muscles that coordinate speech. (57, 66)
    - *sensory aphasia*—inability to comprehend the spoken word, if the auditory word center is affected, and the written word, if the visual word center is involved. The patient will not understand the spoken or written word if there is an involvement of both centers. (57)
- *ataxia*—motor incoordination. (71, 72)
- *aura*—patient's awareness of pending epileptic seizure. (26)
- *cerebrospinal otorrhea*—escape of cerebrospinal fluid from the ear following craniocerebral trauma. It is caused by a fistulous communication between the ventricular system or subarachnoid space and the ear.
- *cerebrospinal rhinorrhea*—escape of cerebrospinal fluid from the nose following craniocerebral trauma. It is caused by a fistulous passage leading from the ventricular system or subarachnoid space to the nose. (80)
- *coma*—state of unconsciousness or deep stupor. (34)
- *convulsion*—paroxysms of involuntary muscular contractions and relaxations. (34)
- *diplegia*—paralysis on both sides of the body.
- *dysarthria*—incoordination of speech muscles affecting articulation. (19)
- *dyskinesia*—abnormal involuntary movement and body posture due to brain lesion. (57)
    - *athetosis*—slow, wormlike, writhing movement, especially in hands and fingers.
    - *ballism*—violent, flinging, shaking, or jerking movements of extremities.
    - *chorea*—quick, explosive, purposeless movements.
    - *dystonia*—abnormal posture from twisting movements, usually of limbs and trunk. (72)
- *euphoria*—sense of well-being associated with mild elation.
- *fasciculation*—involuntary twitchings of groups of muscle fibers. (71, 72)
- *festination*—quick, shuffling steps; accelerated gait seen in Parkinson's disease. (33, 62)
- *hemiparesis*—slight degree of paralysis of one side of the body. (37, 50)
- *hemiplegia*—paralysis affecting one side of the body. (20, 43)

- *hyperesthesia*—increased sensibility to sensory stimuli. (12, 51)
- *nystagmus*—constant movements of the eyeballs, as seen in the brain damage and disorders of vestibular apparatus. (19)
- *paraparesis*—slight paralysis of lower limbs. (12, 37)
- *paraplegia*—paralysis of lower limbs and at varying degrees of lower trunk (39, 66)
- *paresis*—partial paralysis. (71)
- *paresthesia*—abnormal sensation; heightened sensory response to stimuli. (12, 52)
- *scanning speech*—hesitant, slow speech; pronouncing words in syllables.
- *syncope*—fainting. (1, 78)
- *tic*—involuntary, purposeless contractions of muscle groups such as twitching of facial muscles, eye blinking, or shrugging of the shoulders. (25, 35, 77)

Psychiatric Disorders

Origin of Terms

dynamo- (G)—power	*psych-, psycho- (G)*—mind
mania (G)—madness	*schizo- (G)*—division, split
phren- (G)—mind, diaphragm	*soma (G)*—body

General Terms

- *commitment*—legal consignment of a mentally unsound or defective person to an institution.
- *descriptive psychiatry*—system of psychiatry that implies the study of clinical patterns, symptoms, and classification.
- *dynamic psychiatry*—the study of emotional processes, their origins, and their mental mechanisms; implies the study of the active, energy-laden, and changing factors in human behavior and their motivation. Dynamic principles convey the concepts of change, evolution, and progression or regression. (18)
- *ego*—in psychoanalytic theory, one of the three major divisions in the model of the psychic apparatus, the others being the id and superego. The ego represents the sum of certain mental mechanisms, such as perception and memory, and specific defensive mechanisms. The ego serves to mediate between the demands of primitive instinctual drives (the id), or internalized parental and social prohibitions (the superego), and of reality. The compromises between these forces achieved by the ego tend to resolve intrapsychic conflict and serve an adaptive and executive function. As used in psychiatry, the term should not be confused with its common usage in the sense of "self-love" or "selfishness." (5)
- *psychiatry*—the medical science that deals with the origin, diagnosis, prevention, and treatment of mental and emotional disorders. (18)
- *psychodynamics*—predictive science that recognizes unconscious drives in human behavior. (18)
- *psychometry*—psychologic measurement or testing of mental processes and potentials, including psychopathologic variants.

Diagnostic Terms*

- *alcohol-induced organic mental disorders*—includes organic mental disorders attributed to the ingestion of alcohol. Examples of this disorder are: (7)

---

*Substantial material in this section is taken verbatim from *Diagnostic and Statistical Manual of Mental Disorders*, 3rd ed., revised (DSM-III-R). Washington, DC: American Psychiatric Association, 1987. Reprinted with permission.

—*alcohol amnestic disorder*—essential feature is loss of memory caused by vitamin deficiency associated with protracted and heavy use of alcohol. Alcohol amnestic disorder resulting from thiamine deficiency is also known as Korsakoff's disease.

—*alcohol hallucinosis*—vivid auditory hallucinations following cessation or reduction in alcohol ingestion by a person who is alcohol dependent.

—*alcohol intoxication*—dominant feature is maladaptive behavior due to recent consumption of alcohol. This may include such manifestations as overaggressiveness, impaired judgment, or malfunctioning in social or occupational settings. Characteristic physiologic signs include slurred speech, incoordination, unsteady gait, nystagmus, and flushed face.

—*alcohol withdrawal, uncomplicated*—dominant features are coarse tremors of the hands, tongue, and eyelids; nausea and vomiting; malaise or weakness; autonomic hyperactivity, with tachycardia and elevated blood pressure; anxiety; depressed mood and irritability. These symptoms follow the prolonged consumption of alcohol over several days or longer.

—*alcohol withdrawal delirium, delirium tremens*—characteristic feature is a delirium that is caused by recent cessation or reduction in the amount of alcohol consumed. Autonomic hyperactivity such as tachycardia, sweating, and elevated blood pressure is present. Delusions, hallucinations, and agitated behavior usually occur.

—*dementia associated with alcoholism*—loss of mental faculties associated with prolonged and heavy ingestion of alcohol and persisting at least three weeks after cessation of alcohol ingestion.

■ *anxiety disorders*—anxiety or avoidance behavior are the chief features of this disorder. Anxiety is either the predominant disturbance or is experienced if the person attempts to master the symptoms, as in confronting dreaded situations or resisting obsessions or compulsions. Examples of disorders in this category include: (4)

—*generalized anxiety disorder*—the essential feature of this disorder is unrealistic or excessive anxiety and worry (apprehensive expectation) about two or more life circumstances. For example, a patient may worry about possible misfortune to one's child (who is in no danger) and worry about finances (for no good reason), for six months or longer. During this time the person has been bothered by these concerns more days than not.

—*obsessive compulsive disorder, obsessive compulsive neurosis*—essential features of this disorder are recurrent obsessions or compulsions sufficiently severe to cause marked distress, be time consuming, or significantly interfere with the person's normal routine, occupational or social functioning, or relationships with others.

—*obsessions*—persistent ideas, thoughts, impulses, or images that are experienced, at least initially, as intrusive and senseless.

—*compulsions*—repetitive, purposeful, and intentional behaviors that are performed in response to an obsession, according to certain rules, or in stereotyped fashion.

—*panic disorder*—essential features of this disorder are recurrent panic attacks (discrete periods of intense fear or discomfort). A person may experience shortness of breath, smothering sensations, dizziness, unsteady feelings or faintness, choking, palpitations or accelerated heart rate, trembling, shaking, nausea or abdominal distress, and fear of going crazy or doing something uncontrolled during the attack. Most persons usually experience approximately four of the aforementioned symptoms during a panic attack. Panic attacks occur (1) unexpectedly; i.e., did not occur immediately before or on exposure to a situation that almost always causes anxiety and (2) they are not triggered by situations in which the person was the focus of others' attention.

—*post-traumatic stress disorder*—development of characteristic symptoms following a psychologically traumatic incident that is generally outside the range of normal human experience. The symptoms may involve re-experiencing the traumatic incident, a numbing of responsiveness to it, or a reduced participation with others and in activities or contacts with the external world.

■ *dissociative disorders*—the dominant aspect is a sudden, temporary alteration in the normally integrative functions of consciousness, identity, or motor behavior. The alteration may occur consciously, such as no recall of major events. When the alteration occurs in identity, the person may forget his or her present identity or assume a new identity. When a disturbance occurs in motor behavior, there is a concurrent disturbance in consciousness and identity, such as the person wandering about unable to recall identity or major events. Examples of disorders in this category include the following: (5)

—*depersonalization disorder*—key features are the occurrence of one or more episodes of depersonalization that cause social or occupational impairment. The symptoms of depersonalization involve a changing perception and experience of the self, so that the usual sense of reality is temporarily adjusted or lost; for example, the person may feel that his or her extremities have changed in size.

—*multiple personality*—the dominant feature is the presence within the person of two or more distinct personalities, each of whom is dominant at a particular time. Transition from one personality to another is sudden and often associated with psychic tension.

—*psychogenic amnesia*—the dominant feature is the sudden inability to recall important personal information, which is not caused by an organic mental disorder.

—*psychogenic fugue*—the major characteristic is sudden, unexpected travel away from the home or customary work site, with the assumption of a new identity and inability to recall one's previous identity.

■ *eating disorders*—characterized by gross disturbances in eating behavior. Some disorders in this category are: (3)

—*anorexia nervosa*—essential features of this disorder are refusal to maintain body weight over a minimal normal weight for age and height; intense fear of gaining weight or becoming fat, even though underweight; a distorted body image; and amenorrhea (in females). The weight loss is usually accomplished by a reduction in total food intake, often with extensive exercising. There may be frequent use of laxatives or diuretics and also self-induced vomiting.

—*bulimia nervosa*—essential features of this disorder are recurrent episodes of binge eating; a feeling of lack of control over eating behavior during the eating binges; use of laxatives or diuretics; strict dieting or fasting, or vigorous exercise in order to prevent weight gain, and persistent overconcern with body shape and weight. In order to qualify for the diagnosis, the person must have had, on average, a minimum of two binge eating episodes a week for at least three months.

—*pica*—the essential feature is the persistent eating of a nonnutritive substance. Infants with this disorder usually eat paint, plaster, string, hair, or cloth. Older children may eat animal droppings, sand, insects, leaves, or pebbles. Pica usually remits in early childhood but may persist into adolescence or on rare occasion continue through adulthood.

- *mental retardation*—significantly subaverage general intellectual functioning existing concurrently with deficits in adaptive behavior and manifested during the developmental period (period of time between conception and the eighteenth birthday). Significantly subaverage is defined as an intelligence quotient (IQ) of 70 or below on standardized measures of intelligence. The upper limit is intended as a guideline; it could be extended upward through an IQ of 75 or more, depending on the reliability of the intelligence test used. Adaptive behavior refers to the effectiveness or degree with which individuals meet the standards of personal independence and social responsibility expected of their age and cultural group. Three aspects of this behavior are maturation, learning, and/or social adjustment. Four degrees of mental retardation are:
    - *mild mental retardation*—describes degrees of mental retardation when intelligence test scores are 50 or 55 to approximately 70.
    - *mental retardation*—describes degree of retardation when intelligence test scores range from 35 or 40 to 50 or 55.
    - *severe mental retardation*—describes the degree of mental retardation when intelligence test scores range from 20 or 25 to 35 or 40.
    - *profound mental retardation*—describes the degree of mental retardation when intelligence test scores are below 20 or 25. (2)*
- *mood episode (hypomanic, manic, or major depressive)*—mood syndrome that is not caused by a known organic factor and is not part of a nonmood psychotic disorder. (6)
    - *hypomanic episode*—the essential feature of this episode is a distinct period in which the predominant mood is either elevated, expansive, or irritable and there are associated symptoms of the manic syndrome. The disturbance is not severe enough to cause marked impairment in social or occupational functioning or to require hospitalization. The associated features of hypomanic episodes are similar to those of a manic episode except that delusions are never present and all other symptoms tend to be less severe than in manic episodes.
    - *manic episode*—distinct period during which the predominant mood is either elevated, expansive, or irritable, and there are associated symptoms of the manic syndrome. Associated symptoms include inflated self-esteem or grandiosity (which may be delusional), decreased need for sleep, pressure of speech, flight of ideas, distractibility, increased involvement in goal-directed activity, psychomotor agitation, and excessive involvement in pleasurable activities that have a high potential for painful consequences, which are not perceived by the patient. The disturbance during this period is sufficiently severe to cause marked impairment in occupational functioning or in usual social activities or relationships with others, or to require hospitalization to prevent harm to self or others.
    - *major depressive episode*—evidenced by depressed mood or loss of interest or pleasure in all, or almost all, activities, and associated symptoms, for a period of at least two weeks. Associated symptoms include appetite decline, change in weight, sleep disturbance, psychomotor agitation or retardation, decreased energy, feelings of worthlessness or guilt, difficulty in concentrating, recurrent thoughts of death, and suicidal ideation or attempts.
- *mood syndrome (depressive or manic)*—group of mood and associated symptoms that occur together for a minimal duration of time. (6)

---

*American Association on Mental Deficiency. Definitions. In Herbert J. Grossman, ed., *Classification in Mental Retardation*, 1983 revision. Washington, DC: American Association on Mental Deficiency, 1983, pp. 11-26. Reprinted with permission.

■ *mood disorders*—the unifying theme of this group of disorders is disturbance of mood, together with a greater or lesser degree of manic or depressive syndrome, that is not caused by any other physical or mental disorder. Mood may be defined as an enduring emotion influencing or characterizing overall psychic life. (Formerly called affective disorders.)

Types of mood disorders: (6)
  —*bipolar disorders*—the essential feature of this disorder is one or more manic episodes usually accompanied by one or more major depressive episodes. Bipolar disorders may be subclassified as mixed, manic, or depressed, depending on clinical features of the current episode (or most recent episode if the disorder is currently in partial or full remission). The disorder may be classified as to severity of disturbance, e.g., mild, moderate, or severe, with or without psychotic features.
  —*cyclothymia*—the essential feature of this disorder is a chronic mood disturbance of at least two years' duration (one year for children and adolescents). It involves numerous hypomanic episodes and numerous periods of depressed mood or loss of interest or pleasure of insufficient severity or duration to meet the criteria for a major depressive or a manic episode. During the two-year period (one year for children and adolescents), the person is never without hypomanic or depressive symptoms for more than two months. Associated features are similar to those of a manic episode and a major depressive episode, except that there is no marked impairment in social or occupational functioning during the hypomanic episode.
  —*depressive disorders*—one or more periods of depression without a history of either manic or hypomanic episodes.
    —*major depression*—essential feature of this condition is one or more major depressive episodes without a history of either a manic episode or an unequivocal hypomanic episode. Major depression may be classified as a single episode or recurrent. The severity of the episode may be classified as mild, moderate, or severe, with or without psychotic features.
  —*dysthymia*—the essential feature of this disorder is a chronic disturbance of mood involving a depressed mood for most of the day, more days than not, for at least two years. In addition, during these periods of depressed mood there are some of the following associated symptoms: poor appetite or overeating, insomnia or hypersomnia, low energy or fatigue, low self-esteem, poor concentration or difficulty in making decisions, and feelings of hopelessness. During the two-year period, the person is never without depressive symptoms for more than two months. People with dysthymia frequently have superimposed major depression, which is often referred to as "double depression."
■ *organic mental syndromes*—refers to a constellation of psychological or behavioral signs and symptoms without reference to etiology (e.g., organic anxiety syndrome, dementia). Some categories of organic mental syndromes are: (7)
  —*delirium and dementia*—cognitive impairment is relatively global. Essential features of delirium are reduced ability to maintain attention to external stimuli and to appropriately shift attention to new external stimuli and disorganized thinking, such as rambling, irrelevant, or incoherent speech. There may be memory impairment and disorientation to time, place, or person. Total duration is usually brief. The chief feature of dementia is impairment in short-term and long-term memory, associated with impairment in abstract thinking, impaired judgment, and other disturbances of higher cortical function or personality change. Delirium and dementia may coexist.

—*organic delusional syndrome*—the essential feature of this syndrome is prominent delusions that are due to a specific organic factor. The diagnosis is not made if the delusions occur in the context of reduced ability to maintain and shift attention to external stimuli, as in delirium. Although the nature of the delusions varies, persecutory delusions appear to be the most common type.

—*organic personality syndrome*—the essential feature of this syndrome is persistent personality disturbance, either lifelong or representing a change or accentuation of a previously characteristic trait, that results from a specific organic factor. Mild cognitive impairment and irritability may be present, as well as at least one of the following: recurrent outbursts of aggression, marked apathy, and suspiciousness or paranoid ideation.

—*intoxication and withdrawal*—associated with ingestion of or reduction in use of a psychoactive substance; does not meet the criteria for any of the aforementioned syndromes.

■ *personality disorder*—condition marked by maladaptive behavior pattern that is deeply ingrained in the personality. Personality traits are enduring patterns of perceiving, relating to, and thinking about the environment and oneself, and are exhibited in a wide range of important social and personal contexts. When these traits become inflexible and maladaptive and result in significant functional impairment or subjective distress, they constitute personality disorders. Some examples of personality disorders are: (8)

—*paranoid personality disorder*—the essential feature of this disorder is a pervasive and unwarranted tendency, beginning by early adulthood and present in a variety of contexts, to interpret the actions of people as deliberately demeaning or threatening.

—*schizoid personality disorder*—essential features of this disorder are a pervasive pattern of indifference to social relationships and a restricted range of emotional experience and expression, beginning by early adulthood. The person is oversensitive, shy, seclusive, unsociable, eccentric, autistic, and almost always chooses solitary activities.

—*schizotypal personality disorder*—essential features of this disorder are a pervasive pattern of peculiarities of ideation, appearance, and behavior and deficits in interpersonal relatedness, beginning by early adulthood and present in a variety of contexts that are not severe enough to meet the criteria for schizophrenia. Persons with this disorder display inappropriate or constricted affect, appearing silly and aloof; they rarely reciprocate gestures or facial expressions such as nodding or smiling. They are extremely anxious in social situations involving unfamiliar people.

—*antisocial personality disorder*—characterized by persistent refusal to follow the norms of society, usually beginning in childhood or early adolescence and continuing into adulthood. Persons with this disorder tend to be irritable and aggressive and to get repeatedly into physical fights and assaults, including spouse-beating or child-beating. They have no remorse about the effects of their behavior on others, and even feel justified at having hurt or mistreated others.

—*narcissistic personality disorder*—essential features of this disorder are a pervasive pattern of grandiosity (in fantasy or behavior), hypersensitivity to the evaluation of others, and a lack of empathy that begin by early adulthood. Persons with this disorder have a grandiose sense of self-importance. They tend to exaggerate their accomplishments and talents and expect to be noticed as "special" even without appropriate achievement.

—*histrionic personality disorder*—the essential feature of this disorder is a pervasive pattern of excessive emotionality and attention-seeking, beginning in early adulthood. Persons with this disorder constantly seek or demand reassurance, approval, or praise from others and are uncomfortable in situations in which they are not the center of attention. They tend to be dramatic and to draw attention to themselves.

—*avoidant personality disorder*—essential features of this disorder are a pervasive pattern of social discomfort, fear of negative evaluation, and timidity, beginning by early childhood. These persons avoid social or occupational activities that involve significant interpersonal contact. These individuals are very hurt by criticism and are devastated by the slightest hint of disapproval.

—*dependent personality disorder*—the essential feature of this disorder is an overall pattern of dependent and submissive behavior, beginning by early adulthood. Individuals with this disorder find it difficult to make everyday decisions without an excessive amount of advice and reassurance from others. These individuals tend to agree with others even when they believe them to be wrong, for fear of being rejected.

—*obsessive-compulsive personality disorder*—the essential feature of this disorder is a pervasive pattern of perfectionism and inflexibility, beginning in early adulthood. These persons tend to constantly strive for perfection, but adherence to their own overly strict and often unattainable standards frequently interferes with actual completion of tasks or projects. They are stingy with their emotions and material possessions and rarely give gifts or compliments. Decision making is avoided for fear of making a mistake.

—*passive-aggressive personality disorder*—the essential feature of this disorder is a pervasive pattern of passive resistance to demands for adequate social and occupational performance, beginning in early adulthood. At work and in social functioning, these individuals habitually resent and oppose demands to increase or maintain a given level of functioning. These persons become sulky, irritable, or argumentative when asked to do something that they do not want to do and often unreasonably criticize persons in authority.

- *schizophrenia*—severe mental disorder of psychotic depth marked by disturbances in behavior, mood, and ability to think. Altered concept formation may lead to a distortion of reality, delusions, and hallucinations, which tend to be self-protective. Emotional disharmony and bizarre regressive behavior are frequently present. The diagnosis of schizophrenia requires that continuous signs of the illness have been present for at least six months, which includes an active phase with psychotic symptoms. The development of the active phase of the illness is usually preceded by a prodromal phase in which there is a clear deterioration from the previous level of functioning. The American Psychiatric Association distinguishes several types, some of which are listed below. (9)

  —*catatonic type*—marked disturbance in activity with either generalized inhibition (mutism, stupor, negativism, waxy appearance) or by excessive motor activity and excitement, as well as voluntary assumption of inappropriate bizarre postures. During catatonic stupor or excitement, the person needs careful supervision to avoid hurting himself or others.

  —*disorganized type*—features of this type are incoherence, marked loosening of associations or grossly disorganized behavior, and, in addition, flat or grossly inappropriate affect.

—*paranoid type*—marked preoccupation with one or more systematized delusions or with frequent auditory hallucinations related to a single theme. Other features usually associated with this type include unfocused anxiety, anger, argumentativeness, and violence, as well as a stilted, formal quality or extreme intensity in interpersonal interaction.

—*undifferentiated type*—marked by prominent psychotic symptoms (delusions, hallucinations, incoherence, or grossly disorganized behavior) that do not meet the criteria for paranoid, catatonic, or disorganized types.

—*residual type*—this category is used when there has been at least one episode of schizophrenia, but the clinical picture that occasioned the evaluation or admission to clinical care is without prominent psychotic symptoms, though signs of the illness persist. Emotional blunting, social withdrawal, eccentric behavior, illogical thinking, and mild loosening of associations are common.

- *somatoform disorders*—essential features are symptoms suggesting a physical disorder, with no evident organic findings or known physiologic mechanisms and no positive evidence, or with a strong presumption that the symptoms are linked to psychologic factors or conflicts. Examples of these disorders are: (10)

  —*body dysmorphic disorder (dysmorphophobia)*—the essential feature of this disorder is preoccupation with some imagined defect in appearance in a normal-appearing person. Most common complaints involve facial flaws, such as wrinkles, spots on the skin, excessive facial hair, shape of nose, mouth, or eyebrows, and swelling of the face.

  —*conversion disorder (hysterical neurosis, conversion type)*—main feature is an alteration or loss of physical functioning that suggests physical disorder, but which instead is apparently an expression of a psychologic conflict or need. The disturbance is not under voluntary control, and after appropriate investigation, cannot be explained by any physical disorder or known pathophysiologic mechanism.

  —*hypochondriasis (hypochondriacal neurosis)*—predominant disturbance is an unrealistic explanation of physical signs or sensations as being abnormal, leading to an absorbing belief or fear of having a serious disease. This fear may be related to such bodily functions as heartbeat, sweating, peristalsis, or minor coughs. Social and work functioning may be impaired because the person is preoccupied with the disease.

  —*somatization disorder*—essential features of this disorder are recurrent and multiple somatic complaints, of several years' duration, for which medical attention has been sought, but that apparently are not due to any physical disorder. This disorder begins before the age of 30 and has a chronic but fluctuating course. Anxiety and depressed moods are frequent. Antisocial behavior and occupational, interpersonal, and marital difficulties are common.

  —*somatoform pain disorder*—the essential feature of this disorder is preoccupation with pain in the absence of adequate physical findings to account for the pain or its intensity. Associated psychologic factors are evident, but the person refuses to consider these factors in establishing the etiology of the pain complaint. Usually, the person becomes very incapacitated and has to quit work. Frequently, an invalid role is assumed.

Symptomatic Terms

- *aggression*—forceful, self-assertive, attacking action that is verbal, physical, or symbolic.

- *agitation*—chronic restlessness; important psychomotor reaction of emotional stress.
- *ambivalence*—opposing drives or emotions; for example, love and hatred for the same person.
- *anaclitic*—leaning on; refers to dependence of infant on mother, which is abnormal later in life.
- *autism*—form of thinking that seeks to satisfy unfulfilled desires but completely disregards reality factors. (27)
- *blocking*—sudden interruption in the stream of thought.
- *body image*—the conscious and unconscious picture a person has of his or her own body at any moment. The conscious and unconscious images may differ from each other.
- *catalepsy*—diminished responsiveness usually characterized by trancelike states. May occur in organic or psychologic disorders or under hypnosis. (69)
- *catharsis*—wholesome emotional release by talking about problems or repressed feelings.
- *compulsion*—powerful drive to perform ritualistic acts, such as handwashing. (17)
- *confabulation*—fabrication of stories in response to questions about situations or events that are not recalled. (20)
- *cyclothymic*—refers to mood swings out of proportion to stimuli.
- *delirium*—syndrome characterized by clouding of consciousness, incoherence of ideas, mental confusion, bewilderment, hallucinations, and illusions. (70)
- *delusions*—false beliefs resulting from unconscious needs and maintained irrespective of contrary evidence.
    - *—delusions of grandeur*—exaggerated ideas about position and importance.
    - *—delusions of persecution*—false ideas that a person is the target of persecution.
    - *—delusions of reference*—erroneous assumption that casual, unrelated remarks are directed to oneself. (20, 76)
- *dementia*—an irreversible impairment of cognitive intellectual capacities. (76)
- *depersonalization*—loss of sense of identity.
- *dissocial behavior*—the term refers to persons who are not classifiable as antisocial personalities but who follow more or less criminal pursuits, such as racketeers, dishonest gamblers, prostitutes, and dope peddlers; formerly called sociopathic personalities.
- *empathy*—objective insight into the feelings of another person, in contrast to sympathy, which is subjective and emotional.
- *hallucinations*—false sensory perceptions without actual external stimulation. (69)
- *illusions*—falsely interpreted sensory perceptions.
- *incoherence in speech*—illogic flow of ideas that is difficult to comprehend by the listener.
- *libido*—a psychoanalytic term denoting the psychic drive that energizes living.
- *malingering*—a conscious simulation of illness used to avoid an unpleasant situation or for personal gain. (20)
- *mental mechanism*—refers to a number of intrapsychic processes primarily functioning on an unconscious level, such as most of the defense mechanisms. Thinking, memory, and perception are included.
    - *—compensation*—a person's striving to make up for deficiencies.
    - *—conversion*—emotional conflict expressed in somatic symptoms.
    - *—denial*—reality factors denied in an effort to resolve emotional conflict.
    - *—displacement*—tension-reducing mechanism in which an emotional response is transferred from its real source to a more acceptable substitute.

—*dissociation*—group of ideas, memories, and feelings that have escaped from normal consciousness and the control of the person.

—*identification*—unconscious imitation of another.

—*projection*—mental mechanism by which unacceptable desires are disowned and attributed to another.

—*regression*—anxiety-evading mechanism; a readoption of immature patterns of thought, behavior, and emotional responses.

—*repression*—common mechanism that excludes unacceptable desires, impulses, and thoughts from conscious awareness.

—*sublimation*—the channeling of undesirable impulses and drives away from their primitive objectives into activities of a higher order. This defense mechanism is nonpathogenic. (18)

- *obsession*—persistent thought that the person knows is unrealistic.
- *phobia*—any morbid fear. (17)
- *sensory deprivation*—experience of being cut off from usual external stimuli and the opportunity for perception. May occur in various ways, such as through loss of hearing or eyesight, by solitary confinement, by traveling in space. May lead to disorganized thinking, depression, panic, delusions, and hallucinations. (25)
- *somnambulism*—sleepwalking, writing, or performing other acts automatically in a somnolent state without remembering the fact on awakening. (69)

Special Procedures

Terms Related to Neurologic Examination

- *Babinski's reflex*—extension of the great toe with or without plantar flexion of other toes when examiner strokes the sole. A positive Babinski's reflex suggests organic disease of the pyramidal tracts. (71)
- *Brudzinski's sign*—when head is passively flexed on chest, the patient draws up legs reflexively. This occurs in meningeal irritation and meningitis. (42)
- *carotid compression test*—evaluation of cerebral blood flow by compressing the carotid arteries digitally. This may lead to the detection of cerebrovascular insufficiency. An irritable carotid sinus reflex is evoked by unilateral compression. (1)
- *Kernig's sign*—when the patient is supine with thigh flexed on the abdomen, he or she is unable to extend the leg. This sign is present in meningeal irritation and meningitis. (42)
- *Romberg's sign*—inability of ataxic persons to stand steady with their eyes closed and feet together. (37)

Terms Related to Neurologic Studies

- *electroencephalography*—the tracing or recording of the electric current generated in the cerebral cortex by brain waves. Marked irregularities indicate pathologic conditions such as epilepsy, brain tumors, scars, and other disorders. The procedure is an aid to medical diagnosis and treatment. (1, 16, 28)
- *electronystagmography*—electric stimulation of the eyeball to induce nystagmus for the recording of eye movements in nystagmus. (25)
- *facial thermography*—a photographic measurement of skin temperatures of the face. In a controlled environment, the skin temperatures reflect variations in blood flow. The central portion of the supraorbital region is the only skin area of the face that receives its blood supply from the terminal branches of the internal carotid artery. In severe stenosis of the internal carotid artery, the decreased blood flow lowers the skin

temperature in the medial supraorbital region. The cool area is detectable by a thermogram.

- *rheoencephalography*—graphic registration of the changes in conductivity of nerve tissue caused by vascular factors.

Terms Related to Psychometric Tests

- *intelligence tests*—devices set up to determine a person's native intellectual ability, including the level of functioning in various areas. The following tests have been widely accepted: (18, 61)
  - *Stanford-Binet*—shows range of mental ability by age. It is assumed that mental growth stops at age 15.
  - *Wechsler Adult Intelligence Scale*—verbal and performance test designed to measure the intellectual capacity of adults at different age levels.
  - *Wechsler Intelligence Scale for Children*—test devised primarily to classify children according to their intellectual abilities.
- *projective tests*—methods employed to uncover a subject's unconscious attitudes, needs, and relationships to others. When taking a test, the subject projects the pattern of his or her own psychologic life and thus reveals the underlying dynamics of personality structure. Of value are the following: (18)
  - *Minnesota Multiphasic Personality Inventory*—affords insight into various phases of the patient's personality.
  - *Rorschach Personality Test*—attempts to detect conscious or unconscious personality traits and conflicts through eliciting the person's associations to a set of ink blots.
  - *Thematic Apperception Test*—uses 20 pictures to stimulate projective expression of personality traits.

Terms Related to Psychopharmacology

- *antianxiety agents*—drugs that exhibit a central calming effect. They are used in the treatment of mild to moderate anxiety. (47)
- *antidepressants*—psychic energizers that relieve despondency, tension, fatigue, and mental depression. (47, 51)
- *antipsychotic agents*—drugs used in treating psychoses and controlling excitation of the central nervous system. (47)
- *ataractics*—tranquilizing agents widely used in psychiatric disorders such as agitation, aggressive outbursts, psychomotor overactivity, and similar symptoms. They are the same as antianxiety agents. (47)
- *hallucinogens*—chemical agents producing hallucinations, disturbed thought processes, and depersonalization in normal persons.
- *psychedelics*—drugs that apparently expand consciousness and enlarge vision.
- *psychopharmacology*—science dealing with drugs that affect the emotions. (47)
- *psychotogens*—drugs producing psychotic behavior.

Terms Related to Psychotherapy

Psychotherapy may be defined as treatment of emotional and personality problems by psychologic means. The following terms refer to psychotherapeutic techniques. (18)

- *abreaction*—expressive form of psychotherapy that encourages a reliving of repressed emotional stress situations in a therapeutic setting. It releases painful emotions and increases insight.

- *activity therapy*—program of activities prescribed for patients on the basis of psychologic understanding of their specific needs. Types of therapy are:
  - —bibliotherapy
  - —educational therapy
  - —music therapy
  - —occupational therapy
  - —recreational therapy. (18)
- *behavior therapy*—a therapeutic approach that attempts to bring about direct change by helping the person to unlearn maladaptive and destructive behavior and to enhance abilities for socially acceptable and productive behavior. (18)
- *biofeedback*—provision of information to the subject based on one or more of the person's physiologic processes, such as brain-wave activity or blood pressure, often as an essential element of visceral learning. (18)
- *group psychotherapy*—a method of psychotherapy applied to a group. Group leaders help patients to gain insight into their emotional difficulties and conflicts, to understand their causes, and to translate their defensive reactions into acceptable behavior. (18)
- *hypnosis*—a state of semiconscious suggestibility. Through verbal suggestion the patient's attention is withdrawn from other stimuli and focused on the therapist's procedure. Under hypnosis, symptoms are made to disappear. Posthypnotic suggestion is important for successful completion of therapy.
- *milieu therapy*—use of a modified and controlled environment in the treatment of mental disease.
- *narcoanalysis*—psychotherapy is offered under the influence of drugs. (18)
- *persuasion*—a form of psychotherapy that utilizes reasoning and moralizing discussions to change faulty attitudes.
- *play therapy*—psychotherapeutic approach to children who tend to reveal their hidden resentments, feelings, and frustrations in play. An analytic therapist uses the interpretations of play as a guide to treatment.
- *psychoanalysis*—type of insight therapy developed by Sigmund Freud. Psychoanalytic treatment seeks to influence behavior by bringing into awareness unconscious emotional conflicts in an effort to overcome them.
- *rational-emotive therapy*—humanistic type of psychotherapy, highly cognitive and empirical, based on the assertion that a person's rational or irrational beliefs about his or her own self influence actions and outlook on life. By recognizing and changing irrational beliefs, the person gains control over emotional life and recovers mental health.
- *supportive psychotherapy*—therapeutic efforts directed toward a strengthening of the patient's ego to reduce anxiety. The real problem remains unsolved and may become acute again at a crucial moment. (18)
- *transactional analysis*—a type of insight therapy developed by Eric Berne. It seeks to understand the psychologic interaction between patient and therapist.
- *transference*—patient's unconscious reaction to a psychiatrist that is a repetition of an early childhood relationship to a parent, sibling, or significant other. The psychiatrist uses the transfer situation to gain insight into the patient's disturbing emotional conflicts and to plan the psychotherapy accordingly.

Terms Related to Shock Therapy

Several types of shock therapy are employed in psychiatric treatment:
- *electroconvulsive or electroshock treatment*—the use of electric current to cause unconsciousness and/or initiate convulsions. (18)
- *electronarcosis*—narcotic-like state produced as a therapeutic measure.

- *insulin coma therapy*—inducing hypoglycemic reaction by the administration of large doses of insulin.
- *subcoma insulin therapy*—producing drowsiness or somnolence by insulin injection, but no coma.

Abbreviations

General

AESP—applied extrasensory projection
ANS—autonomic nervous system
CA—chronological age; cancer
CBF—cerebral blood flow
CBS—chronic brain syndrome
CNS—central nervous system
CP—cerebral palsy
cps—cycles per second
CR—conditioned reflex
CS—completed stroke
CS—conditioned stimulus
CSF—cerebrospinal fluid
CVA—cerebrovascular accident
CVD—cerebrovascular disease
DCR—direct cortical response
DT—delirium tremens
ECT—electroconvulsive therapy
EEG—electroencephalogram
Ej—elbow jerk
ESP—effective sensory projection; extrasensory perception
EST—electric shock therapy
ICT—insulin coma therapy
IQ—intelligence quotient
Kj—knee jerk
LP—lumbar puncture
LSD—lysergic acid diethylamide
MAO—monoamine oxidase
MS—multiple sclerosis
NREM—no rapid eye movements (sleep)
OBS—organic brain syndrome
PEG—pneumoencephalogram
PNS—peripheral nervous system

REM—rapid eye movements (deep sleep)
SLE—St. Louis encephalitis
SNS—sympathetic nervous system
SR—stimulus response
TIA—transient ischemic attack
TIA-IR—transient ischemic attack— incomplete recovery
UCR—unconditioned reflex

Tests

CAT—Child's Apperception Test
ITPA—Illinois Test of Psycholinguistic Ability
MMPI—Minnesota Multiphasic Personality Inventory
TAT—Thematic Apperception Test
WAIS—Wechsler Adult Intelligence Scale
WISC—Wechsler Intelligence Scale for Children
WPPSI—Wechsler Preschool and Primary Scale of Intelligence

Organizations

AA—Alcoholics Anonymous
AAMD—American Association on Mental Deficiency
APA—American Psychiatric Association
MHA—Mental Health Association
NAMH—National Association of Mental Health
NARC—National Association for Retarded Children
NIMH—National Institute of Mental Health

Oral Reading Practice

Cocaine Abuse and Dependency—A Major Psychiatric Problem

Cocaine is derived from the coca plant and is a stimulant. Among the multiphasic causes that makes the person in our society receptive to the degrading influence of addicting drugs is the perception that cocaine will enhance one's mental and physical performance. Another dimension is the **psychosocial milieu** of many adult users, who seek to drown their problems, relieve their depression, and recapture happiness in a dream world. A study published by the National Institute on Drug Abuse (NIDA) entitled "Cocaine Use in America" supports the view that many cocaine users are people who used marijuana and may have become bored with it.

Teenagers and adolescents who face the burden of peer pressure, as well as the craving for excitement, tend to revolt against legal restrictions in their pursuit of drugs to achieve a "high" (type of euphoria, excitement, and increased energy) and to be relieved of their immediate problems. They appear as easy prey to the allurements of drug peddlers. The President's Commission on Organized Crime reported that for the period of 1978 through 1985, the use of **marijuana** and **hashish** declined steadily among high school students, but within the same group, cocaine use showed a steady, slow rise. Researchers note the presence of more potent forms of cocaine (e.g., a smokable form, **"crack"**) among young people, as the price for it comes down. As cocaine supplies increase, people with less money can afford it. Drug dealers may alter the purity of cocaine by combining it with other local anesthetics, such as **lidocaine, procaine,** and **tetracaine.** The higher purity of cocaine has resulted in increased problems. The inability of the person to abstain from frequent compulsive use of cocaine results in the person developing a psychological dependence on the drug. The **psychological dependence** or habituation is manifested by an irresistible craving, compelling the addict to use the drug as an escape measure from unpleasant situations and as a psychologic crutch for a new lease on life.

Even the **neonate,** who has become drug addicted during **intrauterine** existence because of a cocaine-using mother, begins life physiologically damaged. Dr. Ira Chasnoff, a pediatrician at Northwestern University Medical School in Evanston, IL, and one of the nation's leading authorities on effects of cocaine use in pregnancy, has noted the following defects in infants of mothers who use cocaine:
  —an increased rate of **seizures** soon after birth
  —very jittery, experiencing **rapid mood swings,** and quite sensitive to noise and other external stimuli
  —measures of **fetal distress** appear greater in these infants
  —pronounced smaller head size in comparison with head size of normal infants, suggests **retardation in brain growth** and the possibility of **brain deficits** in the future
  —a higher risk of **sudden infant death syndrome** or **crib death.**

Dr. Chasnoff has documented that cocaine can be passed to the infant from the mother's breast milk and that the cocaine stays in the breast milk up to 60 hours after the mother uses cocaine. Also, he reported that pregnant women using cocaine are more likely than others, to have **spontaneous abortions.** Cocaine-using mothers have a 17.3 percent chance of going into labor prematurely, compared with a 2 percent risk in the general population.

The assumption that cocaine use is "pretty safe" is challenged by reports of death from **respiratory depression, cardiac arrhythmias,** and **convulsions** following cocaine snorting and intravenous use. Cardiac rate and blood pressure increase in a dose-related manner. An increase in body temperature may occur following cocaine use, and large doses of cocaine may induce **lethal pyrexia** or **hypertension.**

Initial abstinence from cocaine use may result in symptoms of **depression** and **guilt, insomnia,** and **anorexia. Lithium** treatment and **tricyclic antidepressant** medications may be of assistance in the long-term treatment of cocaine abuse. Individual and group psychotherapy and family and peer-group support programs are helpful in developing long-range remission from drug usage. (47, 56, 67, 79)

Table 3

Some Conditions Amenable to Neurosurgery

Organs Involved	Diagnosis	Type of Surgery	Operative Procedures
Brain Carotid arteries	Cerebrovascular insufficiency due to atherosclerotic plaque at bifurcation of common carotid artery	Carotid endarterectomy of extracranial lesion	Incision to expose obstructive plaque Peeling out lesion Arterectomy closed by suturing Dacron patch into it to widen artery
Brain Internal carotid artery Middle cerebral artery	Massive thrombotic occlusion of internal carotid artery with embolization of middle cerebral artery, causing cerebral ischemia	Microsurgical anastomosis of temporal artery to middle cerebral artery	Craniectomy or osteoplastic flap Use of operative microscope Creation of surgical union of temporal artery and patent segment of middle cerebral artery to support circulation
Brain Meningeal artery	Rupture of middle meningeal artery Epidural hemorrhage Epidural hematoma	Surgical exploration of subtemporal region Removal of epidural hematoma	Drilling exploratory burr holes Burr hole enlarged for exposure of hematoma Removal of epidural hematoma by suction
Brain Subarachnoid space	Subarachnoid hemorrhage from ruptured aneurysm of internal carotid artery	Ligation of carotid artery Intracranial clipping or ligation of aneurysm	Tying carotid artery in neck Applying clip or ligature to aneurysmal sac
Brain Subdural space	Subdural hematoma of the brain	Drainage of subdural space Craniotomy and excision of hematoma	Evacuation of clot through trephine opening in skull Surgical opening of skull and removal of subdural hematoma
Brain Dura mater	Craniocerebral injury; open, depressed fracture with dural laceration	Decompression, suture of dura mater	Elevation of depressed fracture and repair of dural laceration
Brain Meninges	Meningioma, benign	Craniotomy with excision of meningioma	Opening into skull, osteoplastic flap, removal of tumor

Organs Involved	Diagnosis	Type of Surgery	Operative Procedures
Brain Glial tissue	Primary malignant glioma	Craniotomy with resection of tumor	Opening into skull, osteoplastic flap, removal of tumor
Brain Choroid plexus Ventricles	Obstructive, non-communicating hydrocephalus Nonobstructive communicating hydrocephalus	Ventriculocisternostomy Torkildsen's procedure Ventriculocaval shunt Insertion of Holter or Pudenz valve	Shunting cerebrospinal fluid from third ventricle to cisterna magna by means of plastic catheter Shunting cerebrospinal fluid from lateral ventricle to superior vena cava via jugular vein by insertion of one-way valve
Brain Hypophysis	Pituitary tumor Hyperpituitarism	Stereotaxic cryohypophysectomy	Diamond drill dissection of anterior wall of sella turcica using surgical microscope Accurate placement of cryoprobes for destruction of hypophysis and tumor
Brain Basal nuclei	Paralysis agitans or Parkinson's disease	Stereotaxic thalamotomy	Introduction of radiofrequency electrode through burr hole Electrode carried to surgical target by stereotaxic instrument Destruction of ventrolateral nucleus of thalamus
Brain Trigeminal nerve	Trigeminal neuralgia (tic douloureux)	Retrogasserian neurotomy	Transection of sensory root of trigeminal nerve
Spinal cord	Intractable pain due to any cause	Cordotomy Percutaneous high cervical cordotomy	Transection of pain tracts in spinal cord Stereotaxic method used for locating and interrupting spinothalamic tract in cervical cord
Spinal cord Ganglia	Intractable pain in extremity due to causalgia, Raynaud's disease, or Buerger's disease	Sympathectomy	Removal of sympathetic chain and ganglia
Spinal cord Subarachnoid space	Intractable pain in malignant disease	Alcohol injection as nerve block	Injection of alcohol into subarachnoid space

References and Bibliography

1. Adams, Raymond D., and Martin, Joseph B. Faintness, syncope, and seizures. In Braunwald, Eugene, et al., eds., *Harrison's Principles of Internal Medicine*, 11th ed. New York: McGraw-Hill Book Co., 1987, pp. 64-70.

2. American Association on Mental Deficiency. Definitions. In Grossman, Herbert J., ed., *Classification in Mental Retardation*, 1983 revision. Washington, DC: American Association on Mental Deficiency, 1983, pp. 11-26.

3. American Psychiatric Association. Disorders usually first evident in infancy, childhood, or adolescence. *Diagnostic and Statistical Manual of Mental Disorders*, 3rd ed., revised, DSM-III-R. Washington, DC: American Psychiatric Association, 1987, pp. 27-95.

4. ———. Anxiety disorders (or anxiety and phobic neuroses). Ibid., pp. 235-253.

5. ———. Dissociative disorders (or hysterical neuroses, dissociative type). Ibid., pp. 269-277.

6. ———. Mood disorders. Ibid., pp. 213-233.

7. ———. Organic mental syndromes and disorders. Ibid., pp. 97-163.

8. ———. Personality disorders. Ibid., pp. 335-358.

9. ———. Schizophrenia. Ibid., pp. 187-198.

10. ———. Somatoform disorders. Ibid., pp. 255-267.

11. Antel, Jack P., and Arnason, Barry G. Demyelinating diseases. In Braunwald, Eugene, et al., eds., *Harrison's Principles of Internal Medicine*, 11th ed., New York: McGraw-Hill Book Co., 1987, pp. 1995-2000.

12. Asbury, Arthur K. Numbness, tingling, and other abnormalities of sensation. In Braunwald, Eugene, et al., eds., *Harrison's Principles of Internal Medicine*, 11th ed. New York: McGraw-Hill Book Co., 1987, pp. 99-104.

13. ———. Diseases of the peripheral nervous system. Ibid., pp. 2058-2069.

14. Ballantine, H. Thomas. Neurosurgery for behavioral disorders. In Wilkins, Robert H., and Rengachary, Setti S., eds., *Neurosurgery*, vol. 3. New York: McGraw-Hill Book Co., 1985, pp. 2525-2536.

15. Bay, Janet W., and Dohn, Donald F. Surgical sympathectomy. In Wilkins, Robert H., and Rengachary, Setti S., eds., *Neurosurgery*, vol. 2. New York: McGraw-Hill Book Co., 1985, pp. 1912-1917.

16. Bell, Rodney D. Echoencephalography and evoked response. In Stein, Jay H., ed.-in-chief. *Internal Medicine*, 2nd ed. Boston: Little, Brown & Co., 1987, pp. 2197-2206.

17. Britton, Karen Thatcher, et al. Anxiety disorders. In Braunwald, Eugene, et al., eds., *Harrison's Principles of Internal Medicine*, 11th ed. New York: McGraw-Hill Book Co., 1987, pp. 2089-2093.

18. Brophy, James J. Psychiatric disorders. In Schroeder, Steven A., Krupp, Marcus A., and Tierney, Lawrence M., Jr., eds., *Current Medical Diagnosis & Treatment—1988*, Norwalk, CT: Appleton & Lange, 1988, pp. 621-675.

19. Carter, John E. Ocular manifestations of neurologic disorders. In Stein, Jay H., ed.-in-chief. *Internal Medicine*, 2nd ed. Boston: Little, Brown & Co., 1987, pp. 2167-2177.

20. Cassem, Edwin H. Approach to the patient with mental and emotional complaints. In Braunwald, Eugene, et al., eds., *Harrison's Principles of Internal Medicine*, 11th ed. New York: McGraw-Hill Book Co., 1987, pp. 60-64.

21. Cass, A.M., MD. Personal communications.

22. Comenford, J.F., MD. Personal communications.

23. Cosman, Eric R., and Cosman, Bernard J. Methods of making nervous system lesions. In Wilkins, Robert H., and Rengachary, Setti S., eds., *Neurosurgery*, vol. 3. New York: McGraw-Hill Book Co., 1985, pp. 2490-2499.

24. Cranvioto, Humberto. Neoplasms of peripheral nerves. In Wilkins, Robert H., and Rengachary, Setti S., eds. *Neurosurgery*, vol. 2. New York: McGraw-Hill Book Co., 1985, pp. 1894-1899.

25. Daroff, Robert B. Dizziness and vertigo. In Braunwald, Eugene, et al., eds., *Harrison's Principles of Internal Medicine*, 11th ed. New York: McGraw-Hill Book Co., 1987, pp. 76-79.

26. Davenport, John. Epilepsy. In Stein, Jay H., ed.-in-chief. *Internal Medicine*, 2nd ed. Boston: Little, Brown & Co., 1987, pp. 2145-2150.

27. Delong, G. Robert, and Adams, Raymond D. Developmental and congenital abnormalities of the nervous system. In Braunwald, Eugene, et al., eds., *Harrison's Principles of Internal Medicine*, 11th ed. New York: McGraw-Hill Book Co., 1987, pp. 2027-2035.

28. Dichter, Marc A. The epilepsies and convulsive disorders. In Braunwald, Eugene, et al., eds., *Harrison's Principles of Internal Medicine*, 11th ed. New York: McGraw-Hill Book Co., 1987, pp. 1921-1930.

29. Douglas, R. Gordon, Jr. Picornavirus infections (enterovirus, rhinovirus). In Stein, Jay H., ed.-in-chief, *Internal Medicine*, 2nd ed. Boston: Little, Brown & Co., 1987, pp. 1564-1571.

30. Easton, J. Donald. Cerebrovascular disease. In Stein, Jay H., ed.-in-chief. *Internal Medicine*, 2nd ed. Boston: Little, Brown & Co., 1987, pp. 2155-2157.

31. ———. Cranial trauma. Ibid., pp. 2222-2224.

32. ———. Myelopathies. Ibid., pp. 2228-2230.

33. ———. Degenerative diseases. Ibid., pp. 2242-2244.

34. Easton, J. Donald, and Hart, Robert G. Coma and related disorders. In Stein, Jay H., ed.-in-chief. *Internal Medicine*, 2nd ed. Boston: Little, Brown & Co., 1987, pp. 2135-2140.

35. Edmeads, John G. Headache and facial pain. In Stein, Jay H., ed.-in-chief. *Internal Medicine*, 2nd ed. Boston: Little, Brown & Co., 1987, pp. 2178-2185.

36. Ehni, Bruce L., and Ehni, George. Open surgical cordotomy. In Wilkins, Robert H., and Rengachary, Setti S., eds., *Neurosurgery*, vol. 3. New York: McGraw-Hill Book Co., 1985, pp. 2439-2451.

37. Gilman, Sid. Ataxia and disorders of equilibrium and gait. In Braunwald, Eugene, et al., eds., *Harrison's Principles of Internal Medicine*, 11th ed. New York: McGraw-Hill Book Co., 1987, pp. 91-96.

38. Greenlee, John E. Encephalitis. In Stein, Jay H., ed.-in-chief. *Internal Medicine*, 2nd ed. Boston: Little, Brown & Co., 1987, pp. 2224-2228.

39. Growdon, John H., and Young, Robert R. Paralysis and other disorders of movement. In Braunwald, Eugene, et al., eds., *Harrison's Principles of Internal Medicine*, 11th ed. New York: McGraw-Hill Book Co., 1987, pp. 79-91.

40. Gruber, Allan B. Peripheral nerve disorders. In Stein, Jay H., ed.-in-chief. *Internal Medicine*, 2nd ed. Boston: Little, Brown & Co., 1987, pp. 2231-2238.

41. Hart, Robert C., and Easton, Donald J. Demyelinating diseases. In Stein, Jay H., ed.-in-chief. *Internal Medicine*, 2nd ed. Boston: Little, Brown & Co., 1987, pp. 2244-2249.

42. Harter, Donald H., and Petersdorf, Robert G. Viral diseases of the central nervous system: Aseptic meningitis and encephalitis. In Braunwald, Eugene, et al., eds., *Harrison's Principles of Internal Medicine*, 11th ed. New York: McGraw-Hill Book Co., 1987, pp. 1987-1995.

43. Hershey, Linda A., et al. Magnetic resonance imaging in vascular dementia. *Neurology* 37:29-36, Jan. 1987.

44. Hochberg, Fred, and Pruitt, Amy. Neoplastic diseases of the central nervous system. In Braunwald, Eugene, et al., eds., *Harrison's Principles of Internal Medicine*, 11th ed. New York: McGraw-Hill Book Co., 1987, pp. 1968-1980.

45. Hoffmann, H.L., MD. Personal communications.

46. Janetta, Peter J. Trigeminal neuralgia: Treatment by microvascular decompression. In Wilkins, Robert H., and Rengachary, Setti S., eds., *Neurosurgery*, vol. 3. New York: McGraw-Hill Book Co., 1985, pp. 2357-2362.

47. Judd, Lewis L. The therapeutic use of psychotropic medications. In Braunwald, Eugene, et al., eds., *Harrison's Principles of Internal Medicine*, 11th ed. New York: McGraw-Hill Book Co., 1987, pp. 2099-2105.

48. Judd, Lewis L., and Huey, Leighton. Major affective disorders. In Braunwald, Eugene, et al., eds., *Harrison's Principles of Internal Medicine*, 11th ed. New York: McGraw-Hill Book Co., 1987, pp. 2085-2089.

49. King, Robert B. Medullary tractotomy for pain relief. In Wilkins, Robert H., and Rengachary, Setti S., eds., *Neurosurgery*, vol. 3. New York: McGraw-Hill Book Co., 1985, pp. 2452-2454.

50. Kistler, J. Philip, et al. Cerebrovascular disease. In Braunwald, Eugene, et al., eds., *Harrison's Principles of Internal Medicine*, 11th ed. New York: McGraw-Hill Book Co., 1987, pp. 1930-1960.

51. Maciewicz, Raymond, and Martin, Joseph B. Pain: Pathophysiology and management. In Braunwald, Eugene, et al., eds., *Harrison's Principles of Internal Medicine*, 11th ed. New York: McGraw-Hill Book Co., 1987, pp. 13-17.

52. Mankin, Henry, J., and Adams, Raymond D. Pain in back and neck. In Braunwald, Eugene, et al., eds., *Harrison's Principles of Internal Medicine*, 11th ed. New York: McGraw-Hill Book Co., 1987, pp. 34-42.

53. McCullough, David C. Hydrocephalus: Treatment. In Wilkins, Robert H., and Rengachary, Setti S., eds., *Neurosurgery*, vol. 3. New York: McGraw-Hill Book Co., 1985, pp. 2140-2150.

54. McGillicuddy, John E. Techniques of nerve repair. In Wilkins, Robert H., and Rengachary, Setti S., eds., *Neurosurgery*, vol. 2. New York: McGraw-Hill Book Co., 1985, pp. 1871-1880.

55. Meissner, William W. Theories of personality and psychopathology: Classical psychoanalysis. In Kaplan, Harold I., and Sadock, Benjamin J., eds., *Comprehensive Textbook of Psychiatry*, 4th ed. Vol. 1. Baltimore: Williams & Wilkins, 1985, pp. 307-418.

56. Mendelson, Jack H., and Mello, Nancy K. Commonly abused drugs. In Braunwald, Eugene, et al., eds., *Harrison's Principles of Internal Medicine*, 11th ed. New York: McGraw-Hill Book Co., 1987, pp. 2115-2118.

57. Mohr, Jay P., and Adams, Raymond. Disorders of speech and language. In Braunwald, Eugene, et al., eds., *Harrison's Principles of Internal Medicine*, 11th ed. New York: McGraw-Hill Book Co., 1987, pp. 121-127.

58. Ojeman, Robert G. Extracranial carotid artery atherosclerosis. In Wilkins, Robert H., and Rengachary, Setti S., eds., *Neurosurgery*,

vol. 2. New York: McGraw-Hill Book Co., 1985, pp. 1239-1247.

59. Pruitt, Amy A. Intracranial neoplasms. In Stein, Jay H., ed.-in-chief. *Internal Medicine*, 2nd ed. Boston: Little, Brown & Co., 1987, pp. 2220-2222.

60. Pruitt, Amy A., and Sherman, David G. Systemic cancer and the nervous system. In Stein, Jay H., ed.-in-chief. *Internal Medicine*, 2nd ed. Boston: Little, Brown & Co., 1987, pp. 2250-2254.

61. Pryse-Phillips, William. Psychological testing. In Stein, Jay H., ed.-in-chief. *Internal Medicine*, 2nd ed. Boston: Little, Brown & Co., 1987, pp. 2209-2210.

62. Richardson, Edward P., Jr., et al. Degenerative diseases of the nervous system. In Braunwald, Eugene, et al., eds., *Harrison's Principles of Internal Medicine*, 11th ed. New York: McGraw-Hill Book Co., 1987, pp. 2011-2027.

63. Ropper, Allan H. Trauma of the head and spinal cord. In Braunwald, Eugene, et al., eds., *Harrison's Principles of Internal Medicine*, 11th ed. New York: McGraw-Hill Book Co., 1987, pp. 1960-1968.

64. Ropper, Allan H., and Martin, Joseph B. Diseases of the spinal cord. In Braunwald, Eugene, et al., eds., *Harrison's Principles of Internal Medicine*, 11th ed. New York: McGraw-Hill Book Co., 1987, pp. 2040-2047.

65. Roski, Richard A., and Spetzler, Robert F. Carotid artery ligation. In Wilkins, Robert H., and Rengachary, Setti S., eds., *Neurosurgery*, vol. 2. New York: McGraw-Hill Book Co., 1985, pp. 1414-1432.

66. Rosomoff, Hubert L. Percutaneous spinothalamic cordotomy. In Wilkins, Robert H., and Rengachary, Setti S., eds., *Neurosurgery*, vol. 3. New York: McGraw-Hill Book Co., 1985, pp. 2446-2451.

67. *St. Louis Post-Dispatch*. Researcher warns of cocaine dangers during pregnancy. *St. Louis Post-Dispatch*, p. 1.D, Jan. 19, 1987.

68. Salcman, Michael. Supratentorial gliomas: Clinical features and surgical therapy. In Wilkins, Robert H., and Rengachary, Setti S., eds., *Neurosurgery*, vol. 1. New York: McGraw-Hill Book Co., 1985, pp. 579-590.

69. Schwartz, William J., et al. The sleep-wake cycle and disorders of sleep. In Braunwald, Eugene, et al., eds., *Harrison's Principles of Internal Medicine*, 11th ed. New York: McGraw-Hill Book Co., 1987, pp. 109-114.

70. Sherman, David G. Disorders of the intellect. In Stein, Jay H., ed.-in-chief. *Internal Medicine*, 2nd ed. Boston: Little, Brown & Co., 1987, pp. 2150-2153.

71. Sherman, David G., and Easton, J. Donald. Dizziness and disorders of balance and gait. In Wilkins, Robert H., and Rengachary, Setti S., eds., *Neurosurgery*, vol. 3. New York: McGraw-Hill Book Co., 1985, pp. 2163-2167.

72. Sherman, David G., Easton, J. Donald, and Hart, Robert G. Disorders of muscle tone and movement. In Wilkins, Robert H., and Rengachary, Setti S., eds., *Neurosurgery*, vol. 3. New York: McGraw-Hill Book Co., 1985, pp. 2159-2163.

73. Signor, Roger. Manic-depression work called breakthrough. *St. Louis Post-Dispatch*, p. 6A, Feb. 26, 1987.

74. Tasher, Ronald R. Stereotatic surgery: Principles and techniques. In Wilkins, Robert H., and Rengachary, Setti S., eds., *Neurosurgery*, vol. 2. New York: McGraw-Hill Book Co., 1985, pp. 1912-1917.

75. Tindall, Suzie C. Painful neuromas. In Wilkins, Robert H., and Rengachary, Setti S., eds., *Neurosurgery*, vol. 2. New York: McGraw-Hill Book Co., 1985, pp. 1884-1886.

76. Victor, Maurice, and Adams, Raymond D. Confusion, delirium, amnesia, and dementia. In Braunwald, Eugene, et al., eds., *Harrison's Principles of Internal Medicine*, 11th ed. New York: McGraw-Hill Book Co., 1987, pp. 127-135.

77. Victor, Maurice, and Martin, Joseph B. Diseases of the cranial nerves. In Braunwald, Eugene, et al., eds., *Harrison's Principles of Internal Medicine*, 11th ed. New York: McGraw-Hill Book Co., 1987, pp. 2035-2047.

78. Walsh, Robert A., et al. Faintness and syncope. In Stein, Jay H., ed.-in-chief. *Internal Medicine*, 2nd ed. Boston: Little, Brown & Co., 1987, pp. 2141-2145.

79. *Washington Post*. Many cocaine users graduate from marijuana. *St. Louis Post-Dispatch*, pp. 1D-5D, July 26, 1986.

80. Weinstein, Louis. Diseases of the upper respiratory tract. In Braunwald, Eugene, et al., eds., *Harrison's Principles of Internal Medicine*, 11th ed. New York: McGraw-Hill Book Co., 1987, pp. 1111-1115.

81. Wilkins, Robert H. Trigeminal neuralgia: Introduction. In Wilkins, Robert H., and Rengachary, Setti S., eds., *Neurosurgery*, vol. 3. New York: McGraw-Hill Book Co., 1985, pp. 2337-2344.

82. Williams, Gordon H., and Braunwald, Eugene. Hypertensive vascular disease. In Braunwald, Eugene, et al., eds., *Harrison's Principles of Internal Medicine*, 11th ed. New York: McGraw-Hill Book Co., 1987, pp. 1024-1037.

83. Wilson, Robert F. Preoperative medical evaluation. In Stein, Jay H., ed.-in-chief. *Internal Medicine*, 2nd ed. Boston: Little, Brown & Co., 1987, pp. 2324-2329.

84. Woodburne, Russell T., and Burkel, William E. The nervous system. In *Essentials of Human Anatomy*, 8th ed. New York: Oxford University Press, 1988, pp. 27-40.

Cardiovascular Disorders

Heart and Coronary Arteries

Origin of Terms

a-, an- (G) —without, not
angi-, angio- (G) —vessel
atrio- (L) —chamber, hall
brady- (G) —slow
card-, cardio- (G) —heart
cor- (L) —heart
corona (L) —crown
-emia (G) —blood
endo- (G) —within
epi- (G) —upon, in addition to

hem-, hemo- (G) —blood
my-, myo- (G) —muscle
-pathy (G) —disease
peri- (G) —around, about
-plasty (G) —surgical correction or formation
septum (L) —dividing wall, partition
tachy- (G) —rapid, swift
veno- (L) —vein
ventriculo- (L) —ventricle, belly

Anatomic Terms (Refs. 90, 132, 137)

- *cavities of the heart* —the four heart chambers.
    - *atria (sing. atrium)* —the two chambers that form the base of the heart and receive the venous blood.
    - *ventricles* —the two chambers that lie anteriorly to the atria and propel blood into arteries.

(Fig. 32 shows anterior view of heart.)

- *conduction system of the heart* (Fig. 33) —neuromuscular tissue specialized for the conduction of electric impulses. (Components are arranged in order of function instead of alphabetic order).
    - *sinoatrial node, sinus node (SA node)* —node situated in the wall of the right atrium. It is the pacemaker of the heart, since it transmits impulses to both atria, stimulating them to contract simultaneously.
    - *atrioventricular node (AV node)* —node found in the septum of the heart near the junction of the atria and ventricles. It relays impulses from the atria to the atrioventricular bundle.
    - *atrioventricular bundle, bundle of His* —a bundle of specialized neuromuscular tissue within the atrioventricular septum transmitting impulses from the AV node to the Purkinje fibers.

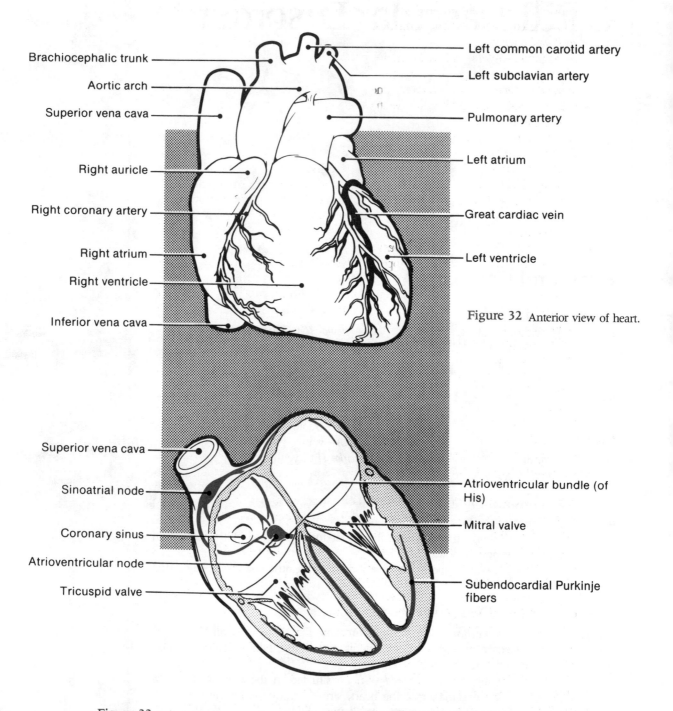

Brachiocephalic trunk

Aortic arch

Superior vena cava

Right auricle

Right coronary artery

Right atrium

Right ventricle

Inferior vena cava

Left common carotid artery

Left subclavian artery

Pulmonary artery

Left atrium

Great cardiac vein

Left ventricle

Figure 32 Anterior view of heart.

Superior vena cava

Sinoatrial node

Coronary sinus

Atrioventricular node

Tricuspid valve

Atrioventricular bundle (of His)

Mitral valve

Subendocardial Purkinje fibers

Figure 33 Schematic diagram of conduction system of heart. Impulses pass from sinoatrial node through both atria, stimulating them to contract. Atrioventricular node is thereby activated and transmits impulses to atrioventricular bundle and its right and left limbs, resulting in contraction of both ventricles.

—*Purkinje fibers*—cardiac muscle fibers of the conduction system that ramify beneath the endocardium and deliver impulses to the ventricular myocardium, initiating contraction of the ventricles.

■ *heart wall and covering:*

—*endocardium*—interior lining of the heart wall.

—*myocardium*—the heart muscle.

—*myocardial sinusoids*—endothelium-lined spaces lying between the myocardial muscle fibers and enabling the ventricular myocardium to absorb blood in a spongelike manner.

—*pericardium*—covering of the heart composed of a fibrous tissue (pericardium fibrosum) and serous tissue (pericardium serosum). The former fits loosely around the heart. The latter consists of a visceral layer or epicardium that adheres closely to the myocardium and a parietal layer that lines the inner surface of the fibrous pericardium. The pericardial cavity is a narrow space between the parietal and visceral layers. It contains a minimal amount of serum that serves as a lubricant.

■ *orifices and valves of the heart and great vessels:*

—*atrioventricular orifices and valves*—openings and cuspid valves between atria and ventricles.

–*mitral valve, bicuspid valve*—valve between left atrium and left ventricle. It contains two endothelial folds or cusps that come together when the ventricle contracts.

–*tricuspid valve*—three endothelial folds or cusps that guard the right atrioventricular orifice.

—*foramen ovale*—opening between the two atria in fetal life. It normally closes after birth.

—*semilunar valves*—half-moon-shaped flaps within the aorta and pulmonary trunk that prevent the blood from flowing back into the ventricles.

■ *sinuses, arteries, and nerves:*

—*aortic sinuses, sinuses of Valsalva*—three dilated spaces of the root of the aorta, related to the three cusps of the aortic valve.

—*coronary arteries*—branches of the ascending aorta arising from the right and left aortic sinuses. The blood vessels with their branches supply the heart muscle and form numerous anastomoses of small arteries and precapillaries. In the event of a sudden occlusion of a major coronary artery, these anastomotic channels may not be able to provide adequate collateral circulation. But if a major coronary artery is slowly occluded, these channels may enlarge and maintain a sufficient blood supply to the heart muscle.

—*coronary sinus*—a short, broad vessel into which most of the veins of the heart empty. It in turn empties into the right atrium.

—*internal thoracic arteries, internal mammary arteries*—blood vessels, usually arising from the subclavian arteries and passing downward on either side of the sternum. They are approximately the same caliber as the coronary arteries. They can be surgically relocated from the chest wall to a coronary artery distal to an obstructing lesion to revascularize the heart muscle.

—*parasympathetic fibers*—preganglionic fibers that reach the heart via the vagus nerve. Ganglia in the heart have postganglionic fibers distributed to both the atria and the ventricles. Impulses slow the heart and depress contractions.

—*sympathetic fibers carried by the cervical and thoracic cardiac nerves to the heart muscle*—fibers involved in control of the heart rate and the force of its contraction. Afferent fibers join the vagus nerve to aid in regulation of blood volume and heart rate.

Diagnostic Terms

- *aneurysm*—dilatation or bulging out of the wall of the heart, aorta, or any other artery. Thrombi may form in the sac, break off, and lead to embolism. The aneurysm may rupture. Ventricular aneurysms are usually complications of coronary atherosclerosis and myocardial infarction.
- *angina pectoris* (12, 14, 38, 39, 80, 127)
    - *classic angina pectoris*—syndrome characterized by short attacks of substernal precordial pain that radiates to the left shoulder and arm. It is more usually associated with S-T segment changes than conduction defects. Electrocardiographic (ECG) findings may show atrioventicular or intraventicular defects of conduction, nonspecific S-T segment changes, previous myocardial scar, or other abnormalities. About 30 percent of the ECG studies are likely to be normal. This condition may be provoked by exertion and relieved by rest.
    - *unstable angina pectoris*—chest pain is more prolonged and severe than in the classic angina and remains unrelieved by rest and nitroglycerine. ECG shows evidence of myocardial ischemia, but infarction or necrosis are absent in the early phase. A favorable prognosis depends on the evolution of the collateral circulation to compensate for the impoverished blood flow of the myocardium or on revascularization surgery, which has been reported to be about 80 percent successful. Untreated patients eventually develop myocardial infarction and die.
    - *variant angina, Prinzmetal's angina*—anginal chest pain at rest, prone to occur on awakening, and tending to be cyclic. The spasm is the predominant factor and is usually but not always located in the proximal right coronary artery, as identified through coronary arteriography studies. Transient S-T segment elevation or other ECG abnormalities may be associated with this syndrome.
- *anomalies, congenital*—gross structural defects of the heart or great intrathoracic vessels arising during fetal development and in selected cases associated with chromosomal abnormalities. (62)
    - *atrial septal defect*—abnormality resulting in a shunting of oxygenated blood from the left into the right atrium. There are wide variations of atrial septal defects in size, position, and shape. Shunting is minimal when the defect is small. A persistent foramen ovale is one of the septal defects that may be encountered. (62)
    - *cor triatriatum*—heart with three atrial chambers due to an obstructing membrane that partitions the left atrium, thus impeding the pulmonary venous circulation, causing pulmonary venous congestion, hypertension, and congestive heart failure. (21)
    - *cor triloculare*—heart composed of three chambers, resulting from the absence of the interatrial or interventricular septum. (62)
    - *isolated pulmonic stenosis, pure pulmonary stenosis*—a narrowing of the pulmonary valve or of the infundibulum associated with an intact ventricular septum. The stenotic defect causes pulmonary outflow tract obstruction. (Infundibulum is the cone-shaped area of the right ventricle from which the pulmonary artery begins.) (21)
    - *patent ductus arteriosus*—persistence of communication between pulmonary artery and aorta after birth. In normal infants, the closure of the ductus takes place during the first six weeks of life. (21, 23, 43)
    - *tetralogy of Fallot*—complex of congenital defects usually considered as having the following four parts. (The first two are essential parts of the complex.)
        - *ventricular septal defect*—malformation of the septum of the ventricles. (21, 43)
        - *pulmonic stenosis*—same as isolated type, except that involvement is associated with other defects. (21)

*—dextroposition of the aorta—*transposition of the aorta to the right. (21)

*—hypertrophy of the right ventricle—*increased size of the ventricle, the body's way of compensating for the added load imposed by the defects. (29)

—*ventricular septal defect—*abnormality allowing oxygenated blood to shunt from the left ventricle to the right ventricle. There are wide variations in size and position.

–isolated absence of the ventricular septum, partial or total; occasionally multiple.

–defect associated with other anomalies. (41, 43, 108)

- *cardiac arrest—*cessation of effective heart action, usually manifested by asystole or ventricular fibrillation. (61)

- *cardiac arrhythmias, cardiac dysrhythmias—*irregularities of heart action, including disturbances of rate, rhythm, and conduction either related or unrelated to other cardiac disease, supraventricular (atrial), or ventricular. Some major arrhythmias that seriously interfere with cardiac or circulatory efficiency are presented. (4, 56, 137, 138)

  —*atrial arrhythmias—*disorders of rhythm having their origin in the SA node. They may be provoked by ischemia, drug toxicity, or atrial distention. If uncontrolled, atrial arrhythmias may become life threatening. (51, 56, 106, 107)

  –*atrial fibrillation—*extremely rapid, vermicular, ineffectual contractions of the atria resulting in irregularity of rhythm in the ventricles. The atrial rate is 350 beats per minute or more. (51, 56, 106, 107, 139)

  –*atrial flutter—*rapid, regular cardiac action of 250 to 350 beats per minute, usually occurring in paroxysms, which are more prolonged than atrial tachycardia. The atrial impulse may produce a rapid ventricular rate or result in an atrioventricular block of varying degree (such as 2:1, 3:1, or 4:1 ratio). (51, 56, 106, 107)

  –*paroxysmal atrial tachycardia (PAT)—*rapid, regular contractions of the atria initiated by an irritable center within the atrium outside the sinoatrial node. Rate is about 160 to 200 beats per minute. Ventricular contractions are in 1:1 ratio with atrial contractions. This arrhythmia (PAT) is practically indistinguishable from nodal paroxysmal tachycardia. The patient may encounter a sudden forceful thump and subsequent attack of palpitation. (4, 106)

  —*atrioventricular nodal arrhythmias—*disorders arising in the atrioventricular node.

  –*atrioventricular nodal rhythm—*pacemaker function assumed by AV node in response to sustained failure of sinoatrial node to send impulses to the atrioventricular node.

  –*premature atrioventricular nodal contractions (PNC)—*arrhythmia caused by irritation of the atrioventricular node, which produces an ectopic stimulus and subsequent premature nodal contractions. Frequent recurrence of PNCs may signal progressive myocardial infarction. (4, 106)

  —*ventricular arrhythmias—*disorders of rhythm arising within the ventricles. (4, 56)

  –*premature ventricular contractions (PVC)—*the most common disturbance of rhythm, frequently an index of myocardial damage and anoxia. If more than six PVCs per minute occur, ventricular efficiency may be seriously impaired. (4, 106, 108)

  –*ventricular tachycardia—*disorder heralding a high degree of irritability, frequently associated with myocardial infarction. The irritable center within the ventricular wall produces a rapid ventricular rate that may change to ventricular fibrillation or ventricular standstill. The rate is 150 to 250 beats per minute or greater, and the rhythm slightly irregular. Sudden dizziness, precordial pain, dyspnea, and weakness are common complaints. (56, 106, 107, 138)

—*ventricular fibrillation* (Figs. 34 and 35)—extremely rapid, nonsynchronous contractions of ventricular muscle bundles; irregularities in rhythm and force result in no ejection of blood from the fibrillating ventricles. It may terminate in ventricular standstill. (56)

—*conduction disturbances*—abnormalities in the cardiac conduction system.

—*atrioventricular block*—delay or obstruction of impulses arising above or within the atrioventricular node.

first-degree heart block—prolongation of atrioventricular conduction time; delay of impulses on their ventricular pathway. Possible causes are increased vagal tone, myocardial ischemia, and drug toxicity. (27, 52, 60)

second-degree or partial heart block—Mobitz type I, benign form: blockage of one atrial beat after six to eight conducted beats and dropping of respective ventricular beat (Wenckebach's pause); Mobitz type II, serious form: not all impulses are transmitted to the bundle of His by the atrioventricular node, resulting in various ratios (2:1, 3:1, 4:1, and others) of atrial contractions. Wrist pulse is 40 to 50 beats per minute. (27, 56, 106, 107)

third-degree or complete block—no atrial impulses are transmitted to the bundle of His by the atrioventricular node. Wrist pulse is 30 to 40 beats per minute as a result of beats initiated within the conduction mechanism of the ventricle. (27, 130)

—*bundle branch block*—obstruction of the wave of excitation in either branch of the atrioventricular bundle. (56, 106, 107)

—*hemiblock*—electrocardiographic patterns that precede or coexist with bundle branch blocks or are precursors of atrioventricular conduction abnormalities. (29, 130)

—*sick sinus syndrome, bradycardia-tachycardia syndrome*—sinoatrial dysfunction of the conduction system of the heart, characterized by abnormal impulse formation or transformation. (52, 56, 60, 107, 139)

—*Stokes-Adams syndrome*—cardiac standstill that occurs with certain forms of heart block, causing syncope and possible fatal convulsions. (7)

—*Wolff-Parkinson-White syndrome*—congenital disorder of atrioventricular conduction that may be associated with recurrent paroxysmal tachycardia, atrial flutter, or other ectopic rhythms. (19, 51, 56, 107)

■ *cardiac tamponade, pericardial tamponade*—compression of the heart by effusion or hemorrhage in the pericardium, which may seriously obstruct the venous inflow to the heart; raise the venous pressure; reduce the cardiac output; and cause hypotension, distention of the neck veins, and orthopnea. (10, 57)

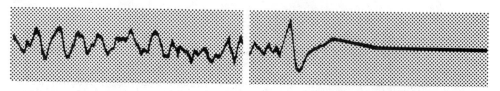

Figure 34 Ventricular fibrillation: life-threatening arrhythmia.

Figure 35 Terminal ventricular fibrillation and ventricular standstill—asystole.

- *cardiomyopathies*—miscellaneous group of heart muscle disorders of unknown etiology. These disorders may be classified as:
    - —*congestive dilatated cardiomyopathy*—marked cardiac enlargement with systolic pump malfunction. Symptoms of congestive heart failure and arrhythmias may be present.
        - –*alcoholic cardiomyopathy*—persons who consume large quantities of alcohol over time may develop a clinical condition similar to idiopathic dilatated cardiomyopathy. Alcoholic cardiomyopathy is the major form of secondary dilatated cardiomyopathy in the western world.
        - –*peripartum cardiomyopathy*—cardiac dilatation and congestive heart failure may develop in the last month of pregnancy or in the first few months after delivery. If the heart size returns to normal after the first episode of congestive heart failure, then subsequent pregnancies may be well tolerated; however, if it remains enlarged, future pregnancies often produce increasing myocardial damage, which may lead to refractory congestive heart failure and finally death.
    - —*hypertrophic cardiomyopathy*—slight to moderate cardiac enlargement with left ventricular hypertrophy. The characteristic feature of this disorder is the asymmetric septal hypertrophy with or without obstruction to ventricular outflow and the presence of a systolic murmur. The most common symptom is dyspnea; however, other symptoms may occur, such as angina pectoris, fatigue, or syncope.
    - —*restrictive cardiomyopathy*—slight cardiac enlargement with endomyocardial scarring and abnormal diastolic function. Interference with the left ventricular filling and emptying cycle may be produced by the presence of infiltrative myocardial fibrosis, amyloid disease, and other disorders. (71, 133)
- *cardiopulmonary arrest*—heart-lung arrest caused by sudden and unexpected cessation of respiration and functional circulation. (61)
- *Chagas' disease*—acute or chronic myocarditis caused by *Trypanosoma cruzi*. Serious arrhythmias and congestive heart failure signal death. The disease is endemic in South and Central America and is fatal in 87 percent of those affected. (29, 130)
- *congestive heart failure*—the heart is unable to pump adequate amounts of blood to tissues and organs. This is generally caused by diseases of the heart causing low cardiac output. It can result from other conditions (anemia, hyperthyroidism) in which the demand for blood is greater than normal and the heart fails despite high cardiac output. In advanced disease, left-sided and right-sided congestive heart failure coexist.
    - —*left-sided heart failure*—failure of the left ventricle precipitated by serious coronary, hypertensive, or valvular heart disease. Except in mitral stenosis, it produces variable degrees of left ventricular dilatation followed by pulmonary congestion and edema, salt and water retention, scanty urinary output, cerebral hypoxia, and coma.
    - —*right-sided heart failure*—failure of the right ventricle characterized by venous congestion of the portal system, with ascites and enlargement of the liver and spleen.
    - —*latent heart failure*—that state in which heart failure is *not* present at rest, but is present during periods of increased stress or after an increase in blood volume.
    - —*compensated heart failure*—that condition in which heart failure was previously present, but in which cardiac output has been returned to (or maintained at) a normal level by compensatory mechanisms or therapy. (91, 104, 105, 108)

- *coronary atherosclerosis*—chronic disorder characterized by lipid deposits that form fibrous fatty plaques within the intima and inner media of the coronary arteries. These plaques are known as atheromas. (12, 79)
- *coronary atherosclerotic heart disease*—the most common heart condition. Progressive thickening of the intima of the coronary arteries leads to occlusion, caused by narrowing of the lumen and intravascular clotting. (41)
- *cor pulmonale*—heart-lung disease characterized by right ventricular hypertrophy caused by pulmonary disorders that increase pulmonary vascular resistance and induce pulmonary hypertension; ventilatory insufficiency is not necessarily impaired.
  - *acute form*—caused by massive pulmonary embolism occurring within hours.
  - *chronic form*—caused by diffuse pulmonary fibrosis, obstructive emphysema, or obstructive vascular disease developing within months. (55, 78)
- *Ebstein's anomaly*—tricuspid insufficiency caused by a spiral-like attachment of a valve leaflet of the tricuspid, resulting in atrial enlargement, defective ventricular filling, right-to-left shunting, other impairments, and variable clinical manifestations such as dyspnea, cyanosis, clubbing of fingers, precordial thrill, and systolic or diastolic murmurs. (42, 62, 70)
- *Eisenmenger's syndrome*—right-to-left shunting of pulmonary circulation, usually recognized first in adolescence and thought to result from an unrepaired congenital defect in infancy. It is manifested by cyanosis, clubbing, chest pain, hemoptysis, syncope, and polycythemia. The clinical course is progressive, and death usually ensues before 50 years of age. (31, 43)
- *endocarditis, bacterial*—acute or subacute infection of the lining of the heart and especially valve leaflets. It is caused by organisms that enter the bloodstream and initiate a bacteremia clinically recognized by fever, fatigue, heart murmurs, spleno-megaly, embolic episodes, and areas of infarction. (17, 30)
- *Libman-Sacks endocarditis*—condition characterized by verrucose lesions found in the endocardium of patients with terminal disseminated lupus erythematosus. (17)
- *Löffler's endocarditis, fibroplastic endocarditis*—marked thickening of the ventricles affecting the underlying heart muscle and mural thrombi, thus diminishing the size of the ventricular cavities. (17, 125)
- *ischemic heart disease*—the prominent feature is a markedly reduced blood supply to the heart muscle, generally due to coronary atherosclerosis. The resultant myocardial ischemia may produce myocardial infarction, heart failure, or angina pectoris. (46, 94)
- *mitral valve prolapse*—slippage of one or more leaflets of the mitral valve into the atrium during ventricular systole, causing stress. The prolapse is associated with a systolic murmur and midsystolic click. The diagnosis is confirmed by auscultation, angiography, and echocardiography. (70, 74)
- *myocardial disease, primary:*
  - *myocarditis*—inflammation of the heart muscle that may result in myocardial fibrosis, followed by cardiac enlargement and congestive heart failure.
  - *myocardosis*—condition characterized by cardiac dilatation, congestive heart failure, and embolization. (12, 25, 125, 132)
- *myocardial disease, secondary*—heart disease associated with noninfectious systemic diseases such as:
  - *amyloidosis*
  - *carcinoidosis*
  - *collagen diseases*
  - *endocrinopathy*
  - *sarcoidosis*
  - *systemic muscular and neurologic disorders* (35, 126, 133)

- *myocardial infarction, acute*—clinical syndrome manifested by persistent, usually intense cardiac pain, unrelated to exertion and often constrictive, followed by diaphoresis, pallor, hypotension, dyspnea, faintness, nausea, and vomiting. The underlying disease is usually coronary atherosclerosis that progressed to coronary thrombosis and occlusion and resulted in a sudden curtailment of blood supply to the heart muscle and myocardial ischemia.
    - *inferior wall infarction, diaphragmatic infarction*—occlusion of the right coronary artery.
    - *lateral wall infarction*—occlusion of the diagonal branch of the left anterior descending artery or left circumflex artery.
    - *posterior wall infarction*—infarction precipitated by occlusive lesions of the right coronary artery or circumflex coronary artery branch. (12, 68, 75, 128)
- *pericarditis*—inflammation of the covering membranes of the heart. Its distinctive feature is pericardial friction rub, a transitory scratchy or leathery sound elicited on auscultation.
    - *constrictive pericarditis, chronic*—disorder characterized by a rigid, thickened pericardium that prevents adequate filling of the ventricles and may lead to congestive heart failure.
    - *purulent pericarditis*—disease caused by pyogenic bacteria, which may be associated with purulent, pericardial effusion. (10, 56, 97)
- *rheumatic heart disease*—involvement of the heart in the course of rheumatic fever and attacking the myocardium, pericardium, and endocardium, with the valvular endocardium as the site of predilection. (109)
- *sudden cardiac death*—unexpected death, either instantaneously or within 24 hours, excluding trauma, suicide, or terminal illness as possible causes. (12, 61)
- *valvular (valvar) heart disease, chronic*—disorder referring to any permanent organic deformity in one or more of the valves. Some examples of this condition are:
    - *aortic insufficiency*—indicates regurgitation of small amounts of blood through the incompetent leaflets during diastole. As the valve deformity increases, larger amounts are regurgitated. The diastolic blood pressure is lowered, and the pulse wave assumes its characteristic contour. The left ventricle progressively enlarges. Left ventricular failure may suddenly occur, with acute pulmonary edema or recurrent paroxysmal nocturnal dyspnea and orthopnea. The murmur of aortic insufficiency may be absent during severe heart failure but may reappear following treatment.
    - *aortic stenosis*—reduction in the valve orifice, interfering with the emptying of the left ventricle. Characteristic signs include a systolic ejection murmur at the aortic area transmitted to the neck and a systolic ejection click at the aortic area. In severe cases, there may be a palpable left ventricular heave, reversed splitting of the second heart sound, and a weak-to-absent aortic second sound. Eighty percent of patients with aortic stenosis are men. (8, 9, 70)
    - *mitral insufficiency*—the mitral leaflets do not close normally during the ventricular systole, and blood is forced back into the atrium and through the aortic valve. This condition is characterized by a pansystolic murmur that is maximal at the apex and radiates to the axilla, a hyperdynamic left ventricular impulse, a brisk carotid upstroke, and a prominent third heart sound. (73)
    - *mitral stenosis*—very common sequela of rheumatic fever, marked by the development of minute vegetations and thrombi that narrow the orifice of the valve leaflets. Calcifications form as the disease progresses. The characteristic sign is a localized, delayed diastolic murmur that is low in pitch and has a duration that varies with the severity of the stenosis and heart rate. (8, 9, 14, 73)

—*tricuspid insufficiency*—affects the right ventricle. This condition may occur in a variety of disorders other than disease of the tricuspid valve itself. The left ventricular overload resulting from left ventricular failure is usually caused by coronary heart disease, hypertensive heart failure, cardiomyopathy, and mitral or aortic stenosis. The tricuspid insufficiency is characterized by a prominent regurgitant systolic wave in the right atrium and in the jugular venous pulse. Regurgitation of blood from the right ventricle to the right atrium may occur during systole, as noted by right ventricular angiography. (73)

—*tricuspid stenosis*—associated with mitral stenosis, this defect reduces the valve to a small, triangular opening that causes resistance in the flow of blood from the right atrium to the right ventricle and leads to congestion of the lungs and liver. Careful examination is required to differentiate the typical diastolic rumble along the lower left sternal border from the murmur of mitral stenosis. Women represent the majority of those affected, and mitral valve disease is usually present. (8, 9, 73, 74, 108, 130)

Operative Terms

■ *biopsy of pericardium*—excision of a small piece of pericardial tissue for microscopic study. (57)

■ *cardiac biopsy*—excision of tissue from the heart for the purpose of diagnosing various disease states. This can be done at the time of the operation or by means of a biotome adapted to an intracardiac catheter. Under fluoroscopic control the biotome is passed through a large peripheral vein into the right atrium and right ventricle for biopsy. Tissue studies aid in the evaluation of the patient's condition before cardiovascular surgery. Biopsy is the primary method of detecting rejection of the transplanted heart. (5, 130)

■ *cardiac massage, open*—emergency thoracotomy and manual compression of the heart 40 to 60 times a minute in an attempt to force blood from the ventricles into the aorta and pulmonary artery. (130)

■ *cardiac transplantation, heart transplantation*—removal of a human cadaver heart for implantation into a recipient who is in irreversible cardiac failure. The procedure includes: a median sternotomy, cannulation of vena cavae, cardiopulmonary bypass, surgical divisions of the ascending aorta, main pulmonary artery, and atria, the excision of donor and recipient hearts, and implantation of donor heart by atrial and vascular anastomoses to recipient. (84, 105, 114, 130)

■ *correction of congenital septal defects:*
    —*atrial septal defect*—closure of defect under direct vision using cardiopulmonary bypass with or without hypothermia. (49)
    —*ventricular septal defect*—repair of defect by:
      –*direct suture* or
      –*use of ventricular patch* such as Dacron patch. Extracorporeal circulation with or without hypothermia is employed. (50, 130)

■ *correction of transposition of the great vessels:* (23, 101)
    —*Blalock-Hanlon operation*—surgical creation of an atrial septal defect as a palliative method, which provides increased intracardiac mixing of the oxygenated and unoxygenated blood.
    —*Mustard's operation*—surgical revision of the atrial septum, transposing the venous return to match the transposed outflow tracts.
    —*Rashkind's operation, atrioseptostomy by balloon catheter*—surgical creation of an atrial septal defect for palliation.

—*Senning's operation, revised technique*—reconstruction of a new atrial septum using the left atrial appendix to invert the atrial flow in transposition of the great arteries.

- *mitral commissurotomy*—separation of the stenotic valve at points of fusion. (33, 122)
- *mitral valve reconstruction*—procedure to relieve mitral valve incompetence, including:
  —*anulus remodeling*—restoring the proper size and shape by prosthetic rings to establish normal valve orifice and function.
  —*chordal fenestration and resection*—improving leaflet motion by resecting fused chordae at triangular portion.
  —*chordal shortening*—shortening chordae by plastic repair of chordae or papillary muscle.
  —*leaflet resection*—resecting abnormal segments in the presence of abnormal leaflets or fibrotic lesions. (33, 122)
- *myocardial revascularization*—operative procedure that supplies the ischemic heart muscle with systemic arterial blood (see Figs. 36 and 37). Various techniques are used, for example:
  —*aortocoronary artery bypass*—revascularization of the heart muscle by attaching autogenous saphenous vein grafts (SVG) to the ascending aorta and the coronary arteries distal to the occlusions. Vascular obstructions are thus bypassed, and adequate blood flow to the heart is immediately restored. Since coronary atherosclerosis frequently involves several vessels, multiple grafts are often employed to safeguard permanent circulatory efficiency.
  —*internal mammary-coronary artery anastomoses*—cardiac revascularization by joining internal mammary artery grafts (IMAG) to one or more coronary arteries to bypass occlusive lesions and relieve myocardial ischemia. Since IMA grafts have proved to be highly patent and stable, they are successfully used when recurrence of disabling angina caused by graft closure or progressive coronary atherosclerosis necessitates reoperative revascularization. Unstable angina may be effectively treated with venous autografts, internal mammary artery autografts, or both.
  —*sequential vein graft for coronary artery bypass*—procedure used for serious coronary disease with multiple vessel narrowing. Complete myocardial revascularization may be achieved by grafting distally to all or any of the following:
  —*posterior descending right coronary artery*
  —*second marginal circumflex artery*
  —*first marginal circumflex coronary arteries or*
  —*diagonal branch and left anterior descending coronary arteries* (Cleveland's technique). (12, 41, 76, 80, 86)
- *pericardiectomy*—incision and partial dissection of the pericardium to relieve the heart from constricting fibrous adhesions. (57, 58)
- *pulmonary banding*—operation performed in infants with congenital defects and large left-to-right shunts at the ventricular level, which are not suitable for immediate complete correction. (130)
- *tetralogy of Fallot:* (62, 83, 99, 130)
  —*palliative operations:*
  -*Blalock-Taussig total repair*—anastomosis of the subclavian artery to the pulmonary artery to shunt some of the systemic circulation into the pulmonary circulation.
  -*pulmonary valvotomy or infundibular resection*—correction of pulmonary stenosis by valvotomy or resection.
  -*Waterston shunt initial repair*—anastomosis between the right pulmonary artery and ascending aorta for palliation of hypoxia in infants with tetralogy.

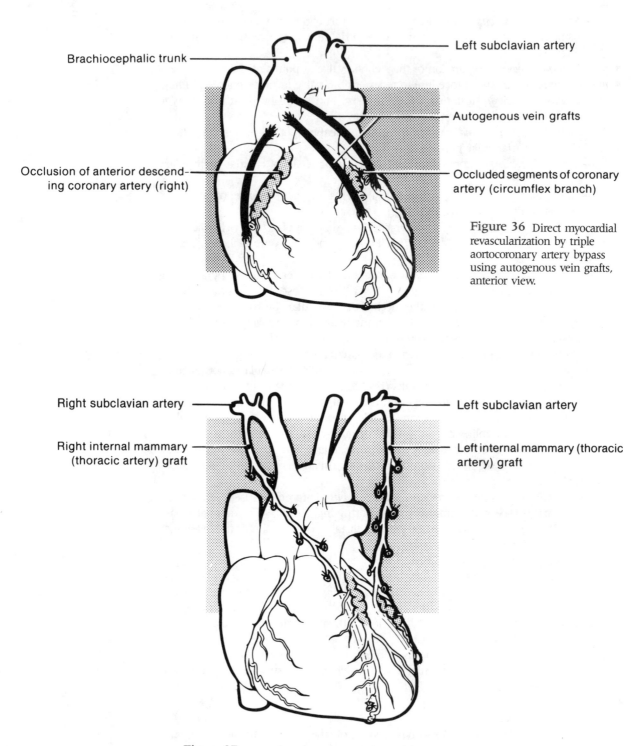

Brachiocephalic trunk

Left subclavian artery

Autogenous vein grafts

Occlusion of anterior descending coronary artery (right)

Occluded segments of coronary artery (circumflex branch)

Figure 36 Direct myocardial revascularization by triple aortocoronary artery bypass using autogenous vein grafts, anterior view.

Right subclavian artery

Right internal mammary (thoracic artery) graft

Left subclavian artery

Left internal mammary (thoracic artery) graft

Figure 37 Internal mammary artery bypass grafts for myocardial revascularization, anterior view.

—*total correction by direct vision*—removal of pulmonary obstruction and closure of ventricular septal defect.

- *tricuspid repair*—remodeling of anulus with prosthetic ring. (99, 122)
- *valve replacement surgery, cardiac*—removal of incompetent or stenotic heart valve and replacement with a
    —*bioprosthesis and homograft:* (8, 33, 40, 122)
        —*Carpentier-Edwards bioprosthesis*—porcine valve preserved in glutaraldehyde.
        pericardial valve—designed to improve hemodynamics in small orifices. The septal bar projection is reduced in this model by mounting techniques that incorporate the bar into an asymmetric anulus. The mounting techniques avoid fixation sutures at the commissures. The design has a flexible stent to reduce stress at the commissures and at the base of the cusps.
        supra-anular porcine valve—design characteristics aim at decreasing the transvalvular gradient and turbulence around the valve, as well as increasing longevity and decreasing calcification incidence.
        —*Hancock bioprosthesis*—consists of the aortic valve of the pig secured to a flexible support with a stellite ring at the anulus to prevent distortion. The frame is covered with fabric and a sewing ring allows the valve to be attached securely to the patient's tissues.
        —*Hancock modified-orifice bioprosthesis*—valve has been modified by removing the right coronary cusp with its muscular shelf and replacing it with a non-coronary cusp (which has no muscle shelf) from another valve.
        —*Ionescu-Shiley bioprosthesis*—valve is composed of three leaflets of bovine pericardium attached to a symmetrical titanium support covered with Dacron fabric.
        —*unstented hemograft valve*—"fresh" hemograft for replacing the aortic valve.
    —*mechanical prosthesis:* (8, 33, 41, 95, 130)
        —*Björk-Shiley prosthesis*—tilting disc valve of pyrolite carbon that is retained by two struts. Other designs of the Björk-Shiley prostheses include:
        convex-concave disc of pyrolite carbon—the inlet strut is formed from the same solid block of alloy as the valve housing and is no longer welded in place; however, the outlet strut is welded.
        monostrut valve with a single outlet strut—the whole valve housing is constructed from one piece of metal alloy, eliminating all welds.
        —*St. Jude Medical prosthesis*—bileaflet valve, made of pyrolytic carbon with no metal parts. The two leaflets open to give central flow, tilting nearly perpendicular to the anulus when the valve opens, eliminating the need for any supporting struts.
        —*Medtronic-Hall prosthesis*—tilting disc prosthesis with pyrolytic carbon disc occluder in a titanium valve housing. The disc is retained by sliding along a central bar that allows the disc to move downstream away from the orifice during opening.
        —*Sutter prosthesis (formerly the Smeloff-Cutter prosthesis)*—caged ball prosthesis with a silicone rubber ball occluder and a titanium retaining cage on each side of the valve seat.
        —*Starr-Edwards prosthesis*—caged ball prosthesis. Both the models for aortic and mitral valve prostheses have a silicone rubber ball occluder with an uncovered stellite alloy cage.
- *valvotomy*—incision into a valve.
    —*mitral valvotomy*—splitting the two commissures (areas of fusion) of the mitral valve to widen its opening.

    *—pulmonary valvotomy—*incising the valve of the pulmonary artery to improve the pulmonary circulation. (8)

- *ventricular aneurysmectomy—*excision of aneurysms, which are nonfunctional areas that weaken the pumping efficiency of the heart. Aneurysms may harbor clots, which can send embolisms to the brain or other vital organs. The procedure may be combined with coronary revascularization using saphenous vein bypass grafts. (41, 130)

Symptomatic Terms

- *anasarca—*massive edema with serous effusion, especially in the right pleural and peritoneal cavities. It occurs in right-sided heart failure and systemic congestion.
- *Aschoff bodies—*nodular lesions of the myocardium, pathognomonic (characteristic) of rheumatic disease.
- *asystole—*cardiac standstill; no contractions of the heart.
- *bradycardia—*slow heart action. (56)
- *cardiac edema—*retention of water and sodium in congestive heart failure due to circulatory impairment.
- *cardiac syncope—*fainting associated with marked sudden decrease in cardiac output. (6)
- *cardiogenic shock—*syndrome related to cardiovascular disease, primarily to myocardial infarction, ventricular failure, severe ventricular arrhythmias, cardiac tamponade, massive pulmonary embolism, and other disorders. The common denominator of shock, irrespective of its cause, is the reduced circulation to the vital organs. It is clinically characterized by mental torpor, reduction of blood pressure and pulse pressure, tachycardia, pallor, cold clammy skin, and signs of congestive heart failure. (1, 68, 124)
- *carotid sinus syncope, vasopressor type—*fainting or clouded consciousness without change in heart rate. It is caused by hyperirritability of the carotid sinus or local disease. (7)
- *coronary risk factors* (see Table 4)—predispose to coronary heart disease (CHD); may or may not be preventable. In addition to the major risk factors tabulated, obesity, a sedentary occupation or lack of physical activity, stress, and competitiveness may lead to heart disease. Oral contraceptives taken over years present a coronary risk, since they adversely affect the lipoprotein metabolism, even after the contraceptive has been discontinued. (38)
- *ischemia—*reduced blood supply to an organ, usually caused by arterial narrowing or occlusion in advanced atherosclerosis.
    *—cerebral ischemia—*local anemia in the brain.
    *—myocardial ischemia—*inadequate blood supply to the heart muscle. (11, 94)
- *murmur—*blowing sound heard on auscultation.
- *palpitation—*subjective awareness of skipping, pounding, or racing heartbeats.
- *postinfarction (Dressler's) syndrome—*develops within the first week or weeks after myocardial infarction. It exhibits the clinical features of a benign form of pericarditis, with or without effusion. (68)
- *sinus rhythm—*normal cardiac rhythm initiated at the sinoatrial node. (56, 139)
- *systole—*rhythmic contractions of the heart, particularly those of the ventricles that pump the blood through the body.
- *tachycardia—*rapid heart action. (56)

Table 4
Coronary Risk Factors of Prime Importance According to Framingham Study*

Risk Factors	Atherogenic Bases	Preventive Aspects
Hyperlipidemia genetic defect	Familial predisposition to hyperlipidemia due to genetic defect	Intake low in cholesterol and saturated fat
Diet induced	High dietary intake of cholesterol and saturated fatty acids	Therapeutic diet rich in polyunsaturated fats and low in cholesterol
Hypertension	Increased peripheral resistance due to vasoconstriction	Reduction of blood pressure by appropriate hypotensive drugs
	If diastolic pressure is greater than 105 mm Hg, coronary risk is four times greater than in normotensive pressure	Life-style conducive to tranquility, and weight loss in obesity
Cigarette smoking	Constriction of coronary arteries by cigarette smokers who inhale nicotine while smoking one or two packs of cigarettes a day	Control of smoking habit over 10-20 years to reduce cardiovascular morbidity and mortality
	Death rate from coronary heart disease 70%-200% higher in smokers than nonsmokers	
Diabetes mellitus	Accelerated process of coronary, cerebral, renal, aortoiliac, and femoropopliteal atherosclerosis in diabetic persons	Careful adherence to treatment regimen to maintain diabetic control
	Wide distribution of microvascular changes in diabetes	

*(3, 37, 38, 92, 130)

Arteries, Capillaries, Veins

Origin of Terms

angi-, angio- (G)—vessel
arterio- (G)—artery
diastole (G)—expansion
hemangio- (G)—blood vessel
phleb-, phlebo- (G)—vein

pulsus (L)—stroke, beat
sclero- (G)—hard
systole (G)—contraction
thrombo- (G)—clot
veno- (L)—vein

Anatomic Terms (Refs. 2, 3, 64, 65, 90)

- *aorta*—the main artery of the trunk.
- *blood pressure:*
    - *systolic*—the force exerted by the blood against the arterial walls at the end of the contraction of the left ventricle.
    - *diastolic*—the force exerted by the blood against the arterial walls at the end of the relaxation of the left ventricle.
- *coats of arteries:*
    - *tunica externa, adventitia*—outer coat.
    - *tunica media*—middle coat.
    - *tunica intima*—inner coat.

Diagnostic Terms

- *acute limb ischemia*—sudden catastrophic interruption of blood flow to an extremity demanding reversal by surgery or clot lysis to save the limb. Vascular disorders such as acute arterial embolization and the deposition of atheromatous plaques associated with bleeding and a relatively rapid thrombus formation precipitate the occlusive event. The limb is waxy, pale, cold, painful, or insensitive to touch and exhibits rigidity or deep muscle tenderness. (46, 130)
- *aneurysm of aorta*—dilatation of a weakened part of the wall of the vessel.
    - *dissecting type*—progressive splitting of the middle coat that may involve the entire circumference of the aorta. When pulsating blood is driven between the media and intima, the tear may rapidly extend the whole length of the aorta, causing excruciating, ripping pain.
    - *fusiform type*—tubular swelling of the walls of the aorta involving the three coats and circumference.
    - *sacculated type*—saclike bulging of a weakened part of the aorta formed by the middle and outer coats. (14, 36, 48, 98, 112)
- *aortic arch syndrome, pulseless disease, Takayasu's syndrome*—group of disorders characterized by occlusion of vessels of the arch of the aorta associated with extremely weak or absent pulses, low blood pressure in upper extremities, and diminished circulation to the brain that may result in neurologic deficit. (14)
- *aortic atresia*—congenital narrowing or absence of the ascending portion of the aorta, usually involving the aortic valve as well. (48, 130)
- *aortic stenosis*—congenital or acquired narrowing of valvar opening into aorta. (14, 73, 119)
- *aortoiliac disease, Leriche's syndrome*—gradual thrombosis of terminal aorta near the bifurcation and extending to the iliac arteries. Claudication and trophic changes may be present. (2, 48)
- *arteriosclerosis*—degenerative, vascular disorder characterized by a thickening and loss of elasticity of arterial walls. It assumes three distinctive morphologic forms:
    - *atherosclerosis*—the most common form, in which an intimal plaque or atheroma is produced by focal lipid deposits. In the beginning the atheroma is soft and pasty. With time the plaque may undergo fibrosis and calcification, or it may ulcerate into the arterial lumen. Ulcerated plaques are prone to cause mural thrombosis and eventually arterial occlusion. Arteriosclerosis and atherosclerosis are frequently used as synonyms.
    - *arteriolosclerosis*—vascular disorder that affects the small arteries and arterioles and seems to be secondary to hypertension.
    - *Mönckeberg's medial calcific sclerosis, medial calcinosis*—vascular disorder in which ringlike calcifications occur in the media of muscular arteries. It is clinically of

little importance, since the medial lesions fail to encroach on the arterial lumen. (2, 3, 12, 130)

- *arteriosclerosis obliterans*—arterial obstruction of extremities, particularly affecting the lower limbs and causing ischemia. (46, 111)
- *carotid occlusive disease*—extracranial and/or intracranial vascular disorder usually caused by atheromatous lesions that obstruct carotid arteries; if progressive, may lead to reduced blood flow in the brain, transient ischemic attacks, cerebrovascular insufficiency, and stroke. (98, 131)
- *coarctation of aorta*—constriction of a segment of the aorta. (23, 108, 112, 123, 130)
- *dilatation of aorta*—abnormal enlargement of the aorta. (112, 121)
- *embolism*—a "throwing in"; blocking of a blood vessel by a clot or other substance brought by the circulating blood. (98)
- *hypertension*—pathologic elevation of the blood pressure. According to the World Health Organization (WHO), the reading consistently exceeds 160/95 mm Hg. (64)
- *hypertensive vascular disease*—sustained high blood pressure associated with cardiovascular, renal, and retinal changes. (64)
- *peripheral arterial insufficiency of extremities*—impaired circulation to the extremities, particularly to the lower limbs. It is characterized by claudication, coldness, pallor, trophic changes, ulceration, and gangrene in the involved extremity. (130)
- *peripheral vascular disease*—any disorder directly affecting the arteries, veins, and lymphatics, except those of the heart. (2, 22, 134)
- *phlebitis*—inflammation of the veins.
- *phlebosclerosis*—hardening of the walls of the veins.
- *Raynaud's disease*—painful vascular disorder characterized by peripheral spasms of the digital arterioles of the fingers and toes, which may result in gangrene. (21, 134)
- *rupture of an aneurysm*—break in the weakened vascular wall of an aneurysm, associated with hemorrhage. (48)
- *subclavian steal syndrome*—a symptom complex of cerebrovascular insufficiency, usually due to segmental atheromatous occlusion of the subclavian artery proximal to the vertebral artery. Since the circulation through the vertebral artery is reversed, the subclavian is said to "steal" cerebral blood. A delay in the arrival time of the radial pulse on the affected side is diagnostic of reversed vertebral artery flow. A localized murmur and a difference in brachial blood pressure are common manifestations. The patient may experience dizziness, vertigo, light-headedness, tinnitus, blurred vision, headache, and ataxia. (48, 54, 113)
- *superior vena cava syndrome*—obstruction of the superior vena cava, clinically recognized by numerous collateral veins distributed over the anterior chest, dilated neck veins, edema, and cyanosis of the upper body. In a Mayo Clinic report, 78 percent of these syndromes were caused by malignancies, and 22 percent by benign conditions, such as thrombosis of superior vena cava or clot formation around central venous catheters. (69, 87)
- *thoracic outlet syndromes*—neurovascular compression syndromes affecting the structures of the thoracic outlet. Offending lesions are detected by angiography. Included are:
    - *cervical rib and scalenus anticus syndrome*—cutoff or torsion of subclavian artery may be present.
    - *scalenus anticus and pectoralis minor syndrome*—cutoff or torsion of subclavian artery and compression or thrombosis of axillary veins may be demonstrated by angiography.
    - *scalenus anticus syndrome and tightness of costoclavicular space*—a ridgelike compression of subclavian artery and venous compression or thrombosis may produce the syndrome. (102, 111, 120)

- *thromboangiitis obliterans, Buerger's disease*—inflammatory, obstructive disease involving primarily the peripheral blood vessels of the lower extremities. (2, 46, 82, 111, 115)
- *thrombophlebitis*—inflammatory reaction of the walls of veins to infection, associated with intravascular clotting. (46)
- *thrombosis*—formation of blood clots in a blood vessel, leading to circulatory obstruction. (98, 111)
- *varicose veins, varicosity*—condition of having distended and tortuous veins, most commonly present in lower extremities. (111, 115)
- *vascular injuries:*
  - —*aortic lacerations*—tears of the aorta occur most frequently at the aortic isthmus, the weakest part of the aorta, and less frequently in the ascending or descending aorta. Traumatic transection of the aorta may be followed by dissection of the entire vessel. (18, 130)
    - —*brachiocephalic lacerations*—these injuries are frequently associated with aortic lacerations, and if multiple and severe, they are life threatening. (18, 130)

Operative Terms

- *anastomosis of blood vessels*—end-to-end union of two different blood vessels or two segments of the same blood vessels after excision of a lesion. (130)
- *aneurysmectomy*—removal of an aneurysm. (36)
- *aneurysm, resection of*—excision of aneurysm and repair of arterial defect by insertion of homograft or prosthesis. (41, 48)
- *aortic aneurysm resection, abdominal*—clamping of aorta and iliac arteries, opening of the aneurysm, removal of thrombus, and reconstruction by means of a preclotted, knitted Dacron graft. (48, 81, 130)
- *abdominal aortic aneurysm wrapping*—suture placement of a Dacron mesh graft across the anterior aspect of the abdominal aneurysm and fitted around the surrounding vessels in order to give the aneurysm firm graft support. The procedure is recommended for poor-risk patients, calcified aneurysms, or aneurysms extending above the renal arteries, and as prophylaxis for small aneurysms. (44)
- *aortofemoral bypass grafting*—procedure of choice for aortoiliac occlusive (Leriche) disease, consisting of appropriate vascular clamping and graft anastomoses, usually end-to-side, below, and above the obstructed segments to bypass circulatory occlusions. The formation of collateral vessels may maintain the circulation in graft failure. (2, 22, 130)
- *aortoiliac replacement grafting*—excision of occluded segments of the aorta and iliac arteries followed by graft replacement. Graft failure is life threatening. (129)
- *arterial homograft*—arteries obtained at autopsies under aseptic technique and preserved by freezing, dry freezing, or using chemicals in a blood vessel bank. They are used for replacing the excised segments of an artery. (22)
- *bypass graft, autogenous*—implantation of an autograft, usually a segment of a saphenous vein to bypass a vascular obstruction such as occlusive lesions of the coronary, femoropopliteal, or carotid-subclavian arteries. The occluded vascular segment is left in place. Circulatory efficiency is usually restored. (22, 46)
- *carotid endarterectomy*—removal of the inner coat (intima) of the carotid artery for occlusive vascular disease. The integrity of the procedure may be evaluated intraoperatively by means of a sterile Doppler probe, real-time B-mode ultrasonography, or operative arteriogram. (2, 22, 46, 98, 103)
- *coarctation of the aorta repair:*
  - —*subclavian flap angioplasty*—suture ligation of the ductus arteriosus followed by the subclavian flap being sutured to the aortic incision.

   *—resection of the coarctation and end-to-end anastomosis—*dissection of the coarctation followed by aorta-to-aorta anastomosis.

   *—resection with insertion of Dacron prosthesis—*dissection of the coarctation followed by insertion of tubular woven Dacron prosthesis. Preclotting of the woven prosthesis is beneficial in preventing bleeding from the cloth interstices. This approach is used where the coarctation is too long for a primary anastomosis to be performed.

   *—aortoplasty with Dacron patch—*resection of the coarctation and application of a diamond-shaped Dacron patch sutured to the aorta. This procedure may be especially appropriate in older patients who have undergone sclerotic changes of the aorta, where it would be hazardous to perform an end-to-end anastomosis.

   *—Vosschulte aortoplasty—*procedure involves a lateral incision across the area of narrowing followed by a transverse suture closure. This approach is best used in patients where the coarctation involves only a lateral shelf and the proximal and distal ends of the aorta are in close proximity.

   *—insertion of Dacron prosthesis—*approach avoids further resection of stenotic area resulting from previous resection and end-to-end anastomosis.* (123)

- *embolectomy—*emboli may be excised directly or removed by retrograde method via femoral arteries by balloon catheter. With balloon deflated, Fogarty catheter is inserted into the vein where the embolus is located. When in proper position, the balloon is inflated. By withdrawing the catheter, the clot is pulled through the incision to the body surface. (2, 48, 67)

- *femoropopliteal arterial reconstruction—*bypass surgery for restoring the circulation in femoral artery occlusion. The obstruction is bypassed using a autogenous saphenous vein, a bioprosthesis such as an umbilical vein, or an inert prosthesis (Dacron or expanded polytetrafluoroethylene [PTFE]). (22, 103, 130)

- *femorotibial bypass grating—*graft from femoral or posterior or anterior tibial or peroneal artery to bypass the obstructed arterial segment. (22, 103, 130)

- *phleborrhapy—*suture of a vein.

- *phlebotomy—*opening of a vein; for example, to reduce high red count in polycythemia vera by bloodletting.

- *profundaplasty, profundoplasty—*reconstruction of the profunda femoris artery enabling relief of intermittent claudication; also may affect limb salvage. (22, 116)

- *shunt for portal hypertension—*method of diverting a large volume of blood from the hypertensive portal system into the normal systemic venous circulation. This operation prevents hemorrhages from esophageal varices which result from portal hypertension. (69) (See Chapter 8.)

- *subclavian steal syndrome operations:*

   *—axillo-axillary bypass graft—*passing the graft subcutaneously in the anterior chest wall with end-to-side anastomosis of the graft to each axillary artery.

   *—carotid-subclavian anastomosis—*joining the carotid and subclavian arteries to improve cerebral blood flow.

   *—carotid-subclavian bypass graft—*implanting an autograft in carotid and subclavian arteries to bypass the occluded segment of the subclavian artery.

   *—subclavian-subclavian bypass—*inserting a knitted, preclotted Dacron graft and anastomosing one end of the graft with the right and the other end with the left subclavian artery, thus creating a crossover bypass of the occluded arterial segment. (48, 54, 130)

---

*John A. Waldhausen and David B. Campbell. Repair of coarctation of the aorta. In Stuart W. Jamieson and Norman E. Shumway, eds., *Cardiac Surgery,* 4th ed. St. Louis: The C.V. Mosby Co., 1986, pp. 371-380. Reprinted with permission.

- *thrombectomy*—removal of a thrombus; for example, from an occluded portal vein. (130)
- *thromboendarterectomy (TEA)*—initial arteriotomy followed by stripping of the diseased intima and subsequent closure of the vessel. Saphenous vein or Dacron patches may be used to prevent narrowing of the lumen following TEA. (22, 130)
- *vein stripping*—surgical procedure to relieve varicosity.
- *venesection*—incision into a vein. (126)

Symptomatic Terms

- *acrocyanosis*—bluish discoloration of fingertips and toes. (46, 111)
- *angiospasm, vasospasm*—involuntary contractions of the muscular coats of blood vessels; spasm of blood vessels. (2, 22)
- *claudication:*
  - *lower extremity claudication*—limping caused by inadequate blood supply and associated with cramping pains in the calf muscles. It is usually relieved by rest and thus is intermittent.
  - *upper extremity claudication, brachial claudication*—inadequate blood supply to an arm causing intermittent or persistent cramping pain. (2, 130, 134)
- *extravasation*—escape of fluid (serum, lymph, blood) into the adjacent tissues.
- *digital*—referring to fingers and toes.
- *digital blanching*—fingers and toes becoming pallid as a result of vasospasm of digital arterioles; seen in Raynaud's disease. (6, 71, 134)
- *ischemia*—local anemia of an organ or part resulting from circulatory obstruction or vasospasm.
- *paroxysmal digital cyanosis*—attacks of cyanosis caused by the interruption of blood flow in palmar and plantar arteries. (6, 7)
- *pedal circulation*—circulation in the foot.
- *pulse*—contractions of an artery that can be felt by a finger.
  - *bigeminal pulse*—coupled beats. (7, 139)
  - *Corrigan's or water-hammer pulse*—strong, jerky beat followed by a sharp decline and collapse of beat. (7)
  - *dicrotic pulse*—arterial beat with weak secondary wave that may be mistaken for two beats. (7)
- *pulse deficit*—difference between apical heart rate and radial pulse rate, found in cardiac disease.
- *shock*—complex syndrome affecting the various body systems, resulting from the inability of cells to metabolize oxygen and needed substrates normally. Classification according to
  - *etiology:*
    - *cardiogenic shock*—phenomenon caused by decreased cardiac output, as in acute myocardial infarction, serious injury or cardiac surgery, ventricular arrhythmias, and ventricular failure.
    - *hypovolemic shock*—syndrome caused by markedly decreased blood volume.
    - *septic shock*—serious state resulting from infections, septicemia, or bacteremia.
    - *other kinds.*
  - *onset:*
    - *early shock*—initial arteriolar or venous constriction, accelerated contractability of the heart, hyperventilation, and other effects.
    - *late shock*—life-threatening impairment of cellular metabolism causing advanced hypovolemia, intravascular clotting, and respiratory failure. (1, 124, 129)

- *vasoconstriction*—a narrowing of the vascular lumen, resulting in decreased blood supply. (31)
- *vasodepression*—collapse caused by vasomotor depression.
- *vasodilatation*—widening of the vascular lumen, increasing the blood supply to a part. (105)
- *vasomotor*—referring to nerves that control the muscular contractions of blood vessels.

Special Procedures

Terms Related to Diagnostic and Therapeutic Procedures

- *actuarial method*—statistical calculation, especially of life expectancy.
- *antistreptolysin-O titer*—diagnostic aid for rheumatic fever that may be used as a screening test in statewide programs. (109)
- *atherogenic index (pl. indices)*—determination of serum lipoproteins by ultracentrifugal analysis used as a possible aid in the detection of factors causing atherosclerosis. (39, 79)
- *automatic implantable cardioverter defibrillator (AICD)*—therapeutic modality designed to detect and cardiovert ventricular tachycardia, as well as providing defibrillation. The AICD is used for individuals who have sustained a life-threatening episode of ventricular tachyarrhythmia or cardiac arrest not associated with acute myocardial infarction. (4, 59)
- *automatic implantable defibrillator (AID)*—therapeutic modality designed to protect high-risk patients from sudden death. The device is capable of monitoring the heart rhythm, detecting ventricular tachycardias, especially fibrillation, and delivering discharges that automatically convert arrhythmia to sinus rhythm. (4, 59)
- *cardiac index*—cardiac output in relation to body size, useful in assessing the cardiovascular status, particularly after open heart surgery. (4, 137)
- *cardiac monitor*—electronic device applied to a patient that reveals the electric activity of the heart by visual and auditory signals and thereby permits the immediate detection of dangerous arrhythmias. (4, 137)
- *cardiac pacing, physiologic*—a normal response to myocardial stimulation initiated at the sinoatrial node, followed by atrial contractions, activation of the atrioventricular node, spread of the impulse through the bundle of His, and subsequent contractions of the ventricles. (137)
- *cardiac pacing, electronic*—substitution of normal cardiac pacing in Stokes-Adams syndrome, ventricular standstill, certain dysrhythmias such as tachyarrhythmias, and in myocardial infarction.
    —*pacemakers in use:*
    —*external cardiac pacemaker*—electronic device for stimulating the ventricles through the closed chest wall in cardiac standstill.
    —*implantable cardiac pacemaker for temporary or permanent use*—electronic device that achieves myocardial stimulation by epicardial or endocardial and unipolar or bipolar electrodes. Recent technical improvements are the reduced size of the pulse generator and a prolonged pacemaker life. (60, 107, 137)
    —*types of pacing:*
    —*demand pacing*—impulse is fired by pacemaker according to patient's need. If QRS complex fails to occur within a given period, pacing impulse is triggered. If QRS complex develops within a certain interval, pacing impulse is withheld. (52, 107, 140)

—*fixed-rate pacing*—impulse is generated at a predetermined rate, irrespective of intrinsic cardiac rhythm. (107)

—*synchronized pacing*—impulse is fired synchronously with the P wave of the patient. One electrode is placed in the atrium, the other in the ventricle. Since the atria are stimulated to pour their entire contents into both ventricles, cardiac function is almost normal and synchronous. A drawback is that a thoracotomy may be needed for a stable epicardial insertion of the atrial electrode. (60, 140)

—*methods of pacing:*

—*epicardial pacing*—asynchronous or synchronous pacing in response to impulses of electrodes firmly attached to the epicardium and to a pulse generator concealed in a subcutaneous pocket.

—*transthoracic pacing*—ventricular stimulation achieved by electrodes inserted through the chest wall into the ventricle. A battery-powered pacer serves as a power source. Since pacing can be quickly initiated, transthoracic pacing is an effective emergency measure for resuscitating patients in cardiac arrest.

—*transvenous pacing*—electrode catheter is introduced into the heart through the jugular or other suitable vein, and its tip is lodged in the right ventricular apex; the battery case is located in a subcutaneous pouch below the clavicle. The rate is fixed, usually 75 impulses per minute. No thoracotomy is required. Transvenous pacing may be used temporarily for myocardial stimulation to control bradycardia and prevent ventricular standstill. (4, 52, 130, 140)

- *cardiopulmonary bypass*—mechanism for diverting the blood around the heart and lungs for the purpose of providing inflow occlusion to the heart. This enables the surgeon to operate on a bloodless heart muscle under direct vision. (32, 63, 100)

- *cardiopulmonary resuscitation*—heart-lung revival achieved by establishing a patent airway and restoring respiratory and circulatory functions by drugs, electric myocardial stimulation, or closed or open chest cardiac compression. (130)

- *cardioversion*—direct current (DC) countershock applied to the chest to convert abnormal rhythms to normal sinus rhythm. (4, 28, 53, 107, 128, 130)

- *central venous pressure (CVP)*—measurement of pressure within the superior vena cava reflecting the pressure of the right atrium and expressed in centimeters of water pressure. CVP provides some index of the adequacy of the pumping action of the heart and of the blood volume in the vessels.

—*Reference values*—usually CVP: 5 to 8 centimeters of water pressure.

—*Increase*—indicative of overload of the right heart in congestive heart failure.

—*Decrease*—suggestive of reduced blood volume and need for fluid replacement. (93)

- *cold cardioplegia*—hypothermic elective cardiac arrest for myocardial protection in patients undergoing intracardiac surgery. Its disadvantage is uneven cooling, since obstructed arterial lesions of the heart are distinctly less cooled. (32, 96, 112)

- *coronary artery perfusion*—introduction of blood into the coronary arteries by catheters during procedures in which the root of the aorta is opened. (11, 130)

- *counterpulsation*—method of supporting the failing myocardium by removing arterial blood during the ejection of the ventricles and returning it to the circulation during diastole. (89)

- *countershock*—use of an external electronic defibrillator to terminate the disorderly electric activity within the heart that provokes the arrhythmia. In ventricular fibrillation, a brief high-voltage shock abruptly stops the chaotic twitching of the ventricular muscle fibers. If effective, the natural cardiac pacemaker regains control and restores normal contractions. (28)

- *defibrillator*—mechanical device for applying electric shock to the closed chest or to the open heart to terminate abnormal cardiac rhythms. (4, 28, 53)
- *diastolic augmentation procedure*—circulatory assistive technique in which a balloon, placed in the aorta, is inflated during diastole and collapsed during systole (phase-shift). This reduces the pressure against which the heart pumps, yet increases diastolic pressure and thus favorably influences coronary flow. (130)
- *direct-current defibrillation*—countershock by a capacitator discharge defibrillator (DC type) instead of the alternating current of the original type of defibrillator (AC type). (4, 53)
- *Doppler blood flowmetry*—modality that utilizes ultrasonic signals permitting transcutaneous auscultation of blood flow. Evaluation of the signal at various levels on the leg and thigh can assist in locating a lesion. (22, 130)
- *elective cardiac arrest, cold anoxic arrest*—standstill of the heart induced by cross-clamping the aorta and by cardiac cooling. The temperature may be lowered by perfusing the coronary arteries with a cold solution, instilling a coolant into the pericardial sac, or applying ice to the myocardium. Cold anoxic arrest provides a motionless, dry operative field conducive to aortic valve surgery and repair of congenital defects. It is the same as cold cardioplegia. (130)
- *exhaled-air ventilation*—artificial respiration using the mouth-to-mouth, mouth-to-nose, or mouth-to-tracheal-stoma method to restore ventilatory lung function. (130)
- *external arteriovenous (AV) shunt*—procedure used to facilitate access to the patient's circulation by cannulation of blood vessels for prolonged hemodialysis. One piece of Silestic tubing is inserted into an artery, the other into an adjacent vein. They are then brought on top of the skin and connected with each other by a removable Teflon connector. (63, 130)
- *external cardiac compression*—the application of rhythmic pressure (60 times per minute) over the lower sternum to compress the heart and produce artificial circulation. (130)
- *extracorporeal circulation*—blood circulating outside of the body, a form of cardiopulmonary bypass. It may be achieved by using a heart-lung machine. (130)
- *heart-lung machine*—apparatus used to substitute for cardiopulmonary function. It permits a direct-vision approach to cardiac lesions requiring corrective surgery. Venous blood returning to the heart is not allowed to enter the right atrium but is sucked away by two tubes, one in each of the main veins. It is then pumped into an artificial lung. Then the oxygen-laden blood enters a reservoir, passes through filters, and is pumped to the patient's arterial system. Many different types of heart-lung machines are now in use. (63, 130)
- *hemodilution*—reduction of normal red cell mass of the blood and its subsequent oxygen content. It may be caused by injury, hemorrhage, or blood dyscrasias, or may be therapeutically used, as in cardiovascular surgery to prime the pump oxygenator systems.
    - —*extreme hemodilution*—total washout achieved by removing most of the blood and replacing it with colloid electrolyte solution that maintains a normal circulating volume and a colloid osmotic pressure of plasma.
    - —*moderate hemodilution*—induced dilution of the normal blood that keeps the volume of the packed red cells (VPRC) greater than 20 percent. It may be used as a primer in cardiopulmonary bypass and in treating shock, polycythemia, and high-viscosity disorders. (32)
- *induced hypothermia*—artificial reduction of the body temperature in an effort to lower the metabolic requirements of the patient, who is then better able to tolerate the interruption of cardiac inflow.

- *intra-aortic balloon counterpulsation*—method of circulatory assistance for left ventricular power failure and cardiogenic shock refractory to adrenergic stimulation. A balloon catheter is inserted in the femoral artery and advanced to the descending thoracic aorta. Circulatory assistance is provided by diastolic counterpulsation, which is monitored by electrocardiographic recordings. Similar procedures have gained wide acceptance. (11, 13, 89, 124)
- *medical electronics*—the use of electronics in medical areas. Electronics refers to the action of charged electric particles in any medium: solid, liquid, or gas.
- *normothermia*—the environmental temperature that maintains body temperature and metabolic requirements at normal levels. (138)
- *oscillation*—movement to and fro.
- *oscillometer*—instrument for measuring any kind of oscillations; for example, those related to blood pressure.
- *oxymetry*—measuring the amount of oxygen in blood by one of a variety of techniques. (130)
- *percutaneous angiographic embolization*—deliberate therapeutic occlusion of a blood vessel by injecting an embolic pharmaceutical agent through an angiographic catheter
    - —to control acute or recurrent bleeding
    - —to close an atriovenous fistula
    - —to occlude an atriovenous malformation *or*
    - —to devascularize bone, kidney, or other tumors. (130)
- *percutaneous transluminal angioplasty*—nonoperative procedure used to dilate a stenosed artery by introducing a double-lumen balloon catheter (usually Grüntzig type) with the balloon deflated into the stenosed artery. After the catheter has crossed the stenotic lesion, the balloon is inflated to enlarge the arterial lumen and the deflated catheter is withdrawn. The procedure has been used to relieve angina pectoris caused by single high-grade coronary artery stenosis and ischemic atherosclerotic disease in the basilar, iliac, or femoral arteries. It is an effective method of treating renovascular hypertension due to renal artery stenosis. (34, 45, 94, 108, 115)
- *perfusion in intracardiac surgery*—method of providing oxygenated blood to the body by a heart-lung machine while interrupting the circulation through the heart. (32, 63)
- *precordial shock*—electric treatment of arrhythmias.
    - —elective procedure for converting certain tachyarrhythmias to normal rhythm. It is known as cardioversion.
    - —emergency procedure for controlling ventricular fibrillation. It is usually referred to as defibrillation. (108)
- *pulmonary artery balloon counterpulsation*—counterpulsation applied to the pulmonary circuit to improve blood flow to the lungs and relieve ventricular failure. (89)
- *pulmonary wedge pressure (PWP)*—measurement of filling pressure of the left heart using an open-ended catheter wedged into a small pulmonary artery. A Swan-Ganz catheter is one such device. The procedure aids in differentiating congestive heart failure, allergic drug response, and fat embolism. (93, 130)
- *sphygmomanometer*—instrument for measuring blood pressure. (65)
- *stethoscope*—instrument for listening to sounds within the body.
- *Swan-Ganz pulmonary artery catheterization*—insertion of balloon-tipped catheter by peripheral venipuncture to catheterize the pulmonary artery and achieve hemodynamic monitoring of critically ill patients. (129)
- *synchronized direct current (DC) countershock*—electric shock producing cardioversion by the use of a synchronized capacitator. DC is the method of choice in converting chronic atrial flutter or fibrillation to normal sinus rhythm. (108)

- *transducer, medical use*—transforms energy into electric signals for monitoring physiologic functions such as blood pressure. (130)
- *treadmill exercise tolerance*—stress test for evaluating the ability of the coronary circulation to meet the metabolic demands of an increasing exercise load. The patient is subjected to graded exercise on the treadmill or bicycle ergometer until the electrocardiogram shows ischemic changes. (26, 97, 117)
- *two-step exercise test, Master's test*—exercise test of coronary reserve. Within 1½ minutes the patient goes up and down 2 steps, 9 inches high, 15 to 25 times. A postexercise electrocardiogram is taken immediately. If it is negative, a 3-minute double two-step test is performed. As soon as the patient experiences pain the exercise is discontinued. (26, 97)
- *Valsalva maneuver*—effective treatment for paroxysmal atrial tachycardia and similar disorders. The patient is instructed to inhale deeply, hold his breath, and then strain down forcefully while slowly counting for 10 seconds. The Valsalva maneuver is also used as a test for cardiac reserve. (7, 77, 104)

Terms Related to Cardiac Catheterization and Coronary Artery Catheterization

- *cardiac catheterization, right side*—a procedure of diagnostic value in detecting various cardiac defects and diseases. A radiopaque cardiac catheter is inserted into an accessible vein and passed into the heart and pulmonary artery. Various techniques may be employed. If the basilic or the cephalic vein is used as a starting point, the catheter passes through the innominate vein and superior vena cava into the right atrium, right ventricle, and pulmonary artery. If the saphenous vein is used, the catheter enters the heart through the inferior vena cava and traces its course through the cardiac chambers and pulmonary artery. Oxygen saturation of the blood in the chambers and the pressure recorded inside determine the defect within the heart, if present. Different indicator techniques aid in the detection and quantitation of shunts. Oxygen data or dye curves may be used for calculation of cardiac output. Although right cardiac catheterization is of great diagnostic value in certain heart lesions, it is incomplete if cineangiography does not accompany the hemodynamic data. (20, 30, 72)
- *cardiac catheterization, left side*—obtaining pressures and blood samples in the left side of the heart can be accomplished in several ways:
  - *catheterization of the left atrium:*
    - *suprasternal or Radner method*—inserting a needle behind the suprasternal notch and directing it downward into the left atrium. The pulmonary artery, aorta, and left ventricle can be entered by the same method.
    - *transseptal or Ross method*—inserting a long needle through a catheter up to the right atrium and then pushing the needle out the catheter and puncturing the atrial septum at the foramen ovale.
      Modifications of this method are:
      Brockenbrough technique—the cardiac catheter itself is slipped over the needle into the left atrium following transseptal puncture with the needle in the catheter.
      Shirey technique—the cardiac catheter is passed in a retrograde manner through the brachial artery cutdown into the aorta, left ventricle, and left atrium.
      In the Radner method, only the pressures may be recorded; in the Brockenbrough or Shirey technique, cineangiograms may be obtained by injection of opaque media through the catheter.
  - *cardiac catheterization of left ventricle:*

–direct puncture of left ventricle—use of a small-gauge needle either through the apex (Brock technique) or through the subxiphoid approach (Lehman technique).

–retrograde method—femoral or arm approach using a percutaneous or cutdown technique, respectively. (20, 30, 72)

- *cardiac pressures*—pressures created by the force of the contraction within the heart chambers on the circulating blood. (20, 30, 72)
- *hemodynamics*—a study of blood circulation and blood pressure. (20, 30, 72)
- *oscilloscope*—an instrument for displaying electric signals, such as those made by blood pressure, electrocardiogram, heart sounds, or other signals, on a cathode-ray tube monitoring screen.
- *selective catheterization of the coronary arteries:*

    —*Judkins' technique*—technique uses percutaneous puncture of femoral artery and introduction of three differently shaped catheters in succession for catheterization of left and right coronary arteries and left ventricular cineangiography.

    Under fluoroscopic or television guidance a catheter is introduced into the common femoral artery and advanced via the aortic arch to the coronary orifice. Catheter manipulation differs for selective left and right coronary artery catheterization. Following contrast injection, rapid direct serial radiography and cinephotofluorography provide coronary visualization, thereby revealing the presence and extent of occlusive arterial heart disease. (20, 30, 47, 72)

    —*Sones' technique*—technique uses approach through the brachial artery following a cutdown. A single catheter is inserted for the catheterization of both coronary arteries and left ventricular cineangiography. Selective catheterization of the coronary arteries is done according to an accepted technique:

    –to assess the potential need for heart surgery in angina pectoris.

    –to evaluate operative results such as: the extent of revascularization following the Vineberg procedure.

    –the patency of aortocoronary saphenous vein grafts or internal mammary artery grafts following bypass surgery.

    –to detect progression of coronary atherosclerotic heart disease leading to graft closure. (20, 30, 47, 72)

Terms Related to Special Recordings of Heart Action

- *apexcardiogram (ACG)*—recording low-frequency vibrations of the precordium when a transducer is placed against the chest wall. The graphic record of the movements reflects the apex beat of the heart. (7, 16)
- *ballistocardiography*—electrographic recording of body movements during the cardiac cycle. (66)
- *bipolar lead*—lead with two electrodes, one negative and one positive. (60)
- *electrocardiogram computer analysis*—a program for processing electrocardiograms automatically according to the revised IBM Bonner-2 (V2MO) computer analysis program. (16)
- *electrocardiography (ECG)*—graphic recording of the electric waves of the cardiac cycle or spread of excitation throughout the heart. It is an invaluable diagnostic aid in the detection of arrhythmias and myocardial damage. (See Fig. 38 for electrocardiographic cycle.) (16)

    —*P wave*—reflects the contraction of the atria.

    —*PR interval*—period in which the impulse passes through the atria and AV node, normally 0.16 to 0.20 seconds.

    —*QRS complex*—waves represent ventricular excitation or depolarization of the ventricular myocardium, normally 0.12 seconds.

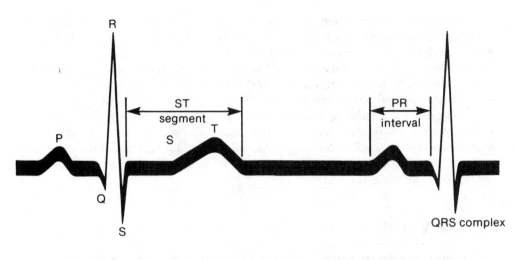

Figure 38 Normal electrocardiographic cycle.

—*Q wave*—downward deflection and beginning of the complex.
—*R wave*—large upward wave.
—*S wave*—second large downward deflection and end of the QRS complex.
—*ST segment*—the interval between the completion of depolarization and recovery of ventricular muscle fibers. The segment may be depressed or elevated in myocardial injury.
—*T wave*—recovery phase following the contraction. Inversion of the T wave usually reflects injury or ischemia of the heart muscle. (19)

- *electrocardiography (ECG)*—techniques:
  —*ambulatory electrographic (Holter) monitoring*—continuous ECG recording of an ambulatory high-risk patient for early assessment and treatment of cardiac ischemia and ventricular arrhythmias or evaluation of response to activity or artificial pacemaker. (136, 137)
  —*His bundle electrography (HBE)*—combined atrial and ventricular ECG, showing the spread of the electric current throughout the heart muscle and separating conduction into two distinct subdivisions:
  –*PH interval*—onset of P wave to His bundle activation or conduction time through both atria.
  –*HR interval*—His bundle activation to onset of QRS complex, termed ventricular activation.
  –*intracardiac electrography (IE)*—adjunct to standard surface ECG using recordings by electrode catheters, percutaneously introduced into the heart via femoral or other suitable veins to assess arrhythmias and conduction disturbances. (19, 24, 25, 27, 66, 137)
- *electrokymography*—recording of the movements of the heart and great vessels by an electrokymograph. (130)
- *kinetocardiography, precordial cardiography*—a method of recording vibrations of the chest wall produced by heart action. (15, 16)
- *phonocardiography*—graphic recording of heart sounds, usually on an oscilloscope for quick scanning, or on a tape recorder for a permanent record. (16)
- *phonocardiography, intracardiac*—sound tracing recorded from within the cardiac chambers through a phonocatheter that has a microphone at the tip. Method seeks to detect minor defects not revealed by cardiac catheterization. (16)

- *plethysmography*—instrumental recording of variations in size of a part or organ caused by fluctuations in the size of the vascular bed. (110)
- *pulse analysis*—use of a special transducer for recording of:
  - —*carotid pulse*—an initial abrupt rise corresponding to the opening of the aortic valve, subsequent brief tidal wave and decline with closing of the aortic valve, and a gradual return to the baseline.
  - —*jugular venous pulse*—accurate reflection of right atrial activity, recording waves of atrial systole, the filling of the right ventricle, and tricuspid function. (65)
- *vectorcardiography*—graphic recording of the direction and magnitude of the instantaneous electric forces of the heart from a cathode-ray tube. A Polaroid photographic camera is frequently used. (19)

Abbreviations

ABE—acute bacterial endocarditis
ACG—angiocardiography; apex cardiogram
AHA—American Heart Association
AMI—acute myocardial infarction
AS—aortic stenosis
ASD—atrial septal defect
ASHD—arteriosclerotic heart disease
ASO—arteriosclerosis obliterans
AV—atrioventricular; arteriovenous
BBB—bundle branch block
BP—blood pressure
CCA—circumflex coronary artery
CCCR—closed chest cardiopulmonary resuscitation
CCU—coronary care unit
CP—cardiopulmonary
CVA—cerebrovascular accident
CVD—cardiovascular disease
CVP—central venous pressure
DCC—direct current cardioversion
DM—diastolic murmur
ECG—electrocardiogram
EKG—electrocardiogram
ESR—erythrocyte sedimentation rate
HBE—His bundle electrocardiogram
Hg—mercury
HLR—heart-lung resuscitation
HVD—hypertensive vascular disease
IABP—intra-aortic balloon pump
IACP—intra-aortic counterpulsation
IASD—interatrial septal defect
IMAG—internal mammary artery graft
IVC—inferior vena cava
IVSD—interventricular septal defect
JVP—jugular venous pulse
LA—left atrium

LAD—left anterior descending (coronary artery)
LHF—left-sided heart failure
LV—left ventricle
LVH—left ventricular hypertrophy
M—murmur
MI—myocardial infarction
mm Hg—millimeter of mercury
MS—mitral stenosis
PA—pulmonary artery
PAC—premature atrial contractions
PAT—paroxysmal atrial tachycardia
PDA—patent ductus arteriosus
PPS—postperfusion syndrome
PVC—premature ventricular contractions
PWP—pulmonary wedge pressure
RA—right atrium
RCA—right coronary artery
RF—rheumatic fever
RHF—right-sided heart failure
RV—right ventricle
RVH—right ventricular hypertrophy
SA—sinoatrial (node)
SBE—subacute bacterial endocarditis
SR—sedimentation rate
SVC—superior vena cava
SVG—saphenous vein graft
TES—treadmill exercise score
TGA—transposition of great arteries
TIA—transient ischemic attack
VC—vena cava
VCG—vectorcardiogram
VHD—valvar (valvular) heart disease
VSD—ventricular septal defect
WPW—Wolff-Parkinson-White (syndrome)

Oral Reading Practice

Coarctation of the Aorta

Coarctation of the aorta, genetically identified as a **chromosomal abnormality,** is one of the most interesting congenital defects amenable to surgery. It consists of a constriction of a segment of the aorta and occurs in two types. The first type is a rare condition in which the aortic obstruction is located proximal to the **ductus arteriosus.** The **lumen** of the aorta is atretic or completely blocked, so that the impairment of the systemic circulation presents a serious problem. This defect is incompatible with life, and the child dies in infancy if corrective surgery cannot be performed.

The other type of coarctation is a common form that yields to surgical intervention. There may be either a narrowing or a complete **stenosis of the aortic lumen** distal to the left subclavian artery and to the insertion of the ductus. The latter is generally **ligamentous** and **obliterated.** The aorta near the constriction appears to be normal in size, but its major proximate branches are generally enlarged. The **intercostal arteries** distal to the obstruction also show an increase in size. The constriction of the aorta is usually limited to a short segment and permits a reasonable life expectancy, if not associated with other cardiovascular defects.

The outstanding diagnostic characteristic of aortic coarctation is high blood pressure in the arms and low blood pressure with a barely perceptible pulse in the legs. The differential diagnosis hinges on this disparity of the blood pressure in the extremities and the diminished or absent **femoral** pulse. Since the oxygenated blood reaches the systemic circulation, the patient's color remains normal. Hypertension may lead to **cerebrovascular accident.** In addition, infection presents a constant threat to the **debilitated** patient, since nutritional deficiency may accompany the impoverished systemic circulation.

When a short aortic segment is constricted, the clinical symptoms are absent or so minimal that they may escape notice, especially in childhood. In adolescence, symptoms of **fatigability,** decreased exercise tolerance, **epistaxis, syncope,** and coldness of the feet tend to develop and cause varying degrees of disability. In untreated cases the life span rarely exceeds the fourth decade. Death may ensue from **rupture** of the aorta, **bacterial endocarditis,** or **congestive heart failure.**

The optimal age for surgical correction is usually within the second decade of life. It is during this period that the aorta has a high degree of elasticity, works with facility, shows little or no evidence of **degenerative** changes, and is in good condition for making a sizable **anastomosis.**

The surgical procedure consists of the removal of the constricted region and an end-to-end anastomosis of the aortic segments. Where no surgical communication of the aortic segments can be created, the left subclavian artery may be joined to the descending aorta. Suitable bypass grafts may be implanted for complex or recurrent coarctations of the aorta.

Postoperatively, progress is spectacular. The blood pressure in upper and lower extremities equalizes, the femoral artery pulsation is present almost immediately, and the circulation is markedly improved. The most dreaded complications are infection of the suture line, resulting in leakage, or dissolution of the anastomosis. (23, 108, 112, 123, 130)

Table 5

Some Cardiovascular Conditions Amenable to Surgery

Organs Involved	Diagnosis	Type of Surgery	Operative Procedures
Heart Pulmonary artery Aorta	Patent ductus arteriosus	Complete division of ductus arteriosus	Obliteration of ductus by dividing ductus and suturing the cut ends
Heart Pulmonary artery Aorta	Complete trans-position of pulmonary artery and of aorta	Blalock-Hanlon operation Closed heart surgery	Right thoracotomy and exposure of interatrial groove Occlusion of vessels, application of Satinsky-type clamp, section of both atria Removal of segment and portion of septum
Heart Atria Septum	Interatrial septal defect	Repair of interatrial septal defect Open method under direct vision	Interatrial septal defect closed by direct suture or patch Extracorporeal circulation
Heart Ventricles Septum	Congenital heart disease Interventricular septal defect with pulmonary hypertension	Banding of pulmonary artery	Pulmonary artery constricted with umbilical tape in instances where direct closure is contraindicated
Heart Ventricles Septum	Interventricular septal defect	Open cardiotomy and repair of inter-ventricular defect under direct vision	Incision into right ventricle and exposure of defect Repair with suture or ventricular patch Extracorporeal circulation with or without hypothermia
Heart Ventricles Pulmonary artery	Tetralogy of Fallot 1. ventricular defect 2. pulmonic stenosis 3. dextroposition of aorta 4. hypertrophy of right ventricle	Shunting operations Blalock's method Potts-Smith's method Brock's operation Total correction of Tetralogy of Fallot Open heart surgery	Joining right or left subclavian to pulmonary artery Anastomosis between pulmonary artery and aorta Removal of pulmonic obstruction Defects totally repaired using suture closure or patch for closure Infundibulum resected to correct pulmonary stenosis Cardiopulmonary bypass with or without hypothermia*

*Vallee L. Willman, MD, Personal communications.

Organs Involved	Diagnosis	Type of Surgery	Operative Procedures
Heart Atria Ventricles	Atherosclerotic heart disease Adams-Stokes syndrome, atrio-ventricular block	Insertion of trans-venous endocardial pacemaker	Catheter electrode passed through incision in jugular vein and lodged in apex of right ventricle Subcutaneous tunnel and pocket constructed Catheter electrode fastened to pacemaker Pacemaker inserted into pocket
Heart Left ventricle	Ventricular aneurysm Left-sided heart failure	Ventricular aneurysmectomy Open heart surgery	Transverse sternotomy with bilateral thoracotomy; heart opened Removal of aneurysm, its sac, and related thrombus Reconstruction of left ventricle and closure of heart Extracorporeal circulation with or without hypothermia
Heart Right atrium	Myxoma of right atrium with progressive right-sided heart failure	Atriotomy with excision of primary cardiac tumor Open heart surgery	Right atrium opened and myxoma removed Use of cardiopulmonary bypass with or without hypothermia
Heart Pericardium	Constrictive pericarditis Adherent pericardium	Pericardiectomy Pericardiolysis	Partial removal of pericardium Breaking up of adhesions
Heart Myocardium Coronary arteries	Obstructive coronary artery disease with myocardial ischemia and angina pectoris	Myocardial revascu-larization by aortocoronary bypass with autogenous grafts of saphenous vein Open heart surgery	Surgical creation of new ostium in ascending aorta and new openings into vessels of aortic arch for implanting proximal ends of vein grafts Anastomoses of distal ends of grafts with coronary arteries to bypass occlusive lesions Extracorporeal circulation with or without hypothermia
Heart Myocardium Coronary arteries	Triple-vessel coronary artery disease Severe, unstable angina pectoris	Sequential or multiple grafts for triple-vessel disease One circular graft used much less frequently	Standard cardiopulmonary bypass procedure Moderate hemodilution and hypothermia or cold cardioplegic solution infused into aortic root for myocardial arrest

Organs Involved	Diagnosis	Type of Surgery	Operative Procedures
Heart Myocardium Coronary arteries (continued)			Sequential or multiple grafts reversed and implanted into anterior aortic arch Creation of four to six coronary artery anastomoses to bypass stenotic lesions and establish complete myocardial revascularization
Heart Myocardium Coronary arteries	Progression of coronary athero-sclerotic heart disease with graft closure and recurrence of disabling angina pectoris	Reoperative revasculari-zation by internal mammary-coronary artery anastomoses	Median sternotomy Pericardium opened Circulatory support as needed Internal mammary artery grafts implanted in coronary branches to bypass occlusions Pump oxygenator primed with colloid electrolyte solution Moderate hemodilution with or without hypothermia
Heart	Advanced occlu-sive coronary artery disease, diffuse myo-cardial damage, irreversible left ventricular failure	Median sternotomy Cardiac homotrans-plantation	Sternal split incision Simultaneous division of aorta, pulmonary artery, and atria followed by excision of donor and recipient hearts Implantation of donor heart by atrial and vascular anastomoses to recipient heart Extracorporeal circulation with or without hypothermia
Heart Pulmonic valve	Pulmonic valvar stenosis	Pulmonic valvotomy Closed method or Open heart surgery	Division and dilatation of valve Extracorporeal circulation if open method used
Heart Mitral valve	Mitral valve incompetence	Mitral valve reconstruction	Anulus remodeling Leaflet resection Chordal shortening Chordal fenestration and resection
Tricuspid valve	Tricuspid incompetence	Tricuspid repair	Remodeling of anulus with prosthetic ring

Organs Involved	Diagnosis	Type of Surgery	Operative Procedures
Heart Mitral valve	Mitral stenosis due to rheumatic carditis	Mitral commissurotomy	Separation of commissure of stenotic valve
	Combined mitral stenosis and mitral insufficiency	Mitral valvoplasty	Suture or plastic repair of valve; use of prosthesis
Heart Aortic valve Mitral valve	Aortic stenosis and insufficiency Mitral stenosis and insufficiency due to rheumatic heart disease	Excision and replacement of aortic valve and mitral valve with Starr-Edwards aortic and mitral prostheses	Removal of calcified cusps of aortic valve and seating of aortic prosthesis Total removal of calcified mitral valve and insertion of mitral valve prosthesis Extracorporeal circulation, coronary artery perfusion, and hypothermia
Aorta	Dissecting aneurysm of thoracic aorta	Resection of aneurysm Replacement with plastic prosthesis	Aneurysm removed and defect bridged with prosthesis
Aorta	Atherosclerotic aortoiliac occlusion	Aortoiliac endarterectomy	Incision into left external iliac artery and removal of plaque Dissection of segmentally obstructed portion of intima of: 1. common iliac arteries near bifurcation of aorta and 2. terminal aorta
Aorta	Aortic coarctation	Excision of coarctation Aortic anastomosis	Removal of constricted area and joining cut ends together with suture
Aorta Renal artery Hypogastric artery	Abdominal aortic coarctation Hypertension Renal artery stenosis	Aortoaortic bypass with renal vessel bypass	Insertion of an end-to-side aortoaortic bypass from the descending thoracic aorta to the distal abdominal aorta, with a 12 mm Dacron graft. The left renal artery is divided distal to the stenotic area and attached directly to the aortic graft. Autogenous graft (hypogastric artery, splenic artery or saphenous vein) may be used to bypass right renal artery. (Also, Dacron prostheses may be used to bypass the right renal artery.*) (121)

*Patrick S. Vaccaro, et al. Surgical correction of abdominal aortic coarctation and hypertension. *Journal of Vascular Surgery* 3:643-648, April 1986. Reprinted with permission.

Organs Involved	Diagnosis	Type of Surgery	Operative Procedures
Aorta	Aortic coarctation	Dacron patch angioplasty	Longitudinal incision extending from the normal aorta below the coarctation to a point above the coarctation on the subclavian artery. A Dacron patch sutured across the coarctation after excision of any intraluminal membrane* (62)
Aorta	Aortic coarctation	Subclavian arterial flap angioplasty	Subclavian artery divided at the apex of the left pleural cavity. The lateral wall of the artery incised with the incision continuing across the coarctation onto normal aorta below. The flap developed via these incision routes are sutured across the coarctation after excision of intraluminal membrane* (62)
Artery	Subclavian steal syndrome	Subclavian-subclavian crossover bypass graft	Extrathoracic approach Subclavian artery cross-clamped Dacron graft anastomosed to vessel and tunneled subcutaneously in tissues of anterior neck Second anastomosis performed
	Left-sided proximal subclavian obstruction	Carotid-subclavian bypass graft	Supraclavicular approach: restoration of blood supply to the brachiocephalic region by using an autogenous saphenous vein graft† (54)

*Elizabeth W. Nugent, William H. Plauth, Jr., Jesse E. Edwards, Robert C. Schlant, and Willis H. Williams. The pathology, abnormal physiology, clinical recognition and medical and surgical treatment of congenital heart disease. In J. Willis Hurst, ed.-in-chief. *The Heart.* Vol. 1. New York: McGraw-Hill Book Co., 1986, pp. 580-726. Reprinted with permission.
†J.A. Mannick. Subclavian steal syndrome. In David C. Sabiston, Jr., ed. *Textbook of Surgery.* 13th ed. Vol. 2. Philadelphia: W.B. Saunders Co., 1986, pp. 1854-1862. Reprinted with permission.

Organs Involved	Diagnosis	Type of Surgery	Operative Procedures
Artery	Occlusive femoropopliteal disease due to atherosclerotic lesions Pregangrenous state	Femoropopliteal arterial reconstruction by the use of reversed autogenous vein graft	Removal of saphenous vein from knee to saphenofemoral junction Vein reversed and attached to patent vessel by end-to-end anastomosis bypassing the obstruction
Artery	Occlusive femoropopliteal disease of the lower extremity	Femoropopliteal arterial reconstruction by use of in situ saphenous vein bypass	Disruption of the venous valves *without* removal of the saphenous vein from its bed, followed by end-to-end anastomosis bypassing obstruction* (76)
Artery	Embolus in femoral artery	Embolectomy	Incision into femoral artery and removal of clot
Veins	Esophageal varices due to portal hypertension	Portacaval anastomosis	Joining the portal vein and the inferior vena cava to create a large shunt
Veins	Varicosity	Vein stripping	Ligation of saphenous vein; incision made and stripper introduced into vein; vein extirpated

*D. Michael Rogers, et al. In situ saphenous vein bypass for occlusive disease in the lower extremity. *The Surgical Clinics of North America* 66:319-331, April 1986. Reprinted with permission.

References and Bibliography

1. Abboud, Francois M. Shock. In Wyngaarden, James B., and Smith, Lloyd H., Jr., eds., *Cecil's Textbook of Medicine*, 18th ed. Philadelphia: W.B. Saunders Co., 1988, pp. 236-250.

2. Barnes, Robert W. The arterial system. In Sabiston, David C., Jr., ed. *Essentials of Surgery*, Philadelphia: W.B. Saunders Co., 1987, pp. 887-932.

3. Bierman, Edwin L. Atherosclerosis and other forms of arteriosclerosis. In Braunwald, Eugene, et al., eds., *Harrison's Principles of Internal Medicine*, 11th ed. New York: McGraw-Hill Book Co., 1987, pp. 1014-1024.

4. Bigger, J. Thomas, Jr. Cardiac Arrhythmias. In Wyngaarden, James B., and Smith, Lloyd H., Jr., eds., *Cecil's Textbook of Medicine*, 18th ed. Philadelphia: W.B. Saunders Co., 1988, pp. 250-274.

5. Billingham, Margaret E., and Tazelaar, Henry D. Cardiac biopsy. In Parmley, William W., and Chatterjee, K., eds., *Cardiology*, vol. 2. Philadelphia: J.B. Lippincott Co., 1988, pp. 1-17.

6. Braunwald, Eugene. The history. In Braunwald, Eugene, ed., *Heart Disease: A Textbook of Cardiovascular Medicine*, 3rd ed. vol. 1. Philadelphia: W.B. Saunders Co., 1988, pp. 1-12.

7. ———. The physical examination. Ibid., vol. 1, pp. 13-40.

8. ———. Valvular heart disease. Ibid., vol. 2, pp. 1023-1092.

9. Braunwald, Eugene. Valvular heart disease. In Braunwald, Eugene, et al., eds., *Harrison's Principles of Internal Medicine*, 11th ed. New York: McGraw-Hill Book Co., 1987, pp. 956-970.

10. ———. Pericardial disease. Ibid., pp. 1008-1014.

11. Braunwald, Eugene, and Sokel, Burton E. Coronary blood flow and myocardial ischemia. In Braunwald, Eugene, ed., *Heart*

Disease: A Textbook of Cardiovascular Medicine, 3rd ed., vol. 2. Philadelphia: W.B. Saunders Co., 1988, pp. 1191-1221.

12. Bulkley, Bernadine Healy. Pathology of coronary atherosclerotic heart disease. In Hurst, J. Willis, ed.-in-chief. *The Heart*, vol. 1. New York: McGraw-Hill Book Co., 1986, pp. 839-856.

13. Carver, Joseph M., and Hatcher, Charles R., Jr. Techniques of using intra-aortic balloon pump. In Hurst, J. Willis, ed.-in-chief. *The Heart*, vol. 2. New York: McGraw-Hill Book Co., 1986, pp. 2021-2024.

14. Cohen, Lawrence S. Diseases of the aorta. In Wyngaarden, James B., and Smith, Lloyd H., Jr., eds., *Cecil's Textbook of Medicine*, 18th ed. Philadelphia: W.B. Saunders Co., 1988, pp. 370-374.

15. Craige, Ernest. Echophonocardiography and noninvasive techniques to elucidate heart murmurs. In Braunwald, Eugene, ed., *Heart Disease: A Textbook of Cardiovascular Medicine*, 3rd ed., vol. 1. Philadelphia: W.B. Saunders Co., 1988, pp. 65-82.

16. Craige, Ernest, and Smith, Damon. Heart sounds: Phonocardiography; carotid, apex, and jugular venous pulse tracings; and systolic time intervals. In Braunwald, Eugene, ed., *Heart Disease: A Textbook of Cardiovascular Medicine*, 3rd ed., vol. 1. Philadelphia: W.B. Saunders Co., 1988, pp. 41-64.

17. Durack, David T. Infective endocarditis. In Wyngaarden, James B., and Smith, Lloyd H., Jr., eds., *Cecil's Textbook of Medicine*, 18th ed. Philadelphia: W.B. Saunders Co., 1988, pp. 1586-1596.

18. Freeach, Robert J., and Baker, William, H. Arterial injuries. In Sabiston, David C., Jr., ed., *Textbook of Surgery*, 13th ed., vol. 2. Philadelphia: W.B. Saunders Co., 1986, pp. 1886-1903.

19. Fisch, Charles. Electrocardiography and vectocardiography. In Braunwald, Eugene, ed., *Heart Disease: A Textbook of Cardiovascular Medicine*, 3rd ed., vol. 1. Philadelphia: W.B. Saunders Co., 1988, pp. 180-222.

20. Franch, Robert H., et al. Techniques of cardiac catheterization including coronary arteriography. In Hurst, J. Willis, ed.-in-chief. *The Heart*, vol. 2. New York: McGraw-Hill Book Co., 1986, pp. 1768-1809.

21. Friedman, William F. Congenital heart disease in infancy and childhood. In Braunwald, Eugene, ed., *Heart Disease: A Textbook of Cardiovascular Medicine*, 3rd ed., vol. 2. Philadelphia: W.B. Saunders Co., 1988, pp. 896-975.

22. Fry, Richard E., and Fry, William J. Aortoiliac, femoral, and popliteal artery occlusive disease. In Hardy, James D., ed., *Hardy's Textbook of Surgery*, 2nd ed. Philadelphia: J.B. Lippincott Co., 1988, pp. 924-942.

23. Gaynor, J. William, and Sabiston, David C., Jr. Patent ductus arteriosus, coarctation of the aorta, aortopulmonary window, and anomalies of the aortic arch. In Sabiston, David C., Jr., ed., *Essentials of Surgery*. Philadelphia: W.B. Saunders Co., 1987, pp. 1061-1076.

24. Goldman, Mervin J. *Principles of Clinical Electrocardiography*, 12th ed. Los Altos, CA: Lange Medical Publications, 1986, pp. 1-15.

25. ———. Normal electrocardiographic complexes. Ibid., pp. 36-57.

26. ———. Coronary artery disease: Myocardial ischemia. Ibid., pp. 142-212.

27. ———. Disturbances of atrioventicular conduction. Ibid., pp. 244-259.

28. ———. Cardiac pacing and defibrillation. Ibid., pp. 323-334.

29. Goldsmith, Robert S. Infectious diseases: Protozoal. In Schroeder, Steven A., Krupp, Marcus A., and Tierney, Lawrence M., Jr., eds., *Current Medical Diagnosis & Treatment—1988*, Norwalk, CT: Appleton & Lange, 1988, pp. 896-923.

30. Grossman, William, and Barry, William H. Cardiac catheterization. In Braunwald, Eugene, ed., *Heart Disease: A Textbook of Cardiovascular Medicine*, 3rd ed. vol. 1. Philadelphia: W.B. Saunders Co., 1988, pp. 242-267.

31. Grossman, William, and Braunwald, Eugene. Pulmonary hypertension. In Braunwald, Eugene, ed., *Heart Disease: A Textbook of Cardiovascular Medicine*, 3rd ed., vol. 1. Philadelphia: W.B. Saunders Co., 1988, pp. 793-818.

32. Guyton, Robert A., and Hatcher, Charles R., Jr. Techniques of cardiopulmonary bypass surgery. In Hurst, J. Willis, ed.-in-chief. *The Heart*, vol. 2. New York: McGraw-Hill Book Co., 1986, pp. 2025-2029.

33. ———. Techniques of valvular surgery. Ibid., pp. 2030-2034.

34. Hall, David Petrie, and Gruentzig, Andreas R. Technique of percutaneous transluminal angioplasty of coronary, renal, mesenteric, and peripheral arteries. In Hurst, J. Willis, ed.-in-chief. *The Heart*, vol. 2. New York: McGraw-Hill Book Co., 1986, pp. 1901-1915.

35. Hall, Robert J., and Cooley, Denton A. Neoplastic heart disease. In Hurst, J. Willis, ed.-in-chief. *The Heart*, vol. 2. New York: McGraw-Hill Book Co., 1986, pp. 1284-1304.

36. Hardy, James D. Aneurysms of the aorta and its branches. In Hardy, James D., ed., *Hardy's Textbook of Surgery*, 2nd ed. Philadelphia: J.B. Lippincott Co., 1988, pp. 943-967.

37. Hopkins, Paul N., and Williams, Roger R.

Identification and relative weight of cardiovascular risk factors. *Cardiology Clinics* 4:3-31, Feb. 1986.

38. Hurst, J. Willis, et al. Atherosclerotic coronary heart disease: Recognition, prognosis, and treatment. In Hurst, J. Willis, ed.-in-chief. *The Heart,* vol. 1. New York: McGraw-Hill Book Co., 1986, pp. 882-1008.

39. Hurst, J. Willis, et al. The history: Past events and symptoms related to cardiovascular disease. In Hurst, J. Willis, ed.-in-chief. *The Heart,* vol. 1. New York: McGraw-Hill Book Co., 1986, pp. 109-122.

40. Jamieson, W.R. Eric, et al. Carpentier-Edwards supra-annular porcine bioprosthesis. *Journal of Thoracic and Cardiovascular Surgery* 91:555-565, Apr. 1986.

41. Jones, Ellis L., and Hatcher, Charles R., Jr. Techniques for surgical treatment of atherosclerotic coronary artery disease and its complications. In Hurst, J. Willis, ed.-in-chief. *The Heart,* vol. 2. New York: McGraw-Hill Book Co., 1986, pp. 2036-2042.

42. Jones, Robert N., and Sabiston, David C., Jr. Ebstein's anomaly. In Sabiston, David C., Jr., ed., *Essentials of Surgery.* Philadelphia: W.B. Saunders Co., 1987, pp. 1153-1155.

43. Kaplan, Samuel. Congenital heart disease. In Wyngaarden, James B., and Smith, Lloyd H., Jr., eds., *Cecil's Textbook of Medicine,* 18th ed. Philadelphia: W.B. Saunders Co., 1988, pp. 303-318.

44. Kartchner, Mark M., and Lovett, Vernon F. Wrapping of abdominal aortic aneurysms: A viable alternative. *The Surgical Clinics of North America* 66:397-401, Apr. 1986.

45. Kent, Kenneth A. Transluminal coronary angioplasty. In Rackley, Charles E., ed., *Advances in Critical Care Cardiology,* Philadelphia: F.A. Davis Co., 1986, pp. 53-66.

46. Kontos, Hermes A. Vascular diseases of the limbs. In Wyngaarden, James B., and Smith, Lloyd H., Jr., eds., *Cecil's Textbook of Medicine,* 18th ed. Philadelphia: W.B. Saunders Co., 1988, pp. 375-389.

47. Leatham, Aubrey, and Leech, Graham J. The first and second heart sounds. In Hurst, J. Willis, ed.-in-chief. *The Heart,* vol. 1. New York: McGraw-Hill Book Co., 1986, pp. 164-176.

48. Lindsay, Joseph Jr., et al. Diseases of the aorta. In Hurst, J. Willis, ed.-in-chief. *The Heart,* vol. 2. New York: McGraw-Hill Book Co., 1986, pp. 1321-1338.

49. Lofland, Gary K., and Sabiston, David C., Jr. Atrial septal defect, ostium primum defect, and atrioventricular canal. In Sabiston, David C., Jr., ed., *Essentials of Surgery,*

Philadelphia: W.B. Saunders Co., 1987, pp. 1076-1081.

50. ———. Ventricular septal defects. Ibid., pp. 1085-1089.

51. Lowe, James E. Surgical treatment of cardiac arrhythmias. In Sabiston, David C., Jr., ed., *Essentials of Surgery,* Philadelphia: W.B. Saunders Co., 1987, pp. 1156-1163.

52. Lowe, James E., and German, Lawrence D. Cardiac pacemakers. In Sabiston, David C., Jr., ed., *Essentials of Surgery,* Philadelphia: W.B. Saunders Co., 1987, pp. 1169-1179.

53. Lown, Bernard, and deSilva, Regis A. Cardioversion and defibrillation. In Hurst, J. Willis, ed.-in-chief. *The Heart,* vol. 2. New York: McGraw-Hill Book Co., 1986, pp. 1741-1746.

54. Mannick, John A. Subclavian steal syndrome. In Sabiston, David C., Jr., ed., *Textbook of Surgery,* 13th ed., vol. 2. Philadelphia: W.B. Saunders Co., 1986, pp. 1854-1862.

55. McFadden, E. Regis, Jr., and Braunwald, Eugene. Cor pulmonale. In Braunwald, Eugene, ed., *Heart Disease: A Textbook of Cardiovascular Medicine,* 3rd ed., vol. 2. Philadelphia: W.B. Saunders Co., 1988, pp. 1597-1616.

56. Marriott, Henry J.L., and Myersburg, Robert J. Recognition of arrhythmias and conduction abnormalities. In Hurst, J. Willis, ed.-in-chief. *The Heart,* vol. 1. New York: McGraw-Hill Book Co., 1986, pp. 433-475.

57. McLaughlin, Joseph S. Surgical disorders of the pericardium. In Sabiston, David C., Jr., ed., *Essentials of Surgery.* Philadelphia: W.B. Saunders Co., 1987, pp. 1045-1053.

58. Miller, Joseph L. Surgical management of pericardial disease. In Hurst, J. Willis, ed.-in-chief. *The Heart,* vol. 2. New York: McGraw-Hill Book Co., 1986, pp. 2008-2013.

59. Mirowski, M. The implantable cardioverter-defibrillator. In Hurst, J. Willis, ed.-in-chief. *The Heart,* vol. 2. New York: McGraw-Hill Book Co., 1986, pp. 1761-1763.

60. Mond, Harry G., and Sloman, J.G. Artificial cardiac pacemakers. In Hurst, J. Willis, ed.-in-chief. *The Heart,* vol. 1. New York: McGraw-Hill Book Co., 1986, pp. 486-506.

61. Myersburg, Robert J., and Castellanos, Agustin. Cardiac arrest and sudden death. In Braunwald, Eugene, ed., *Heart Disease: A Textbook of Cardiovascular Medicine,* 3rd ed., vol. 1. Philadelphia: W.B. Saunders Co., 1988, pp. 742-777.

62. Nugent, Elizabeth W., et al. The pathology, abnormal physiology, clinical recognition, and medical and surgical treatment of congenital heart disease. In Hurst, J. Willis,

ed.-in-chief. *The Heart*, vol. 1. New York: McGraw-Hill Book Co., 1986, pp. 580-726.

63. Olsen, Craig O., and Sabiston, David C., Jr. Cardiopulmonary bypass for cardiac surgery. In Sabiston, David C., Jr., ed., *Essentials of Surgery*, Philadelphia: W.B. Saunders Co., 1987, pp. 1185-1190.

64. Oparil, Suzanne. Arterial hypertension. In Wyngaarden, James B., and Smith, Lloyd H., Jr., eds., *Cecil's Textbook of Medicine*, 18th ed. Philadelphia: W.B. Saunders Co., 1988, pp. 276-293.

65. O'Rouke, Robert. Physical examination of arteries and veins including blood pressure determination. In Hurst, J. Willis, ed.-in-chief. *The Heart*, vol. 1. New York: McGraw-Hill Book Co., 1986, pp. 138-151.

66. Pacher, Douglas L., Gallagher, John J., and Wallace, Andrew G. Techniques of His bundle recordings: Clinical value and indications. In Hurst, J. Willis, ed.-in-chief. *The Heart*, vol. 2. New York: McGraw-Hill Book Co., 1986, pp. 1727-1733.

67. Panetta, Thomas, et al. Arterial embolectomy: A 34-year experience with 400 cases. *The Surgical Clinics of North America* 66:339-353, Apr. 1986.

68. Pasternak, Richard C., et al. Acute myocardial infarction. In Braunwald, Eugene, ed., *Heart Disease: A Textbook of Cardiovascular Medicine*, 3rd ed. vol. 2. Philadelphia: W.B. Saunders Co., 1988, pp. 1222-1313.

69. Perdue, G.D. Jr., and Smith, Robert B., III. Diseases of the peripheral veins and the vena cava. In Hurst, J. Willis, ed.-in-chief. *The Heart*, vol. 2. New York: McGraw-Hill Book Co., 1986, pp. 1727-1733.

70. Perloff, Joseph K. Assessment of structural abnormalities and blood flow. In Hurst, J. Willis, ed.-in-chief. *The Heart*, vol. 1. New York: McGraw-Hill Book Co., 1986, pp. 247-264.

71. Perloff, Joseph K., and Stevenson, Lynne W. Diseases of the myocardium. In Wyngaarden, James B., and Smith, Lloyd H., Jr., eds., *Cecil's Textbook of Medicine*, 18th ed. Philadelphia: W.B. Saunders Co., 1988, pp. 352-362.

72. Peterson, K.L., and Ross, John, Jr. Cardiac catheterization and angiography. In Braunwald, Eugene, et al., eds., *Harrison's Principles of Internal Medicine*, 11th ed. New York: McGraw-Hill Book Co., 1987, pp. 888-896.

73. Rackley, Charles E. Valvular heart disease. In Wyngaarden, James B., and Smith, Lloyd H., Jr., eds., *Cecil's Textbook of Medicine*, 18th ed. Philadelphia: W.B. Saunders Co., 1988, pp. 340-352.

74. Rackley, Charles E., et al. Tricuspid and pulmonary valve disease. In Hurst, J. Wil-

lis, ed.-in-chief. *The Heart*, vol. 1. New York: McGraw-Hill Book Co., 1986, pp. 792-800.

75. Rackley, Charles E., et al. Use of hemodynamic measurements of acute myocardial infarction. In Rackley, Charles E., ed., *Advances in Critical Care Cardiology*, Philadelphia: F.A. Davis Co., 1986, pp. 3-16.

76. Rogers, D. Michael, et al. In situ saphenous vein bypass for occlusive diseases in the lower extremity. *The Surgical Clinics of North America* 66:319-331, Apr. 1986.

77. Ross, John Jr. Cardiac function and circulatory control. In Wyngaarden, James B., and Smith, Lloyd H., Jr., eds., *Cecil's Textbook of Medicine*, 18th ed. Philadelphia: W.B. Saunders Co., 1988, pp. 184-191.

78. Ross, Joseph C., and Newman, John H. Chronic cor pulmonale. In Hurst, J. Willis, ed.-in-chief. *The Heart*, vol. 2. New York: McGraw-Hill Book Co., 1986, pp. 801-816.

79. Ross, Russell. The pathogenesis of atherosclerosis. In Braunwald, Eugene, ed., *Heart Disease: A Textbook of Cardiovascular Medicine*, 3rd ed., vol. 2. Philadelphia: W.B. Saunders Co., 1988, pp. 1135-1152.

80. Rutherford, John D., et al. Chronic ischemic heart disease. In Braunwald, Eugene, ed., *Heart Disease: A Textbook of Cardiovascular Medicine*, 3rd ed., vol. 2. Philadelphia: W.B. Saunders Co., 1988, pp. 1314-1378.

81. Sabiston, David C., Jr. Aortic abdominal aneurysms. In Sabiston, David C., Jr., ed., *Textbook of Surgery*, 13th ed., vol. 2. Philadelphia: W.B. Saunders Co., 1986, pp. 1830-1838.

82. ———. Thrombo-obliterative diseases of the aorta and its branches. Ibid., pp. 1843-1845.

83. Sabiston, David C., Jr. The tetralogy of Fallot. In Sabiston, David C., Jr., ed., *Essentials of Surgery*, Philadelphia: W.B. Saunders Co., 1987, pp. 1089-1094.

84. ———. Cardiac transplantation: The total artificial heart. Ibid., pp. 1127-1128.

85. ———. Congenital lesions of the coronary arteries. Ibid., pp. 1128-1136.

86. Sabiston, David C., Jr. Surgical treatment of coronary artery disease. In Wyngaarden, James B., and Smith, Lloyd H., Jr., eds., *Cecil's Textbook of Medicine*, 18th ed. Philadelphia: W.B. Saunders Co., 1988, pp. 337-340.

87. Salmon, Sydney E. Malignant disorders. In Schroeder, Steven A., Krupp, Marcus A., and Tierney, Lawrence M., Jr., eds., *Current Medical Diagnosis & Treatment—1988*, Norwalk, CT: Appleton & Lange, 1988, pp. 1060-1075.

88. Satler, Lowell F., et al. Thrombolysis in acute myocardial infarction. In Rackley,

Charles E., ed., *Advances in Critical Care Cardiology,* Philadelphia: F.A. Davis Co., 1986, pp. 39-52.

89. Satler, Lowell F., and Rackley, Charles E. Assessment of adequate circulatory assist during intra-aortic balloon counterpulsation. In Rackley, Charles E., ed., *Advances in Critical Care Cardiology,* Philadelphia: F.A. Davis Co., 1986, pp. 141-149.

90. Schlant, Robert C., and Silverman, Mark E. Anatomy of the heart. In Hurst, J. Willis, ed.-in-chief. *The Heart,* vol. 1. New York: McGraw-Hill Book Co., 1986, pp. 16-37.

91. Schlant, Robert C., and Sonneblick, Edmund H. Pathophysiology of heart failure. In Hurst, J. Willis, ed.-in-chief. *The Heart,* vol. 1. New York: McGraw-Hill Book Co., 1986, pp. 319-345.

92. Schneider, Roland E., et al. Risks for arterial hypertension. *Cardiology Clinics* 4:57-66, Feb. 1986.

93. Schroeder, Steven A., and Chatton, Milton J. General care—symptoms and disease prevention. In Schroeder, Steven A., Krupp, Marcus A., and Tierney, Lawrence M., Jr., eds., *Current Medical Diagnosis & Treatment—1988,* Norwalk, CT: Appleton & Lange, 1988, pp. 1-16.

94. Selwyn, Andrew P., and Braunwald, Eugene. Ischemic heart disease. In Braunwald, Eugene, et al., eds., *Harrison's Principles of Internal Medicine,* 11th ed. New York: McGraw-Hill Book Co., 1987, pp. 975-982.

95. Sethia, B., et al. Fourteen years' experience with the Björk-Shiley tilting disc prosthesis. *Journal of Thoracic and Cardiovascular Surgery* 91:350-361, March 1986.

96. Shabetai, Ralph. Diseases of the pericardium. In Wyngaarden, James B., and Smith, Lloyd H., Jr., eds., *Cecil's Textbook of Medicine,* 18th ed. Philadelphia: W.B. Saunders Co., 1988, pp. 362-367.

97. Sheffield, L. Thomas. Exercise stress testing. In Braunwald, Eugene, ed., *Heart Disease: A Textbook of Cardiovascular Medicine,* 3rd ed., vol. 1. Philadelphia: W.B. Saunders Co., 1988, pp. 223-241.

98. Shoor, Perry M., and Fogarty, Thomas J. Arterial embolism. In Hardy, James D., ed., *Hardy's Textbook of Surgery,* 2nd ed. Philadelphia: J.B. Lippincott Co., 1988, pp. 968-973.

99. Sink, James D., and Sabiston, David C., Jr. Tricuspid atresia. In Sabiston, David C., Jr., ed., *Essentials of Surgery,* Philadelphia: W.B. Saunders Co., 1987, pp. 1098-1099.

100. ———. Truncus arteriosus. Ibid., pp. 1100-1102.

101. ———. Transposition of the great arteries. Ibid., pp. 1102-1109.

102. Smith, Robert B., III. Thoracic outlet syndrome. In Hurst, J. Willis, ed.-in-chief. *The Heart,* vol. 2. New York: McGraw-Hill Book Co., 1986, pp. 2057-2062.

103. ———. Technique of surgical treatment of peripheral vascular disease. Ibid., vol. 2, pp. 2057-2062.

104. Smith, Thomas W. Heart failure. In Wyngaarden, James B., and Smith, Lloyd H., Jr., eds., *Cecil's Textbook of Medicine,* 18th ed. Philadelphia: W.B. Saunders Co., 1988, pp. 215-236.

105. Smith, Thomas W. The management of heart failure. In Braunwald, Eugene, ed., *Heart Disease: A Textbook of Cardiovascular Medicine,* 3rd ed., vol. 1. Philadelphia: W.B. Saunders Co., 1988, pp. 485-543.

106. Smith, Warren M., and Gallagher, John J. Mechanisms of arrhythmias and conduction abnormalities. In Hurst, J. Willis, ed.-in-chief. *The Heart,* vol. 1. New York: McGraw-Hill Book Co., 1986, pp. 406-432.

107. Smith, Warren M., and Wallace, Andrew G. Management of arrhythmias and conduction abnormalities. In Hurst, J. Willis, ed.-in-chief. *The Heart,* vol. 1. New York: McGraw-Hill Book Co., 1986, pp. 475-485.

108. Sokolow, Maurice, and Massie, Barry. Heart and great vessels. In Schroeder, Steven A., Krupp, Marcus A., and Tierney, Lawrence M., Jr., eds., *Current Medical Diagnosis & Treatment—1988,* Norwalk, CT: Appleton & Lange, 1988, pp. 189-265.

109. Stollerman, Gene H. Rheumatic and heritable connective tissue diseases of the cardiovascular system. In Braunwald, Eugene, ed., *Heart Disease: A Textbook of Cardiovascular Medicine,* 3rd ed., vol. 2. Philadelphia: W.B. Saunders Co., 1988, pp. 1706-1733.

110. Strandness, D.E., Jr. Doppler methods of arterial and venous disorders. In Hurst, J. Willis, ed.-in-chief. *The Heart,* vol. 2. New York: McGraw-Hill Book Co., 1986, pp. 1974-1977.

111. Strandness, D.E., Jr. Vascular diseases of the extremities. In Braunwald, Eugene, et al., eds., *Harrison's Principles of Internal Medicine,* 11th ed. New York: McGraw-Hill Book Co., 1987, pp. 1040-1046.

112. Symbas, P.N., and Hatcher, Charles R., Jr. Techniques of surgical treatment of diseases of the aorta. In Hurst, J. Willis, ed.-in-chief. *The Heart,* vol. 2. New York: McGraw-Hill Book Co., 1986, pp. 2043-2052.

113. Thompson, Jesse E., and Garrett, Wilson V. Thrombo-obliterative disease of the vessels of the aortic arch. In Hardy, James D., ed., *Hardy's Textbook of Surgery,* 2nd ed. Philadelphia: J.B. Lippincott Co., 1988, pp. 892-906.

114. Thompson, Mark E., et al. Cardiac transplantation. In Parmley, William W., and Chatterjee, K., eds., *Cardiology,* vol. 2.

Philadelphia: J.B. Lippincott Co., 1988, pp. 1-18.

115. Tierney, Lawrence M., and Erskine, John M. Blood vessels and lymphatics. In Schroeder, Steven A., Krupp, Marcus A., and Tierney, Lawrence M., Jr., eds., *Current Medical Diagnosis & Treatment—1988*, Norwalk, CT: Appleton & Lange, 1988, pp. 266-293.

116. Towne, Jonathan B., and Rollins, David L. Profundaplasty: Its role in limb salvage. *The Surgical Clinics of North America* 66:403-414, Apr. 1986.

117. Trinkle, J. Kent, and Crawford, Michael H. The heart: Anatomy, diagnostic modalities, and the pump oxygenator. In Hardy, James D., ed., *Hardy's Textbook of Surgery,* 2nd ed. Philadelphia: J.B. Lippincott Co., 1988, pp. 1031-1044.

118. Ungerleider, Ross M., and Sabiston, David C., Jr. Double outlet right ventricle. In Sabiston, David C., Jr., ed., *Essentials of Surgery,* Philadelphia: W.B. Saunders Co., 1987, pp. 1095-1098.

119. ———. Congenital aortic stenosis. Ibid., pp. 1109-1113.

120. Urschel, Harold G., Jr. Thoracic outlet syndrome. In Hardy, James D., ed., *Hardy's Textbook of Surgery,* 2nd ed. Philadelphia: J.B. Lippincott Co., 1988, pp. 906-911.

121. Vaccaro, Patrick S., et al. Surgical correction of abdominal aortic coarctation and hypertension. *Journal of Vascular Surgery* 3:643-648, Apr. 1986.

122. Van Trigt, Peter, and Sabiston, David C., Jr. Acquired mitral and tricuspid valvular disease. In Sabiston, David C., Jr., ed., *Essentials of Surgery,* Philadelphia: W.B. Saunders Co., 1987, pp. 1142-1153.

123. Waldhausen, John A., and Campbell, David B. Repair of coarctation of the aorta. In Jamieson, Stuart W., and Shumway, Norman E., eds., *Cardiac Surgery,* 4th ed. St. Louis: The C.V. Mosby Co., 1986, pp. 371-380.

124. Weil, Max Henry, et al. Acute circulatory failure (shock). In Braunwald, Eugene, ed., *Heart Disease: A Textbook of Cardiovascular Medicine,* 3rd ed., vol. 1. Philadelphia: W.B. Saunders Co., 1988, pp. 561-580.

125. Wenger, Nanette Kass, et al. Myocarditis. In Hurst, J. Willis, ed.-in-chief. *The Heart,* vol. 2. New York: McGraw-Hill Book Co., 1986, pp. 1158-1179.

126. Wenger, Nanette Kass, et al. Cardiomyopathy and myocardial involvement in ischemic disease. In Hurst, J. Willis, ed.-in-chief. *The Heart,* vol. 2. New York: McGraw-Hill Book Co., 1986, pp. 1181-1248.

127. Willerson, James T. Angina pectoris. In Wyngaarden, James B., and Smith, Lloyd

H., Jr., eds., *Cecil's Textbook of Medicine,* 18th ed. Philadelphia: W.B. Saunders Co., 1988, pp. 323-329.

128. ———. Acute myocardial infarction. Ibid., pp. 329-337.

129. Williams, J. Mark, and Sabiston, David C., Jr. Acquired diseases of the aortic valve. In Sabiston, David C., Jr., ed., *Essentials of Surgery,* Philadelphia: W.B. Saunders Co., 1987, pp. 1137-1153.

130. Willman, Vallee L. Personal communication.

131. Willman, Vallee L., and Peterson, Gary J. Carotid occlusive disease. In Sabiston, David C., Jr., ed., *Textbook of Surgery,* 13th ed., vol. 2. Philadelphia: W.B. Saunders Co., 1986, pp. 1846-1854.

132. Woodburne, Russell T., and Burkel, William E. The heart and pericardium. *Essentials of Human Anatomy,* 8th ed. New York: Oxford University Press, 1988, pp. 364-388.

133. Wynne, Joshua, and Braunwald, Eugene. The cardiomyopathies and myocarditides. In Braunwald, Eugene, ed., *Heart Disease: A Textbook of Cardiovascular Medicine,* 3rd ed., vol. 2. Philadelphia: W.B. Saunders Co., 1988, pp. 1410-1469.

134. Young, Jess R. Diseases of peripheral arteries. In Hurst, J. Willis, ed.-in-chief. *The Heart,* vol. 2. New York: McGraw-Hill Book Co., 1986, pp. 1339-1354.

135. Zaret, Barry L. Nuclear cardiology. In Wyngaarden, James B., and Smith, Lloyd H., Jr., eds., *Cecil's Textbook of Medicine,* 18th ed. Philadelphia: W.B. Saunders Co., 1988, pp. 207-214.

136. Zierler, R.E., and Strandness, D. Eugene, Jr. Diseases of the small arteries of the extremities. In Hardy, James D., ed., *Hardy's Textbook of Surgery,* 2nd ed. Philadelphia: J.B. Lippincott Co., 1988, pp. 985-994.

137. Zipes, Donald G. Genesis of cardiac arrhythmias: Electrophysiological considerations. In Braunwald, Eugene, ed., *Heart Disease: A Textbook of Cardiovascular Medicine,* 3rd ed., vol. 2. Philadelphia: W.B. Saunders Co., 1988, pp. 581-620.

138. Zipes, Douglas P. Management of cardiac arrhythmias: Pharmacological, electrical, and surgical techniques. In Braunwald, Eugene, ed., *Heart Disease: A Textbook of Cardiovascular Medicine,* 3rd ed., vol. 1. Philadelphia: W.B. Saunders Co., 1988, pp. 621-657.

139. ———. Specific arrhythmias: Diagnosis and treatment. Ibid., pp. 658-716.

140. Zipes, Douglas P., and Duffin, Edwin G. Cardiac pacemakers. In Braunwald, Eugene, ed., *Heart Disease: A Textbook of Cardiovascular Medicine,* 3rd ed., vol. 1. Philadelphia: W.B. Saunders Co., 1988, pp. 717-741.

Disorders of the Blood and Blood-Forming Organs

CHAPTER 6

Blood

Origin of Terms

aniso- (G)—unequal, dissimilar
blasto- (G)—germ
cyt-, cyto- (G)—cell
-emia (G)—blood
hem-, hemo- (G)—blood
leuko- (G)—white
megalo- (G)—big, large
micro- (G)—small

myel-, myelo- (G)—marrow
-osis (G)—increase, disease, condition
-penia (G)—deficiency, decrease
-phagia, phagy (G)—to eat
plasmo- (G)—anything formed, plasma
poikilo- (G)—varied, irregular
-poly (G)—many

Hematologic Terms

- *erythroblasts*—immature red blood cells; possess a nucleus and are present in fetal blood.
- *erythrocytes*—red blood cells; mature cells have no nucleus. (34)
- *erythropoiesis*—the production of red blood cells. (47)
- *hematopoiesis, hemopoiesis*—the development of the various cellular elements of the blood—erythrocytes, leukocytes, platelets, and others. (19)
- *hemoglobin*—a chemical component of erythrocytes containing two substances: globin and hematin, an iron pigment responsible for the transport of oxygen to the cells.
- *leukocytes*—white blood cells divided according to structure into granulocytes, lymphocytes, and monocytes. (18)
- *leukocytes of granulocytic series*—the cytoplasm contains granules. This series includes:
    - *polymorphonuclear neutrophils (see Fig. 39)*—cytoplasmic granules stainable with a neutral dye. Schilling's hemogram, or differential leukocyte count, distinguishes four age-groups (see Table 6).
    - *neutrophilic myelocytes*—youngest neutrophils; nucleus round or ovoid-shaped.
    - *neutrophilic metamyelocytes, junge kernige*—immature cells in which the nucleus has become indented.
    - *neutrophilic band or staff cells*—immature nonfilamented cells in which the nucleus is T, V, or U-shaped without division into segments.

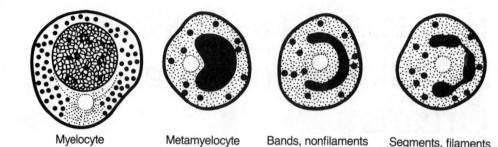

| Myelocyte | Metamyelocyte | Bands, nonfilaments 4% | Segments, filaments 66% |

Figure 39 Developmental phases of neutrophils from immature to mature cells. Eosinophils, basophils, monocytes, and lymphocytes make up the remaining 30% of leukocytes.

    *—neutrophilic lobocytes or polymorphonuclear neutrophils—*filamented mature cells with distinct segmentation.

    *—polymorphonuclear eosinophils—*cytoplasmic granules of cells that take an acid stain.

    *—polymorphonuclear basophils—*cytoplasmic granules of cells that take an alkaline stain. (18, 34)

- *lymphocytes—*leukocytes derived from lymphoid tissue. The cytoplasm contains no or few granules. (18)
- *monocytes—*mononuclear leukocytes. The cytoplasm contains no or few granules. (34)
- *myelopoiesis—*the formation of blood cells and tissue elements from bone marrow. (35)
- *myeloproliferative—*referring to an increased production of myelopoietic cells and tissue.
- *normoblasts—*nucleated red cells that precede normal erythrocytes in the developmental process.
- *normocytes—*normal nonnucleated red blood cells. (19)
- *phagocytes—*two classes of white cells:
      —the *macrophages,* which absorb dead cells and tissues.
      —the *microphages,* which ingest bacteria. (19)
- *plasma—*liquid portion of blood without cellular elements.
- *plasma cells, plasmacytes—*leukocytes, normally absent in blood film, occasionally seen in infection but rarely present in circulating blood. Their function is to synthesize immunoglobulins. (34, 36)
- *platelets, thrombocytes—*round or oval disks that control clot formation and clot retraction. (7, 34)
- *polymorphonuclear—*having nuclei of variable shape. (34)
- *reticulocytes—*immature red cells in intermediary stage of development between nucleate and anucleate forms. They contain a fine intracellular network and are normally present in the blood in small numbers. (34)
- *serum—*liquid portion of the blood after fibrinogen has been consumed in the process of clotting.
- *sideroblasts—*nucleated erythrocytes containing stainable iron granules. (49)
- *siderocytes—*circulating red cells containing stainable iron granules. (34)

Diagnostic Terms

- Conditions primarily affecting the red cells:

—*anemia*—blood disorder characterized by a reduction in erythrocyte count, hemoglobin, and hematocrit, although not all three findings may be present. It is usually a manifestation or a complication of a disease, not a diagnosis. (22, 48)

A condensed version of Wintrobe's etiologic classification of anema is presented:

—*anemia of blood loss*—disorder develops subsequent to an acute or chronic hemorrhage. (22, 48)

—*deficiency factors in red cell production (erythropoiesis):*

  iron deficiency anemia—depletion of body's iron storage, which may be followed by an inadequate production of hemoglobin and a reduction of the oxygen-carrying capacity of the blood. (22, 49)

  megaloblastic anemias—the common denominator is a disordered synthesis of DNA (deoxyribonucleic acid) due to deficiency of vitamin B_{12} or folic acid. Normally dietary vitamin B_{12} interacts with a mucoid secretion of the gastric fundus, the intrinsic factor of Castle. In the absence of this factor, B_{12} cannot be absorbed by the ileum and nutritionally utilized by the body. (4, 12) Folic acid (B_c) deficiency may be caused by malnutrition, malabsorption, increased requirement, or loss of folic acid and defective folate metabolism. (4, 12)

  pernicious anemia—prototype of a megaloblastic anemia, usually associated with marked vitamin B_{12} deficiency caused by failure of gastric mucosa to secrete an intrinsic factor. Laboratory findings reveal a very low red count, often below 2,000,000; a hemoglobin relatively less reduced; and achylia gastrica (absent or diminished gastric juice). Anorexia, sore tongue, weakness, fatigue, a waxy pallor, and neurologic damage are common clinical manifestations. (4, 12)

  sideroblastic anemias—hereditary or acquired anemias exhibiting an excess of iron deposits within normoblasts, usually in association with hypochromia and microcytosis. The anemia may be present at birth but develops more frequently in young adults. The iron overload tends to initiate cardiac arrhythmias and liver fibrosis. Diabetes is frequently associated with sideroblastic anemia. (49)

—*failure of bone marrow:*

  aplastic anemia—marked reduction of red cells, white cells, and platelets (pancytopenia) or a selective reduction of red cells or platelets. Fat cells abound in the bone marrow. Clinical features are pallor, lassitude, bleeding, and purpura. The disease may be idiopathic or caused by toxic drugs or ionizing irradiation. (35)

  Fanconi's syndrome, congenital pancytopenia—idiopathic anemia that develops in early infancy, appears to be hereditary, and is associated with congenital abnormalities of the bones, heart, kidneys, and eyes; microcephaly; and an olive brown skin. The dominant hematologic finding is pancytopenia in which there is a profound depression of the cellular elements of the blood. (35, 46)

—*excessive destruction of erythrocytes:*

  hemolytic anemias—congenital or acquired blood disorders characterized by a shortened life span and an excessive destruction of mature red corpuscles. (26)

  hemolytic disease of the newborn (HDN), erythroblastosis fetalis—reduction of the life span of red cells, usually resulting from a hemolytic reaction of the Rh-positive infant to the sensitized Rh-negative mother. Uncontrolled high bilirubin levels may result in brain damage, evidenced by lethargy, characteristic spasms, and sharp cries. (26)

hereditary elliptocytosis, elliptocytic anemia, ovalocytosis—inherited hemolytic disorder noted for the presence of a large proportion of elliptic-shaped erythrocytes in the circulating blood. Occasionally the disorder seems to be associated with leg ulcers, an enlarged spleen, and abnormalities of the skeleton. Clinical manifestations are uncommon. (26)

hereditary spherocytosis, spherocytic anemia—familial type of hemolytic anemia characterized by the presence of sphere-shaped red cells, reticulocytosis, and increased osmotic fragility. Clinical features may include cholelithiasis, a palpable liver, splenomegaly, nosebleed, and a typical skeletal abnormality, the tower skull.

paroxysmal nocturnal hemoglobinuria—hemolytic disorder characterized by a defect of the red cell membrane that causes enzymatic and serologic abnormalities. The hemolysis ranges from mild to severe. Iron deficiency is present due to the loss of hemoglobin in urine at night. Episodes of fever, chills, and hemoglobinuria signal acute hemolysis. (26, 35)

—*enzyme deficiency and increased red cell destruction:*

glucose-6-phosphate dehydrogenase (G6PD) deficiency—a common erythrocyte metabolic defect or hereditary red-cell enzyme defect. G6PD is necessary for the normal metabolism of erythrocytes. A drug-induced hemolytic anemia develops in G6PD deficiency. Antimalarials, sulfonamides, analgesics and antipyretics are chiefly responsible for the increased red cell destruction. (26)

pyruvate kinase (PK) deficiency—the most common enzymatic deficiency, characterized by varying degrees of chronic hemolytic anemia and accelerated symptoms during stress or intercurrent infection. (26)

—*increased destruction and decreased production of erythrocytes*

—*sickle cell anemia*—genetic abnormality of red blood cells caused by the presence of the gene Hb S* (homozygous genotype). Hemoglobin S produces progressive hemolysis and sickling of cells as the oxygen tension is lowered and deoxygenation increases. The resultant circulatory impairment may lead to vascular occlusions by plugs of sickled red cells, causing thrombosis, infarction, and leg ulcers. The disease is found among American blacks. (26)

—*thalassemias*—group of hereditary, familial anemias of the hypochromic microcytic type caused by a genetic defect that results in a reduced synthesis of adult hemoglobin (Hb A). They comprise:

thalassemia major, Cooley's anemia—the homozygous genotype (both parents transmit defect) usually causes severe anemia, enlargement of the spleen and liver, jaundice, and mongoloid facies.

thalassemia minor—heterogenous genotype (one parent transmits thalassemia trait to offspring) results in mild anemia.

other syndromes of thalassemia. (26, 28)

—*polycythemia*—outstanding characteristics are highly increased red cell mass and hemoglobin concentration. (29)

—*primary polycythemia, polycythemia rubra vera, erythremia*—chronic blood condition of unknown cause characterized by hyperplasia of bone marrow,

---

*Many other abnormal hemoglobins produce sickling without clinical symptoms. Hb S inherited from *one* parent may be asymptomatic.

abnormally high red cell count, hemoglobin and hematocrit that may be associated with a high platelet count, leukocytosis, and leukemia. (29)

—secondary polycythemias—various blood disorders in which tissue hypoxia is a significant feature. The abnormally reduced oxygen supply of the tissues stimulates an excessive production of erythropoietin, which in turn increases bone marrow activity and thus red cell formation. (29)

- Conditions primarily resulting from a defective mechanism of coagulation. The various substances involved in the clotting of the blood are called coagulation factors, designated by Roman numerals I to XIII. According to Wintrobe, factor III, tissue thromboplastin, and factor IV, calcium, are rarely used, and factor VI does not exist. Effective hemostasis is dependent on the integrity of the following factors and cellular components of the blood and the walls of the blood vessels. A final step in the complex coagulation process involves the conversion of fibrinogen to fibrin. The remaining coagulation factors according to the International Nomenclature are:

Factor I—fibrinogen

Factor II—prothrombin

Factor V—proaccelerin, labile factor, accelerator globulin (AcG), thrombogen

Factor VII—proconvertin, stable factor, serum prothrombin conversion accelerator (SPCA)

Factor VIII—antihemophilic factor (AHF) or antihemophilic globulin (AHG), or antihemophilic factor A (AHF-A)

Factor IX—plasma thromboplastin component (PTC) or Christmas factor (CF), or antihemophilic factor B (AHF-B)

Factor X—Stuart factor or Prower factor

Factor XI—plasma thromboplastin antecedent (PTA), antihemophilic factor C (AHF-C)

Factor XII—Hageman factor (HF), glass factor, contact factor

Factor XIII—fibrin-stabilizing factor, Laki-Lorand factor (LLF), fibrinase

——— Prekallikrein, Fletcher factor

——— HMW, Kininogen, high-molecular-weight kininogen, contact activation cofactor (10, 22, 27)

(The last two factors have been recently added and are without Roman numerals.)

Bleeding disorders are present in:

—diffuse intravascular coagulation (DIC), consumption coagulopathy—pathologic clotting that differs from normal coagulation by:

—being a diffuse instead of a local process

—damaging the clotting site instead of giving it protection

—consuming some coagulation factors (fibrinogen, factors V, VIII, XIII), thus predisposing to spontaneous bleeding

—forming fibrin-fibrinogen degradation products (FDP) due to intravascular fibrinogen breakdown, which occurs simultaneously with the pathologic clotting. Alternative names of FDP are:

fibrin-fibrinogen split products

fibrin-fibrinogen related antigens (FR-antigens)

Diagnostic essentials include platelet reduction, prolonged prothrombin time, marked fibrinolysis, and defective clot formation, resulting in diffuse bleeding. Intravascular coagulation with massive hemorrhage may follow trauma, surgery, childbirth, gastrointestinal insult, and other causes. (10, 22, 27)

—Henoch-Schönlein syndrome, anaphylactoid purpura—acquired bleeding abnormality seen primarily in children and characterized by widespread vasculitis

affecting many organs. Purpura is the dominant clinical feature. The syndrome may be accompanied by intussusception, abdominal pain, bleeding from digestive and urinary systems, kidney disease, and bone pain. (10, 22, 27)

—*hemophilia-A, Factor VIII deficiency*—well-known hereditary disease in which a sex-linked trait is transmitted by females, whereas the hemorrhagic disorder develops exclusively in males. In its classic form there is marked deficiency of the antihemophilic factor VIII, leading to spontaneous bleeding episodes. Hemarthroses and hematomas are common complications. (10, 22, 27)

—*hemophilia-B, Factor IX deficiency, Christmas disease*—familial disorder of blood coagulation attributed to a deficiency of the thromboplastin component, factor IX. The clinical picture of the disease hemophilia-B is that of hemophilia-A. (10, 22, 27)

—*hereditary hemorrhagic telangiectasia, Rendu-Osler-Weber syndrome*—congenital defect in the vascular hemostatic mechanism, usually complicated by iron deficiency anemia. Localized dilatations of venules and capillaries are visible on the skin and mucous membranes. Epistaxis is common, and bleeding may occur from digestive, urinary, and respiratory tracts. The elderly tend to develop spiderlike skin lesions. (8, 23)

—*purpura*—disorder characterized by pinpoint extravasations or petechiae and larger skin lesions, the ecchymoses. Bleeding may occur spontaneously, particularly from mucous membranes and internal organs. (8, 23)

—*thrombocytopenia purpura, idiopathic (cause unknown)*—disorder resulting from a marked degree of platelet reduction. Symptoms vary from insignificant purpuric spots to serious bleeding from any body orifice or into any tissue. (9, 22)

—*von Willebrand's disease, pseudohemophilia, vascular hemophilia*—lifelong inherited bleeding disorder affecting both sexes, characterized by Factor VIII deficiency and prolonged bleeding time. Abnormal bruising and bleeding into the skin and mucosa are usually of the purpuric type. (10, 22, 23, 27)

■ *Conditions primarily affecting the white blood cells:*

—*leukemia*—a neoplastic disease that primarily involves the bone marrow and lymphatic and reticuloendothelial systems. It is usually characterized by an overproduction of leukocytes. The more common forms are presented: (39, 46)

—*acute leukemia, stem cell leukemia*—an undifferentiated form of leukemia, since the cells are too young to be identified. Immature leukocytes usually abound in the peripheral blood and bone marrow. The onset is either abrupt or gradual, ushering in fever, pallor, prostration, bleeding, and joint and bone pains. Acute leukemia may occur in differentiated forms such as acute granulocytic, lymphoblastic, myeloblastic, monocytic, basophilic, or eosinophilic leukemia and others, depending on the dominant cell. Anemia and thrombocytopenia may coexist. (39, 46)

—*chronic lymphocytic leukemia*—great excess of lymphocytes, 50,000 to 250,000 white cells, enlargement of lymph nodes and spleen, anemia, and bleeding episodes. (22, 39)

—*chronic myelocytic leukemia*—predominance of myelocytes in blood, white count ranging between 100,000 to 500,000 cells per cubic millimeter of blood, anemia, splenomegaly, pallor, weakness, dyspnea, cachexia, pain, and hemorrhagic tendencies. (See Table 6.) (39)

—*leukemoid reaction*—blood disorder simulating leukemia because of its highly increased white count. (2)

—*leukemic reticuloendotheliosis, hairy cell leukemia*—rare disorder in which an atypical cell with cytoplasmic projections (hair cells) characterizes the blood and

Table 6
Modified Schilling's Hemogram—Differential Leukocyte Count

Type of Count	Percentage									
	Neutrophils									
	Myelo-blasts	Myelo-cytes	Meta-myelo-cytes	Bands, nonfila-ments	Segments, filaments	Total Neutro-phils	Eosin-ophils	Baso-phils	Lympho-cytes	Mono-cytes
Normal Range	—	—	—	2-6	50-70	52-76	1-4	0-1	20-40	2-8
Shift to left; for example, infections	—	—	4	12	69	85	—	—	12	3
Shift to left; for example, chronic myelocytic leukemia	1	4	10	20	40	75	11	9	3	2
Shift to right; for example, pernicious anemia	—	—	—	2	78	80	—	—	16	4

In most infections the differential leukocyte count reveals a shift to the left. Characteristically, a few metamyelocytes (juveniles or junge kernige) and an abnormally high number of bands are found in the blood smear. The more immature the cells are, the more serious is the condition, as may be gleaned from the shift to the left in myelocytic leukemia. In pernicious anemia there is a shift to the right, and the mature neutrophils are polysegmented filaments.

replaces the bone marrow. Leukocytosis and marked splenomegaly are typical findings. (22, 39)

—*leukopenia, granulocytopenia, agranulocytosis*—low white count, less than 5,000 leukocytes per cubic millimeter of blood caused by certain infections, nutritional deficiencies, hematopoietic disorders, chemical agents, and ionizing radiation. (20)

—*neutropenia*—decreased concentration of neutrophils in the blood, predisposing to multiple severe infections. The normal median concentration is 3,650 neutrophils per cubic millimeter of blood. (20)

—*preleukemia*—leukemia suspected but no definitive laboratory evidence to justify the diagnosis. The significant hematologic disorder is the presence of anemia— normochromic or normocytic, hypochromic or microcytic—associated with a low or normal reticulocyte count. Preleukemia occurs in all age-groups, with some predilection for the elderly. The majority of children develop lymphoblastic leukemia; the majority of adults develop myeloblastic leukemia. (38, 46)

■ *Conditions primarily affecting cells produced by myelopoietic tissue of the bone marrow:*

—*chronic granulomatous leukemia (CGL)*—blood disorder that belongs to myeloproliferative syndromes. CGL is chiefly a disorder of stem cell proliferation of the bone marrow. In its terminal phase it mimics acute leukemia or an acute myeloproliferative state. Nearly 90 percent of CGL patients have a typical cytogenetic defect, the Philadelphia (Ph[1]) chromosome, the first classic marker chromosome in human malignant oncology. (39)

—*myeloproliferative disorders*—conditions that have their origin in bone marrow and in varying degrees show an overgrowth of bone marrow cells. Examples are chronic polycythemia vera and granulocytic leukemia. (22)

—*myelosclerosis, myelofibrosis*—the classic form of this myeloprolific disorder reveals a triad of findings: (1) increasing marrow fibrosis, (2) a huge spleen and enlarged liver, and (3) progressive anemia. The patient may experience a dragging sensation and intense pain in the splenic area. (3, 42, 43)

■ *Conditions primarily concerned with an unbalanced proliferation of cells*, usually plasma cells, and associated with an abnormality of immunoglobulins (gamma globulins). (36)

—*amyloidosis*—the presence of amyloid infiltrates in body tissues. Amyloid is a complex substance, principally containing protein and carbohydrates. It is imperfectly understood and undergoing further investigation. (17, 23)

–*primary systemic (or local) amyloidosis*—a plasma cell dyscrasia and genetic metabolic disorder characterized by cardiac and gastrointestinal involvements, arthropathy, peripheral neuropathy, and paresthesias. (17, 36)

–*secondary parenchymatous amyloidosis*—condition usually associated with infection and chronic tissue breakdown of underlying disease, particularly as that seen in multiple myeloma. Amyloid deposits are found in the spleen, kidney, adrenals, liver, lymph nodes, and pancreas. (17, 36)

—*multiple myeloma, plasma cell myeloma*—malignant neoplastic disease characterized by widespread bone destruction, intense bone pain, an excess of atypical plasma cells in the bone marrow, abnormal immunoglobulins, anemia, and recurrent pneumonia or other bacterial infections related to defective antibody synthesis. Renal damage may be associated with elevated calcium levels in blood and urine. (17, 22, 36)

—*Waldenström's macroglobulinemia*—plasma cell dyscrasia in which the production of gamma M globulin is greatly accelerated. Bone marrow findings resemble those of chronic lymphocytic leukemia and multiple myeloma. Anemia and low hemoglobin levels are present in symptomatic disease. The heart, nerves, muscles, and joints may be involved. (17, 22, 36)

Terms Related to Transfusions and Marrow Transplantations

■ *transfusions*—the transfer of blood or its components into the circulating blood of recipients. (21, 22, 30, 45)

—*autologous transfusions*—transfusions prepared from recipient's own blood. They are safe and of particular value to patients who have unusually rare blood types, react severely to homologous blood transfusions, or refuse donor blood on religious grounds. Two forms are used:

–*intraoperative autologous transfusion*—blood salvaged in massive bleeding at surgery and reinfused in patient.

–*predeposit autologous transfusion*—receipt's blood withdrawn weeks before an anticipated need and stored in blood bank. The withdrawal of blood stimulates red cell production. When erythropoiesis is inadequate, iron supplements aid in maintaining the patient's iron storage.

—*homologous transfusions*—donors' blood products obtained before an anticipated need of recipient and deposited in blood bank. Blood preparations are standardized by the *National Institute of Health* (NIH) or *United States Pharmacopeia* (USP) or both.

–*whole blood:*

banked whole blood, citrated whole blood, USP—normal blood collected in acid citrate dextrose (ACD) solution, USP, to prevent coagulation; primarily used for restoring or maintaining blood volume.

heparinized whole blood—normal blood in heparin solution to prevent coagulation; formerly used for priming heart-lung machines to maintain extracorporeal circulation in open heart surgery.

—blood cells:

cytapheresis*—procedure in which one or more cellular elements of the blood (white cells, thrombocytes) are removed from the donor's blood and given to a recipient who has a marked deficiency of these components. The remainder of the blood is retransfused into the donor.

hemapheresis, pheresis—any procedure in which leukocytes, thrombocytes, plasma, or other components are separated from the withdrawn donor blood and transfused into a patient who is deficient in these hemic elements. The donor is reinfused with the remaining part of the blood.

leukapheresis—collection of granulocytes obtained by a blood cell separator or filtration leukapheresis device. The granulocytes are transfused into a patient, usually one with cancer, granulocytopenia, or sepsis, to stimulate bone marrow production of neutrophils. The leukocyte-poor blood is returned to the donor.

leukocyte transfusion, granulocyte transfusion—white cell transfusion used in neutropenia and granulocytopenia, when neutrophils or other granulo-cytes are needed, and in immune deficiency, when cellular immune responses should be evoked. Its therapeutic effect in leukemia and cancer has not been established.

packed red cells—concentrated suspension of red cells (about 70 percent) in acid citrate dextrose (ACD) solution with most of the plasma removed. The procedure is indicated in anemia and hemorrhage, when the oxygen-carrying capacity of the blood needs to be increased.

platelet concentrate—platelet-rich plasma freshly drawn from a single donor or from pooled donors and widely used in thrombocytopenic disorders.

plateletpheresis, thrombocytapheresis—platelet concentration obtained from withdrawn donor blood for transfusing a patient depleted of platelets (thrombocytes) and reinfusing the donor with the remaining platelet-(thrombocyte-) poor blood.

red cells, deglycerolized—frozen and thawed red blood cells with glycerol to prevent cellular damage during freezing and thawing, then removing glycerol before transfusion. Autologous and rare-blood-type transfusion products can be preserved for long periods in frozen blood centers to meet future needs.

—blood proteins and plasma fractions:

antihemophilic human plasma, USP—normal plasma, promptly processed to preserve antihemophilic globulin factor VIII, a component of fresh plasma. It is indicated in the treatment of hemophilia.

cryoprecipitate (Cyro)—commercial product prepared by slowly thawing fresh frozen plasma to form cryoprecipitate rich in antihemophilic factor VIII. Cryo is the treatment of choice in hemophilia and other bleeding disorders.

fresh frozen plasma (FFP)—plasma separated from whole blood and containing all clotting factors; useful as replacement therapy in depletion of coagulation factors. (19)

gamma globulin (IgC)—plasma fraction used for the amelioration of hepatitis and IgC deficiency.

plasma exchange (PE)—the removal of several liters of plasma to rid the blood of unwanted substances, such as large immunoglobulins (IgM).

---

*Cytapheresis—*kytos* (G), cell; *aphairesis* (G), removal of: the linguistically correct derivative. "Pheresis" is abbreviated form used in current medical terminology.

The withdrawn plasma is replaced with normal plasma or suitable fluid, usually Ringer's lactate solution.

plasmapheresis—plasma withdrawn from donor according to prescribed size and frequency of donation for the purpose of transfusing patient in need of plasma fraction therapy. The remaining cells are reinfused into the donor.

plasma protein fraction (PPF)—effective therapeutic agent for hypovolemia. It contains serum albumin (5 percent) and a number of other plasma proteins.

serum albumin—plasma fraction used in the treatment of shock and some protein deficiencies.

transfusion reaction—untoward response to intravenous infusion of a blood preparation. It may be caused by air embolism, allergy, bacterial contaminants, circulatory overload, and hemolysis due to incompatibility of cells. Reactions vary in degree from mild to life threatening; chills, fever, malaise, and headache are common warning signals.

post-transfusion disorders—conditions transmissible through blood transfusions. These disorders include:

acquired immunodeficiency syndrome (AIDS)

cytomegalovirus (CMV)

viral hepatitis, hepatitis B virus, non-A, and non-B hepatitis virus

others. (A few cases of malaria and some isolated cases of brucellosis, filariasis, infectious mononucleosis, and toxoplasmosis also have been reported).

■ *bone marrow transplantation*—bone marrow grafting in hematologic neoplasia, aplastic anemia or leukemia. Bone marrow grafting has been applied in recent years to patients with genetic disorders of hematopoiesis. (1, 35, 37, 41, 44)

—*allogenic marrow transplantation*—bone marrow obtained from:

—*donor related to recipient, matched siblings*—histocompatibility usually present in members of the same family.

—*donor unrelated to recipient*—histoincompatibility frequently present. Infused marrow cells are prone to reject the patient's cells and patient is likely to develop:

graft-versus-host disease (GVHD)—major problem in the transplantation of tissues or organs, occurring when an immunoincompetent host receives histoincompatible lymphocytes. The chief targets of GVHD are the skin, gut, and liver.

histoincompatibility—tissue incompatibility between a donor and recipient.

immunoincompetence—deficient response to antigenic stimulus, congenital or acquired disease, or related to therapy and other causes.

—*autologous marrow transplantation*—aspiration of the patient's own bone marrow before the initiation of aggressive radiotherapy with or without intensive chemotherapy and its infusion when bone marrow toxicity becomes life threatening.

—*isogenic or syngenic marrow transplantation*—marrow grafting between identical twins. Since donor and host have the same tissue antigens, no immunologic barrier to transplantation should be present.

Symptomatic Terms

■ *anisocytosis*—variation in size of red cells, seen in pernicious anemia.
■ *blood dyscrasia*—morbid blood condition.
■ *erythrocytosis*—abnormal increase in red blood cells.

- *erythropenia*—abnormal decrease in red blood cells.
- *fibrinolysis*—dissolution of fibrin; blood clot becomes liquid. (22, 27)
- *hemochromatosis*—intracellular iron overload associated with organic damage.
- *hemolysis*—destruction of red cells and subsequent escape of hemoglobin into blood plasma. (4)
- *leukocytosis*—abnormally high white count. (1)
- *leukopenia*—abnormally low white count.
- *macrocytosis*—abnormally large erythrocytes in the blood.
- *megaloblastosis*—large, usually oval-shaped, embryonic red corpuscles found in bone marrow and blood. (4)
- *microcytosis*—abnormally small erythrocytes present in the blood.
- *neutropenia*—excessively low neutrophil count. (1, 5, 6)
- *neutrophilia*—increase in neutrophils including immature forms, seen in pyogenic infections. (2, 5, 6)
- *pancytopenia*—abnormal reduction of all blood cells: erythrocytes, leukocytes, and platelets. (11)
- *poikilocytosis*—irregularly shaped red cells in the blood, seen in pernicious anemia.
- *proliferation*—increase in reproduction of similar forms or cells.
- *reticulocytosis*—increase in reticulocytes, as seen in active blood regeneration due to stimulation of red bone marrow or in congenital hemolytic anemia and some other anemias.
- *rouleaux formation, pseudoagglutination*—false agglutination in which the erythrocytes appear as stacks of coins. It is seen in plasma cell dyscrasias such as multiple myeloma. (22, 36)
- *thrombocytopenia*—deficiency of thrombocytes or platelets in the circulating blood. (23)
- *thrombocytosis*—excess of thrombocytes or platelets in the circulating blood. (13, 14)

Lymphatic Channels and Lymph Nodes

Origin of Terms

aden-, adeno- (G)—gland
angi-, angio- (G)—vessel
cyt-, cyto- (G)—cell
hist-, histio-, histo- (G)—web, tissue

lymph-, lympho- (L)—lymph, water
-osis (G)—increase, disease, condition
-penia (G)—deficiency, decrease
reticulum (L)—little net

Anatomic Terms (25)

- *histiocytes, histocytes*—tissue cells or macrophages that belong to the reticuloendothelial system and possess phagocytic properties.
- *lymph*—clear or sometimes milky liquid found in lymphatics.
- *lymphatic duct, right*—duct that drains into the right brachiocephalic vein or one of its tributaries.
- *lymphatics (Fig. 40)*—thin-walled vessels widely distributed throughout the body and containing many valves.
- *lymph nodes (Fig. 40)*—encapsulated lymphoid tissue scattered along the lymphatics in chains or clusters.
- *reticuloendothelial system*—system includes highly phagocytic cells, such as macrophages or histiocytes, present in the loose connective tissue of the body, the sinusoids of the lymph nodes, spleen, and liver, as well as in the bone marrow and lungs. It is thought that the function of these cells is:
  —normally the removal of destroyed cells from the circulation and perhaps the storage of iron to be used in the regeneration of erythrocytes.

Figure 40 Main lymphatics and lymph nodes

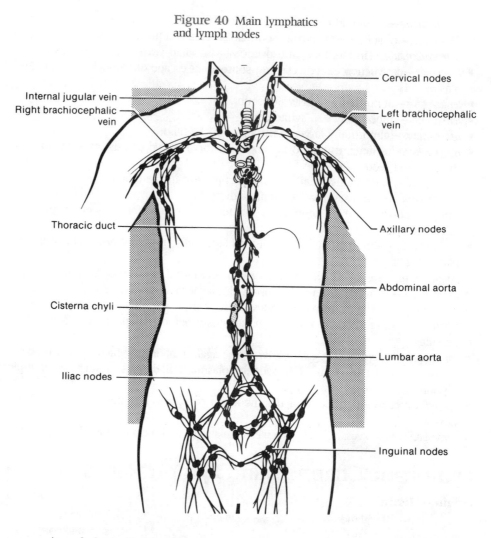

—in pathologic disorders the removal of bacteria, dead tissue, and foreign bodies.

- *thoracic duct*—duct that drains into the left brachiocephalic vein or one of its tributaries.

Diagnostic Terms

- *Burkitt's lymphoma*—a malignant tumor of lymphoid tissue that usually involves the facial bones and abdomen of young children. The etiologic agent is the Epstein-Barr virus. (33)

- *histiocytosis X*—the term refers to three disorders in which there is histiocytic proliferation without the presence of an infective agent or abnormal lipid metabolism.

  —*eosinophilic granuloma of bones*—generally a solitary benign osteolytic lesion containing numerous histiocytes and eosinophils. Sites of predilection are the pelvis, vertebrae, head, and ribs. The lesion occurs in children and adolescents. (15, 16)

  —*Hand-Schüller-Christian disease*—childhood affliction with diffuse bone involvement caused by multiple osteolytic lesions, which may be associated with diabetes insipidus, eczema, exophthalmos, otitis media, respiratory disease, and enlargement of the liver, spleen, and lymph nodes. (15, 16, 40, 44)

—*Letterer-Siwe disease*—histiocytic proliferation present in lymph nodes, spleen, liver, skin, lung, and bones. Pancytopenia occurs frequently, since histiocytes are prone to replace the bone marrow. The disorder is primarily seen before age three and less commonly in older children. (15, 16, 40, 44)

- *Hodgkin's disease*—life-threatening, neoplastic disease producing widespread lymph node involvement, enlargement of the spleen and liver, serious blood disorders, pathologic changes in the bones and other organs, systemic manifestations such as recurrent bouts of fever, night sweats, malaise, and weight loss. Exacerbations and remissions are characteristic of the clinical course. (14, 22, 24, 40, 43, 44)

See Table 7 and Table 8 below.

Table 7
Rye Histopathologic Classification of Hodgkin's Disease (Modified from Lukes and Butler Classification*

Subgroup	Major Histologic Features	Relative Frequency
Lymphocyte predominance	Abundant normal-appearing lymphocyte infiltrate with or without benign histiocytes; occasionally nodular; rare Reed-Sternberg (R-S) cells	5-15%
Nodular sclerosis	Nodules of lymphoid infiltrate of varying size, separated by bands of collagen and containing numerous "lacunar" cell variants of R-S cells	40-75%
Mixed cellularity	Pleomorphic infiltrate of eosinophils, plasma cells, histiocytes, and lymphocytes with numerous R-S cells	20-40%
Lymphocyte depletion	Paucity of lymphocytes with numerous R-S cells, often bizarre in appearance; may have diffuse fibrosis or reticulum fibers	5-15%

*(Reprinted by permission from John H. Glick. Hodgkin's disease. In James B. Wyngaarden, and Lloyd H. Smith, Jr., eds. *Cecil's Textbook of Medicine.* 18th ed. Philadelphia: W.B. Saunders Co., 1988, p. 1016.)

Table 8
Modified Ann Arbor Staging Classification for Hodgkin's Disease*

Stage	Pathologic Status
I	Involvement of a single lymph node region or of single extralymphatic organ or site
II	Involvement of two or more lymph node regions on the same side of the diaphragm or localized involvement of an extralymphatic organ or site and of one or more lymph node regions on the same side of the diaphragm
III	Involvement of lymph node regions on both sides of the diaphragm, which also may be accompanied by involvement of the spleen or by localized involvement of an extralymphatic organ or site or both
III$_1$	Involvement limited to the lymphatic structures in the upper abdomen; that is, spleen, or splenic, celiac, or hepatic portal nodes, or any combination of these
III$_2$	Involvement of lower abdominal nodes; that is para-aortic, iliac, inguinal or mesenteric nodes, with or without involvement of the splenic, celiac, or hepatic portal nodes.
IV	Diffuse or disseminated involvement of one or more extralymphatic organs or tissues, with or without associated lymph node involvement

*(Reprinted by permission from John H. Glick. Hodgkin's disease. In James B. Wyngaarden, and Lloyd H. Smith, Jr., eds. *Cecil's Textbook of Medicine.* 18th ed. Philadelphia: W.B. Saunders Co., 1988, p. 1017.)

- *lymphadenitis*—inflammation of the lymph glands. (43)
- *lymphadenopathy*—any diseased condition of the lymph nodes, such as enlarged lymph nodes due to an unknown cause. (16)
- *lymphangioma*—tumor composed of lymphatics. (25)
- *lymphangitis*—inflammation of the lymphatics.
- *lymphedema*—congenital or acquired disorder of the lymphatics that prevents the removal of tissue fluids by the lymph channels and the absorption of protein and other substances by lymphatic capillaries, resulting in impairment of lymph flow and edema. (25, 43)
- *lymphocytic choriomeningitis (LMC)*—acute (rarely fatal) or mild form of aseptic meningitis caused by the LMC virus. Clinical features of the mild form are weakness, malaise, fever, myalgia, back pain, and sometimes respiratory symptoms. The cell count of the cerebrospinal fluid (CSF) is highly increased. Lymphocytes predominate.
- *lymphomas*—neoplasms that may arise in lymphoid tissue and vary in degree of malignancy. (24, 31)
    - *non-Hodgkin's lymphomas*—neoplasms of B or T lymphocytic lineage are included in this classification. Three classifications of non-Hodgkin's lymphomas are: (1) Rappaport histopathologic classification; (2) Lukes and Collins classification based on the lymphoma's cell origin; and (3) The National Cancer Institute Working Formulation classification, which is proving both clinically useful and immunologically precise. (3, 32, 40)
- *mycosis fungoides, granuloma fungoides*—chronic, progressive, lymphomatous tumor of the skin that tends to ulcerate and ultimately cause death. (15)

Operative Terms

- *biopsy of lymph node*—removal of small piece of lymphoid tissue for microscopic study. (16, 25)
- *lymphadenectomy*—excision of lymph nodes. (25)
- *lymphadenotomy*—incision and drainage of lymph gland. (25)
- *multiple lymph node excision*—removal of metastatic lymph nodes in a certain region, such as the axillary nodal cluster, the periaortic chain, or the pelvic and retroperitoneal nodes. (16)

Symptomatic Terms

- *lymphocytosis*—abnormal increase of lymphocytes in the blood.
- *lymphocytopenia*—deficient number of lymphocytes in the blood. (1, 2)
- *Pel-Ebstein pyrexia*—cyclic fever in Hodgkin's disease and some other disorders, characterized by several days of pyrexia, followed by days or weeks of normal body temperature. The cycle repeats itself. (14)

Spleen

Origin of Terms

aut-, auto- (G)—self
lien-, lieno- (L)—spleen

-oma (G)—tumor
splen- spleno- (G)—spleen

Anatomic Term (13, 24)

- *spleen*—a lymphoid organ located in the left hypochondriac region. It is active in the destruction of red blood cells and the manufacture of lymphocytes and phagocytes.

Diagnostic Terms

- *accessory spleens*—additional spleens, performing the same function as the spleen. The condition is very common. (24)
- *asplenia*—absence of the spleen. (16)
- *chronic congestive splenomegaly, hepatolienal fibrosis, Banti's syndrome*—condition characterized by long-standing congestion and enlargement of the spleen, usually caused by liver disease associated with portal or splenic artery hypertension. Leukopenia, anemia, and gastrointestinal bleeding are common manifestations. (13, 16, 24)
- *hypersplenism, hypersplenic syndrome*—excessive splenic activity associated with highly increased blood cell destruction, leading to anemia, leukopenia, and thrombocytopenia. (16)
- *splenic infarcts*—relatively common lesions usually caused by embolism, thrombosis, or infection. (13, 24)
- *splenic sequestration crisis*—the spleen rapidly enlarges, followed by a quick drop in blood volume and fatal hypovolemic shock. (16)
- *splenitis, lienitis*—inflammation of the spleen. (13, 16, 24)
- *splenoptosis*—downward displacement of the spleen.
- *splenorrhexis*—rupture of spleen due to injury or advanced disease.

Operative Terms

- *splenectomy*—removal of the spleen. (24)
- *splenopexy*—fixation of a movable spleen.
- *splenorrhaphy*—suture of a ruptured spleen. (16)
- *splenotomy*—incision into the spleen.

Symptomatic Terms

- *autosplenectomy*—small, fibrotic spleen in adult with sickle cell anemia. Multiple splenic infarctions result in shrinkage of the organ. (13)
- *splenomegaly, splenomegalia*—enlargement of the spleen. (13, 24)

Abbreviations

Related to Hematology

Ab—antibody
ACD—acid-citrate-dextrose
Ag—antigen
AHF—antihemophilic factor VIII
AHG—antihemophilic globulin factor VIII
bas—basophils
CBC—complete blood count
CF—Christmas factor, factor IX
eos—eosinophils
ESR—erythrocytic sedimentation rate
FDP—fibrin-fibrinogen degradation products
FR—fibrin-fibrinogen related
FSP—fibrin-fibrinogen split products
HAI—hemagglutination-inhibition immunoassay
Hb—hemoglobin
Hb A—adult hemoglobin
Hb F—fetal hemoglobin

Hb S—sickle cell hemoglobin
Hct, Ht—hematocrit
lymph—lymphocytes
MCH—mean corpuscular hemoglobin
MCT—mean circulation time
MCV—mean corpuscular volume
PCT—plasmacrit test
PCV—packed cell volume (hematocrit)
PMN—polymorphonuclear neutrophils
PTA—plasma thromboplastin antecedent, factor XI
PTC—plasma thromboplastin component, factor IX
RBC—red blood count
RES—reticuloendothelial system
SI—saturation index
VI—volume index
VPRC—volume packed red cells
WBC—white blood count

Related to Hematologic Disorders

AIHA—autoimmune hemolytic anemia
ALL—acute lymphoblastic leukemia,
  acute lymphocytic leukemia
AML—acute myeloblastic leukemia
ANLL—acute non-lymphocytic leukemia
CGL—chronic granulomatous leukemia
CLL—chronic lymphocytic leukemia
CML—chronic myelocytic leukemia
DIC—diffuse intravascular coagulation
G6PD—glucose-6-phosphate
  dehydrogenase
GvH, GVHD—graft-versus-host disease
HCD—heavy-chain disease
HCL—hairy cell leukemia
HDN—hemolytic disease of the newborn
HE—hereditary elliptocytosis

HS—hereditary spherocytosis
IMF—idiopathic myelofibrosis
ITP—idiopathic thrombocytopenia
  purpura
NHL—non-Hodgkin's lymphoma
PA—pernicious anemia
PK—pyruvate kinase deficiency
SCA—sickle cell anemia

Related Organizations

AABB—American Association of Blood
  Banks
ACS—Association of Clinical Scientists
ASCP—American Society of Clinical
  Pathologists
ASLM—American Society of Law and
  Medicine

Oral Reading Practice

Hodgkin's Disease

This peculiar and interesting disease is characterized by a painless enlargement of the lymph nodes that is initially confined to one group, frequently located in the cervical region. From there the lymph node involvement spreads to the axillary and inguinal regions and progressively assumes systemic proportions. If **mediastinal spread** and **infiltration** of the lung **parenchyma** and pleura occur, the patient may experience substernal pain, cough, **dyspnea,** and **stridor.**

Retroperitoneal lymph node involvement may lead to the formation of a mass that presses on the stomach and produces a sense of fullness. This type of involvement tends to exert a deleterious effect, resulting in a dislodgment of the kidneys, compression of the **ureters** and **inferior vena cava,** and **infiltrations** into the neighboring structures, the spinal nerves, and **vertebrae. Splenomegaly** and **hepatomegaly** are common signs and may be associated with progressive **anemia, obstructive jaundice,** and **ascites.**

Lesions of Hodgkin's disease are sometimes found in the reproductive system. **Osteolytic** and **osteoplastic** changes may occur in the ribs, vertebrae, femur, and pelvis and cause bone tenderness or intense pain. As the disease progresses to the terminal phase, the patient manifests high fever and a marked degree of **lassitude, debility, pallor,** and **cyanosis.**

The diagnostic feature of Hodgkin's disease is the **Reed-Sternberg cell,** a tumor cell containing irregularly shaped **cytoplasm,** a large **nucleus,** heavy clumps of **chromatin,** and **distinctive nucleoli** surrounded by a clear halo.

In 1902, Pusey reported the remarkable responsiveness of Hodgkin's and non-Hodgkin's lymphomas to **radiotherapy;** however, x-ray machines lacked technical efficiency, delivered inadequate depth dose, and caused painful skin burns. Radiation therapy continued to be a method of choice, but it was not until half a century later that

Kaplan and the Stanford research team obtained dramatic results from the use of **megavoltage radiotherapy. "Mantle" field irradiation** treats cervical, supraclavicular, intraclavicular, axillary, hilar, and mediastinal nodes down to the level of the diaphragm. **"Inverted Y" field irradiation** treats the spleen or splenic pedicle, celiac, para-aortic, iliac, inguinal, and femoral nodes. The **"mantle"** and the **"inverted Y"** fields compose the **total nodal irradiation (TNI)** or **total lymphoid irradiation (TLI).** When the pelvis is omitted from treatment, the terms are called **subtotal nodal irradiation (STNI)** or **subtotal lymphoid irradiation (STLI). Radiation pericarditis** occurs in about six percent of the cases treated with 4400 rad or less to the mantle field and is usually asymptomatic. Another common neurologic complication of radiotherapy is **Lhermitte's syndrome,** characterized by tingling, numbness, or electric sensations and is usually associated with bending of the head. This symptom gradually disappears over a period of several months.

Cyclic combination chemotherapy is the treatment of choice in advanced Hodgkin's disease. Large-scale trials were carried on by the National Cancer Institute over a 17-year period using 198 patients, of whom 159 or 80 percent achieved complete remission. The **MOPP** program of chemotherapy—including **nitrogen mustard** (M); **vincristine,** or **Oncovin** (O); **procarbazine** (P); and **prednisone** (P)—was repeated every four weeks at a minimum of six cycles, inducing remissions and prolongation of life. It is known that the use of **antineoplastic** drugs requires much caution because of their potential toxicity. Alternative regimens are available if the patient is unable to tolerate the prescribed medications. The most widely utilized of these is the ABVD program, which is a combination of **doxorubicin, bleomycin, vinblastine,** and **dacarbazine.** This regime or variations of it has produced remission in some patients where the **MOPP** program of chemotherapy had failed. **Combined radiotherapy** and **chemotherapy** is reserved for advanced Hodgkin's disease that has not been controlled by a single treatment approach.

The most serious untoward effect of aggressive **megavoltage** radiotherapy and chemotherapy is **myelosuppression,** resulting in a reduction of all cellular elements of the blood **(pancytopenia). Granulocytopenia** with its lowered resistance to infection and **thrombocytopenia** with its hemorrhagic tendencies become life-threatening sequelae. The terminal phase of Hodgkin's disease is signalled by lymphopenia, a striking immunologic manifestation heralding a defective response to previously encountered antigens.

A **staging laparotomy** should include a careful abdominal inspection, **splenectomy,** and **sectioning** of the **spleen** in slices one centimeter apart. The procedure is only justifiable if done thoroughly. According to the Ann Arbor Conference, proper staging techniques include a complete history, signs and symptoms, detection of **extranodal** involvement and adenopathy, biopsy of abnormal lymph nodes, **bipedal lymphangiography,** and chest **roentgenography** or **computed tomography.** Bone marrow biopsy is indicated in the presence of bone pain or osseous lesions.

Pathologic staging of the extent of the disease is of practical significance as a guide to the best therapeutic approach. Early diagnosis, improved understanding of **Hodgkin's disease** and the **modality** of treatment adapted to the stage of the disease now give rise to a more favorable prognosis than in the past. As a result of the addition of curative **chemotherapy** to the therapeutic regimen, the national mortality from Hodgkin's disease has fallen 58 percent during the past decade. Approximately 70 percent of all patients with Hodgkin's disease are curable. (14, 22, 24, 40, 43, 44)

Table 9

Some Disorders of the Blood and Blood-Forming Organs Amenable to Surgery

Cells or Organs Involved	Diagnosis	Type of Surgery	Operative Procedures
Red cells Bone marrow	Aplastic anemia	Marrow transplantation Allogenic grafting	Multiple marrow aspirations from iliac bones Intravenous infusion of marrow from histocompatible donor
White cells Bone marrow	Acute lymphoblastic leukemia Acute myelogenous leukemia Chronic myelogenous leukemia	Marrow transplantation Allogenic grafting Isogenic grafting Autologous grafting	Same as above Intravenous infusion of marrow from identical twin Aspiration and storage of patient's own marrow Intravenous infusion of autologous marrow when blast crisis develops
Red cells	Hereditary spherocytosis	Splenectomy	Removal of spleen
Platelets	Thrombocytopenia due to increased platelet destruction	Splenectomy	Removal of spleen
Blood cells Spleen	Congestive splenomegaly with cytopenia	Splenectomy	Removal of spleen
Spleen	Traumatic rupture of spleen	Splenectomy	Removal of spleen
Lymph nodes Spleen	Hodgkin's disease Lymphoma	Exploratory laparotomy and splenectomy	Surgical opening of abdomen with removal of spleen for the purpose of staging before initiating treatments
Lymph nodes	Embryonal cell carcinoma of testis Metastases to lymph nodes	Radical retroperitoneal lymph node dissection (postorchiectomy)	Peritoneal cavity opened; peritoneum reflected off the aorta and vena cava Multiple pelvic and periaortic lymph nodes removed

References and Bibliography

1. Bagby, Grover C., Jr. Leukopenia. In Wyngaarden, James B., and Smith, Lloyd H., Jr., eds., *Cecil's Textbook of Medicine*, 18th ed. Philadelphia: W.B. Saunders Co., 1988, pp. 961-967.

2. ———. Leukocytosis and leukemoid reactions. Ibid., pp. 967-972.

3. Berk, Paul D. Myeloproliferative disorders. In Wyngaarden, James B., and Smith, Lloyd H., Jr., eds., *Cecil's Textbook of Medicine*, 18th ed. Philadelphia: W.B. Saunders Co., 1988, pp. 984-988.

4. Beck, William S. Megaloblastic anemias. In Wyngaarden, James B., and Smith, Lloyd H., Jr., eds., *Cecil's Textbook of Medicine*, 18th ed. Philadelphia: W.B. Saunders Co., 1988, pp. 900-907.

5. Babior, Bernard M. Function of neutrophilis and mononuclear phagocytes. In Wyngaarden, James B., and Smith, Lloyd H., Jr., eds., *Cecil's Textbook of Medicine*, 18th ed. Philadelphia: W.B. Saunders Co., 1988, pp. 951-957.

6. ———. Disorders of neutrophil function. Ibid., pp. 967-972.

7. Bithell, T. Platelets and megarkaryocytes. In Thorup, Oscar A., Jr., ed., *Fundamentals of Clinical Hematology*, 5th ed. Philadelphia: W.B. Saunders Co., 1987, pp. 115-125.

8. ———. Vascular defects and hemorrhage. Ibid., pp. 784-791.

9. ———. Disorders of platelets. Ibid., pp. 792-823.

10. ———. Disorders of blood coagulation. Ibid., pp. 824-876.

11. Clarkson, Bayard. The chronic leukemias. In Wyngaarden, James B., and Smith, Lloyd H., Jr., eds., *Cecil's Textbook of Medicine*, 18th ed. Philadelphia: W.B. Saunders Co., 1988, pp. 988-1001.

12. Colon-Otero, Gerardo, and Wheby, Munsey S. Disorders of cobalamin and folate metabolism. In Thorup, Oscar A., Jr., ed., *Fundamentals of Clinical Hematology*, 5th ed. Philadelphia: W.B. Saunders Co., 1987, pp. 185-211.

13. Faller, Douglas V. Diseases of the spleen. In Wyngaarden, James B., and Smith, Lloyd H., Jr., eds., *Cecil's Textbook of Medicine*, 18th ed. Philadelphia: W.B. Saunders Co., 1988, pp. 1036-1040.

14. Glick, John H. Hodgkin's disease. In Wyngaarden, James B., and Smith, Lloyd H., Jr., eds., *Cecil's Textbook of Medicine*, 18th ed. Philadelphia: W.B. Saunders Co., 1988, pp. 1014-1022.

15. Groopman, Jerome E. Langerhans cell (esoinophilic) granulomatosis. In Wyngaarden, James B., and Smith, Lloyd H., Jr., eds., *Cecil's Textbook of Medicine*, 18th ed. Philadelphia: W.B. Saunders Co., 1988, pp. 1022-1024.

16. Hess, Charles E. Approach to patients with lymphadenopathy or splenomegaly. In Thorup, Oscar A., Jr., ed., *Fundamentals of Clinical Hematology*, 5th ed. Philadelphia: W.B. Saunders Co., 1987, pp. 536-577.

17. ———. Multiple myeloma and other monoclonal gammopathies. Ibid., pp. 721-772.

18. Keeling, Richard P. Differentiation, biochemistry of the granulocyte. In Thorup, Oscar A., Jr., ed., *Fundamentals of Clinical Hematology*, 5th ed. Philadelphia: W.B. Saunders Co., 1987, pp. 90-107.

19. ———. Differentiation, biochemistry, and physiology of the monocyte and macrophage. Ibid., pp. 108-125.

20. ———. Non-neoplastic disorders of granulocytes and monocytes. Ibid., pp. 424-459.

21. Keeling, Richard P., and Alberico, Thomas A. Transfusion therapy. In Thorup, Oscar A., Jr., ed., *Fundamentals of Clinical Hematology*, 5th ed. Philadelphia: W.B. Saunders Co., 1987, pp. 928-983.

22. Linker, Charles. Blood. In Schroeder, Steven A., Krupp, Marcus A., and Tierney, Lawrence M., Jr., eds., *Current Medical Diagnosis & Treatment—1988*, Norwalk, CT: Appleton & Lange, 1988, pp. 294-338.

23. Marcus, Aaron J. Hemorrhagic disorders: Abnormalities of platelet and vascular function. In Wyngaarden, James B., and Smith, Lloyd H., Jr., eds., *Cecil's Textbook of Medicine*, 18th ed. Philadelphia: W.B. Saunders Co., 1988, pp. 1042-1060.

24. Matsumoto, Teruo, and Perlman, Morton H. The spleen. In Sabiston, David C., Jr., ed., *Essentials of Surgery*, Philadelphia: W.B. Saunders Co., 1987, pp. 615-633.

25. McCann, Richard L. The lymphatic system. In Sabiston, David C., Jr., ed., *Essentials of Surgery*, Philadelphia: W.B. Saunders Co., 1987, pp. 634-638.

26. Mohler, Daniel N., and Thorup, Oscar A., Jr. Hemolytic anemia. In Thorup, Oscar A., Jr., ed., *Fundamentals of Clinical Hematology*, 5th ed. Philadelphia: W.B. Saunders Co., 1987, pp. 251-348.

27. Mosher, Deane F. Disorders of blood coagulation. In Wyngaarden, James B., and Smith, Lloyd H., Jr., eds., *Cecil's Textbook of Medicine*, 18th ed. Philadelphia: W.B. Saunders Co., 1988, pp. 1060-1081.

28. Niehuis, Arthur W. The Thalassemias. In Wyngaarden, James B., and Smith, Lloyd H., Jr., eds., *Cecil's Textbook of Medicine*, 18th ed. Philadelphia: W.B. Saunders Co., 1988, pp. 930-936.

29. Niskanen, Eero. Polycythemia. In Thorup,

Oscar A., Jr., ed., *Fundamentals of Clinical Hematology*, 5th ed. Philadelphia: W.B. Saunders Co., 1987, pp. 409-423.

30. Perkins, Herbert A. Blood transfusions. In Wyngaarden, James B., and Smith, Lloyd H., Jr., eds., *Cecil's Textbook of Medicine*, 18th ed. Philadelphia: W.B. Saunders Co., 1988, pp. 947-951.

31. Portlock, Carol S. Introducton to neoplasms of the immune system. In Wyngaarden, James B., and Smith, Lloyd H., Jr., eds., *Cecil's Textbook of Medicine*, 18th ed. Philadelphia: W.B. Saunders Co., 1988, pp. 1007-1009.

32. ———. The non-Hodgkin's lymphomas. Ibid., pp. 1009-1013.

33. ———. Burkitt's lymphoma. Ibid., pp. 1013-1014.

34. Quesenberry, Peter J. Origin of blood cells and architecture of the bone marrow. In Thorup, Oscar A., Jr., ed., *Fundamentals of Clinical Hematology*, 5th ed. Philadelphia: W.B. Saunders Co., 1987, pp. 1-22.

35. ———. Bone marrow failure. Ibid., pp. 349-372.

36. Salmon, Sydney. Plasma cell disorders. In Wyngaarden, James B., and Smith, Lloyd H., Jr., eds., *Cecil's Textbook of Medicine*, 18th ed. Philadelphia: W.B. Saunders Co., 1988, pp. 1026-1036.

37. Schechter, Alan N. Hemoglobin structure and function. In Wyngaarden, James B., and Smith, Lloyd H., Jr., eds., *Cecil's Textbook of Medicine*, 18th ed. Philadelphia: W.B. Saunders Co., 1988, pp. 925-927.

38. Smith, Roy E. Myeloproliferative disorders. In Thorup, Oscar A., Jr., ed., *Fundamentals of Clinical Hematology*, 5th ed. Philadelphia: W.B. Saunders Co., 1987, pp. 394-408.

39. ———. Leukemia. Ibid., pp. 578-615.

40. Stewart, F. Marc, and Hess, Charles E. Malignant lymphomas. In Thorup, Oscar A., Jr., ed., *Fundamentals of Clinical Hematology*,

5th ed. Philadelphia: W.B. Saunders Co., 1987, pp. 616-719.

41. Strob, Rainer. Bone marrow transplantation. In Wyngaarden, James B., and Smith, Lloyd H., Jr., eds., *Cecil's Textbook of Medicine*, 18th ed. Philadelphia: W.B. Saunders Co., 1988, pp. 1040-1042.

42. Talpaz, Moshe, et al. Recent advances in therapy of chronic myelogenous leukemia. In DeVita, Vincent T., Jr., Hellman, Samuel, and Rosenberg, Steven A., eds., *Important Advances in Oncology—1988*, Philadelphia: J.B. Lippincott Co., 1988, pp. 297-321.

43. Tierney, Lawrence M., and Erskine, John M. Blood vessels and lymphatics. In Schroeder, Steven A., Krupp, Marcus A., and Tierney, Lawrence M., Jr., eds., *Current Medical Diagnosis & Treatment—1988*, Norwalk, CT: Appleton & Lange, 1988, pp. 266-293.

44. Tucker, Eugene, MD. Personal communications.

45. Wallerstein, Ralph O. Blood transfusions. In Schroeder, Steven A., Krupp, Marcus A., and Tierney, Lawrence M., Jr., eds., *Current Medical Diagnosis & Treatment—1988*, Norwalk, CT: Appleton & Lange, 1988, pp. 338-341.

46. Weinstein, Howard J. The acute leukemias. In Wyngaarden, James B., and Smith, Lloyd H., Jr., eds., *Cecil's Textbook of Medicine*, 18th ed. Philadelphia: W.B. Saunders Co., 1988, pp. 1001-1007.

47. Wheby, Munsey S. Differentiation, biochemistry, and physiology of the erythrocyte. In Thorup, Oscar A., Jr., ed., *Fundamentals of Clinical Hematology*, 5th ed. Philadelphia: W.B. Saunders Co., 1987, pp. 64-89.

48. ———. Classification, mechanisms, diagnosis, and physiologic effects. Ibid., pp. 163-184.

49. ———. Disorders of iron metabolism. Ibid., pp. 212-250.

Respiratory Disorders

CHAPTER 7

Nose

Origin of Terms

choane (G)—a funnel
concha (L)—a shell
meatus (L)—a passage

osmo- (G)—sense of smell
rhino- (G)—nose

Anatomic Terms (Refs. 23, 72)

- *choana (pl. choanae), posterior aperture*—opening of the nasal cavity into the nasopharynx.
- *concha (pl. conchae), turbinate*—one of the scroll-like bony projections on the lateral wall of the nasal cavity.
- *naris (pl. nares)*—nostril.
- *nasal meatus (pl. meatuses)*—space beneath each concha of the nose.
- *nasal septum*—partition between the two halves of the nasal cavity.
- *nasopharynx*—open chamber located behind the nasal fossa and below the base of the skull.

Diagnostic Terms

- *atresia of choanae*—pathologic closure of posterior nares or congenital absence of the same.
- *coryza*—cold in head. (32)
- *deflection of septum*—deviation of septum (deviation: departure from normal). (23)
- *nasal polyp*—benign lesion that may cause considerable obstruction of the nasal airway. (32)
- *nasal skin cancer*—dermal lesion of the basal cell, squamous cell, epidermoid, or melanoma variety, differing in degree of malignancy and metastatic potential. (23)
- *nasopharyngeal cancer*—usually an epidermoid carcinoma or lymphosarcoma of the nasopharynx, which may spread by direct extension to the meninges, compress cranial nerves, and cause cranial nerve paralyses, ptosis of the eyelid, and eventually loss of sight. Invasion of lymph nodes occurs frequently. The incidence of nasopharyngeal cancer is high among the Chinese and Malaysians and low in Caucasians. (13, 23)

- *nasopharyngitis*—inflamed condition of the nasopharynx. (34, 56)
- *rhinitis*—inflammation of the nasal mucosa.
    - —*allergic rhinitis*—hay fever.
    - —*atrophic*—chronic infection with crust formation and nasal obstruction. (23, 32)
    - —*hypertrophic*—swollen nasal mucosa leading to nasal obstruction. (58)
- *rhinolith*—nasal concretion.

Operative Terms

- *rhinoplasty*—plastic reconstruction of the nose. (23)
- *septal dermoplasty*—excision of septal mucosa in telangiectatic area and its replacement with skin graft or oral mucous membrane to control bleeding. (23)
- *septectomy, submucous resection*—excision of the nasal septum or part of it. (23)
- *transantral ligation of maxillary artery*—the application of vascular clips on the maxillary artery in uncontrolled recurrent epistaxis. (23)
- *turbinectomy*—excision of a turbinate bone.
- *turbinotomy*—surgical incision of a turbinate bone.

Symptomatic Terms

- *anosmia*—absence of sense of smell. (4)
- *epistaxis*—nosebleed. (23, 32)
- *rhinorrhea*—thin, watery discharge from nose. (67)

Paranasal Sinuses

Origin of Terms

antro- (L)—cavity, antrum
ethmoid (G)—sieve
maxilla (L)—jawbone
sinus (L)—hollow
spheno- (G)—wedge, wedge shaped

Anatomic Terms (13, 23, 72)

- *ethmoidal sinus*—collection of small cavities or air cells in the ethmoidal labyrinth between the eye socket (orbit) and nasal cavity.
- *frontal sinus*—air space in the frontal bone above each orbit.
- *maxillary sinus, antrum of Highmore*—large air sinus of the maxillary bone.
- *sphenoidal sinus*—air space, variable in size, in the sphenoid bone. It is divided into right and left halves by a septum.

Diagnostic Terms

- *actinomycosis of sinus*—fungus infection in sinus.
- *pansinusitis*—inflammation of all the sinuses. (34, 61)
- *sinusitis*—inflammation of a sinus or sinuses. (34, 61)

Operative Terms

- *antrotomy*—opening of antral wall.
- *Caldwell-Luc operation*—radical maxillary antrotomy. (23)
- *ethmoidectomy*—excision of ethmoid cells. (23)
- *lavage of sinus*—washing out a sinus for removal of purulent material.

Larynx

Origin of Terms

chondro- (G) —cartilage
cricoid (G) —ringlike
glottis (G) —aperture of larynx
laryngo- (G) —larynx

larynx (G) —voice box
phono- (G) —voice
vox (L) —voice

Figure 41 Larynx, anterior view.

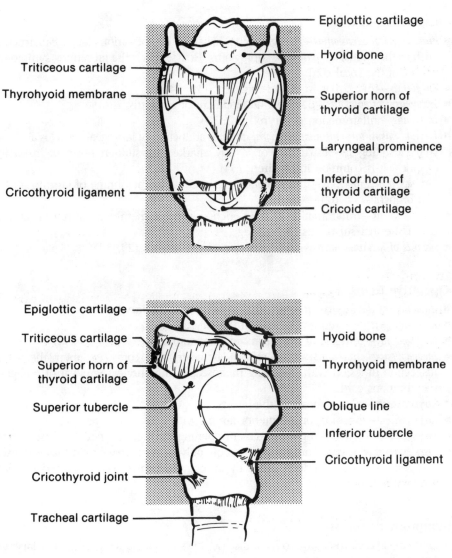

Posterior   Anterior

Figure 42 Larynx, right lateral view.

Anatomic Terms (13, 72)

- *cricoid cartilage*—ring-shaped cartilage of lowest part of larynx.
- *endolarynx*—interior of larynx, divided into a supraglottic portion, the glottis, and a subglottic portion.
- *epiglottis*—thin, leaf-shaped cartilage partially covered with mucuous membrane. It closes the entrance of the larynx during swallowing.
- *glottis*—two vocal folds with the rima glottidis between them.
- *larynx* (Figs. 41 and 42)—tone-producing organ, the voice box, composed of muscle and cartilage. Its interior surface is lined with mucous membrane.
- *rima glottidis*—narrowest portion of laryngeal cavity between the vocal folds.
- *vocal folds, vocal cords*—mucosal folds each containing a vocal ligament and muscle fibers.

Diagnostic Terms

- *endolaryngeal carcinomas*—malignant epithelial tumors of various laryngeal structures such as the glottis, subglottis or supraglottis. Hoarseness is the presenting symptom in cancer of the vocal cord. (13)
- *epiglottitis*—inflammation of the epiglottis. (32, 34)
- *hypoplasia of epiglottis*—defective development of epiglottis. (26)
- *laryngitis*—inflammation of larynx. (32, 39)
- *laryngospasm, laryngismus, laryngeal stridor*—adduction of laryngeal muscles and vocal cords resulting in obstruction of airway, marked by sudden onset of inspiratory dyspnea. It is common in children. (34)
- *laryngotracheobronchitis*—inflammation of the mucous membrane of larynx, trachea, and bronchi. (32, 62)
- *perichondritis*—inflammation of the perichondrium, a membrane of fibrous connective tissue that surrounds the cartilage.
- *stenosis of larynx*—narrowing or stricture of the larynx. (23, 34)

Operative Terms

- *dilatation of the larynx*—instrumental stretching of the larynx.
- *hemilaryngectomy*—removal of half of the larynx.
- *laryngectomy*—removal of the larynx for carcinoma.
- *laryngofissure and cordectomy*—incision between the cords to open the glottis, inspection of lesion with operating microscope, and surgical removal of malignant membranous cord.
- *laryngoplasty*—plastic repair of the larynx.
- *laryngoscopy*—examination of interior larynx with a laryngoscope. (66)
- *laryngostomy*—establishing a permanent opening through the neck into the larynx.
- *laser excision of laryngeal cancer*—method of applying a suitable surgical laser to excise malignant vocal cord lesions, aided by an operating microscope attached to a laser micromanipulator.

Symptomatic Terms

- *aphonia*—loss of voice due to local disease, hysteria, or injury to recurrent laryngeal nerve.
- *dysphonia*—difficulty in speaking, hoarseness.

Trachea

Origin of Terms

bi- (L)—two

steno- (G)—narrow

trachea (G)—windpipe, rough

Anatomic Terms (50, 72)

- *bifurcation*—division into two branches.
- *carina*—ridge between the trachea at the bifurcation.
- *trachea* (see Fig. 43)—windpipe composed of about 18 C-shaped cartilages, held together by elastic tissue and smooth muscle and extending from the larynx to the bronchi.

Diagnostic Terms

- *calcification of tracheal rings*—deposit of calcium in trachea.
- *stenosis of trachea*—contraction or narrowing of lumen of trachea. (59, 62)
- *tracheoesophageal fistula*—communication of esophagus with trachea, a congenital or acquired anomaly.
- *tracheopleural fistula*—communication of trachea with the pleura that may be caused by postoperative injury or pressure necrosis from inflated cuff of a tracheostomy tube. (50)

Operative Terms

- *tracheoplasty*—plastic operation on trachea.
- *tracheoscopy*—inspection of interior of trachea.
- *tracheostomy*—formation of a more or less permanent opening into the trachea, usually for insertion of a tube. Tracheostomy (or laryngostomy) is absolutely imperative before total laryngectomy to establish an open airway. It may be necessary after thyroidectomy and brain or lung surgery to overcome a tracheal obstruction. (32, 50)
- *tracheotomy*—incision into the trachea. (15)

Bronchi

Origin of Terms

bronchiolus (L)—air passage

bronchus (L)—bronchus, windpipe

-plasty (G)—surgical formation

-scope (G)—to examine, to view

Anatomic Terms (73)

- *bronchi, main* (see Fig. 43 p. 165)—the two primary divisions of the trachea, structurally resembling it.
  - —right main bronchus is shorter and more vertical than the left and is therefore more prone to become lodged with foreign bodies when aspirated. Its upper and lower parts provide the air passages for the three lobes of the right lung.
  - —left main bronchus gives rise to two lobar bronchi, which supply the lobes of the left lung.
- *bronchioles, bronchioli (sing. bronchiole, bronchiolus)*—the smaller subdivisions of the bronchial tubes, which do not have cartilage in their walls.

Diagnostic Terms

- *aplasia of bronchus*—undeveloped bronchus.
- *asthma*—disorder characterized by increased responsiveness of the trachea and bronchi to various stimuli, resulting in narrowing of the airways. These changes are reversible either spontaneously or as a result of treatment. Symptoms are variable in intensity and duration, which include wheezing, cough, and dyspnea. Patients with asthma may be classified into two clinical groups: extrinsic and intrinsic.
    - —*extrinsic asthma*—characterized by childhood onset or early adult onset. Periods of intermittent asthma are present. IgE level is raised. Family history of multiple allergies is common. The stimulus in extrinsic asthma is antigenic (dust, pollen, danders).
    - —*intrinsic asthma*—usually occurs in older adults. More continuous presence of asthma prevails. IgE normal or low. Family history of multiple allergies less common. Reversible airway obstruction is caused by various and unrelated stimuli that are nonantigenic (infection, pollution, cold, exercise, and psychogenic causes). (16)
- *bronchial carcinoid*—slowly growing, highly vascular tumor, potentially malignant, usually found in mainstem bronchus as an obstructive endobronchial lesion.
- *bronchiectasis*—dilatation of a bronchus or bronchi, with secretion of large amounts of offensive pus. (29, 44, 62)
- *bronchiectasic*—pertaining to bronchiectasis. (44)
- *bronchiogenic carcinoma*—lung cancer arises in the mainstem bronchus in 75 percent of patients with this malignant tumor. Metastasis occurs readily, since the great vascularity, rich network of pulmonary lymph nodes, and constant lung movements facilitate transport to neighboring and remote structures such as the brain, liver, and other organs. (55, 62)
- *bronchitis*—inflammation of the bronchial mucous membrane. Two types are:
    - —*simple chronic bronchitis*—a syndrome primarily reflecting a chronic productive cough that results from exposure to bronchial irritants in a person without hyper-reactive airways. Clinical criteria establishing simple chronic bronchitis include an excessive amount of mucous; presence of symptoms, mainly cough, on most days for at least three months annually during two or more successive years; and exclusion of bronchiectasis, tuberculosis, or other causes of these symptoms.
    - —*chronic obstructive bronchitis*—develops in a small percentage of individuals suffering from simple chronic bronchitis and results in irreversible narrowing of airways. When the obstruction is in the bronchioles and bronchi and is 2 mm or less in diameter, the term "small airways disease" is used. The condition reflected by chronic obstructive bronchitis is severe and disabling, manifested by increased resistance to airflow, hypoxia, and hypercapnia. (35, 39)
- *bronchopleural fistula*—open communication between a bronchus and the pleural cavity. This may be a complication of pulmonary resection. (28)
- *chronic obstructive diseases*—disorders of respiratory tract resulting from generalized bronchial narrowing and destruction of functional lung tissue. It is usually characterized by impaired expiratory outflow that responds poorly to therapy. The following respiratory disorders have chronic airway obstruction as a dominant feature: (35)
    - —*emphysema, chronic obstructive bronchitis*—severe disabling disorder, with presence of increased resistance to airflow, hypoxia, and usually hypercapnia.
    - —*small airways disease*—chronic obstructive bronchitis combined with simple chronic bronchitis that results in irreversible narrowing of airways. The obstruction occurs in the bronchioles and bronchi, 2 mm or less in diameter.

—*asthma*—recurrent episodes of symptomatic bronchospasm.

—*asthmatic bronchitis*—chronic bronchitis and episodic airway obstruction.

—*chronic asthmatic bronchitis*—persistent airway obstruction, chronic productive cough, and a major problem of episodic bronchospasm.

- *status asthmaticus*—prolonged state of severe asthma. (16)

Operative Terms

- *bronchoplasty*—plastic operation for closing fistula. (53)
- *bronchoscopy*—examination of the bronchi through a bronchoscope. (36, 55, 68)
- *bronchotomy*—incision into a bronchus.
- *YAG laser therapy*—application of the yttrium-aluminum-garnet (YAG) laser beam, which causes the tumor to vaporize on contact. This type of therapy has been used effectively in the treatment of malignant lesions of the trachea and bronchi. (51)

Lungs

Origin of Terms

apex (L)—tip

phthisis (G)—a wasting

pneumo- (G)—air, lung

pulmo-, pulmono- (L)—lung

Anatomic Terms (49, 73)

- *alveoli (sing. alveolus)*—air cells of the lungs in which the exchange of gases takes place.
- *apex of lung*—most superior part of the lung above the clavicle.
- *base of lung*—inferior part of the lung above the diaphragm.

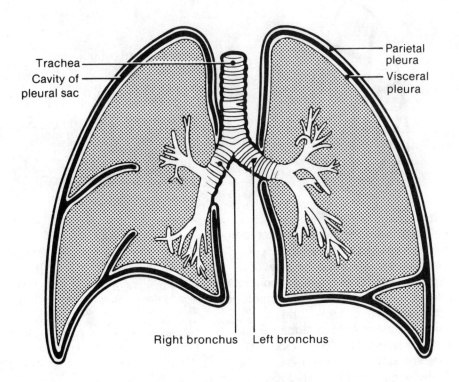

Figure 43   Trachea, bronchi, lungs, and pleural sacs.

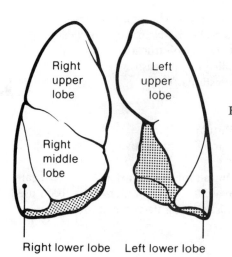

Figure 44 Lobes of lungs.

Figure 45 Bronchopulmonary segments of lungs.

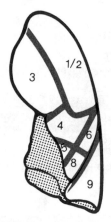

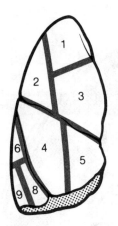

Right lung
1. Apical segment of upper lobe
2. Posterior segment of upper lobe
3. Anterior segment of upper lobe
4. Lateral segment of middle lobe
5. Medial segment of middle lobe
6. Apical segment of lower lobe
7. Medial segment of lower lobe
8. Anterior segment of lower lobe
9. Lateral segment of lower lobe
10. Posterior segment of lower lobe

Left lung
1. Apicoposterior segment of upper lobe
2. (Combined with #1 in left lung*)
3. Anterior segment of upper lobe
4. Superior lingular segment of upper lobe
5. Inferior lingular segment of upper lobe
6. Apical segment of lower lobe
7. Medial segment of lower lobe
8. Anterior segment of lower lobe
9. Lateral segment of lower lobe
10. Posterior segment of lower lobe

*The bronchopulmonary segment (#1) of the upper lobe of the left lung corresponds with the bronchopulmonary segments (#1 and #2) of the upper lobe of the right lung. Neither the medial segment (#7) nor the posterior segment (#10) has an anterior surface that would be visible from the anterior aspect of the lungs and therefore are not depicted in this illustration.

- *bronchopulmonary segment* (see Figs. 44 and 45)—one of the subdivisions of a pulmonary lobe, supplied with a bronchial tube, blood, and lymph vessels. The right lung has 10 segments, and the left lung has 9.
- *bronchopulmonary tree*—the lung compared to a hollow tree upside down in the thorax. The tree trunk is the trachea, kept open and stiffened by C-shaped bars of cartilage. The main bronchi are two large branches that ramify into smaller and smaller ones until they become leaf stems or bronchioles. These in turn form tiny airways, the alveolar ducts, which lead to countless clusters of air cells surrounded by capillaries. There the exchange of gases takes place.
- *hilus*—triangular depression on the medical surface of the lung that contains the hilar lymph nodes and the entrance or exit of blood and lymph vessels, nerves, and bronchi. They form the root of the lung.
- *lobe* (see Figs. 44 and 45)—major division of the lung composed of bronchopulmonary segments.
- *parenchyma*—the functional tissue of any organ; for example; the respiratory bronchioles, alveolar ducts, sacs, and alveoli, which participate in respiration.

Diagnostic Terms

- *abscess of lung*—a localized area of suppuration in the lung with or without cavitation. It is accompanied by necrosis of tissue. (7, 27)
- *acute respiratory failure*—life-threatening condition characterized by excessively high carbon dioxide tension or abnormally low oxygen tension of the arterial blood. It may be caused by blockage of air passages by tenacious secretions from lung infection, by exposure to atmospheric smog or other irritant inhalants, or by brain damage to the respiratory center. (42, 45, 62)
- *adult respiratory distress syndrome (ARDS)*—the essential feature is substantial intrapulmonary right-to-left shunt, a decreased functional residual capacity, and interstitial lung edema. Intubation and ventilation with positive and end-expiratory pressure (PEEP) is used in the treatment of this syndrome. (30, 54)
- *anthracosis*—disease of the lungs caused by the prolonged inhalation of fine particles of coal dust.
- *aplasia of lung*—incomplete development of the lung. (62)
- *asbestosis*—occupational disease caused by protracted inhalation of asbestos particles. (12, 36)
- *atelectasis*—functionless, airless lung or portion of a lung. (62, 64)
- *blast injury*—internal trauma of lungs, ears, and intestines resulting from high-pressure waves following an explosion. It may result in extreme bradycardia, severe cyanosis, dyspnea, hemorrhage, and deafness.
- *byssinosis*—chronic occupational lung disease caused by the inhalation of hemp, flax, or cotton. (62)
- *carcinoma of the lung; primary, secondary, or metastatic*—malignant new growth and the most important of the neoplastic diseases of the lung. Common tumors are:
  - *adenocarcinoma*—tumor containing glandular tissue that may form a mucinous secretion.
  - *oat cell carcinoma, small cell carcinoma*—very malignant tumor, notorious for its early, life-threatening metastases. It is thought to be a variant of bronchial carcinoid.
  - *squamous cell carcinoma*—the most common type of lung cancer, found almost exclusively in men.

Metastatic dissemination may occur to any organ but most frequently involves the liver, brain, adrenal glands and bones. (2, 51, 55)

- *chronic obstructive pulmonary disease (COPD)*—this refers to a class of diseases of uncertain etiology characterized by persistent slowing of airflow during forced expiration. This prolonged airway obstruction can cause disabling progressive respiratory disease, frequently with irreversible functional deterioration and fatal prognosis. (11, 35, 56)
- *histoplasmosis*—fungus disease caused by *Histoplasma capsulatum;* sometimes associated with calcified pulmonary lesions. (18, 27)
- *legionnaires' disease*—*Legionella pneumophila*—the gram-negative bacillus causing this disease, only recently has been described as a result of a dramatic outbreak of respiratory infections in individuals attending an American Legion Convention in Philadelphia. Erythromycin is the drug of choice for the treatment of this disease. Symptoms may include weakness, malaise, anorexia, dry cough, purulent or nonpurulent sputum, pleuritic pain, nausea, headache, vomiting, and diarrhea. High fever, relative bradycardia, dyspnea, confusion, and signs of consolidation are usually present. Pulmonary infiltrates progress to form patchy, localized lesions leading to multilobar lesions and consolidation. (9, 26, 74)
- *pneumoconiosis*—disease of the lungs caused by injury by dust from any source. (62)
- *pneumonia*—inflammation of the lungs with exudation into lung tissue and consolidation. Predominent etiologic agents are pneumococci and mycoplasmas or pleuropneumonia-like organisms (PPLO) and less frequently staphylococci, streptococci, meningococci, viruses, tubercle bacilli, and others. Hospital-acquired (nosocomial) infections are usually caused by gram-negative organisms. (69)
  Various types are:
    - —*bronchopneumonia*—inflammation of bronchioli and air vesicles with scattered areas of consolidation.
    - —*lobar pneumonia*—acute inflammation of one or more lobes of the lung or lungs.
    - —*primary atypical pneumonia*—infection caused by *Mycoplasma pneumoniae,* varying from mild to fatal disease. (8, 43, 67, 70)
- *pneumonitis*—inflammation of the lung; a virus form of pneumonia. (62, 69)
- *pneumonocele, pneumocele*—pulmonary hernia. (66)
- *pulmonary edema*—excess of intra-alveolar and intrabronchial fluid in the lungs, inducing cough and dyspnea; common in left-sided heart failure.
- *pulmonary embolism*—lodgment of a clot or foreign substance in a pulmonary arterial vessel, cutting off the circulation. (24, 33, 57)
- *pulmonary or vesicular emphysema*—overdistention of alveoli and smaller bronchial tubes with air. (65)
- *pulmonary hypertension*—condition caused by increased pressure in the pulmonary artery resulting from obstruction by pulmonary embolism or thrombosis, tuberculosis, emphysema, or pulmonary fibrosis. (57, 62)
- *pulmonary infarction*—necrosis of functional lung tissue (parenchyma) due to loss of blood supply usually caused by embolism. (57)
- *pulmonary thrombosis*—clot formation in any pulmonary blood vessel resulting in circulatory obstruction. (57)
- *pulmonary tuberculosis, phthisis*—a specific inflammatory disease of the lungs caused by tubercle bacillus and characterized anatomically by a cellular infiltration that subsequently caseates, softens, and leads to ulceration of lung tissue; manifested clinically by wasting, exhaustion, fever, and cough. (12, 38, 46)
- *shock lung*—pulmonary changes due to shock, closely resembling severe congestion and edema, both interstitial and intra-alveolar in nature. A shock lung is associated with marked hypoxia, diffuse intravascular coagulation, and formation of microthrombi. (1)

- *siderosis*—chronic respiratory disorder caused by the inhalation of iron oxide, an industrial hazard of arc welding or steel grinding leading to pulmonary irritation, chronic bronchitis, and emphysema. (16)
- *silicosis*—occupational disease due to inhalation of silica dust usually over a period of 10 years or more. (5, 62)

Operative Terms

- *biopsies:*
  - *lung biopsy*—small specimen of lung tissue used for pathologic, bacteriologic, and spectrographic studies to aid diagnosis.
  - *lymph node biopsy*—removal of tissue from scalene or supraclavicular lymph nodes for gross or microscopic examination to aid in the detection of cancer, tuberculosis, or other disease.
  - *percutaneous needle biopsy*—procedure used when tissue diagnosis is needed to plan radiation therapy and chemotherapy. The area to be biopsied is detected by television fluoroscopy. A biopsy needle is inserted through a small skin incision, and cells aspirated are used for cytologic and bacteriologic diagnosis. (19, 48, 49, 66)
- *bronchofiberscopy*—endoscopic examination of the tracheobronchial tree using a flexible bronchofiberscope to view the carina and right and left mainstem of bronchus. A 35 mm camera, attached to the bronchofiberscope, provides photographic documentation. (68)
- *excisional surgery (extirpative, definitive)*—partial or complete removal of the diseased lung. (49)
  - *lobectomy*—removal of a pulmonary lobe.
  - *lung resection, pulmonary resection*—partial excision of the lung, such as:
  - *segmental resection*—removal of a bronchopulmonary segment.
  - *subsegmental resection*—removal of a portion of a bronchopulmonary segment.
  - *pneumonectomy*—removal of an entire lung.
  - *wedge resection*—removal of a triangular portion of the lung, usually a small peripheral lesion, such as a tuberculoma.
- *extrapleural thoracoplasty*—multiple rib resection without entering the pleural space.
  - *primary*—to effect permanent collapse of the diseased lung and cavity closure.
  - *postlobectomy or postpneumonectomy*—to obliterate dead space subject to infection or to reduce empyema space. (49)
- *lung transplantation*—removal of patient's lung with subsequent replacement by implantation of a donor lung. In the past single lung transplantation procedures often threatened by infection and rejection occurrences provided discouraging results. However, several recent changes have greatly improved past results. These include strict adherence to preoperative criteria in selecting one-lung transplant recipients; the advent and availability of cyclosporine for immunosuppression combined with the avoidance of routine postoperative administration of prednisone in the first two or three weeks following transplantation; and a significant change in operative technique, which included the use of omentum (a long fold of membranes attached to the stomach and adjacent organs in the abdomen) to protect and revascularize the bronchial anastomosis. The omentum is wrapped around the ends of the bronchial tube where the new lung has been attached. When the omentum is placed in contact with damaged tissue, it is able to promote the growth of new blood vessels to facilitate the healing process. Patients suffering from various terminal pulmonary diseases and who are unresponsive to medical therapy may be candidates for single lung transplantation. These disorders may include pulmonary fibrosis, chronic

emphysema, cystic fibrosis, bronchiectasis, post-traumatic pulmonary insufficiency, and silicosis.

> —*heart lung transplantation*—removal of patient's heart and lungs with subsequent replacement by implantation of a donor's heart and lungs. Cyclosporine for immunosuppression has been a pivotal improvement in the reduction in morbidity and in the improvement in survival. It has also provided a major element in the revival of heart-lung transplantation procedures. The combined replacement of heart and lungs offers several advantages, e.g., all the diseased tissues are replaced and removed, and since the coronary-bronchial vascular beds are undisturbed, blood is supplied immediately to the tracheal anastomosis. By using endomyocardial biopsy procedures, the clinician can evaluate the rejection factor of both the heart and lung grafts. Those who would benefit from a heart-lung transplantation include children with congenital heart disease complicated either by irreversible vascular disease from prolonged left to right shunting or by marked hypoplasia of pulmonary arteries that makes correction impossible. Patients with moderate to severe pulmonary hypertension could also benefit. (3, 53, 63, 65)

- *pulmonary embolectomy*—removal of lung embolus employing extracorporeal circulation in patients presenting with massive embolus and profound circulatory collapse. (33, 57)

Symptomatic Terms

- *anoxemia*—deficient oxygen tension in arterial blood.
- *anoxia*—oxygen want in tissues and organs.
- *apnea, apnoea*—temporary absence of respiration; also seen in Cheyne-Stokes respiration.
- *bronchial or tubular breathing*—harsh breathing with a prolonged high-pitched expiration that may have a tubular quality. (41, 62)
- *Cheyne-Stokes respiration*—irregular breathing with shallow breaths that increase in depth and rapidity, then gradually decrease and cease altogether. After 10 to 20 seconds of apnea, the same cycle is repeated. (60)
- *cyanosis*—bluish color of skin due to deficient oxygenation.
- *dyspnea, dyspnoea*—difficult breathing. (40, 62)
- *expectoration*—act of coughing up and spitting out material from the lungs, trachea, and mouth.
- *hemoptysis*—expectoration of blood. (38)
- *hiccough, hiccup, singultus*—spasmodic lowering of the diaphragm followed by spasmodic, periodic closure of the glottis.
- *hypercapnia, hypercarbia*—excess of carbon dioxide in the circulating blood, with abnormally high carbon dioxide tension (Pco_2) causing overstimulation of respiratory center. (42)
- *hyperpnea*—respirations with increased rate and depth. (40, 50)
- *hyperventilation, hyperaeration*—excessive movement of air in and out of the lungs. (6, 57)
- *hyperventilation syndrome*—prolonged heavy breathing and long, sighing respirations causing marked apprehension, palpitation, dizziness, muscular weakness, paresthesia, and tetany. The attack may result from biochemical changes in neuromuscular and neurovascular function or from acute anxiety. (14)
- *hypoxia*—oxygen want due to decreased amount of oxygen in organs and tissues. (32, 47)
- *orthopnea, orthopnoea*—breathing possible only when person sits or stands.

- *paroxysmal nocturnal dyspnea (PND)*—attacks of difficult breathing, usually occurring in heart disease at night. (40)
- *rales*—bubbling sounds heard in bronchi at inspiration or expiration. (31, 62)
- *tachypnea*—abnormally rapid breathing. (25)

Thorax Pleura and Mediastinum

Origin of Terms

paries (L)—wall
phren (G)—diaphragm, mind
pleuro- (G)—pleura
pyo- (G)—pus

thorax (G)—breast plate, chest
viscus, viscera (L)—flesh, vital body organ
viscero- (L)—viscera, body organ

Anatomic Terms (12, 17, 72, 73)

- *mediastinum*—the interpleural space containing the pericardium, heart, major vessels, esophagus, and thoracic duct.
- *pleura (pl. pleurae)* (see Fig. 43)—thin sac of serous membrane that is invaginated by the lung and lines the mediastinum and thoracic wall. Each lung has its own pleural sac.
    - *parietal pleura*—the costal, mediastinal, and diaphragmatic parts of the pleura and the cupola, which covers the apex of the lung.
    - *visceral pleura, pulmonary pleura*—pleura that invests the lungs and lines the interlobal fissures.
- *pleural cavity*—potential space between the parietal and visceral pleurae, lubricated by a thin film of serum.
- *thorax, chest*—upper trunk composed of the thoracic vertebrae, sternum, ribs, costal cartilages, and muscles. The thoracic cage protects the vital organs of circulation and respiration as well as other mediastinal structures.

Diagnostic Terms

- *abnormal chest:*
    - *barrel chest*—barrellike appearance of chest on inspiration in advanced emphysema.
    - *flail chest, flapping chest cage*—instability of thoracic cage due to fracture of ribs or sternum or both
    - *pectus carinatum*—keeled chest
    - *rachitic chest*—resembling pigeon breast, as in rickets. (12, 17, 35, 37, 52)
- *empyema of pleura, pyothorax*—pus in pleural cavity.
- *hemothorax*—blood in pleural cavity caused by trauma or ruptured blood vessel. (12, 24, 28)
- *hydropneumothorax*—watery effusion and air in pleural cavity. (12, 27)
- *mediastinitis*—acute or chronic inflammation of the mediastinum. (12, 54)
- *mesothelioma of the pleura*—primary neoplasm arising from the surface lining of the pleura. Approximately three fourths of the pleural mesotheliomas are malignant, and the remaining one fourth present as localized benign tumors. (12, 28, 66)
- *pleural effusion*—excessive formation of serous fluid within the pleural cavity. (12, 37)
- *pleurisy, pleuritis*—inflammation of the pleura. (28)
- *pyopneumothorax*—pus and air in the pleural cavity. (12, 17)
- *spontaneous pneumothorax*—entrance of air into the pleural cavity resulting in a collapse of a lung. (12, 15)

- *tension or valvular pneumothorax*—entrance of air into pleural cavity on inspiration; air exit blocked by valvelike tissue on expiration; enlargement of pleural cavity and collapse of lung as positive pressure increases, resulting in mediastinal shift and depression of diaphragm. (15, 28)
- *tumors of mediastinum*—may not cause patient distress until they become large. Such tumors are often discovered on routine chest x-ray films or fluoroscopy. Biopsy of the mass may prove the best technique to establish a definitive diagnosis. A computed tomography scan of the thorax is the most precise noninvasive technique for detecting mediastinal tumors. Definitive treatment depends on the primary disease and extension of the tumor to other vital organs, such as heart, great vessels, esophagus, air passages, and surrounding nerves. Examples of these tumors are teratomas and neuroblastomas. (12, 17, 52)

Operative Terms

- *artificial or therapeutic pneumothorax*—the introduction of a measured amount of air into the pleural cavity through a needle to give the diseased lung temporary rest.
- *biopsies:*
    - —*mediastinal node biopsy*—resection of small piece tissue from regional lymph node for microscopy and culture.
    - —*pleural biopsy*—aspiration of cells from parietal pleura with biopsy needle for bacteriologic and histologic studies. (12, 17)
- *cervical mediastinotomy*—small incision into the mediastinum in the neck region to obtain biopsy specimen from lymph node for diagnostic evaluation.
- *mediastinoscopy*—examination of the mediastinal organs by a mediastinoscope under direct vision to aid in the diagnosis of disease and in assessing the resectability of bronchogenic carcinoma. (19, 48, 66)
- *pleurectomy:*
    - —*partial*—removal of a portion of the pleura.
    - —*complete*—removal of the entire pleura. This is generally associated with pneumonectomy.
- *pulmonary decortication*—removal of fibrinous exudate or pleural peel from the visceral surface of the imprisoned lung to restore its functional adequacy. (49)
- *thoracostomy, open*—surgical excision of rib segment to create an opening in the chest wall for drainage of the empyema space.

Symptomatic Terms

- *pleural adhesions*—fibrous bands that bind the visceral pleura to the parietal pleura. They may be loose, elastic, and avascular or firm, inelastic, and vascular. (66)
- *pleural effusion*—abnormal accumulation of fluid within the pleural space. (28, 37)
- *pleural exudate*—pus or serum accumulating in the pleural cavity. Fibrinous exudate may lead to the formation of adhesions. (28)
- *pleural peel*—abnormal layer of fibrous tissue adherent to the visceral pleura and underlying diseased lung. The ever-thickening peel may inhibit respiratory function.
- *pleuritic pain, pleurodynia*—sharp, intense pain felt in intercostal muscles. (66)

Special Procedures

- *augmented ventilation*—increased capillary circulation and gas exchange in respiration. The primary goal of assisted or augmented ventilation is to support ventilation until the patient can support ventilation for himself or herself.
    - —*continuous positive airway pressure (CPAP)*—measured in centimeters of H_2O

pressure, this technique may be used when the respiratory drive is normal and the pulmonary disease is not overwhelming.

—*intermittent mandatory ventilation (IMV)*—the patient breathes on his own, but at intervals mandatory respirations are supplied by the ventilator. This procedure permits a gradual weaning from mechanical ventilation to unaided breathing.

—*synchronized intermittent mandatory ventilation (SIMV)*—this is similar to IMV except that mandated breaths are synchronized with the patient's own spontaneous breathing rate. Utilizing the SIMV technique prevents delivery of a mandatory tidal volume from the ventilator on top of spontaneous inspiration.

—*intermittent positive pressure ventilation (IPPV)*—breaths received by bag or by a ventilator without continuous flow of gas through the circuit.

—*positive end-expiratory pressure (PEEP)*—maneuver used to increase the functional residual capacity of the lungs. It affects the airway during expiration, preventing intrathoracic pressures from returning to atmospheric pressure.

—*peak inspiratory pressure (PIP)*—peak positive pressure in centimeters of H_2O given at the top of the inspiration just before expiration. (6, 10, 20, 21, 22, 59, 71)

- *thoracentesis, pleurocentesis*—tapping of the pleural cavity to remove pleural effusion for diagnostic or therapeutic purposes. (12, 37, 48, 57)

Abbreviations

General

ACD—anterior chest diameter

AFB—acid-fast bacillus

A&P—auscultation and percussion

AP—anterior-posterior, anteroposterior
(projection of x-rays)

ARD—acute respiratory disease

ARDS—adult respiratory distress
syndrome

ARF—acute respiratory failure

BCG—bacillus Calmette-Guérin
(vaccine for tuberculosis)

BS—breath sounds

CMV—controlled mechanical ventilation

COPD—chronic obstructive pulmonary
disease

D^1Co_2—diffusion capacity of carbon
monoxide by the lung

FEF—forced expiratory flow

FEV—forced expiratory volume

Fio_2—fraction of inspired oxygen

FRC—functional residual capacity

IMV—intermittent mandatory ventilation

IPPB—intermittent positive-pressure
breathing

IPPV—intermittent positive-pressure
ventilation

IS, ICS—intercostal space

LSB—left sternal border

MBC—maximum breathing capacity

MCL—midcostal line

MSL—midsternal line

OT—old tuberculin

PA—posterior-anterior, posteroanterior

Pao_2—arterial oxygen tension

$Paco_2$—arterial carbon dioxide tension

PEEP—positive end-expiratory pressure

PIP—peak inspiratory pressure

PND—paroxysmal nocturnal dyspnea

PPD—purified protein derivative

PPLO—pleuropneumonia-like organisms

RD—respiratory disease

RM—respiratory movement

RV—residual volume

TB—tuberculosis

TF—tactile fremitus

TLC—total lung capacity

TNM—tumor, nodes, and metastases
(criteria for staging tumors)

URI—upper respiratory infection

VC—vital capacity

VF—vocal fremitus

Organizations

ALA—American Lung Association

ATS—American Thoracic Society

Oral Reading Practice

Legionnaires' Disease

Legionnaires' disease was first described as an acute pneumonia occurring in an outbreak among American citizens attending the Legionnaires' Conference in Philadelphia in 1976. By using **rickettsial** isolation techniques (eggs and animal inoculation) and by **rickettsial** stains, researchers found the organism to be a fastidious gram—negative bacillus.

Another diagnostic method that is valuable in such cases but not widely available at present is direct **immunofluorescent staining** of lung secretions or lung tissue by fluorescent-tagged antibody raised against **antigenic** determinants of the organism. Pneumonia caused by **Legionella pneumophila** is an acute alveolar process. Initially the pulmonary infiltrates are patchy and localized in character; however, these infiltrates progress to **multilobar** involvement and **consolidation.** The lower lobes are the most commonly affected sites. **Pleural effusion** and cavitation also may be present. Symptoms associated with **L. pneumophila** may include weakness, malaise, anorexia, dry cough, small amounts of sputum (either purulent or nonpurulent), chest pain, nausea, headache, vomiting, and diarrhea. Frequent symptoms such as high fever, **bradycardia,** dyspnea, confusion, and signs of consolidation are observed in some cases.

Erythromycin has proved the most effective antibiotic in the treatment of Legionnaires' disease. Other antibiotics, such as **rifampin,** may be used to supplement the erythromycin regime. (9, 26, 74)

Table 10

Some Respiratory Conditions Amenable to Surgery

Organs Involved	Diagnosis	Type of Surgery	Operative Procedures
Nasal septum	Deflection of septum, congenital or post-traumatic	Septectomy or submucous resection	Removal of nasal septum, partial or complete
Nasal mucosa	Mucous polyp	Excision of lesion	Removal of polyp
Maxillary sinus (antrum of Highmore)	Maxillary sinusitis due to streptococcus	Maxillary sinusotomy, antrum window operation	Opening of antrum
Larynx	Papilloma or cyst of larynx	Laryngoscopy with excision of lesion	Endoscopic examination with removal of neoplasm
Larynx Epiglottis Vocal cords	Squamous carcinoma of larynx	Total laryngectomy	Removal of entire larynx

Organs Involved	Diagnosis	Type of Surgery	Operative Procedures
Trachea	Carcinoma of larynx	Tracheostomy (preliminary step to laryngectomy)	Fistulization of trachea
Bronchi	Endobronchial tuberculosis	Bronchoscopy with aspiration of bronchial secretions	Endoscopic examination of bronchi
Broncho-pulmonary segment	Cystic disease of lung, tension air cyst	Segmental resection, lateral segment, middle lobe	Removal of segment, including tension air cyst of lung
Broncho-pulmonary segment	Moderately advanced tuberculosis with cavitation	Segmental resection, upper lobe	Removal of two segments of upper lobe
Bronchus Bronchioli Lung	Bronchiectasis, postinfectional	Lobectomy, middle lobe	Removal of middle lobe of lung
Lobe	Tuberculoma	Wedge resection, upper lobe	Excision of triangular-shaped tuberculoma
Lung	Far-advanced fibrocaseous tuberculosis	Lobectomy, upper lobe	Removal of upper lobe
Visceral pleura	Fibrinous pleurisy, lower lobe	Decortication, lower lobe	Excision of thickened fibrotic lesion of visceral pleura
Lung Visceral pleura	Carcinoma of lung or unilateral far-advanced tuberculosis	Pneumonectomy Pleurectomy	Removal of lung, including visceral pleura
Lung Thorax	Excessive pleural effusion, empyema	Postpneumonectomy thoracoplasty	Multiple rib resection in two stages

References and Bibliography

1. Abdoud, Francois. Shock. In Wyngaarden, James B., and Smith, Lloyd H., Jr., eds., *Cecil's Textbook of Medicine*, 18th ed., vol. 1. Philadelphia: W.B. Saunders Co., 1988, pp. 236-250.
2. Aisner, Joseph. Primary lung cancer. In Rakel, Robert E., ed., *Conn's Therapy—1988*, Philadelphia: W.B. Saunders Co., 1988, pp. 127-131.
3. Baldwin, John C. Lung transplantation. *Journal of the American Medical Association* 259:2286-2287, Apr. 15, 1988.
4. Baloh, Robert W. The special senses. In Wyngaarden, James B., and Smith, Lloyd H., Jr., eds., *Cecil's Textbook of Medicine*, 18th ed., vol. 2. Philadelphia: W.B. Saunders Co., 1988, pp. 2109-2124.
5. Banks, Daniel E. Silicosis. In Rakel, Robert

E., ed., *Conn's Therapy—1988*, Philadelphia: W.B. Saunders Co., 1988, pp. 161-163.

6. Barnes, Thomas A. Mechanical ventilation. In Barnes, Thomas A., ed., *Respiratory Care Practice*, Chicago: Year Book Medical Publishers, Inc., 1988, pp. 216-248.

7. Bartlett, John G. Lung abscess. In Wyngaarden, James B., and Smith, Lloyd H., Jr., eds., *Cecil's Textbook of Medicine*, 18th ed., vol. 1. Philadelphia: W.B. Saunders Co., 1988, pp. 435-438.

8. Baum, Stephen G. Mycoplasmal infections. In Wyngaarden, James B., and Smith, Lloyd H., Jr., eds., *Cecil's Textbook of Medicine*, 18th ed., vol. 2. Philadelphia: W.B. Saunders Co., 1988, pp. 1561-1565.

9. Beaty, Harry N., and Pasculle, A. William. Legionella infections. In Braunwald, Eugene, et al. eds., *Harrison's Principles of Internal Medicine*, 11th ed. New York: McGraw-Hill Book Co., 1987, pp. 620-623.

10. Beauchamp, Richard K. Pulmonary function testing procedures. In Barnes, Thomas A., ed., *Respiratory Care Practice*, Chicago: Year Book Medical Publishers, Inc., 1988, pp. 32-92.

11. Berry, Richard B., and Light, Richard W. Chronic obstructive pulmonary disease. In Rakel, Robert E., ed., *Conn's Therapy—1988*, Philadelphia: W.B. Saunders Co., 1988, pp. 121-127.

12. Brody, Jerome S. Diseases of the pleura, mediastinum, diaphragm, and chest wall. In Wyngaarden, James B., and Smith, Lloyd H., Jr., eds., *Cecil's Textbook of Medicine*, 18th ed., vol. 1. Philadelphia: W.B. Saunders Co., 1988, pp. 466-473.

13. Coleman, John J., III., and Jurkiewicz, M. J. The head and neck. In Sabiston, David C., Jr., ed., *Essentials of Surgery*, Philadelphia: W.B. Saunders Co., 1987, pp. 706-735.

14. Crystal, Ronald G. Interstitial lung disease. In Wyngaarden, James B., and Smith, Lloyd H., Jr., eds., *Cecil's Textbook of Medicine*, 18th ed., vol. 1. Philadelphia: W.B. Saunders Co., 1988, pp. 421-435.

15. Curreri, P. William. Management of the acutely injured person. In Wyngaarden, James B., and Smith, Lloyd H., Jr., eds., *Cecil's Textbook of Medicine*, 18th ed., vol. 1. Philadelphia: W.B. Saunders Co., 1988, pp. 180-199.

16. Daniele, Ronald P. Asthma. In Wyngaarden, James B., and Smith, Lloyd H., Jr., eds., *Cecil's Textbook of Medicine*, 18th ed., vol. 1. Philadelphia: W.B. Saunders Co., 1988, pp. 403-410.

17. Davis, R. Duane, Jr., and Sabiston, David C., Jr. Primary mediastinal cysts and neoplasms. In Sabiston, David C., Jr., ed., *Essentials of Surgery*, Philadelphia: W.B. Saunders Co., 1987, pp. 1020-1036.

18. Deepe, George S., Jr., and Bullock, Ward E. Histoplasmosis. In Rakel, Robert E., ed., *Conn's Therapy—1988*, Philadelphia: W.B. Saunders Co., 1988, pp. 135-138.

19. DeMeester, Tom R., and Albertucci, Mario. Surgical therapy. In Britain, Jacob D., et al., eds., *Lung Cancer: A Comprehensive Treatise*, Orlando: Grune & Stratton, Inc., 1988, pp. 135-147.

20. Douce, F. Herbert. Incentive spirometry and other aids to lung inflation. In Barnes, Thomas A., ed., *Respiratory Care Practice*, Chicago: Year Book Medical Publishers, Inc., 1988, pp. 208-215.

21. Dripps, Robert D., and Eckenhoff, James E. Respiration and respiratory care. In *Introduction to Anesthesia: The Principles of Safe Practice*, 7th ed. Philadelphia: W.B. Saunders Co., 1988, pp. 441-467.

22. ———. Inhalation therapy and pulmonary physiotherapy. Ibid., pp. 469-476.

23. Farmer, Joseph C. Otolaryngology. In Sabiston, David C., Jr., ed., *Essentials of Surgery*, Philadelphia: W.B. Saunders Co., 1987, pp. 686-705.

24. Fedullo, Peter F. Pulmonary embolism. In Rakel, Robert E., ed., *Conn's Therapy—1988*, Philadelphia: W.B. Saunders Co., 1988, pp. 154-158.

25. Fishman, Alfred P. Pulmonary hypertension. In Wyngaarden, James B., and Smith, Lloyd H., Jr., eds., *Cecil's Textbook of Medicine*, 18th ed., vol. 1. Philadelphia: W.B. Saunders Co., 1988, pp. 293-303.

26. Fraser, David W. Legionellosis. In Wyngaarden, James B., and Smith, Lloyd H., Jr., eds., *Cecil's Textbook of Medicine*, 18th ed., vol. 2. Philadelphia: W.B. Saunders Co., 1988, pp. 1570-1572.

27. Hill, Ronald C., and Sabiston, David C., Jr. Lung abscess and fungal infections. In Sabiston, David C., Jr., ed., *Essentials of Surgery*, Philadelphia: W.B. Saunders Co., 1987, pp. 984-988.

28. ———. Disorders of the pleura and empyema. Ibid., pp. 988-992.

29. ———. Bronchiectasis. Ibid., pp. 992-994.

30. Holman, William L., and Sabiston, David C., Jr. Thoracic outlet syndrome. In Sabiston, David C., Jr., ed., *Essentials of Surgery*, Philadelphia: W.B. Saunders Co., 1987, pp. 1010-1012.

31. Hopewell, Philip. Critical care medicine. In Wyngaarden, James B., and Smith, Lloyd H., Jr., eds., *Cecil's Textbook of Medicine*, 18th ed., vol. 1. Philadelphia: W.B. Saunders Co., 1988, pp. 482-501.

32. Jackler, Robert K., and Kaplan, Michael J. Ear, nose and throat. In Schroeder, Steven A., Krupp, Marcus A., and Tierney, Lawrence M., Jr., eds., *Current Medical Diagnosis & Treatment—1988*, Norwalk, CT: Appleton &

Lange, 1988, pp. 110-131.

33. Lyerly, H.K., and Sabiston, David C., Jr. Pulmonary embolism. In Sabiston, David C., Jr., ed., *Essentials of Surgery*, Philadelphia: W.B. Saunders Co., 1987, pp. 945-968.

34. Massie, F. Standford. Pediatric pulmonary medicine. In Crapo, James D., Hamilton, Michael A., and Edgman, Susan, eds., *Medicine & Pediatrics in One Book*, St. Louis: The C.V. Mosby Co., 1988, pp. 144-158.

35. Matthay, Richard A. Chronic airway disease. In Wyngaarden, James B., and Smith, Lloyd H., Jr., eds., *Cecil's Textbook of Medicine*, 18th ed., vol. 1. Philadelphia: W.B. Saunders Co., 1988, pp. 410-419.

36. ———. Abnormalities of lung aeration. Ibid., pp. 419-421.

37. Mentzer, Robert M., and Wyatt, David A. Pleural effusion and empyema (thoracis). In Rakel, Robert E., ed., *Conn's Therapy—1988*, Philadelphia: W.B. Saunders Co., 1988, pp. 139-141.

38. Moran, Jon F. The surgical treatment of pulmonary tuberculosis. In Sabiston, David C., Jr., ed., *Essentials of Surgery*, Philadelphia: W.B. Saunders Co., 1987, pp. 994-998.

39. Mufson, Maurice A. Viral pharyngitis, laryngitis, croup, and bronchitis. In Wyngaarden, James B., and Smith, Lloyd H., Jr., eds., *Cecil's Textbook of Medicine*, 18th ed., vol. 2. Philadelphia: W.B. Saunders Co., 1988, pp. 1757-1758.

40. Murray, John F. Introduction. In Wyngaarden, James B., and Smith, Lloyd H., Jr., eds., *Cecil's Textbook of Medicine*, 18th ed., vol. 1. Philadelphia: W.B. Saunders Co., 1988, pp. 390-394.

41. ———. Respiratory structure and function. Ibid., pp. 395-403.

42. ———. Respiratory failure. Ibid., pp. 473-481.

43. Neu, Harold C. Bacterial pneumonia. In Rakel, Robert E., ed. *Conn's Therapy—1988*; Philadelphia: W.B. Saunders Co., 1988, pp. 146-149.

44. Newth, Christopher. Bronchiectasis. In Wyngaarden, James B., and Smith, Lloyd H., Jr., eds., *Cecil's Textbook of Medicine*, 18th ed., vol. 1. Philadelphia: W.B. Saunders Co., 1988, pp. 438-440.

45. Peters, Jay I., and Jordan, J. Michael. Acute respiratory failure. In Rakel, Robert E., ed., *Conn's Therapy—1988*, Philadelphia: W.B. Saunders Co., 1988, pp. 115-119.

46. Prichard, John G., and Raliegh, James W. Tuberculosis and other myobacterial diseases. In Rakel, Robert E., ed., *Conn's Therapy—1988*, Philadelphia: W.B. Saunders Co., 1988, pp. 167-174.

47. Ravitch, Mark M., and Steichen, Felicien M. The chest wall. In *Atlas of General Thoracic Surgery*, Philadelphia: W.B. Saunders Co.,

1988, pp. 10-87.

48. ———. Diagnostic and therapeutic procedures. Ibid., pp. 161-187.

49. ———. Pulmonary resections. Ibid., pp. 189-291.

50. ———. The trachea. Ibid., pp. 293-331.

51. Sabiston, David C., Jr. Carcinoma of the lung. In Sabiston, David C., Jr., ed., *Essentials of Surgery*, Philadelphia: W.B. Saunders Co., 1987, pp. 998-1010.

52. ———. Disorders of the chest wall. Ibid., pp. 1012-1019.

53. Salvatierra, Oscar Jr., Melzer, Juliet, and Feduska, Nicholas J. Organ transplantation. In Way, Lawrence W., ed., *Current Surgical Diagnosis & Treatment*, 8th ed., Norwalk, CT: Appleton & Lange, 1988, pp. 1164-1178.

54. Schulak, James A., and Corry, Robert J. Surgical complications. In Sabiston, David C., Jr., ed., *Essentials of Surgery*, Philadelphia: W.B. Saunders Co., 1987, pp. 201-223.

55. Scoggin, Charles H. Pulmonary neoplasms. In Wyngaarden, James B., and Smith, Lloyd H., Jr., eds., *Cecil's Textbook of Medicine*, 18th ed., vol. 1. Philadelphia: W.B. Saunders Co., 1988, pp. 457-466.

56. Selecky, Paul A., and Young, Stephen L. Adult pulmonary medicine. In Crapo, James D., Hamilton, Michael A., and Edgman, Susan, eds., *Medicine & Pediatrics in One Book*; St. Louis: The C.V. Mosby Co., 1988, pp. 96-143.

57. Senior, Robert M. Pulmonary embolism. In Wyngaarden, James B., and Smith, Lloyd H., Jr., eds., *Cecil's Textbook of Medicine*, 18th ed., vol. 1. Philadelphia: W.B. Saunders Co., 1988, pp. 442-450.

58. Shapiro, Gail G. Allergic rhinitis due to inhalant factors. In Rakel, Robert E., ed., *Conn's Therapy—1988*, Philadelphia: W.B. Saunders Co., 1988, pp. 642-648.

59. Smith, Peter K., and Sabiston, David C., Jr. Physiologic aspects of respiratory function and management of respiratory insufficiency in surgical patients. In Sabiston, David C., Jr., ed., *Essentials of Surgery*, Philadelphia: W.B. Saunders Co., 1987, pp. 969-980.

60. Smith, Thomas W. Heart failure. In Wyngaarden, James B., and Smith, Lloyd H., Jr., eds., *Cecil's Textbook of Medicine*, 18th ed., vol. 1. Philadelphia: W.B. Saunders Co., 1988, pp. 215-236.

61. Stankiewicz, James A. Sinusitis. In Rakel, Robert E., ed., *Conn's Therapy—1988*, Philadelphia: W.B. Saunders Co., 1988, pp. 164-165.

62. Stauffer, John L. Pulmonary diseases. In Schroeder, Steven A., Krupp, Marcus A., and Tierney, Lawrence M., Jr., eds., *Current Medical Diagnosis & Treatment—1988*, Norwalk, CT: Appleton & Lange, 1988, pp. 132-188.

63. The Toronto Lung Transplant Group. Experience with single-lung transplantation for pulmonary fibrosis. *Journal of the American Medical Association* 259:2258-2262, April 15, 1988.

64. Todd, Thomas R. Atelectasis. In Rakel, Robert E., ed., *Conn's Therapy—1988*, Philadelphia: W.B. Saunders Co., 1988, pp. 119-121.

65. Turcotte, Jeremiah. Transplantation. In Sabiston, David C., Jr., ed., *Essentials of Surgery*, Philadelphia: W.B. Saunders Co., 1987, pp. 224-267.

66. Turley, Kevin. Thoracic wall, pleura, mediastinum and lung. In Way, Lawrence W., ed. *Current Surgical Diagnosis & Treatment*, 8th ed., Norwalk, CT: Appleton & Lange, 1988, pp. 276-316.

67. Turner, Ronald B. Viral respiratory infections. In Rakel, Robert E., ed., *Conn's Therapy—1988*, Philadelphia: W.B. Saunders Co., 1988, pp. 149-150.

68. Ungerleider, Rosa M., and Sabiston, David C., Jr. Bronchoscopy. In Sabiston, David C., Jr., ed., *Essentials of Surgery*, Philadelphia: W.B. Saunders Co., 1987, pp. 980-983.

69. Washington, John A., II. Techniques for noninvasive diagnosis of lower respiratory tract infections. *The Journal of Critical Illness* 3:97-103, Jan. 1988.

70. Welliner, Robert C. Viral and mycoplasmal pneumonia. In Rakel, Robert E., ed., *Conn's Therapy—1988*, Philadelphia: W.B. Saunders Co., 1988, pp. 150-152.

71. Wiezalis, Carl P. Intermittent positive-pressure breathing. In Barnes, Thomas A., ed., *Respiratory Care Practice*, Chicago: Year Book Medical Publishers, Inc., 1988, pp. 201-207.

72. Woodburne, Russel T., and Burkel, William E. The head and neck. In *Essentials of Human Anatomy*, 8th ed. New York: Oxford University Press, 1988, pp. 79-128.

73. ———. The chest. Ibid., pp. 346-406.

74. Yu, Victor L. Legionellosis (pontiac fever and legionnaires' disease). In Rakel, Robert E., ed., *Conn's Therapy—1988*, Philadelphia: W.B. Saunders Co., 1988, pp. 152-154.

Digestive Disorders

CHAPTER 8

Oral Cavity and Salivary Glands

Origin of Terms

bucca (L)—cheek
cheilo- (G)—lip
dento- (L)—tooth
gingiva (L)—gum
glossa (G)—tongue
labium (L)—lip
lingua (L)—tongue

mandible (L)—lower jaw
odonto- (G)—tooth
parotid (G)—beside the ear
sialo- (G)—salvia
staphylo- (G)—bunch of grapes
stoma (G)—mouth
uvula (L)—little grape

Anatomic Terms (Refs. 7, 111)

- *alveolus*—bony tooth socket.
- *hard palate, bony palate*—anterior part of roof of mouth.
- *soft palate*—posterior part of palate, partially separating the oral from the nasal part of the pharynx.
- *uvula*—small, cone-shaped, downward projection from the free lower edge of the soft palate in midline.
- *oral cavity*—the mouth. The oval-shaped cavity consists of two parts: 1) an outer, smaller part—the vestibule and 2) an inner, larger part—the mouth cavity proper.
    - *vestibule, vestibulum oris*—slitlike space, bounded externally by the lips and cheeks and internally by the gums and teeth.
    - *mouth cavity proper*—bounded laterally and ventrally by the alveolar arches and their contained teeth. Dorsally, it communicates with the pharynx by a constricted aperture termed the isthmus faucium. It is roofed in by the hard and soft palates, with the majority of the floor being formed by the tongue.
- *tongue*—located in the floor of the mouth, within the curve of the body of the mandible. The tongue assists in the mastication and deglutition of food. It serves as an important organ of speech and is the primary organ of the sense of taste.
- *papillae of tongue*—projections of the corium, thickly distributed over the anterior two thirds of its dorsum, giving to this surface its characteristic roughness. The various types of papillae represented are the vallate papillae, fungiform papillae, filiform papillae, and papillae simplices.

- *frenulum linguae*—mucous membrane between the floor of the mouth and the tongue in the midline, which is raised into a distinct vertical fold.
- *lips, labia oris*—two fleshy folds that surround the rima or orifice of the mouth. Externally the lips are covered by integument and internally by mucous membrane, between which are located the orbicularis oris muscle, the labial vessels, nerves, areolar tissue, fat, and many small labial glands.
- *frenulum*—median fold of mucous membrane that connects the inner surface of each lip in the midline to the corresponding gum.
- *gums, gingivae*—consists of dense fibrous tissue connected to the periosteum of the alveolar processes and surrounds the necks of the teeth.
- *tooth, teeth*—three portions of the tooth are:
  - *crown*—projects from the gum.
  - *root*—embedded in the alveolus.
  - *neck*—constricted portion between the crown and the root.

  The 20 teeth of the first set are termed the deciduous or milk teeth. The 32 teeth of the second set are termed the permanent teeth.
- *salivary glands:* (101, 111)
  - *major salivary glands*—three pairs of glands with ducts opening into the oral cavity. They secrete saliva, which moistens, dissolves, and transports food and produces a starch-splitting enzyme, amylase.
    - *parotid gland and duct (Stensen's duct)*—located below the ear.
    - *sublingual gland*—and 10 to 30 ducts situated on the floor of the mouth beneath the tongue; some of the ducts join to form the larger sublingual duct (duct of Bartholin), which opens into the submandibular duct.
  - *submandibular gland (formerly called submaxillary gland) and duct (Wharton's duct)*—situated mainly below the mandible.
  - *minor salivary glands*—numerous small glands in the tongue, cheeks, and lips.

Diagnostic Terms

- *oral cavity:*
  - *ankyloglossia*—tongue tie. (10)
  - *aphthous stomatitis*—small ulceration of the mucous membrane of the mouth. (8, 103)
  - *Behcet's syndrome*—presents as a recurrent oral ulceration, usually indistinguishable from aphthous ulceration. The ulceration occurs in clusters, and associated genital ulceration, iritis, and conjunctivitis may be seen also. (8)
  - *benign mucous membrane pemphigoid*—recurrent painful bullae that desquamate and leave a large, ulcerated area in the oral cavity. (9)
  - *candidiasis, pseudomembranous candidiasis (thrush)*—curdlike, creamy patches in the mouth caused by overgrowth of *Candida albicans*. Pain, fever, and lymphadenopathy may be present. The fungal growth is prone to occur when antibiotics, corticosteroids, or cytostatic therapy or active illness upsets the normal flora.
    - *pseudomembranous candidiasis (thrush)*—favors the buccal mucosa, palate, and tongue areas.
    - *atrophic candidiasis*—occurs when the condition of pseudomembranous candidiasis is not treated, or it may occur as a complication to drug therapy, e.g., broad-spectrum antibiotics, immunosuppressive agents, and/or cytostatic agents. (61, 103)
  - *cavity of tooth, dental caries*—localized progressive decay or loss of tooth structure. In addition to decay, other causes may be attrition, abrasion, erosion, or developmental defects. (4, 103)

—*chilitis, cheilitis*—inflammation of the lips.

—*cleft lip, harelip*—congenital anomaly of upper lip consisting of a vertical fissure, often associated with cleft palate. (42)

—*cleft palate*—congenital fissure of the roof of the mouth due to nonunion of bones. (42)

—*epulis, giant cell epulis*—peripheral giant cell granulomatous lesion of the gingiva that develops in response to trauma or hemorrhage. (108)

—*gingivitis*—inflammation of the gums. (4)

—*glossitis*—inflammation of the tongue. (61, 103)

—*herpangina*—coxsackie A viral infection, although coxsackie B and echoviruses may be infecting agents also. Ulcerating vesicles appear on the anterior of the tonsillar soft palate, uvula, and tonsils. (108)

—*periapical abscess*—abscessed tooth caused by dental decay and leading to infection of the pulp. (61, 103)

—*periodontal disease*—dental disorders characterized by inflammation of the gums, destruction of alveolar bone, degeneration of periodontal ligament, and accumulations of microorganisms and plaque on tooth surfaces. Food, bacteria or calcifications located between the gums and teeth areas (dental pockets) may cause the formation of pus (pyorrhea). (61, 103)

—*squamous cell carcinoma*—most frequently occurring malignant neoplasm of the oral cavity. It usually presents as an infiltrative lesion with a fissurelike ulceration. Metastasis develops early and spreads to contralateral side and mandible. (61, 103, 106)

—*torus palatinus*—benign overgrowth of the hard palate. Bony, asymptomatic lesions may be present along the inner aspect of the mandible. (106)

—*Vincent's infection, acute necrotizing gingivitis, trench mouth*—painful inflammatory condition of the gums, usually associated with fever, ulcerations, bleeding, and lymphadenopathy. (61)

■ *salivary glands:*

—*carcinoma of a salivary gland*—malignant neoplasm arising from the glandular epithelium of a salivary gland. (46, 54, 106)

—*epidemic parotitis, mumps*—painful, swollen viral disorder of the parotid gland. Exposure to this disease occurs 14-21 days prior to acute phase onset. Fever and malaise may be present, as well as swelling and tenderness of the sublingual and submandibular glands. (101, 110)

—*parotitis*—inflammation of parotid gland. (4)

—*ptyalith, sialolith*—stone in salivary gland. (101)

—*sialadenitis*—inflammation of a salivary gland. (54, 61)

—*sialolithiasis*—calculi forming in the major ducts of the submandibular (formerly called the submaxillary), sublingual, and parotid glands. (101, 106)

Operative Terms

■ *oral cavity:*

—*cheiloplasty*—plastic repair of lip.

—*cheilostomatoplasty*—plastic repair of lip and mouth for cleft lip. (42)

—*clipping of frenulum (frenum) linguae*—clipping of membranous fold below the tongue to relieve tongue tie.

—*glossectomy, complete*—removal of entire tongue, generally done for carcinoma. (22)

—*glossectomy, partial; hemiglossectomy*—resection of the tongue. (22)

—*glossorrhaphy*—suture of injured tongue.

—*lip reconstruction*—repair of lip that may be done following resection of malignant lesion of lip. (22)

—*oral cavity cancer resection*—removal of cancerous tumor, usually followed by immediate reconstruction, either by direct primary closure of oral cavity defect, local tongue flap, or other procedure. (106)

—*palatoplasty*—repair of cleft palate. (42)

—*periapical tissue biopsy*—microscopic tissue study of the periapex (around the root of a tooth) to determine the benign or malignant character of the pathologic process. (61)

—*radical neck dissection*—total removal of all metastatic lesions in the cervical region, together with the primary cancer. This includes lymph nodes, lymphatics, veins (such as the jugular), surrounding muscle, fascia, and fat, which constitute the repository for metastatic dissemination of the primary cancer. Neck dissection may be combined with glossectomy, laryngectomy, and thyroidectomy, as well as resection of the mandible, palate, and maxilla, depending on the extent of the malignant involvement. (22, 42)

—*stomatoplasty*—plastic repair of mouth.

- *salivary glands*

—*sialadenectomy*—removal of a salivary gland.

—*sialolithotomy*—incision of salivary gland and removal of a stone. (106)

—*subtotal parotidectomy*—partial resection of parotid gland with removal of benign tumor. (42)

—*total parotidectomy*—wide excision of malignant tumor and gland, sometimes including metastatic lesions. (42)

Symptomatic Terms

- *glossodynia*—painful tongue caused by a chronic inflammatory process of lingual papillae. (61)
- *halitosis*—offensive odor of breath. (70)
- *leukoplakia of the mouth*—white patches on the mucous membrane of the tongue and buccal mucosa. (61, 103)
- *ptyalism, salivation*—excessive secretion of saliva.

Pharynx and Esophagus

Origin of Terms

esophagus (G)—food-carrier, gullet
fauces (L)—throat

pharynx (G)—throat
tonsilla (L)—almond, tonsil

Anatomic Terms (28, 92, 111)

- *crypts*—follicles or pits in tonsils.
- *esophagus*—a 23 to 25 centimeter long muscular canal extending from the pharynx to the stomach.

—*abdominal esophagus*—portion of the esophagus that lies in the esophageal groove on the posterior surface of the left lobe of the liver.

—*cervical esophagus*—portion of esophagus in the neck.

—*thoracic esophagus*—portion of esophagus that passes through the thorax.

- *lower esophageal sphincter*—area of high pressure between the distal esophagus and stomach.

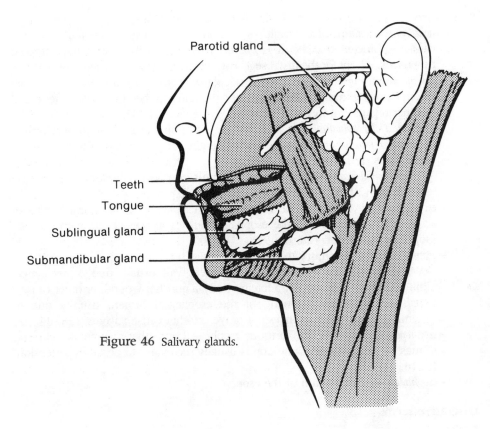

Figure 46 Salivary glands.

- *upper esophageal sphincter*—area of increased intraluminal pressure between the distal esophagus and stomach.
- *palatine tonsil, faucial tonsil*—collection of lymphoid tissue lodged in the tonsillar fossa on either side of the oval part of the pharynx.
- *pharyngeal recess, fossa of Rosenmüller*—deep recess located behind the ostium of the auditory tube.
- *pharyngeal tonsil*—collection of lymphoid tissue located in the posterior wall of the nasal part of the pharynx. During childhood, this tonsil may become hypertrophied into a considerable mass, at which time, it is termed "adenoid."
- *pharynx*—fibromuscular tube lined with mucous membrane and divided into oral, nasal, and laryngeal parts. It extends from the nose and mouth to the esophagus and serves as a common pathway for food and air.

Diagnostic Terms

- *pharynx:*
    - —*adenoids*—enlarged pharyngeal tonsils. (4)
    - —*adenotonsillitis*—bacterial-viral disorder characterized by abnormal oropharyngeal or nasopharyngeal microflora caused by streptococci, adenoviruses, or other organisms. (54)
    - —*hypertrophy of tonsils*—enlarged palatine tonsils. (4)
    - —*peritonsillar abscess, quinsy*—localized collection of pus around the tonsil. (55)
    - —*pharyngitis*—inflammation of pharynx. (54)
    - —*tonsillitis*—inflammation of the tonsils, especially the palatine tonsils. (4, 54)

- *esophagus:*
    - —*achalasia, dilatation of esophagus*—common disorder caused by failure of the cardiac sphincter to relax. It is characterized by a dilated and hypertrophid esophagus, except for the distal segment, which may be atrophied. (28, 61, 92)
    - —*carcinoma of esophagus*—malignant neoplasm, commonly an epidermoid carcinoma, arising from the epidermis or squamous epithelium; metastatic spread to other organs is a frequent occurrence. (28, 32, 61, 84, 92)
    - —*diverticula of esophagus (sing. diverticulum)*—outpouchings of esophageal wall.
    - —*pulsion or true diverticula*—consists of bulging of the mucosa through weakened parts of the esophageal wall.
    - —*traction or false diverticula*—result from pull exerted by diseased neighboring structures. (20, 61, 70, 84, 92)
    - —*esophageal reflux ulceration*—ulceration of the esophagus resulting from reflux of acid-peptic secretions into the esophagus due to incompetence of the gastro-esophageal sphincter. (28, 61, 92)
    - —*esophageal trauma*—injury to the esophagus.
    - —*esophageal perforation*—hole in the esophageal wall, usually due to mechanical injury through ingestion of a foreign body, a gunshot wound, or other causes.
    - —*esophageal stricture*—narrowing of the esophageal lumen, usually due to chemical injury, such as ingestion of lye or other caustic agents. (28, 84, 92)
    - —*esophageal varices*—swollen, tortuous esophageal veins that may burst and result in massive hemorrhage. Condition is usually secondary to portal hypertension. (3, 16, 93)
    - —*esophagitis*—inflammation of the esophagus. (92)

Operative Terms

- *pharynx:*
    - —*adenotonsillectomy*—removal of adenoids and tonsils. (51)
    - —*pharyngeal flap operation, pharyngeal flap augmentation*—conservative palate repair that permits an essentially normal maxillary and dental arch development, thus preventing facial and oral deformities and the hypernasality of cleft palate speech. (108)
- *esophagus:*
    - —*bougienage for esophageal stricture*—dilatation of the esophagus with bougies, flexible instruments resembling sounds, used to diagnose and treat strictures of tubular passages. A safe procedure is to insert the bougies by the retrograde method through a gastrostomy and pull them through the esophagus and the stricture and out through the gastrostomy. (28, 79, 92)
    - —*esophageal diverticulectomy*—excision of diverticulum and closure of resulting defect. (70)
    - —*esophagojejunostomy*—formation of a communication between the esophagus and jejunum.
    - —*esophagoplasty*—reconstruction or plastic repair of esophageal defect. (28)
    - —*esophagoplasty with reversed gastric tube*—physiologic method of esophageal replacement using the patient's own stomach to avoid immune reactions caused by rejection of transplants. (28)
    - —*esophagorrhaphy*—suture of injured or ruptured esophagus.
    - —*fundic patch operation*—surgical procedure for repair of ruptured esophagus or acid-peptic stricture and in the treatment of advanced achalasia. (79, 84)
    - —*fundoplication*—operative procedure to relieve gastroesophageal reflux of large amounts of acid-peptic juice to restore gastroesophageal competence. (28, 54, 79, 84)

—*Heller esophagomyotomy*—incision into the circular muscle fibers of the distal esophagus to relieve achalasia. (21, 28)

—*radical resection for esophageal cancer*—excision of tumor-bearing portion of esophagus and regional lymph nodes, followed by restoration of continuity by anastomosis or interposition of loop of colon or jejunum. (28)

—*resection for esophageal stricture*—removal of extensive narrow segment, followed by colonic bypass. The right colon, with terminal ileum and ileocecal valve, is tunneled into the neck and anastomosed with the proximal esophagus. The operation is indicated when chronic stricture is unresponsive to bougienage. Sometimes, a gastric tube is used as a means of reconstruction. (28, 79)

Symptomatic Terms

- *aphagia*—inability to swallow.
- *deglutition*—swallowing. (28)
- *dysphagia*—difficulty in swallowing. (79, 92)
- *regurgitation*—backflow of gastric contents into the mouth. (79, 84)

Stomach

Origin of Terms

fundus (L)—base
gastr-, gastro- (G)—stomach
pyloro- (G)—gatekeeper, pylorus

ruga (L)—fold, crease
sphincter (G)—binder

Anatomic Terms (60, 91, 92, 112)

- *antrum, gastric*—distal nonacid secreting segment of the stomach or pyloric gland region that produces the hormone gastrin.
- *body of stomach*—largest portion of the stomach, between the antrum and fundus. (See Table 11, p. 188 for various stomach types.)
- *cardia*—small area of the stomach near the esophagogastric junction.
- *cardiac orifice*—opening at the junction of the esophagus with the stomach.
- *curvatures of stomach:*
    - *lesser*—right and superior margin of the stomach.
    - *greater*—left and inferior margin of the stomach.
- *fundus of stomach*—enlarged portion to the left located above the level of the cardiac orifice.
- *omenta (sing. omentum)*—peritoneal sheets connecting the stomach with other viscera, such as the liver, spleen, and transverse colon.
- *pyloric part of stomach*—distal segment of the stomach, including:
    - the antrum or pyloric gland area
    - the pyloric canal
- *pyloric sphincter*—circular muscle around the pylorus.
- *pylorus*—opening between stomach and duodenum.
- *rugae (sing. ruga)*—irregular folds of the mucous membrane of the stomach in which gastric glands are embedded.

Diagnostic Terms

- *gastric malignant neoplasms:* (60, 61, 69, 91, 92)
    - *carcinoma*—usually adenocarcinoma, a malignant new growth of the glandular epithelium. These neoplasms develop mainly along the lesser curvature of the stomach.

> —*lymphoma*—tumors arising from lymphoid tissue. These tumors may be found at any site in the stomach but favor the posterior wall, lesser curvature of the body, and antrum.
>
> Some types of lymphoma are:
> —*Non-Hodgkin's lymphoma*
> —*round cell lymphosarcoma*
> —*reticulum cell lymphosarcoma*
> —*Hodgkin's lymphoma*
> —*plasmacytoma*
> —*malignant smooth muscle tumors of the stomach*—nonepithelial malignant lesions involving the stomach. Some types of this tumor are:
> —*leiomyosarcoma*
> —*leiomyoblastoma**
> —*Other mesenchymal tumors of the stomach that occur rarely are:*
> —*angiosarcoma*
> —*hemangiopericytoma*
> —*Kaposi's sarcoma*
> —*liposarcoma*
> —*linitis plastica (leather-bottle type of stomach)*—occurs at the pylorus and spreads toward the cardia. The pylorus canal becomes constricted by the overgrowth of fibrous tissue, resulting in dilatation of the stomach in its proximal part. When this occurs, the disorder is termed chronic scirrhous carcinoma of the pylorus. This type of cancer is confined to the wall of the stomach for a long period of time and its growth progresses slowly. Metastases usually occurs late in the disease process. Finally, the stomach is transformed into a leathery rigid tube that is incapable of being distended; hence its capacity is limited to a few ounces.

- *gastric polyps*—lesions that project above the surface of the surrounding mucosa or submucosa. Most polyps are sessile; however, the larger polyps may be pedunculated. When the major portion of the gastric mucosal surface reflects numerous polypoid lesions, the disorder is termed "diffuse polyposis." Most of the polyps or benign tumors that occur in the stomach may be classified as follows: (60, 69, 92)
  > —*epithelial polyps:*
  > —*hyperplastic (regenerative) polyps*
  > —*adenomatous polyps*
  > —*mesenchymal or mesothelial polyps:*
  > —*leiomyomas*
  > —*fibromas*
  > —*neurogenic tumors*
  > —*lipomas*
  > —*vascular tumors*
  > —*others:*
  > —*aberrant pancreatic tissue polyps*
  > —*inflammatory pseudotumors*
  > —*hemartomas*
  > —*Peutz-Jeghers polyps*
- *gastric ulcers*—localized erosions of gastric mucosa that may result from digestive action of acid gastric secretion. Secondary involvement of muscle tissue may occur. (38, 61, 89, 92)

---

*(The World Health Organization has termed this lesion epitheloid leiomyoma. These two terms are used interchangeably.)

—*chronic gastric ulcer*—chronic peptic ulceration, characteristically involving the non-acid-secreting antral area and seldom the acid-forming parietal cell region of the stomach.

—*stress ulcer, stress erosive gastritis*—presence of single or multiple ulcerative lesions of the fragile mucosa of the stomach in response to a stressful situation, such as trauma, major surgery, head injury, alcoholic excesses, or increased steroid secretion. A gastric erosion represents a partial disruption of the epithelium, while an ulcer represents penetration through the muscularis mucosae. Superficial erosions rarely cause massive bleeding; however, deeper lesions may penetrate the large arteries that transverse the submucosa and massive bleeding may occur.

- *gastritis*—acute or chronic inflammation of the gastric mucosa. (60, 61, 69, 71, 88, 90, 91)

—*acute hemorrhagic gastritis*—the most severe form of aspirin-induced gastritis and a frequent cause of upper gastrointestinal hemorrhage.

—*atrophic gastritis*—chronic inflammatory process in which atrophic changes of the gastric mucosa are usually irreversible and progressive.

—*hyperplastic gastropathy*—predominant feature is hyperplasia (number of normal cells increased) rather than hypertrophy (number of cells enlarged) or inflammation. Some syndromes associated with hyperplastic gastropathy:

—*Ménétrier's disease*—usually interpreted as a synonym for protein-losing gastropathy. Originally Ménétrier's disease was concerned with the premalignant nature of the gastric lesion and not with its relation to protein loss.

—*mixed or combined type of hyperplastic gastropathy*—presents as a hyperplasia of mucous and specialized glandular cells and may be associated with hypersecretion of pepsin and acid without protein loss. Usually there are no clinical symptoms.

—*mucous cell or foveolate (pitted) type*—seen in Ménétrier's disease; characterized by hyperplasia of the mucous-secreting cells of the surface epithelium and foveolar pits. Hypochlorhydria and loss of albumin into gastric secretions, leading to hypoproteinemia and edema, may be associated with Ménétrier's disease.

—*Zollinger-Ellison syndrome*—excessive gastric secretion rapidly worsening, with refractory or recurrent peptic ulceration and hyperplasia of pancreatic islet cells; may result from an ulcerogenic tumor in the pancreas.

- *gastrocele*—hernia of the stomach, such as diaphragmatic gastric hernia.
- *gastrocolitis*—inflammation of the stomach and colon.
- *gastroduodenitis*—inflammation of the stomach and duodenum.
- *gastroenteritis*—inflammation of the stomach and intestine. (39, 92)
- *gastroptosis*—downward displacement of the stomach.
- *hiatal hernia, hiatus hernia*—protrusion of part of the stomach through the esophageal opening of the diaphragm. (84)
- *hypertrophic pyloric stenosis, congenital*—condition seen in the newborn characterized by an overgrowth of muscle fibers that markedly diminishes the lumen of the pyloric canal and gives rise to obstruction. (82, 92)
- *Mallory-Weiss syndrome*—longitudinal lacerations of the gastroesophageal mucosa causing upper gastrointestinal bleeding. (20, 60, 70)
- *Peutz-Jeghers syndrome*—mucocutaneous pigmentation and gastrointestinal polyposis. The polyps are usually large, pedunculated, and lobulated. The syndrome may involve the stomach, small intestine, and colon. (66)

Table 11
Gastric Types in Relation to Architectural Structures of Individuals

Type of Stomach	Description of Type of Stomach	Tonicity of Stomach	Graphic Description
Hypersthenic— individual stocky short	Stomach high, wide above, narrow below, transverse position, pylorus to the right	Hypertonic Increased tone	
Sthenic— individual well-built	Stomach tubular in shape, as wide above as it is below, pylorus to the right, well above umbilicus	Orthotonic Normal tone	
Hyposthenic— individual more slender	Stomach longer, narrower at the top; tendency to sag below greater curvature near umbilicus; pylorus swinging to the left	Hypotonic Decreased tone	
Asthenic— individual still more slender	Stomach sags far down below umbilicus, being almost collapsed above, expanding into large sac below	Atonic Weak tone	

Operative Terms

- *anastomosis*—surgical formation of a passage or opening between two hollow viscera or vessels; for example, gastrojejunostomy. (59, 60, 105)
- *antrectomy, gastric*—removal of the gastrin-producing pyloric gland area of the stomach. (105)
- *gastrectomy*—partial or subtotal removal of the stomach. Total gastrectomy with jejunal interposition has been advocated for Zollinger-Ellison syndrome. (60, 91, 105)
- *gastric resection*—removal of 50 to 75 percent of the stomach, combined with one of the following procedures: (59, 60, 105)
    —*gastroduodenal anastomosis, Billroth I*—joining the resected stomach to the duodenum.
    —*gastrojejunal anastomosis, Billroth II*—joining the remaining stomach to the jejunum by either the:
    —*Polya technique*—anterior anastomosis, large stoma
      or
    —*Hofmeister technique*—posterior anastomosis, small stoma
- *gastrojejunostomy*—creation of a communication between the stomach and jejunum. (60, 69)
- *gastrostomy*—external fistulization of the stomach. This may be done for the purpose of maintaining nutrition. (79)
- *pyloromyotomy, Fredet-Ramstedt operation*—incision of the hypertrophic pyloric muscle down to the mucosa. (82)
- *pyloroplasty*—revision of pyloric stoma. Procedures of choice are usually those of Finney and Heinecke-Mikulicz. (60, 91)

- *repair of hiatus hernia*—several different methods are used, either by the transthoracic or transabdominal approach; for example, freeing the esophagus at the cardia and attaching the region of the esophagogastric junction to the defect in the diaphragm. (79)
- *vagotomy, gastric*—the surgical interruption of vagal impulses to the pyloric gland area (antrum) and the gastric parietal cell region. (105)
- *vagotomy, selective gastric*—vagal denervation restricted to the parietal cell mass of the stomach. (60, 91, 105)
- *vagotomy and antrectomy*—surgical destruction of vagal impulses and excision of the gastric antrum for removing the major stimuli to acid production in gastric and duodenal ulcers. (91, 105)

Symptomatic Terms

- *achlorhydria*—absence of hydrochloric acid in the gastric juice. (61)
- *achylia gastrica*—absent or reduced gastric secretion due to atrophy of the mucosa of the stomach. (108)
- *anorexia*—loss of appetite. (104)
- *bulimia*—alternate cramming of food and induced vomiting. (104)
- *cyclic vomiting*—periodic vomiting.
- *dumping syndrome*—symptoms occurring after meals following gastrectomy. The patient experiences sweating, flushing, warmth, faintness, and sometimes diarrhea. (61)
- *dyspepsia*—imperfect digestion. (61)
- *epigastric pain*—pain over the pit of the stomach.
- *eructation*—belching. (104)
- *hematemesis*—vomiting blood. (61, 69, 84)
- *hyperchlorhydria*—excessive amount of hydrochloric acid in the gastric juice.
- *hypochlorhydria*—deficient amount of hydrochloric acid in the stomach. (88)
- *hypergastrinemia*—highly increased serum gastrin levels, found in Zollinger-Ellison syndrome and pernicious anemia. (71, 89, 90, 91)
- *intrinsic factor, Castle's intrinsic factor*—factor normally present in gastric mucosa and gastric juice and required for absorption of vitamin B_{12}. It is absent in pernicious anemia. (108)
- *polyphagia*—excessive food intake.
- *pyrosis*—heartburn. (84)

Small and Large Intestines

Origin of Terms

appendix (L)—appendage
cecum (L)—blind gut
colon (G)—large intestine
duodenum (L)—twelve, duodenum
enter-, entero- (G)—intestine

ileo- (L)—ileum
jejuno- (L)—jejunum
procto- (G)—anus
recto- (L)—rectum
vermiform (L)—shape of worm

Anatomic Terms (85, 92, 112)

- *small intestine*—proximal portion of intestine from pylorus to ileocecal junction.
    - *—duodenum*—first part of small intestine; extends from pylorus to jejunum.
    - *—jejunum*—second part of small intestine; extends from duodenum to ileum.
    - *—ileum*—third part of small intestine; extends from jejunum to cecum.

—*mesentery*—peritoneal fold that carries the blood supply and attaches the jejunum and ileum to the posterior abdominal wall.

■ *large intestine*—distal portion of intestine, including cecum, appendix, colon, rectum, and anal canal.

—*anus*—outlet or orifice of anal canal.

—*appendix vermiformis*—an intestinal diverticulum projecting from cecum 3 to 13 cm and ending blindly.

—*cecum*—blind pouch of large intestine at and below level of ileocecal junction.

—*colon*—large intestine from cecum to rectum, including the ascending colon, transverse colon, descending colon, and sigmoid or pelvic colon.

—*flexures of colon:*

—*right colic flexure, formerly hepatic flexure*—bend of colon near liver.

—*left colic flexure, formerly splenic flexure*—bend of colon near spleen.

—*mesocolon*—mesentery attaching the colon to the posterior abdominal wall.

Diagnostic Terms

■ *appendicitis*—inflammation of the appendix. (72, 83, 92)

■ *colitis:* (6, 85, 92)

—*granulomatous colitis*—transmural involvement of colon presenting granulomas and fissures.

—*ischemic colitis*—spontaneous reduction of the arterial blood flow of large intestine associated with abrupt onset of abdominal pain, frequent bloody stools, and radiographic changes of colon.

—*mucous colitis*—inflammatory condition marked by large amount of mucus in stool.

—*ulcerative colitis*—inflammation and multiple erosions of the intestinal mucosa leading to hemorrhage and perforations, clinically noted for frequent evacuations of watery, purulent, and bloody stools.

■ *congenital megacolon, Hirschsprung's disease*—excessive enlargement of the colon associated with an absence of ganglion cells in the narrowed bowel wall distally. The aganglionic segment of the colon is the pathologic lesion. (92)

■ *diverticulitis*—inflammation of a diverticulum or diverticula. Diverticulitis results from perforation of one or more diverticula. Small or large perforations may occur. Perforated diverticula are usually surrounded by areas of inflammation and suppuration. Larger perforations may cause pericolic or pelvic abscesses. Muscular enlargement of the colonic wall is usually present. (77, 92)

■ *diverticulosis*—presence of diverticula in the intestinal tract.

■ *duodenal ulcer*—circumscribed erosion of duodenal wall that may involve its full thickness and that is usually located near the pylorus. (61)

■ *dysentery*—inflammation of the intestinal mucosa characterized by frequent small stools, chiefly of blood and mucus. It is caused by specific bacillus or ameba. (108)

■ *fissure, anal; fissure in ano*—tear in anal mucosa that may become ulcerated, infected, spastic, scarred, and painful. (24, 61)

■ *fistula:*

—*anal fistula, fistula in ano*—abnormal communication between anal canal or lower rectum and skin near anus.

—*fecal fistula*—abnormal passage from intestine to the body surface or another hollow viscus.

—*high-output gastrointestinal fistula*—fistula that produces a minimum of 200 ml of gastrointestinal drainage in 24 hours, including salivary, gastric, pancreatic, and biliary secretions rich in enzymes and electrolytes. Consequently there is a significant energy loss. (76)

- *enteritis*—inflammation of the intestine. (66)
- *hemorrhoids, piles*—dilated varicose veins of the anal canal and at the anal orifice. (92)
- *ileitis*—inflammation of the ileum.
- *intestinal malabsorption syndromes*—disorders resulting from a faulty absorption of fat-soluble vitamins, proteins, carbohydrates, and minerals associated with copious excretion of fatty stools (steatorrhea). (27, 30, 66, 85, 92)
    - *adult celiac disease, gluten enteropathy, celiac sprue*—genetic predisposition to gluten (protein of wheat, cereals) intolerance characterized by malnutrition, chronic diarrhea, edema, and muscle wasting, occurring within the third to sixth decades of life.
    - *childhood celiac disease, gluten enteropathy, celiac sprue*—same as adult disease, except that it develops in infancy and causes retarded growth.
    - *Crohn's disease of small intestine*—nutritional malabsorption due to damaged mucosa, fistulas, strictures, and decreased surface for absorption.
    - *short bowel syndrome, short gut syndrome*—syndrome characterized by malabsorption of fat-soluble vitamins and depletion of fluid and electrolytes.
    - *Whipple's disease*—rare disorder characterized by malabsorption of lipids (fat) with resultant steatorrhea, diarrhea, abdominal distress, fever, anemia, lymph node involvement, and bouts of arthralgia.
- *intestinal obstruction, ileus*—obstruction of small intestine associated with variable symptoms: abdominal distention, colicky pain, nausea, vomiting, obstipation, or diarrhea. Interference with the blood flow to the obstructed intestine demands emergency surgery. (66, 75)
    - *adynamic (paralytic) ileus*—paralysis of intestinal muscles, absence of bowel sounds. It may be caused by electrolyte imbalance or operative handling of intestine.
    - *dynamic (mechanical) ileus*—intestinal occlusion from adhesions, strangulated hernia, volvulus, intussusception, emboli or thrombi. (108)
- *intussusception*—telescoping of intestine; usually ileum slips into cecum, which leads to intestinal obstruction. (85, 92)
- *Meckel's diverticulum*—congenital pouch or sac that usually arises from the ileum and may cause strangulation, intussusception, or volvulus. (77, 92)
- *mesenteric artery thrombosis, bowel infarction*—vascular syndrome initiated either by a slowly developing or a sudden occlusion of the superior mesentery artery in advanced atherosclerosis or following dissecting aneurysm or the use of oral contraceptives. (52, 61)
- *multiple polyposis*—polyps or tumors derived from mucous membrane; scattered throughout intestine and rectum; may undergo malignant degeneration. (24, 92)
- *perforated viscus*—ruptured internal organ due to advanced disease, malignancy, trauma, drugs, or a gunshot or stab wound. It may be complicated by hemorrhage, shock, and peritonitis. (85)
- *proctitis*—inflammation of rectum. (24)
- *prolapse of rectum*—downward displacement of rectum, seen in infants and elderly people. (85)
- *rectal cancer*—malignant tumor of the rectum or rectosigmoid. (85)
- *rectocele*—herniation of rectum into vagina.
- *volvulus*—twisting of the bowel upon itself, leading to obstruction. (85)

Operative Terms

- *abdominal perineal resection*—combined laparotomy and perineal operation for partial or complete removal of colon and rectum. (85)

- *appendectomy*—removal of appendix. (83)
- *cecectomy*—excision of cecum. (24)
- *cecostomy*—external fistulization of the cecum for intestinal obstruction. (85)
- *colectomy*—either segmental colon resection or removal of entire colon. (24, 85)
- *colon resection and end-to-end anastomosis*—excision of involved colon with or without adjacent lymph glands; joining segments of colon. (85)
- *colostomy*—formation of an abdominal anus by bringing a loop of the colon to the surface of the abdomen in an attempt to control fecal discharge. Another procedure is to bring the proximal segment of the colon to the skin, as in abdominoperineal resection. (17, 85)
- *diverticulectomy*—removal of diverticulum, including resection of involved bowel. (72)
- *endorectal ileoanal anastomosis*—procedure aimed at preserving anorectal function with removal of all disease. Functioning is enhanced by incorporating an ileal reservoir proximal to the ileoanal anastomosis. Some types of pouches or reservoirs are:
    - —*"S" type*
    - —*"J" type*
    - —*"H" type* (6, 24)
- *hemorrhoidectomy*—removal of hemorrhoids. (24, 85)
- *ileostomy*—external fistulization of ileum for fecal evacuation, often done with total colectomy for ulcerative colitis.
- *jejunoileal bypass*—creation of a bypass of a considerable portion of the small intestine by joining the proximal jejunum to the terminal ileum and the distal end of the bypassed segment of the cecum. The procedure reduces the absorptive capacity of the small intestine and induces weight loss. Various techniques are used to control morbid obesity and hyperlipidemia. (18, 41, 95)
- *operations for aganglionic megacolon (Hirschsprung's disease)* (108)
    - —*modified Duhamel procedure*—side-to-side anastomosis of colon and rectum.
    - —*modified Soave procedure*—endorectal pull-through of ganglionated bowel to anus.
- *proctocolectomy, total*—removal of the entire rectum and resection of the colon, which may be done as emergency procedure for colonic perforation from ulcerative colitis. (24, 85)
- *proctoplasty*—plastic repair or reconstruction of rectum or anus. (24, 85)
- *reduction of intussusception*—normal intestinal continuity restored either by barium enema or, if unsuccessful, by laparotomy. (85)
- *reduction of volvulus*—manipulation of twisted bowel segment to ease or correct obstruction. Decompression of the twisted bowel segment by proctoscope, rectal tube, or flexible colonoscope usually results in a spontaneous untwisting of the involved segment. (85)
- *sphincterotomy, lateral internal*—effective procedure for the control of an anal fissure using a small circular incision that is closed by suture and avoids fecal soilage. (24)
- *tube cecostomy*—surgical decompression of the colon by tube drainage of the cecum. (85)

Symptomatic Terms

- *borborygmus*—rumbling or splashing sound of bowels.
- *colic*—spasm of any tubular hollow organ associated with pain. (30)
- *diarrhea*—frequency of bowel action, soft or liquid stools. (6, 30)
- *fecalith*—a fecal concretion.
- *melena*—black stool, also black vomit from blood.
- *obstipation*—extreme constipation, often due to obstruction.

- *pruritus ani*—itching sensation around the anus. (85)
- *steatorrhea*—increased fat content in feces as in malabsorption syndrome or in pancreatitis. (5)

Liver, Biliary System, Pancreas, Peritoneum

Origin of Terms

angi-, angio- (G)—vessel
bile (L)—bile, gall
celio- (G)—abdomen, belly
chol-, chole-, cholo- (G)—bile, gall
cholecyst (G)—gallbladder
cyst-, cysti-, cystido-, cysto- (G)—sac, bladder
endo- (G)—within
hepat-, hepato- (G)—liver
ictero- (G)—jaundice
jejuno- (L)—jejunum
laparo- (G)—abdominal wall, loin, flank
necro- (G)—death, dead
pancreatico-, pancreato- (G)—pancreas
peri, (G)—around
scirrho- (G)—hard
sclero- (G)—hard
-scopy (G)—examine, inspection
-stomy (G)—creation of an artificial opening

Anatomic Terms (2, 93, 97, 112)

- *bile duct*—duct formed by union of common hepatic duct and cystic duct; carries bile into duodenum.
- *common hepatic duct*—duct formed by union of right and left hepatic ducts, which receive bile from liver.
- *cystic duct*—passageway for bile from gallbladder to bile duct.
- *gallbladder*—pear-shaped, saclike organ that serves as a reservoir for bile.
- *pancreas*—large endocrine and exocrine gland, its right extremity or head lying within the duodenal curve, its left extremity or tail ending near the spleen.
- *pancreatic duct*—main passageway for pancreatic juice containing enzymes; runs from left to right and empties into duodenum.
- *pancreatic islets, islets of Langerhans*—clusters of cells producing the hormone insulin.
- *pancreatic juice*—clear secretion, 1,000 to 2,500 ml of fluid per day, composed of water, electrolytes, proteins, and enzymes.
- *peritoneum*—sac of serous membrane composed of a parietal peritoneum that lines the abdominal wall and a visceral peritoneum that invests most viscera and holds them in position.
- *portal circulation*—venous blood collected by the portal vein from the gastrointestinal canal, spleen, gallbladder, and pancreas enters the liver, passes through sinusoids, and leaves the liver by the hepatic veins to pour into the inferior vena cava.
- *sphincter of bile duct (of Oddi)*—circular muscle fibers around the end of the bile duct.
- *sphincter of hepatopancreatic ampulla*—circular muscle fibers around end of ampulla (the union of the bile duct and main pancreatic duct).
  (See Fig. 47 for anatomic overview of digestive tract.)

Diagnostic Terms

- *liver*
    - *acute yellow atrophy of liver*—any severe form of hepatitis marked by shrinkage and necrosis of liver. (93, 108)
    - *Budd-Chiari syndrome*—rare disease characterized by occlusion of hepatic veins, usually accompanied by ascites, hepatomegaly, and pain in abdomen. Caval venogram provides delineation of caval webs and occluded hepatic veins. Percutaneous liver biopsy may aid in revealing central lobular congestion. As the disease progresses, bleeding varices and hepatic coma may develop. (16, 61, 81)
    - *cirrhosis of the liver*—organ diffusely nodular and firm. Stages of nodular development may include: (15, 93)
        - *macronodular cirrhosis*—features large nodules, measuring several centimeters in diameter.
        - *micronodular cirrhosis*—features nodules measuring one millimeter in diameter or less.
        - *presence of both macronodular and micronodular cirrhosis*—features the mixture of both small and large nodules.
        - *biliary cirrhosis*—obstructive form is characterized by chronic jaundice and liver failure due to obstruction and inflammation of bile ducts. (15)
    - *fatty liver*—abnormal lipid increase in the liver, probably related to reduced oxidation of fatty acids or decreased synthesis and release of lipoproteins, causing inadequate lipid clearance from the liver. (93)
    - *hemochromatosis*—excess of iron absorption and presence of iron-containing deposits (hemosiderin) in liver, pancreas, kidneys, adrenals, and heart. It may be associated with hepatic enlargement and insufficiency and esophageal bleeding from varices. (93, 99)
    - *hepatic calculi*—stones originating in extrahepatic biliary tract or solely in the liver. They are also found in liver cysts. (61)
    - *hepatic coma, cholemia*—peculiar syndrome characterized by slow or rapid onset of bizarre behavior, disorientation, flapping tremors of extended arms, and hyperactive reflexes, and later lethargy and coma. It seems to be caused by intoxication with ammonia, a product of protein digestion that the diseased liver fails to convert into urea. (80)
    - *hepatic encephalopathy*—serious complication of advanced liver disease probably caused by cerebral toxins, including ammonia, certain amines, and fatty acids. It is clinically manifested by personality changes and impaired intellectual ability, awareness, and neuromuscular functioning. (55, 61, 93)
    - *hepatic failure, fulminant*—clinical syndrome caused by extensive necrosis of the liver, which may be induced by hepatotoxic drugs and may lead to progressive encephalopathy and a fatal prognosis. (61, 67, 93)
    - *hepatic injury, drug-induced*—liver injury may be:
        - *cholestatic*—injury mimicking obstructive jaundice; for example, due to the use of chlorpromazine, erythromycin, steroids, and oral contraceptives.
        - *cytotoxic*—injury leading to severe hepatocellular jaundice and severe liver necrosis and failure; for example, due to the use of isoniazid, methyldopa, halothane, and tetracycline. (33, 108)
    - *hepatic necrosis*—destruction of functional liver tissue. (93)
    - *hepatic trauma*—liver injury resulting from blunt trauma or penetrating wounds.
    - *hepatitis, viral*—acute or chronic inflammation of the liver caused by the hepatitis virus A, B, delta, and non-A, non-B. (62, 63, 64, 93)

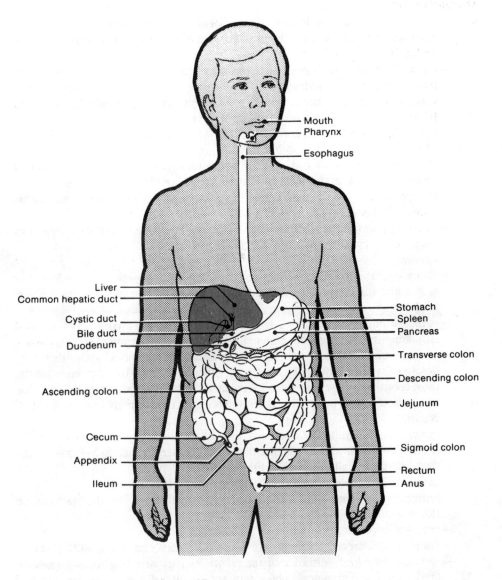

Figure 47 Scheme of digestive tract.

—*hepatoma*—tumor of the liver. (11, 56)

—*hepatorenal syndrome*—combined liver and kidney failure; usually caused by serious injury to the liver associated with hemorrhage, shock, and acute renal insufficiency. (55, 93)

—*liver abscess:* (33, 56, 61, 81, 95)

    —*amebic abscess*—localized hepatic infection by *Entamoeba histolytica;* a common complication of intestinal amebiasis.

    —*pyogenic abscess*—circumscribed area of suppuration. Infection brought to liver via portal vein, hepatic artery, or bile ducts.

—*malaria*—an infection caused by protozoa of the genus *Plasmodium.* The species commonly affecting humans are: (93)

    —*Plasmodium malariae*—causes quartan malaria.

—*Plasmodium vivax and P. ovale*—causes benign tertian malaria.

—*Plasmodium falciparum*—is the most virulent type and causes malignant tertian malaria.

—*polycystic liver disease*—cystic degeneration of the liver usually associated with congenital polycystic kidneys. (33)

—*portal hypertension*—a portal venous pressure greater than 20 mm Hg associated with splenomegaly, increased collateral circulation, varicosity, bleeding, and ascites. It may result from:

—*intrahepatic block*—block within the liver, *or*

—*extrahepatic block*—block within the portal vein. (16, 50, 93)

—*primary carcinoma of the liver*—hepatocellular tumor clinically manifested by an enlarged tender liver, ascites, jaundice, splenomegaly, edema, fever, and hepatic bruit. (93, 108)

—*secondary carcinoma of the liver*—metastatic malignant neoplasm, usually from lung, breast, or gastrointestinal cancer. (11, 93)

■ *biliary system:*

—*biliary stricture*—contraction of a biliary duct that is prone to develop after gallbladder surgery and is evidenced by profuse drainage of bile or obstructive jaundice. (57)

—*carcinoma of the gallbladder*—adenocarcinoma is the most common type, and remaining types originate either in squamous or mesothelial cells; early invasion of adjacent structures. Three kinds of adenocarcinoma that predominate are mucinous, papillary, and scirrhous. Scirrhous carcinomas are the most common and spread rapidly. Papillary carcinomas are more slow growing and present as polypoid filling defects, while mucinous carcinomas are the least occurring kind. (78, 93, 96)

—*cholangitis*—inflammatory disease of bile ducts. (29)

—*cholecystitis*—inflammatory disease of the gallbladder, frequently associated with the presence of gallstones. (23, 49, 93, 96)

—*choledocholithiasis*—gallstones in the biliary ducts. (51, 61, 74)

—*cholelithiasis, biliary calculi*—the presence of gallstones in the gallbladder. (57, 93)

—*empyema of gallbladder*—pus in the gallbladder. (93)

—*hydrops of gallbladder*—distention of gallbladder with clear fluid. (82, 92)

—*sclerosing cholangitis*—disorder of unknown etiology resulting in a progressive fibrotic and inflammatory obliteration of the intrahepatic and extrahepatic biliary tree. In later stages of the disorder, secondary biliary cirrhosis associated with varices, ascites, and splenomegaly develops. The bile duct becomes irregularly thickened by the dense fibrosis, which may pervade the surrounding tissue as well. Death may result from chronic end-stage liver disease or variceal hemorrhage. (6, 93, 96)

■ *pancreas:*

—*pancreatitis*—inflammation of the pancreas. All or part of the pancreas may be involved.

—*acute pancreatitis*—inflammation of the pancreas. Its pathologic process is caused by irritation from enzyme activity, which results in pancreatic edema and vascular engorgement. The main tissue alterations in this disorder are acinar cell necrosis associated with an intense acute inflammatory reaction, and foci of necrotic fat cells. The physical and biochemical changes in the acinar cells affect synthesis, storage, and discharge of pancreatic digestive enzymes. In the initial disease process, pancreatic digestive enzymes are discharged from injured acinar cells into the blood and abdominal cavity. Clinical findings may include epigastric pain, nausea, vomiting, sweating, weakness, abdominal pain or distention, and fever. (2, 25, 97, 113)

—*acute hemorrhagic pancreatitis, acute hemorrhagic pancreatic necrosis*—major medical emergency apparently caused by the destructive lytic action of pancreatic enzymes, clinically manifested by a sudden onset; acute abdomen, agonizing, constant pain, catastrophic peripheral vascular collapse, and shock. (97, 108)

—*chronic pancreatitis*—inflammatory disorder of the pancreas associated with permanent destruction of pancreatic tissue. When most of the pancreatic function declines, malabsorption and steatorrhea develops as well as diabetes, which requires insulin treatment. Chronic abdominal pain and pancreatic calcifications also may be present. Many persons suffering from chronic pancreatitis may have bouts of recurrent acute pancreatic inflammation that may require hospitalization. This condition has been described as relapsing or recurrent chronic pancreatitis. (5, 26, 97)

—*Other types of pancreatitis include:*

—*alcoholic pancreatitis*—caused by the ingestion of alcohol. It may result from an episode of binge drinking in the form of acute pancreatitis or from chronic alcohol ingestion, resulting in chronic pancreatitis. Individuals with chronic alcoholic pancreatitis appear at greater risk for the development of other diseases that affect their survival, such as extrapancreatic carcinoma, head and neck cancer, hepatic cirrhosis, and peptic ulceration. (2, 25, 51, 53)

—*gallstone pancreatitis*—presents as acute pancreatitis associated with gallstones, in which no other etiology is identified. It is caused by the migration of the gallstones through the ampulla of Vater. Acute gallstone pancreatitis is associated with an increased incidence of jaundice or hyperbilirubinemia. (2, 25, 51, 53, 74, 96)

—*postoperative pancreatitis*—development of acute pancreatitis following operative procedures on the biliary tree, particularly those involving the sphincter of Oddi. Those individuals who have had prior episodes of acute pancreatitis are at greater risk to develop postoperative pancreatitis. Clinical findings that help to establish this diagnosis include an abnormal amount of postoperative abdominal pain, vomiting or large volumes of nasogastric aspirate with elevated plasma enzyme levels, or elevated urinary amylase excretion. (2, 25)

—*pancreatic fibrosis, cystic fibrosis of pancreas, mucoviscidosis*—hereditary, familial disease seen in children and adolescents and characterized by a more or less extensive involvement of the exocrine glands, especially those secreting mucus and sweat. (35)

—*pancreatic pseudocyst*—fibrous capsule containing pancreatic juice with high levels of pancreatic enzymes, especially amylase. (2, 113)

—*diabetes mellitus*—the most significant pancreatic disease, in which pathogenic alterations of the islet cells cause a depletion of the insulin stores. (41) (See Chapter 12.)

—*pancreatic tumors:*

—*carcinoma of pancreas*—highly malignant tumor, usually derived from glandular epithelium and involving the head of the pancreas. (97, 113)

—*islet cell tumors*—neoplasms originating from the islets of Langerhans. They tend to induce hyperinsulinism, which in turn produces hypoglycemia. Islet cell lesions may be benign, malignant, and/or metastasizing. (97, 113)

■ *peritoneum:*

—*ascites*—collection of fluid within the peritoneal cavity. (86)

—*hemoperitoneum*—blood within the peritoneal cavity. (31)

—*hernia*—rupture or protrusion of a part from its normal location; for example, an intestinal loop through a weakened area in the abdominal wall.

  —location:

   –femoral—organ passes through femoral ring.

   –inguinal—organ protrudes through inguinal canal.

   –umbilical—hernia occurs at the naval.

  —types:

   –incarcerated—hernia causes complete bowel obstruction.

   –incisional—hernia complicates surgical intervention.

   –strangulated—hernia cuts off circulation so that gangrene develops if emergency operation is not performed. (65, 94)

—*peritonitis*—inflammation of peritoneum. (50, 86, 108)

Operative Terms

- *liver:*

  —*biopsy of liver*—removal of small piece of tissue for microscopic study. (1, 87)

  —*hepatic lobectomy*—removal of a lobe of the liver. (14, 87)

  —*hepatotomy*—incision into liver substance.

  —*liver transplantation*—orthotopic liver replacement in which a healthy liver is implanted after the person's diseased liver has been removed. After the hemograft has been implanted, suprahepatic and intrahepatic anastomoses are performed, followed by portal vein and biliary reconstruction. (19, 73)

  —*shunts for portal hypertension, portal decompression, portosystemic decompression*—surgical method of diverting a considerable amount of blood of the hypertensive portal system into the normal systemic venous system to prevent or treat variceal hemorrhages. (37)

  —*mesocaval shunt*—surgical communication of the side of the superior mesenteric vein and the upper end of the inferior vena cava for thrombosis of the portal vein. (37)

  —*portacaval shunt*—anastomosis of portal vein to vena cava for intrahepatic block. (102)

  —*splenorenal shunt*—splenectomy followed by an anastomosis between the splenic artery and renal artery for extrahepatic block due to thrombosis of the portal vein. (114)

- *biliary system:*

  —*cholecystectomy*—removal of the gallbladder. (40, 57)

  —*cholecystojejunostomy*—anastomosis between the gallbladder and jejunum to bypass the obstruction in the biliary ductal system.

  —*cholecystostomy*—surgical creation of a more or less permanent opening into the gallbladder. This operation is indicated where removal of the gallbladder would be unduly hazardous. (40)

  —*choledochoduodenostomy*—surgical joining of the common bile duct to the duodenum. (36, 40)

  —*choledocholithotomy*—incision into bile duct for removal of gallstones.

  —*choledochoplasty*—plastic repair or reconstruction of bile duct.

  —*Roux-en-Y procedures*—jejunal loop or limb, surgically used to:

   –bypass extensive trauma to the biliary ductal system by constructing a choledochojejunostomy.

   –decompress a choleductal cyst or the biliary tract by performing a cholecystojejunostomy.

—anastomose both ends of the completely transected pancreas following pancreatic injury, thus accomplishing a pancreaticojejunostomy. (2, 57, 58, 78)

—*sphincteroplasty (Oddi)*—plastic repair of stenotic sphincter of Oddi.

- *pancreas:*
  —*pancreatectomy*—partial or total removal of pancreas; for example, for islet cell tumor.

  —*pancreatoduodenectomy*—pancreatoduodenal resection indicated in major injury to the duodenum, pancreas, and adjacent viscera that precludes the salvage of these organs. (78, 113)

  —*pancreatojejunostomy*—anastomosis of pancreas to jejunum; may be done for carcinoma of the ampulla of Vater. (2, 58)

  —*sphincteroplasty (Vater)*—plastic repair of ampulla of Vater for alleviating ampullary obstruction by biliary stones and chronic pancreatitis. (2)

  —*Whipple operation, Whipple pancreaticoduodenostomy*—extensive resection for pancreatic cancer or serious injury, including the head, tail, and portions of the body of the pancreas, together with the duodenum, part of the bile duct, and stomach. The remaining pancreas is anastomosed to the bile duct, jejunum, and stomach. (2, 78)

- *peritoneum:*
  —*exploratory laparotomy*—surgical opening of abdomen for diagnostic purposes.

  —*hernioplasty, herniorrhapy*—repair of hernia. (65, 94)

  —*incision and drainage of abscess*—opening and draining peritoneal, retroperitoneal, or subphrenic abscess.

Symptomatic Terms

- *alopecia, pectoral and axillary*—absence of hair on chest and axillae (armpits) in liver damage.
- *arterial spiders, spider nevi*—cutaneous vascular lesions occurring on face, neck, and shoulders in advanced hepatic disease, as well as in malnutrition and pregnancy. Each lesion consists of a central arteriole from which small vessels radiate. (68)
- *caput medusae*—dilatation of the abdominal veins around the umbilicus seen in severe portal hypertension with liver damage. (93)
- *cholestasis*—impaired or obstructed bile flow. (93)
- *fetor hepaticus*—musty, sweet odor to the breath, characteristic of hepatic coma. (68, 100)
- *flapping tremor, liver flap*—involuntary movements, elicited in the extended hand by supporting the patient's forearm. It consists of bursts of quick, irregular movements at the wrist similar to waving goodbye. The protruded tongue and dorsiflexed feet may likewise be affected. Flapping tremors occur in severe liver disease and signal impending hepatic coma. (80)
- *hepatic bruit*—vascular bruit over liver, a blowing sound or murmur heard on auscultation, probably caused by pressure of enlarged liver on aorta. (108)
- *hyperammoniemia*—excessive amount of ammonia in the blood, as in hepatic coma. (108)
- *icterus, jaundice*—yellow discoloration of skin, sclera (white of eyes), membranes, and secretions due to excess bilirubin in the blood. (98)
- *palmar erythema, liver palms*—bright or mottled redness of the palms and fingertips seen in liver disease. Palmar erythema also occurs in malnutrition and rheumatoid arthritis. (108)

Special Procedures

Terms Related to Gastrointestinal Endoscopies

■ *endoscopy with flexible fiberscope*—visualization of a hollow organ using an endoscope with a tip for remote control and a biopsy channel for tissue sampling and histologic study of lesion. (6, 17, 24, 32, 85, 108, 109, 115)

  —*colonoscopy, colonofiberoscopy*—method of examining the colon by using a colonic fiberscope with a four-way controlled tip to facilitate transversing the flexures of the sigmoid and transverse colon under fluoroscopic guidance. It may permit the removal of polyps up to the ascending colon.

  —*duodenoscopy*—the introduction of a flexible duodenoscope into the first part of the duodenum, for visualization and cannulation of papilla of Vater. Contrast material is injected into the orifice of the ampulla through a minute cannula to obtain a retrograde cholangiogram or pancreatogram.

  —*esophagogastroduodenoscopy*—endoscopic examination of the entire esophagus, stomach, and duodenum, with all mucosal surfaces visualized and photographic recording of visualized abnormalities. Esophagogastroduodenoscopy is used in the evaluation of acid-peptic disorders, malignancy, and gastrointestinal bleeding.

  —*fiberoptic gastroscopy*—use of an end-viewing fiberscope as the usual method of choice for visualizing the esophagus, stomach, antrum, pylorus, duodenal bulb, and an anastomosis after surgery. In addition to the fiberoptic light source, the scope contains a channel for biopsies, for suction and air or water instillation, and for endoscopic photography.

  —*peritoneoscopy*—procedure for visualization of the peritoneal cavity using a peritoneoscope with a fiberoptic light source. It is possible to perform a percutaneous liver biopsy under direct vision, to photograph the lesions, to irrigate the peritoneal cavity, to aspirate ascitic fluid for cytoanalysis, and to finally arrive at a diagnosis of obscure abdominal disease by peritoneoscopy.

  —*proctosigmoidoscopy*—endoscopic procedure for visualization of benign and malignant lesions of the rectosigmoid. It permits excisional biopsy of small lesions such as polyps and segmental biopsy of large ones for diagnosis.

■ *endoscopic retrograde cholangiopancreatography*—combined endoscopic and radiologic procedure that employs a specialized lateral viewing fiberoptic endoscope one centimeter in diameter to visualize the upper gastrointestinal tract and papilla of Vater. Under visual control the pancreatic or biliary duct system is cannulated for the retrograde injection of radiopaque contrast media. An instrument channel of 1.6 cm provides passage of biopsy instruments, cannulating catheters, electrosurgical devices, and baskets or balloons for endoscopic manipulations. This mechanism signals a new advance in the diagnosis and treatment of pancreatic disease. Other technology currently under investigation includes the ultrasound-equipped endoscope for transmitting images within the abdominal cavity and laser therapy for the treatment of intraluminal lesions of the biliary tree and pancreas. In the past, the pancreas was an illusive organ because of its retroperitoneal position and the hazards associated with surgical exploration and biopsy. (25, 32, 108, 115)

Terms Related to Miscellaneous Procedures

■ *balloon tamponade*—emergency procedure to control bleeding from esophageal varices using a Boyce or Linton modification of the Sengstaken-Blakemore tube, which permits aspiration of secretions. (3, 50, 67)

- *endoscopic sclerotherapy*—procedure that involves the use of a rigid or flexible endoscope to directly inject the esophageal varices with a sclerosant. Usually, repeated injections are required to achieve variceal obliteration. Endoscopic sclerotherapy techniques may be used to stabilize the patient so that subsequent elective portosystemic shunt surgery can be employed. (50, 67)
- *transhepatic embolization of varices*—percutaneous insertion of a catheter through the liver and into the portal vein. The coronary vein is cannulated and a sclerosing agent is infused to obliterate the varices. The advantage of this technique is that a single application of variceal therapy is sufficient and repeated injections are not required to achieve variceal obliteration. (13, 50, 67)
- *esophageal manometric studies*—these studies measure intraesophageal pressure variations. The intraluminal esophageal balloons were used to measure changes in early studies; however at present, most studies employ small fluid-filled catheters attached to external transducers, which are in turn connected to amplifiers and a pen recording system. Another system becoming available utilizes sub-miniature electrical transducers for the direct recording of intraesophageal pressures. Two other tests that may be performed in conjunction with esophageal manometric studies are: (21, 28, 79)
    - *acid perfusion test*—perfusion with water is begun for several minutes followed by perfusion, which is switched to 0.1 normal hydrochloric acid at a rate of 4 to 7 cc's per minute. The test serves as a method to differentiate pain of esophageal origin from true angina.
    - *pH measurements*—measurements of esophageal pH using a long gastrointestinal electrode that provides direct and objective evidence of gastroesophageal reflux.
- *exchange transfusion*—exchange of equal volume of blood using a closed transfusion circuit for the purpose of lowering plasma bilirubin levels in cases at high risk for neurotoxicity. Fresh blood is used, and electrolytes are added as needed. (34, 108)
- *hyperalimentation*—long-term intravenous nutrition with an amino acid-glucose infusate using disposable tubing and infusion pump to maintain a constant infusion rate. A large intravenous catheter is inserted through a central vein, and its proper position is radiographically confirmed. Hyperalimentation should be reserved for patients with severe digestive abnormalities. (107)
- *pneumatic dilatation of the lower esophageal sphincter (LES)*—forceful dilatation of LES with a bag dilatator for reinstituting peristalsis and relaxing the sphincter in early achalasia. (21)

Abbreviations

Related Primarily to Tests

BA — barium
BAO — basal acid output
BSP — bromsulphalein
CCF — cephalin cholesterol flocculation
CEA — carcinoembryonic antigen
COH — carbohydrate
GI — gastrointestinal

HAA — hepatitis Australia antigen, hepatitis associated antigen
LAP — leucine aminopeptidase
MAO — maximal acid output
PP — postprandial (following a meal)
SAFP — serum alpha-fetoprotein

Related to Time Schedule for Medications

	Latin	English
ac	ante cibos	before meals
bid	bis in die	twice a day
hs	hora somni	at bedtime
pc	post cibos	after meals
po	per os	by mouth
prn	pro re nata	as necessary
qh	quaque hora	every hour
qid	quater in die	four times a day
stat	statim	immediately
tid	ter in die	three times a day

Oral Reading Practice

Malignant Neoplasms of the Oral Cavity

Carcinomas of the mouth include malignant tumors of the lips, tongue, and floor of the oral cavity. **Neoplastic** growth may be preceded by gradual development of irregular, white, raised patches known as **leukoplakia.** This condition starts as a chronic, painless inflammation of the **oral mucosa.** It is usually considered a premalignant lesion. Although **etiology** is unknown, the relationship of tobacco and leukoplakia is a well established fact, since leukoplakia seen in heavy smokers tends to disappear after smoking has been discontinued. The white patches are caused by a **keratinization** of the **epithelium.** Fissuring or **ulceration** in a leukoplakic area may be a diagnostic sign that malignant changes are in progress.

Tumors of the upper lip are generally **basal cell carcinomas,** which tend to invade adjacent structures but rarely metastasize. Prompt treatment is imperative.

Carcinoma of the lower lip may show a widespread involvement of the **epidermoid (squamous cell)** type. In its early phase, a fissure, flat ulcer, or chronic leukoplakia readily forms a **fungating** mass, malignant in character.

Carcinoma of the tongue begins as a fissure ulcer with raised borders. Pain is not present until the cancer may have progressed and metastasized. The areas of **induration** are prone to extend with time. Spontaneous bleeding occurs from ulcerating crevices and is distressing to the patient. With increasing **infiltration** the movement of the tongue becomes restricted. Metastatic **adenopathy** may develop early or late and generally involves the **cervical** and **submaxillary** lymph nodes.

Any ulcer or new growth of the lips, tongue, or floor of the mouth that does not heal with treatment in three weeks should be **biopsied.** Suspicious lesions must receive prompt attention, since progression to inoperability occurs before the patient feels pain.

The treatment of choice in carcinoma of the mouth is surgical removal of the lesion with or without irradiation or, if inoperable, **palliative** radiotherapy alone. For cancer of the lip a V-excision of the malignant lesion may be done to provide relief from discomfort and overcome disfigurement. Some surgeons treat metastatic cancer of the tongue with preoperative **supervoltage** radiotherapy to reduce the size of the tumor and subsequent **hemiglossectomy,** partial **mandibulectomy,** and cervical lymph node **dissection.** (22, 43, 44, 45, 47, 48)

Table 12
Some Digestive Conditions Amenable to Surgery

Organs Involved	Diagnosis	Type of Surgery	Operative Procedures
Lip	Cleft lip	Cheiloplasty	Plastic repair of lip
Lip (lower)	Squamous cell carcinoma of lower lip	Eslander operation for carcinoma of the lower lip	V-excision of lesion-defect filled by flap from upper lip
Lip (upper)	Squamous cell or basal cell carcinoma of upper lip	Eslander operation for carcinoma of the upper lip	V-excision and replacement of operative defect by triangular flap from lower lip
Tongue	Epidermoid carcinoma and/or metastatic cervical adenopathy	Partial glossectomy Radical neck dissection or Cautery excision with radon seed implantation in selected cases	Wide excision of malignant lesion, including removal of the jugular vein, muscles of the neck, and submaxillary and cervical lymph nodes
Parotid gland	Parotid tumor	Resection of parotid gland and tumor under direct vision	Y-shaped incision and dissection for skin flaps Partial removal of parotid gland with tumor, keeping facial nerve intact
Parotid gland Facial nerve	Parotid tumor widely infiltrating, facial nerve embedded in tumor	Total parotidectomy Elective excision of facial nerve	Removal of entire gland and tumor, including main trunk of facial nerve with plexus
Palate	Cleft palate	Staphylorrhaphy Palatoplasty	Suture of cleft palate Reconstruction of cleft palate
Floor of the mouth	Squamous cell carcinoma	Excision of lesion and/or Radiation therapy	Removal of neoplasm and/or irradiation
Tonsils, palatine	Hypertrophy of tonsils Chronic tonsillitis	Tonsillectomy	Removal of tonsils
Tonsils, pharyngeal	Adenoids	Adenoidectomy	Removal of adenoids
Esophagus	Esophageal lesion	Esophagoscopy with biopsy	Direct visualization of the esophagus with removal of bits of tissue
Esophagus	Diverticulum of esophagus	Diverticulectomy	Extirpation of the diverticulum

Organs Involved	Diagnosis	Type of Surgery	Operative Procedures
Esophagus Stomach	Carcinoma of esophagus of the midthoracic portion	Radical resection of the carcinomatous segment of the esophagus Esophagogastric anastomosis or inter-position of segment of bowel	Excision of malignant lesion and regional lymph nodes Anastomosis of remaining esophagus and stomach or use of bowel segment as substitute
Esophagus Stomach	Recurrent hiatus hernia	Repair of hiatus hernia, abdominal or thoracic approach	Direct vision reduction; sac sutured to undersurface of diaphragm; inclusion of gastric wall in fixation
Stomach Pyloric muscle	Congenital hyper-trophic stenosis of pyloric sphincter	Pyloromyotomy Fredet-Ramstedt operation	Section of hypertrophic pyloric muscle down to mucosa
Stomach	Gastric carcinoma, resectability unknown	Exploratory laparotomy	Opening abdomen to determine operability of lesion
Stomach Duodenum Jejunum	Early carcinoma of stomach Malignant gastric lesion in upper stomach	Subtotal gastrectomy Gastroduodenostomy or Gastrojejunostomy or Esophagojejunostomy	Partial removal of stomach, including lymph glands Joining remaining portion of stomach and duodenum Joining remaining portion of stomach and jejunum Transthoracic approach and esophagojejunal anastomosis
Stomach Duodenum Jejunum	Chronic or recur-rent gastric ulcer with obstruction or hemorrhage	Gastric resection Billroth I or Billroth II Polya modification or Hofmeister modification	Partial removal of stomach and gastroduodenal anastomosis or gastrojejunal anastomosis using anterior approach or posterior approach
Stomach Duodenum	Duodenal ulcer	Selective vagotomy Mucosal antrectomy	Complete vagal denervation of the stomach Excision of entire gastrin-secreting antral mucosa
Duodenum	Progressive duodenal ulcer with obstruction or hemorrhage	Complete bilateral vagotomy Pyloroplasty	Section of vagus nerve fibers before they enter stomach Surgical repair of pyloric muscle

Organs Involved	Diagnosis	Type of Surgery	Operative Procedures
Duodenum Jejunum	Large duodenal perforation	Surgical reconstruction of perforated duodenum	Excision of duodenal ulcer Full-thickness jejunal pedicle graft for closure of large duodenal defect
Jejunum Ileum	Morbid obesity Hyperlipidemia	Jejunoileal bypass	Division of jejunum a few inches distal to ligament of Treitz, and ileum a few inches proximal to ileocecal valve End-to-end anastomosis to restore continuity Closure of distal jejunum Implantation of proximal ileum into transverse colon or into left colon
Ileum Colon	Regional enteritis	Resection of involved ileum and colon Enteroanastomosis	Radical extirpation of bowel involved in regional enteritis Surgical joining of remaining parts
Colon Ileum	Chronic ulcerative colitis with hemorrhage	Permanent ileostomy with total colectomy	Surgical creation of ileal stoma for fecal drainage and removal of colon
Cecum Colon	Intestinal obstruction Cancer of left colon	Cecostomy Gibson's technique Transverse colostomy	Creation of communication between cecum and body surface for fecal drainage Diversion of fecal content to the body surface
Appendix	Appendicitis	Appendectomy	Removal of appendix
Colon Rectum	Aganglionic megacolon (Hirschsprung's disease)	Modified Duhamel procedure or Modified Soave procedure	Side-to-side colorectal anastomosis Endorectal pull-through of ganglionated bowel to anus
Rectosigmoid	Rectal hemorrhage, cause unknown	Rectosigmoidoscopy	Endoscopic examination of the rectosigmoid
Rectosigmoid	Carcinoma of rectum and low sigmoid	Abdominoperineal resection Miles' operation	Sectioning of bowel above the tumor; creation of permanent colostomy; removal of bowel above and below tumor; excision of anus

Organs Involved	Diagnosis	Type of Surgery	Operative Procedures
Rectum	Hemorrhoids, internal anal or external	Hemorrhoidectomy	Removal of hemorrhoids
Peritoneum	Hernia, inguinal femoral umbilical ventral	Hernioplasty	Surgical repair of hernia
Liver	Hepatic necrosis Hepatic failure Hepatic coma	Exchange transfusion (fresh blood)	Construction of arteriovenous shunt Priming exchange-transfusion circuit Exchange of equal volume of blood
Gallbladder	Cholecystitis Cholelithiasis	Cholecystectomy	Removal of gallbladder
Bile duct	Benign stricture bile duct	Repair of biliary stricture by end-to-end anastomosis of bile duct	Excision of constricted part and surgical communication of the two ends of bile duct

References and Bibliography

1. Afroudakis, A.P. Biopsy of the liver. In Gitnick, Gary, ed., *Principles and Practice of Gastroenterology and Hepatology*, New York: Elsevier, 1988, pp. 1475-1498.
2. Anderson, D.K. The pancreas. In Sabiston, David C., Jr., ed. *Essentials of Surgery*, Philadelphia: W.B. Saunders Co., 1987, pp. 587-614.
3. Arthur, M.J.P., and Wright, Ralph. Medical management of bleeding varices. In Blumgart, L.H., ed., *Surgery of the Liver and Biliary Tract*, vol. 2. New York: Churchill Livingstone, Inc., 1988, pp. 1345-1355.
4. Balogh, Karoly. The head and neck. In Rubin, Emanuel, and Farber, John L., eds., *Pathology*, Philadelphia: J.B. Lippincott Co., 1988, pp. 1260-1303.
5. Banks, P.A. Chronic pancreatitis. In Gitnick, Gary, ed., *Principles and Practice of Gastroenterology and Hepatology*, New York: Elsevier, 1988, pp. 778-815.
6. Bayless, T.M. Ulcerative colitis. In Gitnick, Gary, ed., *Principles and Practice of Gastroenterology and Hepatology*, New York: Elsevier, 1988, pp. 461-496.

7. Beaven, D.W., and Grooks, S.E. The normal tongue. In *Color Atlas of the Tongue in Clinical Diagnosis*, Ipswich, England: Year Book Medical Publishers, Inc., 1988, pp. 13-35.
8. ———. Ulcers of the tongue. Ibid., pp. 93-104.
9. ———. Vesiculo-bullous diseases of the tongue. Ibid., pp. 140-147.
10. ———. Tongue changes in congenital and developmental abnormalities. Ibid., pp. 203-215.
11. Bengmark, S., et al. Metastatic tumors of the liver. In Blumgart, L.H., ed., *Surgery of the Liver and Biliary Tract*, vol. 2. New York: Churchill Livingstone, Inc., 1988, pp. 1179-1190.
12. Bengmark, S., et al. Arterial ligation and temporary dearterialization. In Blumgart, L.H., ed., *Surgery of the Liver and Biliary Tract*, vol. 2. New York: Churchill Livingstone, Inc., 1988, pp. 1219-1236.
13. Bengmark, S., et al. Percutaneous transhepatic occlusion of esophageal varices. In Blumgart, L.H., ed., *Surgery of the Liver and*

Biliary Tract, vol. 2. New York: Churchill Livingstone, Inc., 1988, pp. 1379-1383.

14. Blumgart, L.H. Liver resection—liver and biliary tumors. In Blumgart, L.H., ed., *Surgery of the Liver and Biliary Tract,* vol. 2. New York: Churchill Livingstone, Inc., 1988, pp. 1251-1280.

15. Boyer, Thomas D. Cirrhosis of the liver. In Wyngaarden, James B., and Smith, Lloyd H., Jr., eds., *Cecil's Textbook of Medicine,* 18th ed. Philadelphia: W.B. Saunders Co., 1988, pp. 842-847.

16. ———. Major sequelae of cirrhosis. Ibid., pp. 847-852.

17. Bresalier, R.S., et al. Colorectal cancer. In Gitnick, Gary, ed., *Principles and Practice of Gastroenterology and Hepatology,* New York: Elsevier, 1988, pp. 497-523.

18. Buchwald, Henry, et al. Management of morbid obesity and hyperlipidemia (metabolic surgery). In Hardy, James D., ed., *Hardy's Textbook of Surgery,* 2nd ed. Philadelphia: J.B. Lippincott Co., 1988, pp. 744-760.

19. Calne, R.Y., and Williams, R. Orthotopic liver transplantation. In Blumgart, L.H., ed., *Surgery of the Liver and Biliary Tract,* vol. 2. New York: Churchill Livingstone, Inc., 1988, pp. 1509-1517.

20. Castell, Donald O. Introduction—esophagus. In Gitnick, Gary, ed., *Principles and Practice of Gastroenterology and Hepatology,* New York: Elsevier, 1988, pp. 3-7.

21. ———. Disorders of esophageal motility. Ibid., pp. 28-41.

22. Coleman, John J., III, and Jurkiewicz, M.J. The head and neck. In Sabiston, David C., Jr., ed., *Essentials of Surgery,* Philadelphia: W.B. Saunders Co., 1987, pp. 706-735.

23. Cuschieri, A. Acute cholecystitis. In Blumgart, L.H., ed., *Surgery of the Liver and Biliary Tract,* vol. 1. New York: Churchill Livingstone, Inc., 1988, pp. 531-540.

24. Dent, Thomas L., et al. The colon, rectum, and anus. In Hardy, James D., ed., *Hardy's Textbook of Surgery,* 2nd ed. Philadelphia: J.B. Lippincott Co., 1988, pp. 582-636.

25. DiMagno, E.P. Acute pancreatitis. In Gitnick, Gary, ed., *Principles and Practice of Gastroenterology and Hepatology,* New York: Elsevier, 1988, pp. 759-777.

26. ———. Diagnosis of chronic pancreatitis and pancreatic ductal adenocarcinoma. Ibid., pp. 829-849.

27. Dobbins, W.O., III. Whipple's disease. In Gitnick, Gary, ed., *Principles and Practice of Gastroenterology and Hepatology,* New York: Elsevier, 1988, pp. 426-438.

28. Duranceau, André, and Lafontaine, Edwin. The esophagus. In Sabiston, David C., Jr.,

ed., *Essentials of Surgery,* Philadelphia: W.B. Saunders Co., 1987, pp. 363-387.

29. Ellison, E.C., and Carey, L.C. Cholangitis: nonsuppurative and suppurative. In Blumgart, L.H., ed., *Surgery of the Liver and Biliary Tract,* vol. 1. New York: Churchill Livingston, Inc., 1988, pp. 925-932.

30. Farmer, R.G. Crohn's disease. In Gitnick, Gary, ed., *Principles and Practice of Gastroenterology and Hepatology,* New York: Elsevier, 1988, pp. 601-621.

31. Fitts, Charles T. The retroperitoneum: Tumors, cysts, abscesses and other conditions. In Hardy, James D., ed., *Hardy's Textbook of Surgery,* 2nd ed. Philadelphia: J.B. Lippincott Co., 1988, pp. 771-777.

32. Fleischer, David. Neoplasms of the esophagus. In Gitnick, Gary, ed., *Principles and Practice of Gastroenterology and Hepatology,* New York: Elsevier, 1988, pp. 58-77.

33. Flint, Lewis M., Jr., and Polk, Hiram C., Jr. Liver injury, abscess, cysts, and tumors. In Hardy, James D., ed., *Hardy's Textbook of Surgery,* 2nd ed. Philadelphia: J.B. Lippincott Co., 1988, pp. 663-676.

34. Freilic, Howard, and Gollan, John. The metabolism of bilirubin and its congenital disorders. In Gitnick, Gary, ed., *Principles and Practice of Gastroenterology and Hepatology,* New York: Elsevier, 1988, pp. 1135-1152.

35. Gleghorn, E.E., and Thaler, M.M. Congenital and inherited disorders of the pancreas. In Gitnick, Gary, ed., *Principles and Practice of Gastroenterology and Hepatology,* New York: Elsevier, 1988, pp. 722-740.

36. Gliedman, M.L. Choledochoduodenostomy—technique. In Blumgart, L.H., ed., *Surgery of the Liver and Biliary Tract,* vol. 1. New York: Churchill Livingston, Inc., 1988, pp. 669-672.

37. ———. Mesocaval shunt—technique. Ibid., pp. 1469-1478.

38. Graham, D.Y. Gastric ulcer. In Gitnick, Gary, ed., *Principles and Practice of Gastroenterology and Hepatology,* New York: Elsevier, 1988, pp. 164-174.

39. Graham, D.Y., and Estes, M.K. Viral infections of the intestine. In Gitnick, Gary, ed., *Principles and Practice of Gastroenterology and Hepatology,* New York: Elsevier, 1988, pp. 566-578.

40. Ham, J.M. Cholecystectomy. In Blumgart, L.H., ed., *Surgery of the Liver and Biliary Tract,* vol. 1. New York: Churchill Livingston, Inc., 1988, pp. 559-568.

41. Hanna, P.D. Diseases of the liver in obesity and diabetes. In Gitnick, Gary, ed., *Principles and Practice of Gastroenterology and Hepatology,* New York: Elsevier, 1988, pp. 1308-1324.

42. Heckler, Frederick R. Principles of plastic and reconstructive surgery. In Hardy, James D., ed., *Hardy's Textbook of Surgery,* 2nd ed. Philadelphia: J.B. Lippincott Co., 1988, pp. 1171-1186.

43. Henk, K.M. Clinical presentation and diagnosis. In Henk, J.M., and Langdon, J.D., eds., *Malignant Tumors of the Oral Cavity,* London: Edward Arnold Publishers, 1985, pp. 43-52.

44. ———. Classification and staging. Ibid., pp. 71-79.

45. ———. Surgery. Ibid., pp. 90-97.

46. ———. Malignant tumors of the minor salivary glands. Ibid., pp. 204-210.

47. ———. Metastases to the oral cavity. Ibid., pp. 211-214.

48. ———. Premalignant lesions. Ibid., pp. 214-223.

49. Hermann, R.E., and Grundfest-Broniatowski, S. Chronic cholecystitis. In Blumgart, L.H., ed., *Surgery of the Liver and Biliary Tract,* vol. 1. New York: Churchill Livingston, Inc., 1988, pp. 541-550.

50. Hoefs, John C. Portal hypertension. In Gitnick, Gary, ed., *Principles and Practice of Gastroenterology and Hepatology,* New York: Elsevier, 1988, pp. 1225-1267.

51. Howard, John M. Gallstone pancreatitis. In Howard, John M., Jordan, George L., and Reber, Howard A., eds., *Surgical Diseases of the Pancreas,* Philadelphia: Lea & Febiger, 1987, pp. 265-283.

52. Hoyumpa, A.M. Ischemic disorders of the bowel. In Gitnick, Gary, ed., *Principles and Practice of Gastroenterology and Hepatology,* New York: Elsevier, 1988, pp. 538-556.

53. Imrie, C.W. Gallstone acute pancreatitis. In Blumgart, L.H., ed., *Surgery of the Liver and Biliary Tract,* vol. 1. New York: Churchill Livingston, Inc., 1988, pp. 551-558.

54. Ippoliti, Andrew. Inflammatory and infectious esophageal disorders. In Gitnick, Gary, ed., *Principles and Practice of Gastroenterology and Hepatology,* New York: Elsevier, 1988, pp. 42-57.

55. Jackler, Robert K., and Kaplan, Michael J. Ear, nose and throat. In Schroeder, Steven A., Krupp, Marcus A., and Tierney, Lawrence M., Jr., eds., *Current Medical Diagnosis & Treatment—1988,* Norwalk, CT: Appleton & Lange, 1988, pp. 110-131.

56. Johnson, George Jr., and Nuzum, C. Thomas. The liver, gallbladder and biliary tract. In Hardy, James D., ed., *Hardy's Textbook of Surgery,* 2nd ed. Philadelphia: J.B. Lippincott Co., 1988, pp. 663-676.

57. Jones, R. Schott. Gallbladder and biliary tract. In Hardy, James D., ed., *Hardy's Textbook of Surgery,* 2nd ed. Philadelphia: J.B. Lippincott Co., 1988, pp. 676-694.

58. Jordan, George L., Jr. Pancreatic resection for pancreatic cancer. In Howard, John M., et al., eds., *Surgical Diseases of the Pancreas,* Philadelphia: Lea & Febiger, 1987, pp. 666-714.

59. Jordan, George L., Jr. Malabsorption syndromes. In Hardy, James D., ed., *Hardy's Textbook of Surgery,* 2nd ed. Philadelphia: J.B. Lippincott Co., 1988, pp. 563-569.

60. Jordan, Paul H., Jr. Stomach and duodenum. In Hardy, James D., ed., *Hardy's Textbook of Surgery,* 2nd ed. Philadelphia: J.B. Lippincott Co., 1988, pp. 514-539.

61. Knauer, C. Michael, and Silverman, Sol, Jr. Alimentary tract and liver. In Schroeder, Steven, Krupp, Marcus A., and Tierney, Lawrence M., Jr., eds., *Current Medical Diagnosis & Treatment—1988,* Norwalk, CT: Appleton & Lange, 1988, pp. 342-428.

62. Koretz, R. L. Viral hepatitis. In Gitnick, Gary, ed., *Principles and Practice of Gastroenterology and Hepatology,* New York: Elsevier, 1988, pp. 1161-1178.

63. ———. Chronic hepatitis. Ibid., pp. 1192-1204.

64. ———. The serology of viral hepatitis. Ibid., pp. 1460-1464.

65. Kortz, Warren J., and Sabiston, David C. Hernias. In Sabiston, David C., Jr., ed., *Essentials of Surgery,* Philadelphia: W.B. Saunders Co., 1987, pp. 639-654.

66. Levine, Barry A., and Aust, J. Bradley. Surgical disorders of the small intestine. In Sabiston, David C., Jr., ed., *Essentials of Surgery,* Philadelphia: W.B. Saunders Co., 1987, pp. 429-460.

67. Liberman, David A., and Melnyk, Clifford S. Gastrointestinal hemorrhage. In Gitnick, Gary, ed., *Principles and Practice of Gastroenterology and Hepatology,* New York: Elsevier, 1988, pp. 1542-1563.

68. Lindsay, K. L. Fulminant hepatic failure. In Gitnick, Gary, ed., *Principles and Practice of Gastroenterology and Hepatology,* New York: Elsevier, 1988, pp. 1217-1224.

69. MacDonald, Walter C. Gastric tumors. In Gitnick, Gary, ed., *Principles and Practice of Gastroenterology and Hepatology,* New York: Elsevier, 1988, pp. 239-252.

70. McCallum, Richard W., et al. Structural disorders of the esophagus. In Gitnick, Gary, ed., *Principles and Practice of Gastroenterology and Hepatology,* New York: Elsevier, 1988, pp. 8-27.

71. McCarthy, Denis M. Hypergastrinemic peptic ulcer disease. In Gitnick, Gary, ed., *Principles and Practice of Gastroenterology and Hepatology,* New York: Elsevier, 1988, pp. 204-221.

72. McIlrath, Donald C. Surgical disorders of the vermiform appendix and Meckel's di-

verticulum. In Sabiston, David C., Jr., ed., *Essentials of Surgery,* Philadelphia: W.B. Saunders Co., 1987, pp. 461-470.

73. Memsic, L.D.F., and Busuttil, Ronald W. Liver transplantation. In Gitnick, Gary, ed., *Principles and Practice of Gastroenterology and Hepatology,* New York: Elsevier, 1988, pp. 1431-1446.

74. Metcalf, Amanda M., and Maher, James W. Anatomy and physiology. In Hardy, James D., ed., *Hardy's Textbook of Surgery,* 2nd ed. Philadelphia: J.B. Lippincott Co., 1988, pp. 540-544.

75. ———. Small bowel obstruction. Ibid., pp. 545-550.

76. ———. Small bowel trauma, fistula, and radiation injury. Ibid., pp. 551-554.

77. ———. Miscellaneous other small bowel disorders. Ibid., pp. 570-573.

78. Moody, Frank G. Neoplastic disorders. In Gitnick, Gary, ed., *Principles and Practice of Gastroenterology and Hepatology,* New York: Elsevier, 1988, pp. 998-1009.

79. Moody, Frank G., and Roth, Jack A. The esophagus and diaphragmatic hernias. In Hardy, James D., ed., *Hardy's Textbook of Surgery,* 2nd ed. Philadelphia: J.B. Lippincott Co., 1988, pp. 485-513.

80. Ockner, Robert K. Clinical approach to liver disease. In Wyngaarden, James B., and Smith, Lloyd H., Jr., eds., *Cecil's Textbook of Medicine,* 18th ed. Philadelphia: W.B. Saunders Co., 1988, pp. 808-809.

81. Orloff, M.J. Budd-Chiari syndrome and veno-occlusive disease. In Blumgart, L.H., ed., *Surgery of the Liver and Biliary Tract,* vol. 2. New York: Churchill Livingstone, Inc., 1988, pp. 1425-1554.

82. Pandol, Stephen J. Structural abnormalities of the stomach and duodenum. In Gitnick, Gary, ed., *Principles and Practice of Gastroenterology and Hepatology,* New York: Elsevier, 1988, pp. 101-115.

83. Pass, Harvy I., and Hardy, James D. The appendix. In Hardy, James D., ed., *Hardy's Textbook of Surgery,* 2nd ed. Philadelphia: J.B. Lippincott Co., 1988, pp. 574-581.

84. Pope, Charles E. Diseases of the esophagus. In Wyngaarden, James B., and Smith, Lloyd H., Jr., eds., *Cecil's Textbook of Medicine,* 18th ed. Philadelphia: W.B. Saunders Co., 1988, pp. 679-688.

85. Ramming, Kenneth P. Diseases of the colon and rectum. In Sabiston, David C., Jr., ed., *Essentials of Surgery,* Philadelphia: W.B. Saunders Co., 1987, pp. 471-512.

86. Rector, William G. Ascites. In Gitnick, Gary, ed., *Principles and Practice of Gastroenterology and Hepatology,* New York: Elsevier, 1988, pp. 1268-1281.

87. Reintgen, Douglas S., and Sabiston, David

C., Jr. The liver. In Sabiston, David C., Jr., ed., *Essentials of Surgery,* Philadelphia: W.B. Saunders Co., 1987, pp. 513-550.

88. Richardson, Charles T. Gastritis. In Wyngaarden, James B., and Smith, Lloyd H., Jr., eds., *Cecil's Textbook of Medicine,* 18th ed. Philadelphia: W.B. Saunders Co., 1988, pp. 689-692.

89. ———. Peptic ulcer—pathogenesis. Ibid., pp. 692-696.

90. ———. Zollinger—Ellison syndrome. Ibid., pp. 708-709.

91. Ritchie, Wallace P., Jr., and Perez, Alice R. Stomach and duodenum—surgical anatomy, physiology, and pathology. In Sabiston, David C., Jr., ed., *Essentials of Surgery,* Philadelphia: W.B. Saunders Co., 1987, pp. 406-427.

92. Rubin, Emanuel, and Farber, John L. The gastrointestinal tract. In Rubin, Emanuel, and Farber, John L., eds., *Pathology,* Philadelphia: J.B. Lippincott Co., 1988, pp. 628-721.

93. ———. The liver and biliary system. Ibid., pp. 722-807.

94. Rushton, Fred W. Abdominal wall hernias. In Hardy, James D., ed., *Hardy's Textbook of Surgery,* 2nd ed. Philadelphia: J.B. Lippincott Co., 1988, pp. 784-800.

95. Sabiston, David C., Jr. Surgical management of morbid obesity. In Sabiston, David C., Jr., ed., *Essentials of Surgery,* Philadelphia: W.B. Saunders Co., 1987, pp. 427-428.

96. Sarr, Michael G., and Cameron, John L. The biliary system. In Sabiston, David C., Jr., ed., *Essentials of Surgery,* Philadelphia: W.B. Saunders Co., 1987, pp. 551-586.

97. Scarpelli, Dante G. The pancreas. In Rubin, Emanuel, and Farber, John L., eds., *Pathology,* Philadelphia: J.B. Lippincott Co., 1988, pp. 808-831.

98. Schiff, Eugene R. Jaundice. In Gitnick, Gary, ed., *Principles and Practice of Gastroenterology and Hepatology,* New York: Elsevier, 1988, pp. 1586-1598.

99. Schlarschmidt, Bruce F. Inherited, infiltrative, and metabolic disorders involving the liver. In Wyngaarden, James B., and Smith, Lloyd H., Jr., eds., *Cecil's Textbook of Medicine,* 18th ed. Philadelphia: W.B. Saunders Co., 1988, pp. 838-842.

100. ———. Acute and chronic hepatic failure and hepatic transplantation. Ibid., pp. 852-856.

101. Schow, Sterling R. Diseases of the salivary gland. In Peterson, Larry J., ed., *Contemporary Oral and Maxillofacial Surgery,* St. Louis: The C.V. Mosby Co., 1988, pp. 455-469.

102. Shields, R. Technique of portacaval shunt.

In Blumgart, L.H., ed., *Surgery of the Liver and Biliary Tract,* vol. 2. New York: Churchill Livingstone, Inc., 1988, pp. 1455-1461.

103. Silverman, Sol J. Oral medicine. In Wyngaarden, James B., and Smith, Lloyd H., Jr., eds., *Cecil's Textbook of Medicine,* 18th ed. Philadelphia: W.B. Saunders Co., 1988, pp. 674-679.

104. Sleisnger, Marvin H. Introduction— gastrointestinal disease. In Wyngaarden, James B., and Smith, Lloyd H., Jr., eds., *Cecil's Textbook of Medicine,* 18th ed. Philadelphia: W.B. Saunders Co., 1988, pp. 656-662.

105. Thirlby, Richard C. Peptic ulcer—surgical therapy. In Wyngaarden, James B., and Smith, Lloyd H., Jr., eds., *Cecil's Textbook of Medicine,* 18th ed. Philadelphia: W.B. Saunders Co., 1988, pp. 703-706.

106. Thornton, James W., and Argenta, Lewis C. Lesions of the mouth, tongue, jaws, and salivary glands. In Hardy, James D., ed., *Hardy's Textbook of Surgery,* 2nd ed. Philadelphia: J.B. Lippincott Co., 1988, pp. 267-282.

107. Toskes, Phillip P. Malabsorption. In Wyngaarden, James B., and Smith, Lloyd H., Jr., eds., *Cecil's Textbook of Medicine,* 18th ed. Philadelphia: W.B. Saunders Co., 1988, pp. 733-745.

108. Tucker, Eugene, MD. Personal communication.

109. Vennes, Jack A. Gastrointestinal endoscopy. In Wyngaarden, James B., and Smith, Lloyd H., Jr., eds., *Cecil's Textbook of Medicine,* 18th ed. Philadelphia: W.B. Saunders Co., 1988, pp. 668-674.

110. Wilfert, Catherine M. Mumps. In Wyngaarden, James B., and Smith, Lloyd H., Jr., eds., *Cecil's Textbook of Medicine,* 18th ed. Philadelphia: W.B. Saunders Co., 1988, pp. 1778-1780.

111. Woodburne, Russell T., and Burkerl, William E. The head and neck. In *Essentials of Human Anatomy,* 8th ed. New York: Oxford University Press, 1988, pp. 179-323.

112. ———. The abdomen. Ibid., pp. 407-508.

113. Yeo, Charles J., and Cameron, John L. The pancreas. In Hardy, James D., ed., *Hardy's Textbook of Surgery,* 2nd ed. Philadelphia: J.B. Lippincott Co., 1988, pp. 695-725.

114. Zeppa, R. Distal splenorenal shunt. In Blumgart, L.H., ed., *Surgery of the Liver and Biliary Tract,* vol. 2. New York: Churchill Livingstone, Inc., 1988, pp. 1463-1468.

115. Zfass, Alvin M. Endoscopy of the bowel. In Gitnick, Gary, ed., *Principles and Practice of Gastroenterology and Hepatology,* New York: Elsevier, 1988, pp. 669-677.

Urogenital Disorders

CHAPTER 9

Kidneys

Origin of Terms

calyx (G)—cup

cortex (L)—rind, outer portion

medulla (L)—marrow, inner portion

nephr-, nephro- (G)—kidney

ren (L)—kidney

Anatomic Terms (Refs. 16, 37, 53)

- *kidneys* (Fig. 48)—paired, bean-shaped organs situated behind the peritoneum on either side of the lumbar spine. Their function is to preserve the ionic balance of the blood and extract its waste products.
- *nephron, renal tubule* (Figs. 49 and 50)—the functional unit of the kidney, composed of:
    - *glomerular capsule, Bowman's capsule*—double layered envelope of epithelium that encloses a capillary tuft. It filters water and solutes out of the blood into the tubule.
    - *glomerulus (pl. glomeruli)*—capillary cluster or tuft involved in the initial phrase of urine formation.
    - *renal corpuscle*—both glomerular capsule and glomerulus.
    - *secretory tubule*—tubule that completes urine formation and is functionally divided into a proximal tubule, a thin segment, and a distal tubule or thick segment.
    - *collecting tubule*—tubule that conveys urine to the renal pelvis.
- *renal cortex*—outer portion of the kidney.
- *renal medulla*—inner portion of the kidney containing the renal pyramids, which contain collecting tubules and parts of the secretory tubules.
- *renal papillae*—apices of the pyramids that indent the calices.
- *renal pelvis*—funnel-shaped enlargement of the ureter as it leaves the kidney. It contains:
    - *calices (formerly calyces; sing. calyx)*—cuplike indentations in the kidney pelvis. The collecting tubules open into the calices.
    - *hilus*—notch on the medial surface of the kidney through which the ureter and blood vessels enter or leave the kidney.

Figure 48 Longitudinal section of kidney.

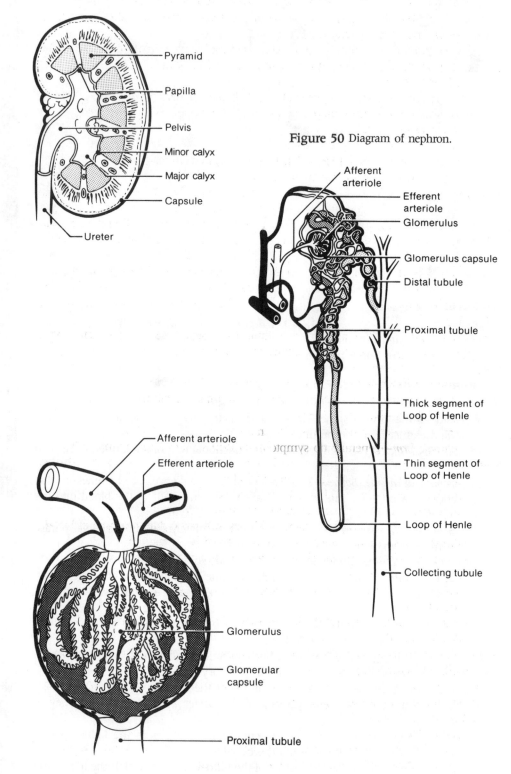

Pyramid

Papilla

Pelvis

Minor calyx

Major calyx

Capsule

Ureter

Figure 50 Diagram of nephron.

Afferent arteriole

Efferent arteriole

Glomerulus

Glomerulus capsule

Distal tubule

Proximal tubule

Thick segment of Loop of Henle

Thin segment of Loop of Henle

Loop of Henle

Collecting tubule

Afferent arteriole

Efferent arteriole

Glomerulus

Glomerular capsule

Proximal tubule

Figure 49 Structure of renal corpuscle.

Diagnostic Terms

- *acute tubular necrosis of kidney, acute reversible renal failure*—a cellular necrosis affecting the renal tubules following shock, trauma, nephrotoxic damage, transfusion reaction, septicemia, and other causes. (1, 19)
- *arteriolar nephrosclerosis*—renal disorder characterized by an intimal thickening of the afferent glomerular arterioles, resulting in a narrowing of the arteriolar lumen and reduced blood supply to nephrons. (14)
    - —*benign type*—common nephropathy with benign hypertension.
    - —*malignant type*—uncommon nephropathy with malignant hypertension.
- *congenital anomalies of kidneys:*
    - —*agenesis*—absence of one kidney.
    - —*dysplasia*—multicystic kidney forming an irregular mass.
    - —*ectopy*—displaced kidney, usually low in position.
- *glomerulonephritis*—form of nephritis involving the renal glomeruli of both kidneys. There is evidence that the glomeruli may be injured by antigen-antibody complexes that develop from the immune responses to streptococcal infection. Common clinical findings include hypertension; headache; malaise; puffiness around the eyes; oliguria; and blood, protein, and casts in the urine. (11, 12, 14)
- *Goodpasture's syndrome, antiglomerular basement membrane nephritis*—acute glomerulonephritis associated with severe diffuse lung disease, hemorrhagic and inflammatory, involving the basement membranes of the glomeruli and lungs. Recovery is rare. (12, 14)
- *heriditary nephritis, Alport's syndrome*—familial glomerulonephritis associated with defective hearing and sight. Renal failure may be the final event in males. (12)
- *infections of the kidney:*
    - —*abscess of kidney*—usually a focal suppuration of the cortex.
    - —*perinephric abscess, perinephritis*—infection around the kidney.
    - —*pyelonephritis*—bacterial kidney infection.
        - –*acute form*—commonly caused by gram-negative enteric bacilli
        - –*chronic form*—generally no symptoms of urinary infection present. (27)
- *injuries to the kidney*—uncommon pathologic lesions usually caused by athletic, occupational, and traffic accidents. They include:
    - —*avulsion*—separation of kidney from blood supply.
    - —*contusions*—simple bruising of functional tissue of kidney.
    - —*ecchymoses*—black and blue spots of kidney substance due to escape of blood.
    - —*fissures*—slits in renal capsule or pelvis; may cause hematuria.
    - —*hematoma*—local mass of clotted blood, which may develop especially after injury to renal pelvis.
    - —*lacerations*—tears may involve renal pelvis and renal capsule and result in severe hematuria.
    - —*rupture*—extensive tear of the kidney may be the cause of massive bleeding and death. (22, 53)
- *interstitial nephritis*—renal disease in which the interstitial connective tissue is involved. Its acute form appears to be a reaction to systemic infection or drug sensitivity; its chronic form exhibits a diffuse interstitial fibrosis and widespread atrophy of the renal tubules. (12, 14, 27)
- *neoplasms of the kidney:*
    - —*benign tumors:*
        - –*cortical adenoma*—small nodule or papillomatous growth originating in the renal tubule and embedded in the renal cortex.
        - –*lipomas*—common soft-tissue tumors that may appear with smooth muscle,

abnormal blood vessels, or alone. Renal lipomas usually arise from the areas of the renal capsule or from perirenal adipose tissue.

—*renomedullary interstitial cell tumor, medullary fibroma*—most common of the benign mesenchymal tumors of the kidney. These tumors develop from medullary interstitial cells and appear as small, unencapsulated, grayish white round nodules. (8, 16)

—*malignant tumors:*

—*embryoma, nephroblastoma, Wilms' tumor*—neoplasm common in children, infrequent in adults; may form huge abdominal mass that exerts pressure on functional renal tissue and metastasizes to the lungs, liver, bones, and brain.

—*mesenchymal tumors*—large malignant soft-tissue tumors that arise from areas of the renal capsule and renal pelvis.

—*renal cell carcinoma, hypernephroid carcinoma, Grawitz tumor*—tumor clinically manifested by a palpable mass, hematuria, and pain in the costovertebral region. Widespread metastases are common. (8, 16)

- *nephrolithiasis, renal calculi*—stones in the kidney, generally in the pelvis and calices. They may be caused by renal tubular syndromes, enzyme disorders, hypercalcemia, increased uric acid, and other factors. (14, 15, 48)
- *nephropathy*—any disease of the kidney, such as:

    —*acute hyperuricemia*—disorder resulting from a sudden high increase of serum uric acid level prone to occur in patients receiving massive antineoplastic therapy for lymphoma or leukemia.

    —*hypercalcemia*—abnormal increase in serum calcium associated with hypercalciuria, renal calculi, and pyelonephritis. In its early phase polyuria and tubular injury are present; in its late phase there is progressive renal insufficiency.

    —*hypercalcemia crisis*—serum calcium 15 to 20 mg/dl (formerly mg/100 ml) or more; may lead to renal failure. (Normal laboratory range for serum calcium is 8.5 to 10.3 mg/dl.)

    —*potassium depletion*—inability of kidneys to concentrate urine because of the potassium deficiency. (12, 13, 36)

- *nephroptosis*—a movable, floating kidney that is displaced downward.
- *nephrotic syndrome*—clinical state characterized by massive edema, excessive loss of protein in urine, and low albumin blood levels. It may develop during the course of glomerulonephritis, a collagen disease, toxic drug reaction, or specific allergy. (12, 36)
- *obstructive uropathy*—obstruction occurring anywhere along the urinary tract, from the renal pelvis to the external urethral meatus, causing changes in renal function, volume of urine, and amount of protein and sediment in urine. Obstructive lesions include renal, ureteral, vesical, and urethral calculi, strictures, and prostatic lesions, all of which may lead to hydronephrosis and renal failure. (11, 12, 40)
- *renal artery occlusion*—acute blockage of renal artery due to embolus, thrombus, or other cause. The kidney is deprived of its blood supply when the occlusion is complete. Renal infarction and renal failure are rare complications. (53)
- *renal calcinosis, nephrocalcinosis*—scattered foci of calcification within functional renal tissue. (36)
- *renal cystic disease:*

    —*acquired cystic disease of kidney (ACDK)*—uremic, multiple cystic disease acquired by patients with end-stage renal disease or dialysis. Long periods of dialysis increase the occurrence of ACDK. Cysts vary in size but are usually small in appearance. In contrast to polycystic disease, the outline of the kidney is maintained because of the small cyst size. The cysts develop in the cortex, medulla, and in the area between the cortex and medulla. Complications may include gross hematuria, tumors (adenoma or adenocarcinoma), abscess, calculus, etc.

—*polycystic disease of the kidney*—hereditary disorder that usually occurs bilaterally. Kidneys appear enlarged and are studded with various sized cysts. Cysts scattered throughout the parenchyma tend to compress the adjacent parenchyma, destroy it by ischemia, and occlude normal tubules. It is thought that cysts originate because of a failure of union of the collecting tubules and the convoluted tubules of some nephrons. Polycystic kidney disease also may involve other organs, such as the liver and pancreas. (12, 23, 36)

—*simple cyst of the kidney*—hereditary kidney disease presenting various cystic lesions of the medulla or cortex. They may be simple, multilocular, solitary cysts, and of the dermatoid type or similar to that of the polycystic kidney, with the only difference being in degree. They may replace and compress normal renal tissue and can be associated with cystic disease of the liver and pancreas. (12, 23, 36)

—*sponge kidney*—papillae and calices appear enlarged, with small cystic cavities within the pyramids. Usually, small calculi occupy the cysts. The condition is asymptomatic and is discovered when the patient has an urogram. (12, 14)

- *renal failure and related disorders:*
  —*azotemia*—biochemical abnormality characterized by impaired renal function, an increase of blood urea nitrogen, and creatinine associated with retention of nitrogenous wastes in the blood. When clinical manifestations are present in addition to the biochemical abnormality, uremia is the proper term. (2)

  —*renal failure, acute*—clinical state marked by a sudden decrease in glomerular filtration rate and cessation of renal function subsequent to severe kidney damage due to toxins, disease, or trauma. Renal tubular necrosis is a dominant characteristic. The lumen of the renal tubules is occluded by debris, usually containing protein, epithelial cells, and hemoglobin. If the initial oliguric phase is followed by a diuretic phase, the patient recovers. Residual damage is common. (1, 14)

  —*renal failure, chronic*—clinical state resulting from irreversible, slowly progressive renal disorder, such as chronic glomerulonephritis or pyelonephritis, drug toxicity, systemic disease, or urinary tract obstruction. Marked glomerular damage, as evidenced by electrolyte imbalance and retention of nitrogenous wastes, signals a fatal prognosis. (2)

  —*uremia*—syndrome resulting from greatly reduced excretory function in progressive bilateral kidney disease. The failure to remove metabolic waste end products from the urine, the subsequent retention of these products in the blood and tissue compartments, and their potential cumulative action as toxins are major components in the development of morbid conditions associated with the syndrome of uremia. Clinical symptoms vary widely, from lassitude and depression in the early phase to anuria, uremic frost, and peripheral neuropathy in the terminal phase. (2, 14, 41)

- *renal hypertension, renovascular hypertension*—high blood pressure of the kidney resulting from marked thickening of arteriolar walls or stenosis of renal artery by atheromatous plaques and thrombi. It is not known why the ischemic kidney elevates the blood pressure. (16, 35)

- *renal medullary necrosis, renal papillary necrosis*—tissue death of renal papillae and medulla, usually a complication of pyelonephritis. (35)

- *renal tuberculosis*—degeneration of kidney substance due to infection with tubercle bacilli.

- *renal vein thrombosis*—occlusion of the renal vein by a thrombus, which may result in the elevation of the renal pressure, excessive proteinuria, and other manifestations of the nephrotic syndrome. A complete occlusion of the renal vein may be complicated by a hemorrhagic infarction of the kidney. (23)

Operative Terms

- *nephrectomy*—excision of kidney, primarily for advanced calculous pyonephrosis, hydronephrosis, or malignant tumor. (6, 33, 36)
- *nephrolithotomy*—incision into kidney for removal of stones. (36)
- *nephrolysis*—surgical destruction of renal adhesions.
- *nephropexy*—surgical fixation of a displaced kidney.
- *nephrorrhaphy*—suture of an injured kidney.
- *nephrostomy*—surgical creation of a renal fistula for drainage. (15, 48)
- *nephrotomy*—incision into kidney. (5)
- *nephroureterectomy*—removal of ureter and kidney for tumor of the renal pelvis or for malignant tumor of the ureter.
- *pyelolithotomy*—incision into renal pelvis for removal of calculi. (36)
- *pyeloplasty*—plastic repair of renal pelvis. (16)
- *pyelotomy*—incision into renal pelvis.
- *renal biopsy:*
    - *—open renal biopsy*—through an incision made below the tip of and parallel to the 12th rib, the muscle and fascia are divided and a wedge of tissue is excised from the kidney for histopathologic studies.
    - *—percutaneous renal biopsy*—removal of renal tissue by a pronged biopsy needle. The procedure is usually performed under fluoroscopic control. It aids in the diagnosis and prognosis of renal disease and also serves as a guide in designating the appropriate therapy. (3, 12, 14, 51)
- *renal transplantation, kidney transplantation*—a form of replacement surgery in which a healthy donor kidney is implanted in a patient after irreversibly diseased kidneys have been removed. The renal homograft may be obtained from a living donor or from a cadaver of a person who met with a fatal accident. Bilateral nephrectomies are imperative in the presence of renal infection or severe hematuria, since invariably the donor transplant will develop the disease of the collateral recipient's kidney if only one kidney has been removed. After the donated homograft is placed extraperitoneally, vascular anastomoses to the iliac vessels and hypogastric artery are performed, and an opening is surgically created between a ureter and the bladder (ureteroneocystostomy). (33, 50)
- *surgery for renovascular hypertension*—operative procedures for the restoration of normal blood flow to the kidney, including:
    - —bypass grafting for unilateral or bilateral renal artery stenosis.
    - —excision of occluded lesion of renal artery followed by end-to-end anastomosis.
    - —renal endarterectomy or surgical removal of intimal plaques from renal artery, with or without patch grafting. (16, 33, 35, 50)

Symptomatic Terms

- *anuria*—total suspension of urine due to renal failure or blockage of urinary tract. (1, 14)
- *Dietl's crisis*—recurrent attacks of lumbar and abdominal pain, nausea, and vomiting, caused by ureteral kinking or by vascular tension in cases of hypermobile kidney. (21)
- *renal insufficiency, renal shutdown, lower nephron nephrosis*—severe disturbance of excretory kidney function in renal disease or following surgery or trauma. Anuria may develop from blood transfusions, overhydration, and electrolyte imbalance. (14)

- *renal pain*—various degrees from dull, aching to severe, stabbing, or throbbing pain in lumbar region. (16, 21)
- *uremic frost*—powdery deposit of urea on the skin due to the excretion of urea through perspiration.

Ureters

Origin of Terms

hydr-, hydro- (G)—water
junction (L)—joining
pyelo- (G)—pelvis, tub
pyo- (G)—pus

-stomy (G)—surgical creation of an artificial opening
uretero- (G)—ureter, duct

Anatomic Terms (16, 37, 53)

- *ureter*—muscular, distensible tube lined with mucous membrane. It carries urine from each kidney to the bladder.
- *ureteric orifice*—opening of the ureter at the outer, upper angle of the trigone (base) of the urinary bladder.
- *ureteropelvic junction*—meeting point between ureter and renal pelvis.
- *ureterovesical junction*—meeting point between ureter and urinary bladder.

Diagnostic Terms

- *calculus in ureter*—ureteral stone causing obstruction. (10, 40)
- *congenital malformations of the ureter*
    - *duplication of ureters*—the most common ureteral abnormality.
      There are two kinds:
      complete duplication—both ureters enter bladder on the same side.
      incomplete duplication—ureters join supravesically.
    - *ectopic ureteral orifice*—displaced opening, a developmental defect seen more frequently in women than men. It may result in incontinence.
    - *incomplete ureter*—embryonic development ceased before ureter reached kidney. Kidney may be absent or multicystic.
    - *stricture of ureter*—abnormal narrowing of the duct, usually occurring at the ureteropelvic junction or at the ureterovesical orifice. It may be complicated by ureteral dilatation.
    - *ureterocele*—cystic protrusion or ballooning sacculation of the lower end of the ureter into the bladder. It may be intravesical or ectopic. Usually, intravesical ureteroceles are involved with single ureters, and ectopic ureteroceles are involved with duplicated ureters. (10)
- *hydroureter*—ureter overdistended with urine due to obstruction.
- *injuries to ureter*—uncommon pathologic states that may result from external trauma, be associated with pelvic fractures, or occur inadvertently during surgery. A penetrating wound from a bullet may perforate a ureter and result in leakage of urine into the peritoneal cavity. (22)
- *obstruction of ureter*—blocking of ureter, usually resulting from pressure. It interferes with passage of urine. (10, 14)
- *occlusion of ureter*—complete or partial closure of ureter.
- *pyoureter*—infection in the ureter, generally secondary to infection of the bladder or kidney.
- *ureteritis*—inflammation of the ureter. (27)

Operative Terms

- *ureteral resection*—local excision of benign ureteral lesion. (41)
- *ureterectomy*—partial or complete removal of ureter.
- *ureterocystostomy, ureteroneocystostomy*—reimplantation of ureter into bladder.
- *ureterolithotomy*—incision into ureter for removal of calculi.
- *ureterolysis*—freeing the ureter from adhesion to relieve secondary obstruction.
- *ureteropelvioplasty*—plastic operation at the ureteropelvic junction. (41)
- *ureteropyelostomy*—anastomosis of ureter and renal pelvis.
- *ureterostomy, cutaneous*—transplantation of ureter to skin.
- *ureteroureterostomy*—operation of joining portions of the same ureter. The urine is diverted by a linear ureterotomy. An oblique oval anastomosis is developed to ensure that healing occurs at different planes and that strictures do not occur. This procedure is performed in cases where the ureter has been severed, either deliberately or accidentally. (16, 53)
- *ureterovesicoplasty*—corrective surgery for persistent reflux by repair of the ureterovesical junction. (41)

Symptomatic Terms

- *ureteral colic*—excruciating, stabbing pain usually caused by the passage of a stone or large clot into the ureter. It may be accompanied by prostration, diaphoresis, shock, and collapse. (21)
- *ureteral spasm*—contraction of ureter, frequently resulting from painful overdistention of ureter by a stone. (36)

Bladder and Urethra

Origin of Terms

cysto- (G)—bladder, sac
trigone (G)—triangular area
urethro- (G)—bladder, urethra
vesical (L)—bladder

Anatomic Terms (16, 37, 46, 53)

- *bladder, urinary*—a hollow, muscular, distensible organ. It serves as a temporary reservoir for urine.
- *bulbourethral glands, Cowper's glands*—these two glands are located posterolaterally to the membranous urethrea. The glands are above the bulb of the penis within the fibers of the sphincter urethra muscle. The ducts of these glands open into the ventral wall of the proximal part of the spongy urethra.
- *detrusor urinae muscle*—muscular network with bundles of muscle fibers running in various directions, intermingling, and decussating. Their contraction effects the expulsion of urine from the bladder.
- *neck of bladder*—lowest angle of bladder.
- *vesical sphincter*—thickened detrusor muscle fibers that surround the bladder neck.
- *vesicouterine*—peritoneum extending between the bladder and the uterus.
- *trigone*—triangular internal surface of the posterior wall of the bladder.
- *urethra*—fibromuscular channel of communication between the urinary bladder and external urethral orifice.
    - *female urethra*—passageway for urine.
    - *male urethra*—passageway for urine and seminal fluid.
      It is composed of:
    - *prostatic portion*—passes through prostate.

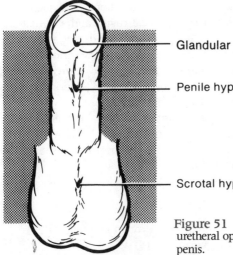

Glandular hypospadias

Penile hypospadias

Scrotal hypospadias

Figure 51 Hypospadias. Various abnormal locations of the uretheral openings are shown on the ventral surface of the penis.

−*membranous portion*−passes through pelvic and urogenital diaphragms.
−*spongy portion*−passes through the penis.
- *urethral glands of Littre*−mucus-producing glands that are most dense on the dorsal surface of the spongy urethra.

Diagnostic Terms

- *atony of bladder*−enormous distention of bladder associated with reduced expulsive force. It occurs in some diseases of the central nervous system.
- *bladder neck obstruction*−blockage of the lumen of the bladder outlet, resulting in overdistention of the urinary bladder, frequency, dysuria, persistent pyuria, retention with overflow and urinary backflow, dilatation of the ureters, renal pain and stone formation. The obstruction may be caused by:
  - −*contracture of vesical outlet, congenital or acquired*−form of urethral stricture. The bladder may be narrowed by hypertrophic muscle, fibrous tissue, or chronic inflammatory disease.
  - −*obstructive lesions of vesical outlet*−blood clots, calculi, diverticula, and tumors, especially prostatic enlargement. (40, 44)
- *calculus (pl. calculi) of bladder*−bladder stone. (46)
- *cord bladder*−bladder dysfunction due to injury or lesion of spinal cord. Residual urine, incontinence, and vesicoureteral reflux are usually present. (43, 46)
- *cystitis, acute or chronic*−inflammation of bladder due to infection. (21, 46)
- *exstrophy of bladder*−congenital absence of the lower abdominal and anterior vesical walls with eversion of the bladder; absence of closure or formation of the anterior one half of the bladder. It is often associated with epispadias. (44, 46)
- *hypospadias* (Fig. 51)−congenital abnormality resulting in a defect in the ventral wall of the spongy urethra, so that it is open for a greater or lesser distance. The glandular and penile types of hypospadias occur because of failure of fusion of the urogenital fold. In the glandular type the prepuce is usually deformed, and its frenulum may be absent. Scrotal hypospadias occurs from failure of the labioscrotal swellings to fuse. (4, 24)
- *injuries to:*
  - −*urinary bladder*−direct trauma to the distended bladder may cause vesical

compression or rupture. A bony spicule of a fractured bone may pierce the bladder, blood and urine will spill into the peritoneal cavity, and a hematoma may form. Accidental perforation of the bladder may occur during surgery.

—*urethra, bulb of spongy urethra*—injury to these sites may be more serious than to the bladder, including contusions, lacerations, and rupture associated with extravasation of urine and blood and formation of hematoma. Shearing injuries or straddle injuries may be complicated by urethral stricture. (22)

- *interstitial cystitis, submucous fibrosis of bladder, Hunner's ulcer*—bladder disorder predominantly seen in middle-aged women. Fibrosis of the vesical wall reduces the bladder capacity, which is clinically manifested by frequency, nocturia, distention of the bladder, and suprapubic tenderness or pain. (44)
- *megalocystis, megabladder*—enormous dilatation of urinary bladder.
- *neoplasms:*
    - —*benign*—papilloma, polyp, and others.
    - —*malignant*—transitional cell carcinoma, epidermoid carcinoma, and others. The diagnosis is usually confirmed by cystoscopy. (8)
- *neurogenic bladder*—two main types:
    - —*flaccid atonic type*—condition caused by lower motor neuron lesion due to trauma, ruptured intervertebral disk, meningomyelocele, or other disorders and resulting in vesical dysfunction. The bladder has a large capacity, low intravesical pressure, and a mild degree of trabeculation (hypertrophy) of the bladder wall.
    - —*spastic automatic type*—condition caused by upper motor neuron lesion due to injury, multiple sclerosis, or other factors. The bladder capacity is reduced, the intravesical pressure is high, and there is marked hypertrophy of the bladder wall and spasticity of the urinary sphincter. (46, 53)
- *prolapse of bladder*—downward displacement of the bladder. (45)
- *stress incontinence*—inability to retain urine under any tension and when sneezing, coughing, or laughing. (43, 44)
- *stricture of urethra*—narrowing of lumen of urethra due to infection or trauma.
- *stricture of vesicourethral orifice*—narrowing of the opening between the bladder and urethra. (40)
- *syphilis of bladder and urethra*—venereal infection due to *Treponema pallidum*.
- *Trichomonas infection*—parasitic infection that may occur in the bladder and male urethra. (40)
- *trigonitis*—inflammation of the trigone, the triangular base of the bladder. (20)
- *urethritis, acute or chronic*—inflammation of urethra, which may be due to gonococcic infection. (45)
- *vesical fistulas*—pathologic openings of bladder leading to adjacent organs.
    - —*vesicoenteric fistula*—sinus tract between bladder and intestine.
    - —*vesicorectal fistula*—fistulous connection between bladder and rectum.
    - —*vesicovaginal fistula*—pathologic opening between bladder and vagina. (44)

Operative Terms

- *cold-punch transurethral resection of the vesical neck*—endoscopic procedure for relief of bladder neck obstruction using a cold-punch resectoscope for transurethral resection of tumor tissue, calcareous deposit, or cicatrix. The Kaplan resectoscope permits:
    - —fiberoptic illumination
    - —magnification and sharp visualization of surgical area
    - —the free flow of irrigation fluid
    - —controlled movement of the knife (41, 46)
- *cystectomy*—excision of bladder.

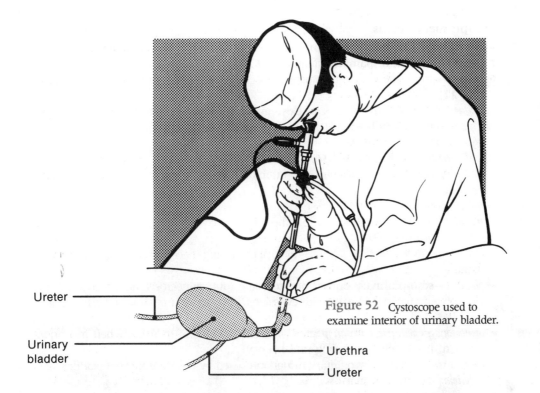

Ureter

Urinary
bladder

Figure 52 Cystoscope used to
examine interior of urinary bladder.

Urethra

Ureter

—*partial*—resection of bladder.

—*complete*—removal of entire viscus. (44)

- *cystolithotomy*—incision into bladder for removal of stones.
- *cystoplasty*—surgical repair of the bladder.
- *cystorrhaphy*—suture of a ruptured or lacerated bladder.
- *cystoscopy* (Fig. 52)—endoscopic examination of the bladder. (49)
- *cystostomy*—surgical creation of a cutaneous bladder fistula for urinary drainage. (49)
- *meatotomy*—incision of urinary meatus to increase its caliber. (41)
- *suprapubic vesicourethral suspension, Marshall-Marchetti repair*—elevation and immobilization of the bladder neck and urethra by suturing them to the pubis and rectus muscles for establishment of urinary control. (16, 44)
- *transurethral resection of the bladder neck*—endoscopic resection of the bladder neck for removal of inelastic tissue using the transurethral approach. (44)
- *urethroscopy, panendoscopy*—endoscopic examination of the male urethra or distal female urethra using a special panendoscope. (44)
- *urinary diversion operations for incapacitated bladder:*
    —*ileal conduit, ureteroileostomy*—transplantation of both ureters to an isolated segment of the ileum. The urine drains through an external ileal stoma into a bag glued to the skin. Candidates for an elective ileal conduit may be children with bladder exstrophy and incontinence, adults with neurogenic bladders caused by injury or neurologic disease, or victims of a vesical carcinoma. In malignancy and persistent bladder infection a cystectomy is done with an ileal conduit.
    —*sigmoid bladder, neobladder, colocystoplasty*—replacement of bladder by creating a substitute bladder. A sigmoid segment is isolated, and the ureters and urethra are implanted in the segment. The cecum may also be used for urinary diversion. (16, 31, 32, 34)

Symptomatic Terms

- *albuminuria, proteinuria*—albumin or protein in urine.
- *dysuria*—difficult or painful urination. (16, 21)
- *enuresis*—incontinence or involuntary discharge of urine when asleep at night. (16, 21)
- *frequency of urination*—voiding at close intervals, more often than every two hours. This is normal in infancy. (16, 21)
- *glycosuria*—sugar in urine.
- *hematuria*—blood in urine. (16, 21)
- *hesitancy*—dysuria due to nervous inhibition or to obstruction of vesical outlet. (16, 21)
- *micturition*—urination. (21)
- *nocturia*—frequent voiding during the night; may be due to renal inability to concentrate urine. (16, 21)
- *obstruction in bladder or urethra*—blockage causing backflow of urine and renal damage.
- *oliguria*—scanty urinary output due to acute tubular necrosis, advanced fluid and electrolyte imbalance, organic kidney lesions, obstructive uropathy, and other causes. (1, 21)
- *orthostatic proteinuria, benign postural proteinuria*—protein in urine when in upright position; no proteinuria during recumbency.
- *overflow incontinence*—involuntary urination caused by overdistention of bladder. (21)
- *polyuria*—excessive urinary output.
- *pyuria*—pus in the urine. (16)
- *residual urine*—inability to empty bladder at micturition, resulting in urinary retention and vesical overdistention. (21)
- *spinal shock*—sequela of transverse injury to cord. It may cause autonomous bladder paralysis and later automatic voiding. (43, 46)
- *suprapubic discomfort*—uncomfortable sensation that may be due to interstitial cystitis, ulceration of the vesical mucosa, or other disorders. It is usually present when the bladder fills and disappears when the bladder empties.
- *tenesmus of vesical sphincter*—painful spasm at the end of micturition.
- *trabeculation, vesical*—hypertrophy involving all muscle layers of the bladder. It may occur in benign prostatic hypertrophy. (40)
- *ureteral pain*—usually acute, colicky pain radiating from renal pelvis to groin; may be due to a stone pressing against the ureteral wall. (14)
- *urethral discharge*—clear, thin, mucoid or purulent, scanty or profuse excretion from the urethra.
- *urgency*—intense need to urinate. (16, 21)
- *urinary retention*—inability to expel urine. This may be acute or chronic, complete or incomplete. It is frequently caused by obstruction of urinary outflow due to a stone, stricture, tumor, and similar blocks. (21)
- *vesicoureteral reflux*—backflow of urine into kidney, usually caused by bladder neck obstruction. It may result in severe renal damage. (41)

Special Procedures

Terms Related to Bladder Studies

- *cystometrogram*—graphic record of pressure reactions while the patient's bladder is being filled with water. Bladder capacity, residual urine, and sensory responses are checked. In cord bladders sensations are absent. (39)

- *cystometry*—measurement of intravesical pressure during filling of the urinary bladder with fluid. (43, 46)

Terms Related to Dialysis Studies

- *dialysis*—the passage of solutes back and forth across a semipermeable membrane placed between two solutions. Each solute moves toward the fluid in which its concentration is lower. Dialysis is used in acute renal failure to remove urea from the body and terminate electrolyte imbalance. Hemodialysis and peritoneal irrigation are the methods of choice. (2)
- *intermittent hemodialysis*—circulation established outside the body with the renal dialyzer one to three times a week, depending on the patient's residual kidney function. An arteriovenous fistula is surgically created, or an artery and vein are cannulated, permitting the repetitive use of hemodialysis. The blood of the patient who is connected to the renal dialyzer passes into a coil of semipermeable membrane immersed in a bath of rinsing fluid. This membrane substitutes for the glomerular membrane. The concentration of solutes in the blood differs from that in the bath to promote a solute transfer through the semipermeable membrane, which restores the electrolyte balance. After the solute exchange is completed, the blood reenters the patient's vein. (2)
- *hemodialysis*—a life-sustaining procedure in irreversible renal failure, since it removes excess water and the end-products of protein metabolism and corrects acidosis as well as electrolyte imbalance.
- *peritoneal dialysis, peritoneal lavage, intermittent method*—perfusion of the peritoneum using commercially prepared electrolyte solutions, special catheters, and a closed system of infusion and drainage in the treatment of renal failure. The peritoneum functions basically as an inert semipermeable membrane, permitting the exchange of solutes in both directions.
- *prophylactic dialysis*—the use of peritoneal dialysis to prevent renal failure. (2)

Terms Related to Nonsurgical Procedures

- *fine needle aspiration cytology*—specimen is obtained via suction through a small-bore (21, 22, or 23 gauge) needle. Computed technology scanning, fluoroscopic studies, or ultrasonic techniques enhance the visualization and localization of lesions. The cytologic specimen is placed on slides and stained by either the Romanowsky method (usually the May-Grünwald-Giemsa stain) or the Papanicolaou (Pap) method. The procedure aids the physician in planning further therapy or diagnostic studies. (15, 48)
- *percutaneous extraction of renal calculi, nephrolithotripsy*—under fluoroscopic control or under direct vision with a nephroscope, a nephrostomy tract can be established, subsequently dilatated to allow for stone manipulation and removal. The lithotripsy probe passes easily through a 26 F nephroscope. When the probe is in direct contact with the stone, electrical or sonic energy is transmitted through the probe to break up the stone. Small stones can be removed via the nephroscope, and larger stones by means of a stone basket or forceps. Another disintegrative method applicable to kidney stones is:
    - —*extracorporeal shock wave lithotripsy (ESWL)*—pulverizes kidney stones by bombarding them with shock waves, which are produced outside the body, focused at the kidney stones and transmitted by body tissues. Patients are immersed in water, since water serves at the medium through which the shock waves are transmitted by body tissues. Shock waves produce a selective disintegrative effect on kidney stones because of their high acoustical impedance compared to the brittle makeup of surrounding tissues. Periodic fluoroscopic monitoring of

the treatment ensures that the stone is still in the shock wave's focal point. As the treatment progresses, video monitors may be employed to display the gradual pulverization of the kidney stone. (15, 16, 29, 53)

- *transcatheter embolization*—therapeutic introduction of an inert embolic or sclerosing substance into a vessel to occlude it. Superselective engagement of branch vessels or use of an occlusive balloon catheter assists in preventing occurrence of inadvertent embolization of the distant organs. Occlusion of the vascular supply of the kidney makes possible early ligation of the renal vein. This ligation may prevent dissemination of tumor cells when the kidney and the tumor are subsequently mobilized. Transcatheter embolization with radioactive particles can create an interstitial infarct implant capable of delivering high doses of radiation to a tumor. This procedure can be used for reducing tumor size and thus making the inoperable tumor operable. (15)

Male Genital Organs

Origin of Terms

balano- (G)—glans
didymos (G)—testis, twin
orchido- (G)—testis (pl. testes)
semen (L)—seed
vaso- (L)—vessel, duct

Anatomic Terms (see Fig. 53) (16, 37, 53)

- *penis*—highly vascular organ containing three erectile tissue components. The distal end is the glans penis, over which is folded the prepuce, or foreskin. The penis serves as the outlet for urine stored in the bladder (urination). During sexual intercourse its role is to deposit seminal fluid or semen in the vagina of the female (ejaculation).
- *prostate*—organ composed of smooth muscle and fibrous and glandular tissue and divided into two lateral lobes and one medial lobe. An extension of the urinary bladder, the prostate is connected to the prostatic urethra and ejaculatory ducts. Its secretion, a type of milky alkaline fluid, is part of the seminal fluid.
- *scrotum*—sac of loose, redundant skin containing testes and epididymides.
- *testes (sing. testis)*—paired male reproductive glands lying in the scrotum and divided into lobules by septa that are inward extensions of the outer covering. The lobules contain threadlike coils, the seminiferous tubules. The testes produce spermatozoa, a minute part of the seminal fluid, and androgen, the male hormone responsible for the secondary sex characteristics. Three ducts share in the transport of spermatozoa on each side:
  - *epididymis (pl. epididymides)*—structure lying on top and at the side of the testis and composed of head, body, and tail. It stores spermatozoa before they are emitted. The greatly coiled duct of the epididymis, about six meters in length, merges into the ductus deferens.
  - *ductus deferens, vas deferens*—duct conveying spermatozoa from the epididymis to the ejaculatory duct.
  - *ejaculatory duct*—duct formed by union of the ductus deferens with the duct of the seminal vesicle. Its fluid is carried into the urethra.
- *tunica vaginalis testis*—double-layered serous sheath partially covering the testis and epididymis. An abnormal collection of serum between the layers is termed hydrocele.

Diagnostic Terms

- *actinomycosis*—fungus disease that may affect the genital organs. (42)
- *adenocarcinoma*—malignant tumor of glandular epithelium. It most commonly involves the prostate, less commonly the other genital organs. Metastases to bone

Figure 53 Male reproductive organs.

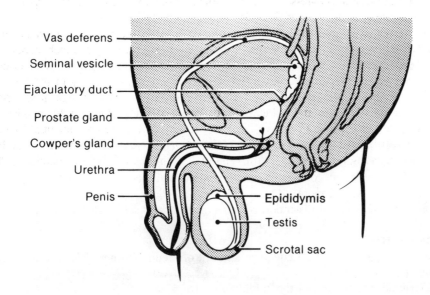

occur frequently. Knowledge of the stage and grade of adenocarcinoma of the prostate may be helpful in treatment of this particular disease entity:

  —*Stage A₁: well-differentiated, unifocal adenocarcinoma*

  —*Stage A₂: diffuse, moderate to poorly differentiated*

  —*Stage B₁: adenocarcinoma with less than two-centimeters involvement of one lobe*

  —*Stage B₂: adenocarcinoma involving more than one lobe*

  —*Stage C: tumor extending through the prostate capsule or into seminal vesicle*

  —*Stage D₁: lymphatic metastasis confined to pelvis*

  —*Stage D₂: metastasis outside of pelvis, usually involving bone or lymph nodes* (8, 16, 53)

- *anorchism*—absence of testes.
- *balanitis*—inflammation of the glans penis.
- *chordee of penis*—painful downward curvature of the penis as a result of a congenital anomaly (hypospadias) or urethral infection (gonorrhea). (28)
- *cryptorchism*—improperly descended testis, descent arrested. (25, 26, 53)
- *ectopy of testis*—testis outside the path of normal descent. (25)
- *epididymitis*—inflammation of the epididymis. (27)
- *hydrocele:*
    —*tunica vaginalis*—collection of fluid within the tunica of the testis.
    —*spermatic cord*—collection of fluid along the spermatic cord, usually within the inguinal canal. (25)
- *hypertrophy of prostate, benign*—diffuse enlargement of the prostate, frequently seen in elderly men. The gland interferes with micturition and eventually results in hydronephrosis and dilatation of ureters. (8, 16)
- *orchitis*—inflammation of the testes. (26, 27)
- *paraphimosis*—foreskin retracted behind the glans, with subsequent edema preventing restoration to normal position. (24)
- *phimosis*—stenosis of the orifice of the prepuce or foreskin. It may be congenital or due to infection. The opening may be pinpoint or absent. (16, 24)
- *polyorchism, polyorchidism*—more than two testes present. (25)
- *prostatitis*—inflammation of the prostate gland. (27)

- *syphilis*—venereal diseases due to *Treponema pallidum*. Involvement of genital organs is common. (20)
- *testicular tumors*—usually malignant neoplasms seen in young adults 18 to 35 years of age, less frequently in children, and rarely in other age-groups. They include:
    - *choriocarcinoma*—malignant tumor secreting chorionic gonadotropin.
    - *embryonal carcinoma*—aggressive, lethal, testicular neoplasm that is highly invasive and readily spreads to lymph nodes and internal organs.
    - *seminoma*—common testicular germ cell tumor.
    - *teratoma, differentiated*—benign cystic dermoid containing multiple tissues, including hair and teeth.
    - *teratocarcinoma*—malignant testicular tumor composed of various poorly differentiated tissues. (8)
- *tuberculosis*—systemic, contagious disease caused by tubercle bacilli. Involvement of genital organs is infrequent. (42)
- *varicocele*—swelling and distention of veins of spermatic cord. (25, 26, 30)

Operative Terms

- *circumcision*—removal of an adequate amount of prepuce to permit exposure of the glans. (24)
- *epididymectomy*—excision of the epididymis. (16, 53)
- *excision of hydrocele*—evacuation of serous fluid or removal of serous tumor from tunica vaginalis.
- *orchiectomy, orchectomy, orchidectomy*—removal of testis. (16, 53)
- *orchiopexy*—suturing an undescending testis in the scrotum.
- *orchioplasty*—plastic repair of a testis.
- *prostatectomies:*
    - *perineal prostatectomy*—removal of prostate through an incision in the perineum.
    - *retropubic prostatectomy*—a form of extravesical removal of prostate with partial or complete resection of gland.
    - *suprapubic prostatectomy*—removal of gland through an opening into the bladder from above.
    - *transperineal urethral resection of the prostate*—endoscopic resection of prostate combined with perineal urethrotomy to avoid the formation of a postoperative urethral stricture.
    - *transurethral cryogenic prostatectomy*—use of special endoscope and freezing technique for destruction of prostatic tumor.
    - *transurethral prostatectomy*—removal of obstructing glandular tissue using a special endoscope and electrocautery. (8, 16, 52, 53)
- *vasectomy*—removal of a short segment of the vas deferens and ligation of the severed ends. (26)
- *vasoligation*—tying the vas deferens with ligature to produce sterility or to prevent epididymitis.
- *vasovasotomy, epididymovasostomy*—anastomosis of the vas deferens to epididymis to produce fertility by circumventing the obstructive lesion in the vas deferens. (26, 30, 47, 55, 56)

Symptomatic Terms

- *azoospermia*—semen without living spermatozoa, causing infertility in the male. (38)
- *dragging inguinal pain*—pain may be caused by enlargement of the testes.
- *edematous swelling*—enlargement of an organ or part resulting from its infiltration with an excessive amount of tissue fluid.

- *lumbosacral pain*—pain felt in the small of the back. (39)
- *mucopurulent discharge*—drainage of mucus and pus.
- *oligospermia*—scanty production and expulsion of spermatozoa. (26)
- *prodromal pain*—initial pain signaling that a more severe attack is approaching.
- *prostatism*—urinary difficulty resulting from obstruction at the bladder neck by hypertrophy of prostate gland or other causes.
- *strangury*—painful urination, drop by drop, due to spasmodic muscular contraction of bladder and urethra.

Abbreviations

General

ADH—antidiuretic hormone
A/G Ratio—albumin/globulin ratio
BPH—benign prostatic hypertrophy
BUN—blood, urea, nitrogen
Cysto.—cystoscopic examination
ERPF—effective renal plasma flow
GBM—glomerular basement membrane
GFR—glomerular filtration rate
GU—genitourinary
ICU—intensive care unit
IVP—intravenous pyelogram
KUB—kidney, ureter, bladder
NPO—nothing by mouth
pH—hydrogen ion concentration

PRA—plasma renin activity
PSP—phenolsulfonphthalein
RER—renal excretion rate
RPF—renal plasma flow
UA—urinalysis
UTI—urinary tract infection
VMA—vanillylmandelic acid

Other

ESWL—extracorporeal shock-wave
　　　 lithotripsy
PNL—percutaneous nephrolithotomy
TUR—transurethral resection

Oral Reading Practice

Hydronephrosis

This condition is a by-product of mechanical obstruction of the urinary tract. When the interference with the outflow of urine is below the bladder, as in **urethral stricture** or **hypertrophy** of the prostate gland, **bilateral hydronephrosis** develops. When above the bladder, as in **unilateral, ureteral stricture, calculus,** or **neoplasm,** the condition affects only one kidney. In addition, pressure from tumors, adhesions, or the **pregnant uterus** outside the urinary tract may interfere with the flow of urine and lead to **hydronephrosis. Congenital anomalies** of the **ureter** or **urethra** may also be responsible for this condition.

There are various degrees of **dilatation** of the **renal pelvis** and ureter. In the initial phase of the disease the pathologic changes are slight. As the condition progresses, the amount of fluid increases, the **papillae** assume a flattened appearance, the **renal cortex** becomes thinned, and the pyramids of the medulla undergo atrophic changes. The kidney resembles a hollow shell filled with fluid. In extreme cases several liters of fluid may accumulate in the renal pelvis, leading to a complete loss of physiologic capacity. If the **hydronephrosis** is unilateral, the healthy kidney undergoes compensatory hypertrophic changes to adapt itself to the increased functional work load. In this case renal insufficiency does not develop. However, in the presence of advanced bilateral hydronephrosis, the downhill clinical course is steady and terminates in fatal uremia.

The fluid in the kidney differs from normal urine in its reduced content of urea. Since it is locked up in the renal shell and unable to escape to its proper destination, it easily becomes a breeding place for invading bacterial organisms. Another deleterious **sequela** of fluid retention in the kidney is the formation of **renal calculi,** which adds insult to injury and completes the physiologic destruction of the organ.

In the early phase of hydronephrosis symptoms may be absent or so mild that they escape notice. As the condition progresses, the kidney becomes palpable, tender, and painful. With unrelieved obstruction continued over weeks, the only symptom may be a dull pain. If intermittent obstruction occurs, attacks of pain develop periodically and are accompanied by oliguria, which is promptly reversed to **polyuria** when the obstruction is abolished. Should the damaged kidney become infected, **leukocytosis,** fever, and **pyuria** signal the onset of **pyonephrosis.**

The treatment of hydronephrosis consists in removing the cause of obstruction, such as the ureteral stricture, or compressing **prostatic** or vesicular tumor. If done early, the kidney may be saved. In advanced cases the presence of irreparable damage demands the excision of the diseased organ, since it serves no useful function and is a constant threat of focal infection. (34, 40, 46)

Table 13
Some Urogenital Conditions Amenable to Surgery

Organs Involved	Diagnosis	Type of Surgery	Operative Procedures
Kidneys	Chronic glomeru-lonephritis, preterminal Irreversible renal failure	Renal homotransplan-tation, including: a. bilateral nephrectomy b. revascularization of homograft c. ureterocystostomy	Removal of both kidneys Extraperitoneal donor homo-grafting with vascular anastomoses to iliac and hypogastric vessels Creation of opening between ureter and bladder
Kidney	Nephroptosis	Nephropexy	Fixation or suspension of movable or displaced kidney
Kidney	Post-traumatic fistula of kidney	Nephrorrhaphy	Suture of kidney
Kidney Ureter	Calculous anuria due to acute ureteral obstruction	Nephrostomy Pyelostomy	Creation of communication between the kidney and skin for drainage
Ureter	Calculus in ureter associated with renal obstruction	Ureterolithotomy	Incision into ureter with removal of calculus
Ureter	Postinfectional stricture of ureter	Ureteroplasty	Plastic repair of ureter
Renal pelvis	Calculus in renal pelvis, small	Pyelolithotomy	Removal of calculus from renal pelvis

Organs Involved	Diagnosis	Type of Surgery	Operative Procedures
Bladder	Diverticulum of bladder	Diverticulectomy of urinary bladder	Local excision of diverticulum
Bladder	Cystocele	Cystoplasty	Plastic repair of cystocele
Bladder	Hemorrhage from urinary bladder	Cystoscopy with evacuation of blood clots	Endoscopic examination of the bladder
Bladder	Early carcinoma of urinary bladder, no metastasis	Partial cystectomy with wide local excision of tumor	Removal of bladder wall, including the carcinoma and surrounding cuff of normal bladder wall
Bladder	Papilloma encroaching on ureteral orifice	Suprapubic cystostomy with excision of tumor Ureterocystostomy	Surgical opening of the bladder above the symphysis pubis and removal of tumor Anastomosis of ureter to bladder and reimplantation of ureter into bladder
Bladder	Rupture of bladder due to injury	Cystorrhaphy	Suture of bladder
Bladder Ureters	Bladder neck obstruction, vesicoureteral reflux	Bladder neck reconstruction (Y-V plasty) Ureteroneocystostomy	Surgical bladder neck revision and reimplantation of ureters into bladder to correct vesicoureteral reflux
Bladder Ureters	Neurogenic bladder associated with vesical calculi and recurrent pyelonephritis	Ureteroileostomy (Ileal conduit)	Transplantation of both ureters to isolated segment of ileum for conveying urine to external stoma
	Carcinoma of bladder Exstrophy of bladder	Cystectomy	Removal of bladder in vesical malignancy and uncontrolled infection
Bladder Ureters Urethra	Carcinoma of bladder	Cystectomy Colocystoplasty (neobladder or sigmoid bladder)	Excision of urinary bladder Creation of new bladder by isolating sigmoid segment and implanting ureters and urethra in segment
Prostate	Hypertrophy of prostate	Transurethral resection of prostate cryosurgery of prostate	Partial removal of prostate using special endoscope and electrocautery or localized freezing of prostate

Organs Involved	Diagnosis	Type of Surgery	Operative Procedures
Prostate Seminal vesicles Vasa deferentia	Carcinoma of prostate	Retropubic prostatectomy Radical perineal prostatectomy	Radical extravesical removal of prostate Removal of prostate, seminal vesicles, and vasa deferentia through perineal incision
Testis Spermatic cord	Torsion of spermatic cord complicated by testicular gangrene	Orchiectomy Orchiopexy	Removal of testis Scrotal fixation of testis
Testes	Advanced carcinoma of the prostate gland with bone metastases	Orchiectomy, bilateral (castration for androgen control)	Removal of both testes
Testis	Undescended testis, unilateral	Orchioplasty Orchiopexy	Surgical transfer of testis to scrotum

References and Bibliography

1. Amend, William J.C., Jr., and Vincenti, Flavio G. Oliguria: acute renal failure. In Tanagho, Emil A., and McAninch, Jack W., eds., *Smith's General Urology*, 12th ed. Norwalk, CT: Appleton & Lange, 1988, pp. 526-529.
2. ————. Chronic renal failure & dialysis. Ibid., pp. 530-532.
3. Andrioli, Gerald L., and Catalona, William Jr. Fine needle aspiration cytology. *The Urologic Clinics of North America* 14:657-661, Nov. 1987.
4. Conte, Felix A., and Grumbach, Melvin M. Abnormalities of sexual differentiation. In Tanagho, Emil A., and McAninch, Jack W., eds., *Smith's General Urology*, 12th ed. Norwalk, CT: Appleton & Lange, 1988, pp. 602-626.
5. Forsham, Peter H. Disorders of adrenal glands. In Tanagho, Emil A., and McAninch, Jack W., eds., *Smith's General Urology*, 12th ed. Norwalk, CT: Appleton & Lange, 1988, pp. 473-492.
6. Fowler, Jackson E., Jr. Nephrectomy in metastatic renal cell carcinoma. *The Urologic Clinics of North America* 14:749-756, Nov. 1987.
7. Goldstein, Irwin. Penile revascularization. *The Urologic Clinics of North America* 14:905-813, Nov. 1987.
8. Johnson, Douglas E., et al. Tumors of the genitourinary tract. In Tanagho, Emil A., and McAninch, Jack W., eds., *Smith's General Urology*, 12th ed. Norwalk, CT: Appleton & Lange, 1988, pp. 330-434.
9. Kay, Robert. Ureterocalicostomy. *The Urologic Clinics of North America* 15:129-137, Feb. 1988.
10. Kogan, Barry A. Disorders of the ureter and ureteropelvic junction. In Tanagho, Emil A., and McAninch, Jack W., eds., *Smith's General Urology*, 12th ed. Norwalk, CT: Appleton & Lange, 1988, pp. 538-551.
11. Kogan, Barry A., and Hattner, Robert S. Radionuclide imaging. In Tanagho, Emil A., and McAninch, Jack W., eds., *Smith's General Urology*, 12th ed. Norwalk, CT: Appleton & Lange, 1988, pp. 142-153.
12. Krupp, Marcus A. Diagnosis of medical renal diseases. In Tanagho, Emil A., and McAninch, Jack W., eds., *Smith's General Urology*, 12th ed. Norwalk, CT: Appleton & Lange, 1988, pp. 514-525.
13. ————. Appendix: Normal laboratory values. Ibid., pp. 679-683.
14. Krupp, Marcus A. Genitourinary tract. In Schroeder, Steven A., Krupp, Marcus A., and Tierney, Lawrence M., Jr., eds., *Current Medical Diagnosis & Treatment—1988*, Norwalk, CT: Appleton & Lange, 1988, pp. 533-570.

15. Lange, Erich K. Interventional uroradiology. In Tanagho, Emil A., and McAninch, Jack W., eds., *Smith's General Urology,* 12th ed. Norwalk, CT: Appleton & Lange, 1988, pp. 111-124.

16. Linehan, W. Marston. The urogenital system. In Sabiston, David C., Jr. ed., *Essentials of Surgery,* Philadelphia: W.B. Saunders Co., 1987, pp. 826-855.

17. Lue, Tom F. Male sexual dysfunction. In Tanagho, Emil A., and McAninch, Jack W., eds., *Smith's General Urology,* 12th ed. Norwalk, CT: Appleton & Lange, 1988, pp. 666-678.

18. Malloy, Terrence R., and Wein, Alan J. Laser treatment of bladder carcinoma and genital condylomata. *The Urologic Clinics of North America* 14:121-126, Feb. 1987.

19. Mansberger, Arlie R., Jr. Acute renal failure. In Hardy, James D., ed., *Hardy's Textbook of Surgery,* 2nd ed. Philadelphia: J.P. Lippincott Co., 1988, pp. 59-66.

20. Mayer, Bruce M., and Berger, Richard E. Sexually transmitted diseases in man. In Tanagho, Emil A., and McAninch, Jack W., eds., *Smith's General Urology,* 12th ed. Norwalk, CT: Appleton & Lange, 1988, pp. 262-274.

21. McAninch, Jack W. Symptoms of disorders of the genitourinary tract. In Tanagho, Emil A., and McAninch, Jack W., eds., *Smith's General Urology,* 12th ed. Norwalk, CT: Appleton & Lange, 1988, pp. 29-37.

22. ———. Injuries to genitourinary tract. Ibid., pp. 302-318.

23. ———. Disorders of the kidneys. Ibid., pp. 493-513.

24. ———. Disorders of the penis & male urethra. Ibid., pp. 568-581.

25. ———. Disorders of the testes, scrotum, & spermatic cord. Ibid., pp. 589-597.

26. McClure, R. Dale. Male infertility. In Tanagho, Emil A., and McAninch, Jack W., eds., *Smith's General Urology,* 12th ed. Norwalk, CT: Appleton & Lange, 1988, pp. 637-662.

27. Meares, Edwin M., Jr. Nonspecific infections of the genitourinary tract. In Tanagho, Emil A., and McAninch, Jack W., eds., *Smith's General Urology,* 12th ed. Norwalk, CT: Appleton & Lange, 1988, pp. 196-245.

28. Montague, Drogo K. Correction of chordee: The Nesbit procedure. *The Urologic Clinics of North America* 13:167-174, Feb. 1986.

29. Newman, Daniel M., et al. Extracorporeal shock-wave lithotripsy. *The Urologic Clinics of North America* 14:114-120, Feb. 1987.

30. Pryor, John L., and Howards, Stuart S. Varicocele. *The Urologic Clinics of North America* 14:499-513, Aug. 1987.

31. Rowland, Randall G., et al. Alternative tech-

niques for a continent urinary reservoir. *The Urologic Clinics of North America* 14:797-804, Nov. 1987.

32. Sagalowsky, Arthur I. Technique of the continent ileal bladder: Camey procedure. *The Urologic Clinics of North America* 14:643-651, Aug. 1987.

33. Salvatierra, Oscar Jr., and Feduska, Nicholas J. Renal transplantation. In Tanagho, Emil A., and McAninch, Jack W., eds., *Smith's General Urology,* 12th ed. Norwalk, CT: Appleton & Lange, 1988, pp. 533-537.

34. Skinner, Donald G., et al. An update on the Koch pouch for continent urinary diversion. *The Urologic Clinics of North America* 14:789-795, Nov. 1987.

35. Sosa, R. Ernest, and Vaughn, E. Darracott, Jr. Renovascular hypertension. In Tanagho, Emil A., and McAninch, Jack W. eds., *Smith's General Urology,* 12th ed. Norwalk, CT: Appleton & Lange, 1988, pp. 627-636.

36. Spirnak, J. Patrick, and Resnick, Martin I. Urinary stones. In Tanagho, Emil A., and McAninch, Jack W., eds., *Smith's General Urology,* 12th ed. Norwalk, CT: Appleton & Lange, 1988, pp. 275-301.

37. Tanagho, Emil A. Anatomy of the genitourinary tract. In Tanagho, Emil A., and McAninch, Jack W., eds., *Smith's General Urology,* 12th ed. Norwalk, CT: Appleton & Lange, 1988, pp. 1-15.

38. ———. Embryology of the genitourinary system. Ibid., pp. 16-28.

39. ———. Physical examination of the genitourinary tract. Ibid., pp. 40-45.

40. ———. Urinary obstruction & stasis. Ibid., pp. 168-180. (70)

41. ———. Vesicoureteral reflux. Ibid., pp. 181-195.

42. ———. Specific infections of the genitourinary tract. Ibid., pp. 246-261.

43. ———. Urodynamic studies. Ibid., pp. 452-472.

44. ———. Disorders of the bladder, prostate & seminal vesicles. Ibid., pp. 552-567.

45. ———. Disorders of the female urethra. Ibid., pp. 582-588.

46. Tanagho, Emil A., and Schmidt, Richard A. Neuropathic bladder disorders. In Tanagho, Emil A., and McAninch, Jack W., eds., *Smith's General Urology,* 12th ed. Norwalk, CT: Appleton & Lange, 1988, pp. 435-451.

47. Thomas, Anthony J., Jr. Vasoepididymostomy. *The Urologic Clinics of North America* 14:527-538, Aug. 1987.

48. Thüroff, Joachim A. Percutaneous antegrade endourology. In Tanagho, Emil A., and McAninch, Jack W., eds., *Smith's General Urology,* 12th ed. Norwalk, CT: Appleton & Lange, 1988, pp. 125-141.

49. ———. Retrograde instrumentation of the

urinary tract. Ibid., pp. 154-167.

50. Turcotte, Jeremiah G., et al. Immunobiology and transplantation of kidney. In Hardy, James D., ed., *Hardy's Textbook of Surgery,* 2nd ed. Philadelphia: J.B. Lippincott Co., 1988, pp. 187-213.

51. Wajsman, Zev, and Klimberg, Ira. Needle aspiration and needle biopsy procedures. *The Urologic Clinics of North America* 14:103-113, Feb. 1987.

52. Walsh, Patrick C. Preservation of sexual function in the surgical treatment of prostatic cancer—An anatomic surgical approach. In DeVita, Vincent T., Hellman, Samuel, and Rosenberg, Steven A., eds., *Important Advances in Oncology.* Philadelphia: J.B. Lippincott Co., 1988, pp. 161-170.

53. Weems, W. Lamar. Urology. In Hardy, James D., ed., *Hardy's Textbook of Surgery,* 2nd ed. Philadelphia: J.B. Lippincott Co., 1988, pp. 1265-1291.

54. Williams, Richard D. Urologic laboratory examinations. In Tanagho, Emil A., and McAninch, Jack W., eds., *Smith's General Urology,* 12th ed. Norwalk, CT: Appleton & Lange, 1988, pp. 46-56.

55. Xie-Yang, Zhu, and Yong, Xiong, Shi. Vasovasostomy with use of medical needle as a support. *The Journal of Urology* 39:43-54, Jan. 1988.

56. Yarbo, E. Scott, and Howards, Stuart S. Vasovasostomy. *The Urologic Clinics of North America* 14:515-526, Aug. 1987.

Gynecologic Disorders

Vulva and Vagina

Origin of Terms

aden-, adeno- (G)—gland(s)
-cele (G)—hernia, protrusion, tumor
colpo- (G)—vagina
fistula (L)—pipe, tube
hymen (G)—membrane
labia (L)—lips

-oma (G)—tumor
-osis (G)—condition, increase
-rhaphy (G)—suture
vagina (L)—sheath
vulva (L)—covering

Anatomic Terms (Refs. 4, 15)

- *perineum*—space between vulva and anus.
- *Skene's glands*—urethral glands in female.
- *vagina*—musculomembranous tube that connects the uterus with the vulva. It is the lower part of the birth canal.
- *vulva, pudendum*—external female genital organ. Some of the vulvar structures of gynecologic importance are the following:
    - —*clitoris*—small body of erectile tissue that enlarges with vascular congestion.
    - —*hymen*—membranous fold that partially covers the vaginal opening in a virgin.
    - —*labia majora (sing. labium majus)*—two raised folds of adipose and erectile tissue covered on their outer surface with skin.
    - —*labia minora (sing. labium minus)*—two small folds covered with moist skin lying between labia majora.
    - —*vestibular glands (greater), Bartholin's glands*—two small ovoid or round glands that secrete mucus. They lie deep under the posterior ends of the labia majora.
    - —*vestibule of vagina*—space between the labia minora that contains the vaginal and urethral orifices and openings of greater vestibular glands.

Diagnostic Terms

- *atresia of:*
    - —*vagina*—congenital absence of vagina.
    - —*vulva*—congenital absence of vulva. (42)

- *Bartholin's adenitis*—inflammation of Bartholin's glands, generally due to gonococcus. (1, 34)
- *Bartholin's retention cysts*—tumors, retaining glandular secretions. They tend to undergo suppuration and form abscesses. (17, 19, 35)
- *carcinoma of vagina*—usually:
  - —*clear-cell type*—cancer characterized by glands and tubules lined by clear cells (hobnail cells) clustering in solid nests and containing glycogen. It occurs in adolescents and young women.
  - —*epidermoid type*—cancer arising from epidermal cells. It occurs in women over 50 years of age. Cells are devoid of glycogen.

  Other forms of vaginal cancer are rare. (20)
- *carcinoma of vulva*—usually a squamous cell cancer that begins with a small nodule, later undergoes ulceration and may become invasive. It is the third most common cancer of the female organs. (20)
- *condylomas*—warty growths scattered over vulva. (19)
- *fistula:*
  - —*rectovaginal*—opening between rectum and vagina.
  - —*vesicovaginal*—opening between bladder and vagina. (5)
- *kraurosis of vulva*—excessive shrinkage and atrophy of vulva, commonly seen during postmenopause. (19)
- *leukoplakia of vulva*—whitish plaques on vulva that tend to form cracks and fissures. Condition results in leukoplakia vulvitis. (19)
- *vaginitis*—inflammation of vagina.
  - —*gonorrheal*—gonococcal infection due to *Neisseria gonorrhoeae*.
  - —*mycotic, monilial*—due to fungus infection.
  - —*senile*—due to atrophic changes; occurs in elderly women.
  - —*Trichomonas*—due to infection with *Trichomonas vaginalis*. (19, 34)
- *vulvar dystrophies*—disorders of epithelial growth and nutrition resulting in changes of the superficial cell layers of the vulva. The International Society for the Study of Vulvar Disease recommends that:
  - —the terms atrophic dystrophy, kraurosis, leukoplakia, leukoplakic vulvitis, hyperplastic vulvitis, and neurodermatitis be deleted and:
  - —histiopathologic definitions be adopted as follows:
    - —*hyperplastic dystrophy of vulva with atypia*—atypical hyperplasia or dystrophy, mild, moderate, or severe, depending on the vulvar alterations.
    - —*without atypia*—the presence of epithelial hyperplasia
    - —*lichen sclerosus*—thinning of the vulvar epithelium with the dermis being characteristically accellular. (19, 34, 35)
- *vulvar Paget's disease*—form of vulvar cancer in situ, recurrent, noninvasive, spreading slowly, and presenting a discrete eruption that is initially velvety, soft, and red and later eczemoid and weepy with white plaques scattered about in the well-localized lesion. Pruritus and burning are distressing symptoms. The presence of Paget's cells in the lesion confirms the diagnosis. (20, 34)
- *vulvovaginitis*—inflammation of the vulva and vagina. (15, 19, 31)

Operative Terms

- *colpectomy*—removal of vagina.
- *colpocleisis*—closure of vagina, one indication being prolapse of vagina following total hysterectomy.
- *colpomicroscopy*—use of the colpomicroscope, which affords higher magnification than a colposcope in studying the superficial cervical epithelium for cytologic diagnosis. (21)

- *colpoperineoplasty*—repair of rectocele.
- *colpoperineorrhaphy*—suture of vagina and perineum. (6)
- *colporrhaphy*—suture of vagina.
    - *—anterior*—repair of cystocele.
    - *—posterior*—repair of rectocele. (15)
- *colposcopy*—examination of the vagina and cervix uteri, usually with a binocular microscope that allows the study of tissues under direct vision by magnifying the cells; makes possible colpophotography and the colposcopic selection of target biopsy sites. (21, 37)
- *colpotomy*—incision into the vagina to induce drainage. (15)
- *episioplasty*—plastic repair of the vulva.
- *excision of Bartholin's gland*—removal of the gland. (15)
- *marsupialization of Bartholin's gland cyst*—incision and drainage of the cyst and partial excision of the cyst wall followed by suture of the cyst lining to the surrounding surface epithelium. Lubrication is preserved, since the gland is not removed. (35)
- *vulvectomy:*
    - *—simple vulvectomy*—removal of the vulvae, which may be done for vulvar carcinoma in situ.
    - *—radical vulvectomy*—total removal of the vulvae with or without dissection of the regional lymph nodes. (15)

Symptomatic Terms

- *leukorrhea*—abnormal cervical or vaginal discharge of white or yellowish mucus. (1)
- *pruritus vulvae*—severe itching of vulva. (1)

Uterus and Supporting Structures

Origin of Terms

cervix (L)—neck
cyst-, cysto- (G)—sac, cyst
fundus (L)—base
hyster-, hystero- (G)—womb
leio- (G)—smooth
meno- (G)—menses

metr-, metro (G)—uterus
ostium (L)—small opening
-rhea (G)—flow
-rhage (G)—hemorrhage, excessive flow
trachelo- (G)—neck
uterus (L)—womb

Anatomic Terms (4, 15)

- *cul-de-sac, rectouterine pouch, Douglas' pouch*—pocket between the rectum and posterior uterus, formed by an extension of the peritoneum.
- *ligaments of uterus:*
    - *—broad ligaments*—double-layered peritoneal sheets that extend from the side of the uterus to the lateral pelvic wall.
    - *—round ligaments*—two fibromuscular bands, one on each side arising anteriorly from the fundus, passing through the inguinal canal, and inserting into the labia majora.
- *myometrium*—muscular wall of uterus.
- *uterus (nonpregnant)* (see Figs. 54 and 55)—pear-shaped, thick-walled, muscular organ, situated in the pelvis between the urinary bladder and the rectum. It is about three inches (7.5 cm) long and two inches (5 cm) wide in its upper segment. It is divided into:
    - *—body of uterus*—main part extending from fundus to isthmus of uterus.

Figure 54 Uterus, uterine tubes, and ovaries (schematic).

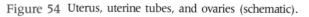

Uterine tube

Ovarian ligament

Isthmus of tube

Fundus
of uterus

Isthmus
of uterus

Ovary

Corpus luteum

Broad ligament

Cervix of uterus

Ostium of uterus

Vagina

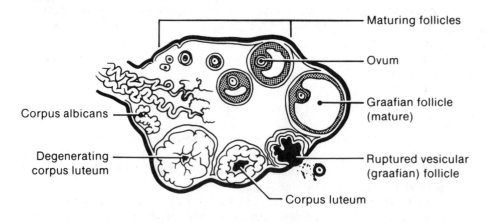

Maturing follicles

Ovum

Graafian follicle
(mature)

Ruptured vesicular
(graafian) follicle

Corpus albicans

Degenerating
corpus luteum

Corpus luteum

Figure 55 Normal ovulatory cycle.

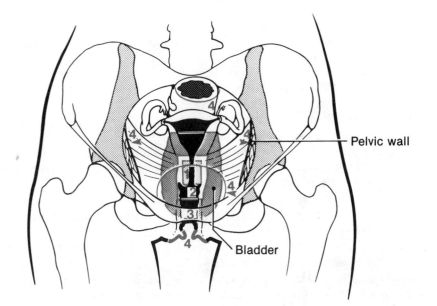

Figure 56 Clinical stages of cervical cancer.

Stage 1—The cancer is exclusively limited to the uterine cervix.

Stage 2—The cancer has spread beyond the cervix but has not reached the pelvic wall.

Stage 3—The cancer involves the lower third of the vagina or extends to the pelvic wall.

Stage 4—The cancer has spread to the mucous membrane of the rectum and bladder or has extended beyond the true pelvis.

—*body cavity, uterine cavity*—triangular space within the body.

—*endometrium*—mucous membrane lining the body cavity.

—*cervix of uterus*—lower part of uterus extending from isthmus of vagina.

—*cervical canal*—passageway between uterine cavity and vagina.

—*ostium of uterus, external os*—opening of cervix into vagina.

—*fundus of uterus*—superior dome-shaped portion of uterus above the openings of the uterine tubes into the body cavity of uterus.

—*isthmus of uterus*—constriction of uterus between body and cervix.

Diagnostic Terms

■ *disease of the cervix uteri:*

—*carcinoma of the cervix*—malignant cervical lesion that may present as an ulceration or tumor associated with excessive and irregular uterine bleeding and a leukorrheic vaginal discharge.

—*adenocarcinoma*—highly malignant cancer assuming a glandular pattern.

—*squamous cell or epidermoid carcinoma*—most frequent form arising from squamous epithelium.

Terms adopted by the International Federation of Gynecology and Obstetrics:

—*invasive carcinoma*—cancer of cervix, including the four stages presented in Fig. 56.

    —microinvasive carcinoma—Stage 1A preclinical cancer characterized by early stromal invasion. Diagnosis is based on microscopic examination from biopsy specimen.

    —preinvasive carcinoma—Stage O intraepithelial carcinoma, carcinoma in situ. (5, 21, 22)

  —*cervicitis*—inflammation of the cervix uteri.

    —acute—typically due to acute gonorrheal infection.

    —chronic—common condition caused by low-grade infection.

    —endocervicitis—inflammation of the mucous membrane of the cervix uteri.

    —erosion of cervix—red area produced by the replacement of squamous epithelium by columnar epithelium.

    —eversion of cervix, ectropion—rolling outward of a swollen mucous membrane resulting from chronic cervicitis. It may be associated with lacerations, cysts, and erosions.

    —polyps of cervix—soft, movable, pedunculated tabs that bleed readily. (18, 23)

- *diseases and malfunctions of the corpus uteri:*

    —adenomyosis—endometrial invasion of the myometrium, which may be associated with dysmenorrhea and excessive uterine bleeding. (11)

    —dysfunctional uterine bleeding—bleeding from the uterine endometrium unrelated to anatomic lesions of the uterus. It may result from an irregular production of estrogen and/or progesterone by the ovary and may occur during puberty, the reproductive period of life, or during menopause. (47)

    —endometriosis—aberrant endometrial tissue found in various pelvic and abdominal organs. (34, 45)

    —endometritis—inflammation of mucous membrane lining the corpus uteri. (7)

    —parametritis—cellulitis of the tissue adjacent to the uterus. (7)

    —perimetritis—pelvic peritonitis. (7)

- *displacements of the uterus:*

    —anteflexion—corpus uteri abnormally bent forward.

    —prolapse, procidentia, descensus uteri—downward displacement of the uterus, which may protrude from the vagina.

    —retroflexion—corpus uteri abnormally bent backward.

    —retroversion—corpus uteri abnormally turned backward with cervix directed toward symphysis pubis. (35)

- *neoplasms of the uterus:*

    —benign tumors, including:

    —endometrial polyps—small, projecting lesions that may be sessile, multiple, and resemble cystic hyperplasia. (47)

    —leiomyomas, myomas—benign smooth muscle tumors, erroneously referred to as fibroids, forming single and multiple, large or small, firm, encapsulated masses that may be:

    —intraligamentous—myoma protrudes into broad ligament.

    —intramural—myoma is embedded in myometrium.

    —submucous—sessile or pedunculated; myoma is located beneath the endometrium and may bleed profusely. (11, 34)

    —malignant tumors, including:

    —adenocarcinoma of the corpus uteri—endometrial cancer, characteristically affecting the postmenopausal woman in two ways: (1) *as a circumscribed lesion*—small portion of endometrium is diseased, although myometrial invasion may be extensive, and (2) *as a diffuse type*—the entire endometrium is involved; ulcerations and necrotic areas are present. (24)

Endometrial cancer may result from prolonged estrogen stimulation with inadequate progesterone or without progesterone and from other causes. (24)
—*leiomyosarcoma*—neoplasm usually arises from the uterine wall, recurs readily after removal, and metastasizes to bone, brain, and lung. (25)

Operative Terms

- *Cold conization, cold knife cone biopsy of uterine cervix*—cold knife removal of lining of cervical canal for locating the site of abnormal exfoliative cells in the absence of a visible lesion. The procedure is valuable in the detection of preinvasive lesions, cancer in situ, and occult cancer. (15, 21)
- *culdocentesis*—surgical puncture of the cul-de-sac used as diagnostic procedure whenever intraperitoneal bleeding is suspected, for example, in ectopic pregnancy. (15, 16)
- *culdoscopy*—endoscopic examination of the rectouterine pouch (cul-de-sac) and pelvic viscera to detect whether or not endometriosis, adnexal adhesions, tumors, or ectopic pregnancy are present or to determine the cause of pelvic pain, sterility, or other disorders. (15)
- *dilatation and curettage*—instrumental expansion of the cervix and scraping of the uterine cavity to remove:
    - —endocervical tissue and endometrial tissue for diagnosis.
    - —placental tissue to control bleeding, as in an incomplete abortion.
    - —small submucous myoma, polyp, or other lesion in the management of uterine bleeding. (15)
- *electrocautery of endocervix*—removing the mucous lining of the cervical canal by a high-frequency current to control chronic cervicitis. The procedure is also used to repair an incompetent cervix so that successful pregnancy may be achieved. (11, 17)
- *hysterectomy*—removal of the uterus.
    - —*partial or subtotal excision*—for example, supracervical removal.
    - —*total hysterectomy*—excision of entire uterus and cervix.
    - —*radical, Wertheim's operation*—removal of entire uterus and dissection of regional lymph nodes.
    - —*vaginal hysterectomy*—removal of the uterus by the vaginal approach. (33)
- *hysteroscopy, fiberoptic*—endoscopic examination for intrauterine diagnosis or therapy by:
    - —*endometrial biopsy*
    - —*identification of uterotubal junction, submucous myomas, polyps, and septa*
    - —*detection and lysis of intrauterine adhesions*
    - —*female sterilization*
    Special features are the use of carbon dioxide or hyperviscosity dextran and the Storz hysteroscope (4 mm), which permits microphotography of the endometrium. (33)
- *laparoscopy*—endoscopic visualization of abdominal organs, especially the pelvic viscera: the uterus, tubes, and ovaries. The procedure is of diagnostic value in primary and secondary amenorrhea, polycystic ovarian syndrome, unruptured ectopic pregnancy, pelvic inflammatory disease, and other disorders. (15, 17, 32)
- *myomectomy:*
    - —*abdominal approach*—removal of intramural myoma or myomas from the uterus.
    - —*vaginal approach*—removal of cervical myoma from uterine cervix. (15)
- *panhysterectomy, total hysterectomy*—removal of entire uterus, including the cervix. (15, 33)
- *suspension of uterus*—correction of retrodisplacement of the uterus.

     —*Baldy-Webster procedure*—creation of a surgical opening for the passage of the round ligaments, which are then sutured to the back of the uterus.

     —*modified Gilliam procedure*—surgical shortening of the round ligaments through the internal inguinal ring. This allows the stronger portion of the round ligament to bring the uterus forward. (35)

- *trachelectomy, cervicetomy*—removal of uterine cervix.
- *tracheloplasty, Sturmdorf procedure*—cone or core excision of endocervix; cervical canal covered with mucosal flap. (17)

Symptomatic Terms

- *amenorrhea*—absence of menstruation for three months or more.
  —*primary amenorrhea*—no menstrual cycle initiated by age 18.
  —*secondary amenorrhea*—menstrual cycle ceased after initial menarche. (46)
- *cryptomenorrhea*—menses occur, but there is no external manifestation; due to obstructive lesion of lower genital canal. (47)
- *dysmenorrhea*—painful menses. There are two types:
  —*primary dysmenorrhea*—menstrual distress is a functional disturbance, precipitated by emotional tension. It is prevalent in adolescence but may occur later in life.
  —*secondary dysmenorrhea*—menstrual pain has an organic basis; onset is usually after adolescence. (34, 47)
- *hypermenorrhea, menorrhagia*—abnormal premenopausal bleeding due to irregular endometrial shedding, endometrial polyposis, uterine myoma or hypertrophy, or a bleeding disorder. (47)
- *hypomenorrhea*—diminished bleeding and number of days in menstrual period. (47)
- *metrorrhagia*—irregular bleeding from uterus caused by hormone imbalance, not menses; sometimes induced by estrogen administration or hypothyroid state or caused by myoma, cervical and endometrial cancer, polyposis, or other disorders. (47)
- *oligomenorrhea*—infrequent menstrual bleeding; interval of cycles is over 38 days but less than three months. (1, 47)
- *polymenorrhea*—recurrent uterine bleeding within 24 days related to an exceptionally short cycle or the interruption of the cycle by psychic or physical trauma. (43, 47)
- *premenstrual syndrome (PMS)*—complex disorder recurring monthly before menstruation, characterized by fluid retention, weight gain, agitation or depression, mood swings, and fatigue. The symptoms increase progressively in some and suddenly in others. (34, 43)

Ovaries and Uterine Tubes

Origin of Terms

albus (L)—white	*-itis (G)*—inflammation
ampulla (L)—little jug	*oophor-, oophoro- (G)*—ovary, bearing eggs
fimbria (L)—fringe	*ovi-, ovo (L)*—egg
infundibulum (L)—funnel	*salpingo- (G)*—tube

Anatomic Terms (4, 15)

- *ova (sing. ovum)*—female reproductive cells.
- *ovaries (sing. ovary)* (see Figs. 54 and 55)—two female reproductive glands producing ova after puberty.
  —*ovarian follicle*—small excretory structure of the ovary. The primary ovarian

follicle is immature, consisting of a single layer of follicular cells. The vesicular ovarian or graafian follicle develops, ruptures, and discharges the ovum. It also secretes the follicular hormone, estrogen.

—*corpus luteum*—small, yellow body formed in ruptured ovarian follicle. It secretes the corpus luteum hormone, progesterone.

—*corpus albicans*—white body that develops from corpus luteum. It leaves a pitlike scar on ovary.

■ *uterine tubes, fallopian tubes, oviducts*—two muscular canals about four inches (10 cm) long that provide a passageway for the ovum to the uterus and a meeting place for the ovum and spermatozoon in fertilization. An ovum entering the tube through the abdominal opening of the fimbriated infundibulum passes through the:

—*ampulla*—wider, thinner-walled, longest part of the tube.

—*isthmic portion*—interstitial portion of the tube, narrower and thicker-walled than the ampulla.

—*uterine part*—tube within the myometrium.

—*uterine opening*—entrance into the uterine cavity.

Diagnostic Terms

■ *abscess, tubo-ovarian*—localized suppuration of uterine tube and ovary. (17)

■ *Brenner tumor*—peculiar, usually benign ovarian tumor containing epithelial cell nests within a matrix of fibrous tissue. It may undergo mucinous transformation or increased epithelial proliferation, as seen in malignancy. (28, 35)

■ *cyst of ovary*—fluid-containing tumor of the ovary.

—*graafian follicle cyst*—retention cyst appearing on the ovary as a fluid-filled bleb, resulting from the inability of the partially formed follicle to reabsorb.

—*corpus luteum cyst*—functional ovarian enlargement, resulting from the fluid increase by the corpus luteum following ovulation.

—*endometrial ovarian cyst*—cyst formed by ectopic endometrial tissue and filled with decomposed blood due to bleeding into the cystic cavity. This cyst may be attached to other pelvic structures.

—*theca lutein cyst*—cyst, prone to occur in both ovaries, is filled with straw-colored or serosanguineous fluid and may rupture. It develops in the presence of hydatidiform mole, choriocarcinoma, and excessive therapy with chorionic gonadotropin. (27, 34)

■ *cystadenoma of ovary*—silent tumor, nonproductive of hormone, constituting 70 percent of ovarian neoplasms.

—*mucinous cystadenoma*—multilocular, large-sized cysts, lined with active mucin-secreting cells. Cysts may rupture, releasing mucinous cells that may transplant and grow on the omentum and the peritoneum. When this condition leads to a continuing collection of mucin in the peritoneum, it is termed "pseudomyxoma peritonei."

—*serous cystadenoma*—encapsulated multilocular glandular cyst filled with thin, yellowish fluid and growing in size, but not to great excess. (26, 27, 28, 35)

■ *dehiscence of wound, burst abdomen, evisceration, wound disruption*—bursting open of a sutured wound, followed by protrusion of intestine through the incision, a serious surgical complication; also dehiscence of a graafian follicle. (3)

■ *dysgerminoma*—germ cell tumor occurring in small girls or in first decades of life, exhibiting variability in size and malignancy. The tumor may be associated with streak ovaries, rudimentary gonads seen in chromosome aberration. (13, 29)

■ *hydrosalpinx*—uterine tube distended by clear fluid. (15)

■ *infertility, female*—temporary or permanent inability to conceive or become pregnant after a year of sexual exposure, dependent on multiple etiologic factors such as:

—anovulation

—defects of the luteal phase

—the condition of the cervix

—the status of the uterine tubes

—immunologic responses

—chromosomal aberrations, e.g., Turner's syndrome or Klinefelter's syndrome

—male factors, e.g., high viscosity of semen, low sperm motility, and low volume of semen. (39, 44)

Associated terms include:

—*primary infertility*—pregnancy never achieved.

—*secondary infertility*—at least one previous conception has occurred, but presently, the couple is not able to achieve pregnancy.

—*sterility*—total inability to conceive. (9, 39, 44)

- *Meig's syndrome*—solid, fibromatous, unilateral tumor of the ovary associated with hydrothorax and ascites. Other pelvic tumors may also form pleural and peritoneal effusions, which promptly disappear with surgical removal of the tumor. (30)

- *oophoritis acute and chronic*—inflammation of the ovary or ovaries.

- *pelvic inflammatory disease*—broad term, including pelvic inflammations caused by gonococcal, streptococcal postabortal infections as well as intestinal parasites; multiple infectious organisms may coexist. (7)

- *polycystic ovarian syndrome, Stein-Leventhal syndrome*—symptom complex characterized by bilateral enlarged ovaries containing multiple follicular microcysts. Amenorrhea, infertility, obesity, hypertension, and hirsutism (hairiness) are common symptoms. (12, 47)

- *pyosalpinx*—pus in the uterine tube.

- *ruptured tubo-ovarian abscess*—breaking open of the abscess and escape of purulent drainage into the peritoneal cavity. (7)

- *salpingitis, acute and chronic*—inflammation of the uterine tube or tubes. (17, 34)

- *torsion of ovarian pedicle*—twisting of the pedicle of an ovarian cyst resulting in circulatory disturbance and sharp persistent pain. (29)

Operative Terms

- *adnexectomy*—removal of uterine adnexa, the tubes, and ovaries.

- *complete ovarian ablation*—surgical removal of the entire ovary.

- *oophorectomy, ovariectomy:*

    —partial removal of an ovary.

    —complete removal of one ovary.

    —castration; bilateral, complete removal of ovaries. (3, 34)

- *oophoropexy*—fixation of a displaced ovary.

- *oophoroplasty*—plastic repair of an ovary.

- *ovarian wedge resection*—removal of a triangular wedge of the ovary for the purpose of stimulating ovarian activity in anovulation and infertility. (46)

- *panhysterectomy and bilateral salpingo-oophorectomy*—removal of complete uterus, both tubes and ovaries. (15)

- *salpingectomy*—partial or complete removal of the uterine tubes. (15)

- *salpingolysis*—the breaking up of peritubal adhesions that damage the fimbriated end of the tube. This procedure is considered an effective means of correcting infertility. (14, 15)

- *salpingo-oophorectomy*—removal of tubes and ovaries. (15)

- *tubal implantation*—correction of the cornual block and implantation of the unobstructed tubes into the uterine cavity, to restore tubal patency following sterilization surgery.

- *tubal insufflation, uterotubal insufflation, Rubin test*—procedure used for diagnostic and therapeutic purposes:
    - —to detect whether the tubes are blocked or patent.
    - —to relieve tubal obstruction by dislodging mucous plugs and breaking up adhesions at the fimbriated ends of the tubes. Successful pregnancy may follow. (44)
- *tubal ligation*—tying the tubes to prevent pregnancy; sterilization surgery. (33, 40)
- *tuboplasty, salpingoplasty*—reconstructive tubal surgery for the correction of infertility. The constricted or occluded end of the uterine tube is excised, and the distal portion of the tube is reimplanted into the uterus. Recently the use of cone-shaped, spiral stents has been advocated as an effective method of maintaining tubal patency. (15)

Symptomatic Terms

- *anovulation*—absence of ovulation due to cessation or suspension of menses. (44)
- *menopause*—cessation of menses and reproductive period of life. (48)
- *ovulation*—expulsion of an ovum from the ruptured graafian follicle. (15)
- *septic shock*—sudden hypotension, renal dysfunction, peripheral blood pooling, and metabolic acidosis caused by gram-negative bacteremia due to septic abortion, puerperal sepsis, or pelvic infection. (16, 34)

Special Procedures

Cytologic Studies for Gynecologic Conditions

- *cytopathologic studies*—these include cytogenetic, cytologic, and hormonal evaluations of gynecologic disorders. The specimen for study is usually obtained by microbiopsy. (21)
- *cytogenetic studies*—these deal with chromosomal structure of cells and aid to clarify issues of hermaphroditism, intersexuality, and antenatal sex determination. (6)
- *cytologic studies*—the detection of tumors of the cervix and endometrium in the preinvasive state when proper treatment can be instituted. Several methods have been devised to obtain smears for cytologic diagnosis. (8, 15, 21, 22, 36, 41, 49)
    - —*Papanicolaou's method (Pap smear)*—employs a curved glass pipette with a rubber bulb for aspirating vaginal fluid with its cellular components. The smear technique is based on the fact that vaginal and uterine epithelia, as with all epithelial tissue, undergo continual exfoliation or shedding of cells. Similarly, tumors that reach the lining surface may exfoliate cells, which fall into the vagina and become mixed with the vaginal secretion. Experts in exfoliative cytology recognize incompletely developed malignant cells, which gradually and progressively change from a benign preinvasive, preclinical stage to an early invasive and late malignant stage.
    - —*hormonal studies*—cytopathologic evaluation for detecting abnormal cytohormonal patterns, which may suggest the presence of functional ovarian neoplasms, endocrine or breast tumors, and endometrial or tubal lesions.
    - —*microbiopsy*—the cellular specimen obtained for tissue examination by the pathologist.

Terms Related to Fertility Studies

- *biopsy:*
    - —*endometrial biopsy and histologic study*—method of determining evidence of ovulation. If absent, the ovarian factor is thought to be the cause of sterility. The

biopsy, however, does not indicate whether the ovary is primarily or secondarily involved.

—*ovarian biopsies, bilateral*—removal of ovarian tissue for the detection of the cause of infertility, evaluation, and resumption of ovarian function. Large ovarian biopsies with use of Palmer biopsy forceps may be done under laparoscopic control. (44)

- *hysterosalpingography*—roentgenography of the uterus and uterine tubes following injection of opaque material. (44)
- *laparoscopy*—endoscopic examination of pelvic and reproductive organs for diagnostic appraisal and/or therapeutic control. (28, 32, 33, 38)
- *tubal insufflation (Rubin test)*—tubal patency test in reproductive failure. Blocked tubes are a cause of sterility. (44)

Other Tests

- *culture for Neisseria gonorrhoeae*—use of Thayer-Martin (TM) medium in cultures for the detection of the gonococcus. (7, 17, 18)
- *dark-field examination*—most specific means of direct demonstration of *Treponema pallidum*, obtained from moist lesions of primary, secondary, or relapsing syphilis. (16, 17, 18)
- *serologic tests for syphilis*—tests that utilize either nontreponemal or treponemal antigens:
    —nontreponemal antigen tests:
      —flocculation tests:
        –Venereal Disease Research Laboratories (VDRL) test
        –Rapid plasma reagin (RPR) test
      —complement fixation tests:
        –Wassermann test
        –Kolmer test
    —treponemal antibody tests:
      —Fluorescent treponemal antibody absorption (FTA-ABS) test
      —*T pallidum* immobilization (TPI) test
      —*T pallidum* complement fixation (TPCF) test
      —*T pallidum* hemagglutination (TPHA) test (16, 17, 18)
- *Schiller test*—test helpful in the detection of superficial cancer, particularly that of the cervix. Normal epithelium is rich in glycogen and stained deeply by iodine solution. Cancerous epithelium has almost no glycogen and takes no stain. The test has its limitations. (21)

Abbreviations

General Terms

CIS—carcinoma in situ
D&C—dilatation and curettage
FSH—follicle-stimulating hormone
GC—gonorrhea
Gyn—gynecology
HPO—hypothalamic-pituitary-ovarian
IUD—intrauterine device
LMP—last menstrual period

MH—marital history
PID-pelvic inflammatory disease

Organizations

ACOG—American College of Obstetricians and Gynecologists
ACS—American College of Surgeons
FIGO—International Federation of Gynecology and Obstetrics

Oral Reading Practice

Toxic Shock Syndrome

Toxic shock syndrome is a severe illness with the sudden onset of high fever, vomiting, diarrhea, and myalgia. Usually **hypotension** develops in severe cases and shock occurs. An **erythematous** rash (sunburnlike) is noted during the acute phase of the illness. Approximately ten days after onset, **desquamation** of the skin occurs, particularly in the area of the palms and soles of the feet. There may be disorientation or alterations in consciousness without focal neurologic signs when fever and hypotension are absent.

The Centers for Disease Control in Atlanta, Georgia investigated this phenomenon as well as the factors underlying the almost exclusive occurrence of toxic shock in menstruating women. Ninety percent of toxic shock syndrome occurred during the menstrual cycle. Although toxic shock syndrome is generally related to menstruation, the Centers of Disease Control found a small precent of toxic shock syndrome was noted following childbirth by vaginal delivery and cesarean section and in association with therapeutic abortions; infected surgical wounds; lymphadenitis; deep abscesses; and subcutaneous lesions such as burns, abrasions, lacerations, furuncles, and insect bites.

The investigators found that a significant portion of the women used a single brand of tampon during the menstrual period and that the *Staphylococcus aureus* isolated from the toxic shock syndrome patients was found to be resistant to penicillin and ampicillin in 95 percent of the cases.

The Centers for Disease Control recommended that women who use tampons and wish to reduce their risk status to this disease do the following: (1) use tampons intermittently during the menstrual period, and (2) immediately remove and discontinue tampon use and consult a physician if a high fever, vomiting, or diarrhea develop during the menstrual period. The Centers recommended that proper management of suspected toxic shock syndrome should include a vaginal examination with removal of any retained tampons, with cervical cultures for the detection of *S. aureus*. Physicians are recommended to employ fluid replacement and use **beta-lactamase-resistant antistaphylococcal antibiotics,** since evidence supports the efficacy of these antibiotics in preventing recurrences. Also women who have had toxic shock syndrome episode should not use tampons, at least until the *S. aureus* has been eradicated from the vagina.

Toxic shock syndrome is a serious disease that primarily affects previously healthy young women of childbearing age. The syndrome resembles **Kawasaki's** disease **(mucocutaneous lymph node syndrome)** in several respects: fever, rash, with subsequent desquamation, and cardiac involvement. However, the shock prominent in toxic shock syndrome is not usually seen in Kawasaki's disease, and the character of the rash is different in these two diseases: **maculopapular** in Kawasaki's disease and nonpapular, diffuse **erythroderma** in toxic shock syndrome. **Azotemia** and **thrombocytopenia** are rarely seen in Kawasaki's disease and are common in toxic shock syndrome. (1, 10, 34)

Table 14

Some Gynecologic Conditions Amenable to Surgery

Organs Involved	Diagnosis	Type of Surgery	Operative Procedures
Hymen	Imperforate hymen	Hymenectomy	Excision of hymen
Clitoris	Hypertrophy of clitoris	Excision of hyper-trophied clitoris	Removal of hypertrophied clitoris and creation of normal looking genitalia
Bartholin's glands	Recurrent Bartholin's gland abscess and cyst	Excision of Bartholin's gland cyst	Removal of entire Bartholin's gland
Bartholin's glands	Chronic bartho-linitis and cyst of Bartholin's gland	Marsupialization of Bartholin's gland cyst	Partial excision of cyst wall Suture of cyst lining to the surrounding surface epithelium
Vulva	Carcinoma in situ	Excision of vulva with split-thickness graft	Removal of carcinoma in situ and abnormal vulva epithelium and replacement with normal epithelium via split-thickness skin graft
Vulva	Leukoplakia of vulvae	Vulvectomy	Removal of vulvae
Vagina Bladder	Vesicovaginal fistula	Vesicovaginal fistula repair	Permanent closure of vesico-vaginal fistula
Vagina Bladder	Urinary stress incontinence	Marshall-Marchetti-Krantz operation	Surgical elevation and fixation of bladder neck and urethra by suture applications, using Cooper's ligament and conjoined tendon for suspension
Vagina Perineum	Rectocele	Posterior repair	Excess vaginal mucosa is exised; plication of perirectal and levator muscles over the anterior rectal wall, providing support to the perineal body, the posterior vaginal wall, and the pelvic floor
Bladder Urethra	Cystocele Urinary stress incontinence	Anterior repair, Kelly plication	Construction of firm shelf of periurethral tissue to support bladder and urethra

Organs Involved	Diagnosis	Type of Surgery	Operative Procedures
Urethra Vagina	Urethrovaginal fistula Urinary stress incontinence	Urethrovaginal fistula repair	Excision of scarred, devascularized tissue surrounding fistula; approximation of healthy margins of tissue with multilayers by closing and bringing source of blood supply to base of urethra to cover fistula
Vagina Cervix Uterus	Carcinoma of vagina, cervix, uterus	Radical Wertheim hysterectomy with bilateral pelvic lymph node dissection	Removal of uterus, upper vagina, and all perimetric tissues to the pelvic wall; common iliac and upper hypogastric vessels are stripped of all lymphatic-bearing tissue
Cervix uteri	Benign erosion of cervix Neoplasia of cervix	Cryosurgery	Freezing techniques
Uterus	Irregular bleeding of undetermined cause	Dilatation and curettage	Scraping of endometrial lining
Uterus	Prolapse of uterus	Manchester operation	Amputation of cervix uteri, tubes, and ovaries
Cervix uteri	Chronic cervicitis	Conization	Removal of mucous lining of cervical canal by high-frequency current
Uterine tubes	Hydrosalpinx	Salpingectomy	Removal of uterine tube
Uterine tubes	Fallopian tube obstruction	Fimbrioplasty	Opening of the obstructed uterine tube, salvaging functions of the fimbriae to allow entry and transport of sperm
Ovary	Polycystic ovary syndrome (Stein-Leventhal disease)	Wedge resection of the ovary	Removal of triangular wedge of ovary for stimulating ovarian activity in anovulation and infertility

References and Bibliography

1. Barclay, David L. Benign disorder of the vulva and vagina. In Permoll, Martin L., and Benson, Ralph C., eds., *Current Obstetric & Gynecologic Diagnosis & Treatment*, 6th ed. Norwalk, CT: Appleton & Lange, 1987, pp. 618-656.

2. Bernaschek, Gerhard, et al. Vaginal sonography versus human chorionic gonadotropin

in early detection of pregnancy. *American Journal of Obstetrics & Gynecology* 158:608-612, March 1988.

3. Burnett, Lonnie S. Gynecologic history, examination, and operations. In Jones, Howard W., III, Wentz, Anne Colston, and Burnett, Lonnie S., eds., *Novak's Textbook of Gynecology*, 11th ed. Baltimore: Williams & Wilkins, 1988, pp. 3-39.

4. ———. Anatomy. Ibid., pp. 40-67.

5. ———. Relaxations, malposition, fistulas, and incontinence. Ibid., pp. 455-478.

6. Butler, Merlin G., et al. Genetics and cytogenetics. In Jones, Howard W., III, Wentz, Anne Colston, and Burnett, Lonnie W., eds., *Novak's Textbook of Gynecology*, 11th ed. Baltimore: Williams & Wilkins, 1988, pp. 101-139.

7. Cartwright, Peter S. Pelvic inflammatory disease. In Jones, Howard W., III, Wentz, Anne Colston, and Burnett, Lonnie S., eds., *Novak's Textbook of Gynecology*, 11th ed. Baltimore: Williams & Wilkins, 1988, pp. 507-525.

8. Cherkis, Richard C., et al. Significance of normal endometrial cells detected by cervical cytology. *Obstetrics & Gynecology* 71:242-250, Feb. 1988.

9. Coulam, Carolyn B. Investigating unexplained infertility. *American Journal of Obstetrics & Gynecology* 158:1374-1381, June 1988.

10. Emancipator, Kenneth, et al. Analytical versus clinical sensitivity and specificity in pregnancy testing. *American Journal of Obstetrics & Gynecology* 158:613-616, March 1988.

11. Entman, Stephan S. Uterine leiomyoma and adenomyosis. In Jones, Howard W., III, Wentz, Anne Colston, and Burnett, Lonnie S., eds., *Novak's Textbook of Gynecology*, 11th ed. Baltimore: Williams & Wilkins, 1988, pp. 443-454.

12. Eshel, Alex, et al. Pulsatile luteinizing hormone—releasing hormone therapy in women with polycystic ovary syndrome. *Fertility and Sterility* 49:956-960, June 1988.

13. Gallion, Holly H., et al. Ovarian dysgerminoma: Report of seven cases and review of the literature. *American Journal of Obstetrics & Gynecology* 158:591-595, March 1988.

14. Gomel, Victor, and Rowe, Timothy C. Microsurgery in gynecology. In Permoll, Martin L., and Benson, Ralph C., eds., *Current Obstetric & Gynecologic Diagnosis & Treatment*, 6th ed. Norwalk, CT: Appleton & Lange, 1987, pp. 979-990.

15. Haney, A.F. Gynecologic surgery. In Sabiston, David C., Jr., ed., *Essentials of Surgery*. Philadelphia: W.B. Saunders Co., 1987, pp. 802-825.

16. Hemsell, David L., et al. Pelvic infections and sexually transmitted diseases. In Permoll, Martin L., and Benson, Ralph C., eds., *Current Obstetric & Gynecologic Diagnosis & Treatment*, 6th ed. Norwalk, CT: Appleton & Lange, 1987, pp. 715-741.

17. Hill, Edward C. Benign disorders of the uterine cervix. In Permoll, Martin L., and Benson, Ralph C., eds., *Current Obstetric & Gynecologic Diagnosis & Treatment*, 6th ed. Norwalk, CT: Appleton & Lange, 1987, pp. 643-669.

18. Jawetz, Ernest. Spirochetes and other spiral microorganisms. In Jawetz, Ernest, et al., eds., *Review of Medical Microbiology*, 17th ed. Norwalk, CT: Appleton & Lange, 1987, pp. 293-300.

19. Jones, Howard W. Benign disease of the vulva and vagina. In Jones, Howard W., III, Wentz, Anne Colston, and Burnett, Lonnie S., eds., *Novak's Textbook of Gynecology*, 11th ed. Baltimore: 11th ed. Baltimore:eWilliams & Wilkins, 1988, pp. 570-596.

20. ———. Malignancies of the vulva and vagina. Ibid, pp. 599-622.

21. ———. Cervical intraepithelial neoplasia. Ibid., pp. 643-678.

22. ———. Invasive cancer of the cervix. Ibid., pp. 679-715.

23. ———. Endometrial hyperplasia. Ibid., pp. 716-727.

24. ———. Endometrial carcinoma. Ibid., pp. 728-760.

25. ———. Sarcoma of the uterus. Ibid., pp. 761-772.

26. ———. Tumors of the tube, paraovarium, and uterine ligaments. Ibid., pp. 773-781.

27. ———. Ovarian cysts and tumors. Ibid., pp. 782-791.

28. ———. Epithelial ovarian cancer. Ibid., pp. 792-830.

29. ———. Germ cell tumors of the ovary. Ibid., pp. 831-848.

30. ———. Sex cord-stromal tumors of the ovary. Ibid., pp. 849-862.

31. Kaufman, Raymond H. Establishing a correct diagnosis of vulvovaginal infection. *American Journal of Obstetrics & Gynecology* 158:986-990, April 1988.

32. Levinson, John M. Laparoscopy in gynecology. In Permoll, Martin L., and Benson, Ralph C., eds., *Current Obstetric & Gynecologic Diagnosis & Treatment*, 6th ed. Norwalk, CT: Appleton & Lange, 1987, pp. 817-821.

33. Malinak, L. Russell, and Wheeler, James M. Therapeutic gynecologic procedures. In Permoll, Martin L., and Benson, Ralph C., eds., *Current Obstetric & Gynecologic Diagnosis & Treatment*, 6th ed. Norwalk, CT: Appleton & Lange, 1987, pp. 822-840.

34. Margolis, Alan J., and Greenwood, Sadja. Gynecology and obstetrics. In Schroeder, Steven A., Krupp, Marcus A., and Tierney,

Lawrence M., Jr., eds., *Current Medical Diagnosis & Treatment—1988*, Norwalk, CT: Appleton & Lange, 1988, pp. 447-495.

35. Newton, Michael, and Lurain, John R., III. Gynecologic surgery. In Hardy, James D., ed., *Hardy's Textbook of Surgery*, 2d ed. Philadelphia: J.B. Lippincott Co., 1988, pp. 1306-1338.

36. Rubin, Stephen C., et al. Peritoneal cytology as an indicator of disease in patients with residual ovarian carcinoma. *Obstetrics & Gynecology* 71:851-853, June 1988.

37. Schneider, A., et al. Colposcopy is superior to cytology for detection of early genital human papillomavirus infection. *Obstetrics & Gynecology* 71:236-241, Feb. 1988.

38. Seifer, David B., et al. Follicular aspiration: A comparison of an ultrasonic endovaginal transducer with fixed needle guide and other retrieval methods. *Fertility and Sterility* 49:462-467, March 1988.

39. Speirs, Andrew L. The changing face of infertility. *American Journal of Obstetrics & Gynecology* 158:1390-1394, June 1988.

40. The American Fertility Society. The American Fertility Society classifications of adnexal adhesions, distal tubal occlusion, tubal occlusion secondary to tubal ligation, tubal pregnancies, müllerian anomalies and intrauterine adhesions. *Fertility and Sterility* 49:944-955, June 1988.

41. Waeckerlin, Ronald W., et al. Correlation of cytologic, colposcopic, and histologic studies with immunohistochemical studies of human papillomavirus structural antigens in an unselected patient population. *American Journal of Obstetrics & Gynecology* 158: 1394-1402, June 1988.

42. Wentz, Anne Colston. Congenital anomalies and intersexuality. In Jones, Howard W., III, Wentz, Anne Colston, and Burnett, Lonnie S., eds., *Novak's Textbook of Gynecology*, 11th ed. Baltimore: Williams & Wilkins, 1988, pp. 140-186.

43. ———. Dysmenorrhea, premenstrual syndrome, and related disorders. Ibid., pp. 240-262.

44. ———. Infertility. Ibid., pp. 263-302.

45. ———. Endometriosis. Ibid., pp. 303-327.

46. ———. Amenorrhea, evaluation and treatment. Ibid., pp. 351-377.

47. ———. Abnormal uterine bleeding. Ibid., pp. 378-396.

48. ———. Management of menopause. Ibid., pp. 397-442.

49. Wentz, Anne Colston, and Cartwright, Peter S. Recurrent and spontaneous abortion. In Jones, Howard W., III, Wentz, Anne Colston, and Burnett, Lonnie S., eds., *Novak's Textbook of Gynecology*, 11th ed. Baltimore: Williams & Wilkins, 1988, pp. 328-350.

Obstetrical, Fetal, and Neonatal Conditions

CHAPTER 11

The Obstetrical Period

Origin of Terms

contra- (L)—against, opposite
ec- (G)—out
ecto- (G)—outside
gravida (L)—pregnancy
multi- (L)—many

nulli- (L)—none
pelvis (L)—basin
placenta (L)—cake
primi- (L)—first
pueri- (L)—child

General Terms

- *basal body temperature*—body temperature taken under basal conditions before arising in the morning. Relatively lower levels are present in the preovulatory phase than in the postovulatory phase. (Ref. 43)
- *blighted ovum*—impregnated ovum that has ceased to grow within the first trimester.
- *contraception*—voluntary prevention of pregnancy. (44, 46)
- *gestation*—intrauterine development of infant.
    - —*embryonic period*—approximately the first trimester.
    - —*fetal period*—approximately the second and third trimesters. (7, 22)
- *gravida*—pregnant woman. (39, 43)
- *high-risk gravida*—there are multiple reasons for considering a pregnant woman a high-risk patient. She may be too young or too old or underweight or overweight, and may have diabetes, hypertension, urinary infection, rubella, hepatitis, Rh incompatibility, alcoholic or narcotic addiction, or other health hazards. By identifying the problem during early gestation, appropriate treatment may be instituted to protect the mother and growing fetus. (3, 22)
- *high-risk neonate*—newborn in need of resuscitation due to abnormally brief or prolonged gestation, too low or too high birth weight, defective Apgar score, fetal diseases, congenital anomalies, chromosomal aberrations, and a host of maternal factors. (2, 32)
- *immature fetus*—weighs 500-1000 grams and has completed 20 weeks of gestation to less than 28 weeks of gestation. (32, 43)
- *mature infant*—a live-born infant who has completed 38 weeks of gestation and with weight of 2500 grams or more. (32, 43)

- *multipara*—woman who has given birth to two or more children. (39)
- *natural childbirth*—childbirth in a normal physiologic manner without anesthetic or instruments. The woman participates actively and consciously in her delivery.
    —*Read's method, childbirth without fear*—antenatal program for mothers-to-be, including education, psychologic conditioning, abdominal breathing methods, exercises, and relaxation techniques preparatory to the three stages of labor. The natural childbirth preparation is focused on eliminating the fear-tension-pain syndrome.
    —*psychoprophylactic method as practiced by Lamaze, childbirth without pain*—verbal analgesia based on antenatal training of the expectant mother. Words are used as therapeutic agents to create in the woman's mind a chain of conditioned reflexes applicable to childbirth (Pavlov's second system). The mother-to-be learns to give birth: to breathe, push and relax effectively and to bring forth the child in a mentally alert state. The couple's united efforts make childbirth without pain a victory for both, since the husband plays an active part in the entire program. (22, 39)
- *natural family planning*—method based on the recognition of the fertile period of the menstrual cycle.
    —*calendar rhythm*—a method of determining the approximate time of ovulation related to the length of a series of a woman's menstrual cycles. It is assumed that:
    —ovulation takes place within a range of 12 to 16 days before menstruation.
    —the maximal survival of the ovum is about 48 hours.
    —the maximal survival of the sperm is about 72 hours.
    Rhythm refers, in obstetrics, to the alternating periods of sterility and fertility. Since fertility depends on the availability of the ovum, pregnancy may be avoided by practicing continence a few days before and after ovulation.
    —*ovulation method, Billings method*—study of the mucous pattern of fertility to predict the fertile period of the menstrual cycle. After menstruation a mucous discharge of sticky, cloudy secretion appears and lasts about six days. It is followed by a peak symptom of lubricative, clear, slippery mucus resembling egg white, which is present for one or two days. Typically ovulation takes place within this phase. After the peak symptom another kind of mucus forms. It is so thick, viscoid, and tenacious that the sperm cannot penetrate it. Conception may be avoided by practicing abstinence from the onset of the mucous discharge until four days after the appearance of the peak symptom.
    —*temperature method*—the recognition of body temperature changes during the normal menstrual cycle with a rise of temperature occurring following ovulation. The infertile period includes a preovulatory and postovulatory phase. Exact temperature recording during the postovulation phase may pinpoint the fertile period. After a temperature elevation for three consecutive days, the fertilization of the ovum is no longer possible. (22, 39, 44)
- *parturient*—woman in labor. (39)
- *perinatology*—the study of the infant before, during, and after birth.
- *postmature infant*—one that has completed 42 weeks or more of gestation. (32, 43)
- *premature infant*—infant with birth weight of 1000-2500 grams or less at birth and a gestation of 28 weeks to less than 38 weeks. (32, 43)
- *primipara*—woman who has delivered her first child after the period of viability. (39)
- *teratogens*—noxious agents: actinic, infectious, chemical, mechanical, or nutritional, capable of disrupting normal gestation, with subsequent antenatal death or resulting in the birth of a misshapen, deformed neonate. (26)

- *teratology*—the study of disfiguring malformations caused by arrested embryonic growth and fetal development of organs or structures. (26)
- *trimester of pregnancy*—division of the pregnancy into a little less than 13 weeks or three calendar months each. (39)

Anatomic Terms (16, 17, 26, 27, 28, 39, 40)

- *pelvis (pl. pelves)*—bony ring adapted to childbearing in female. It is composed of sacrum, coccyx, and hip bones.
    - *false pelvis*—bounded posteriorly by lumbar vertebrae; serves to support pregnant uterus.
    - *true pelvis*—bounded posteriorly by sacrum, of practical significance in child-bearing.
    - *pelvic brim, pelvic inlet*—upper opening into true pelvic cavity.
    - *pelvic outlet*—the lower opening of the pelvis.
    - *promontory of the sacrum*—the upper projecting part of the sacrum.
- *placenta*—vascular structure that provides nutrition for the fetus.
- *secundines, afterbirth*—fetal membranes and placenta; their expulsion occurs in third stage of labor.

Diagnostic Terms

- *abortion*—expulsion of the products of conception, resulting in termination of the fetus. Abortions are less often performed after 20 weeks' gestation. Currently, medical beliefs indicate that viability begins at about 24 weeks. This means that the physical development of the fetus—as in development of the lung structure—is sufficient to sustain life outside the womb. Recent Supreme Court rulings (July 1989) require physicians to test for the viability of a fetus at 20 weeks, or two-thirds of the way through the second trimester of pregnancy. In the future, state legislatures may be the battleground where further debate will occur regarding fetal viability and fetal-viability testing. Again, viability has to do with *physical* ability to survive outside the womb. This ability, however, is increasingly difficult to relate to stages of gestation, given developing technologies for dealing with the prematurely born. The question of physical viability, of course, does not address the more crucial question of when human life begins and the extent to which unborn human life has rights.
    - *habitual abortion*—three or more consecutive, spontaneous abortions.
    - *imminent, threatened abortion*—vaginal bleeding, with or without pain, and cervical dilatation, usually terminating in expulsion of fetus.
    - *incomplete abortion*—fetal expulsion with retention of total or partial placenta and subsequent bleeding.
    - *induced abortion*—voluntary expulsion of fetus, brought about by mechanical means or drugs.
    - *inevitable abortion*—rupture of membranes associated with cervical dilatation and followed by fetal expulsion.
    - *missed abortion*—fetus dead, but retained in utero for days or weeks.
    - *septic abortion*—abortion with fever without any other known cause for temperature elevation, usually referred to as septic. Patients who have had interference, even if afebrile, may have a septic abortion. A foul-smelling vaginal discharge is a dominant feature. (11, 22)
- *atony of the uterus* (see Fig. 57)—loss of uterine muscle tone, usually caused by prolonged labor, resulting in excessive uterine hemorrhage, unrelated to retained products or cervical lacerations, following the completion of the third stage of labor. (16, 31)

- *ectopic pregnancy*—fertilized ovum implanted outside of uterine cavity: in tube, ovary, or free in abdomen attached to a viscus. (22)
- *hyperemesis gravidarum*—severe nausea and vomiting during the first months of pregnancy, which may cause dehydration and serious metabolic disturbances in mother and fetus. (22, 30, 43)
- *hypertensive disorders of pregnancy*—high blood pressure of 140/90 and above, preceding pregnancy or developing during gestation or in early puerperium. Proteinuria, edema, convulsions, and coma may be present.
    - *—eclampsia*—major disorder of pregnancy and puerperium manifested by high blood pressure, convulsions, renal dysfunction, headache, edema, and severe cases of coma.
    - *—preeclampsia*—usually a disorder of a first pregnancy but may also occur in multiparas who are severely hypertensive or diabetic. Characteristically there is an upward trend in high blood pressure, sudden and excessive weight gain related to fluid retention, and kidney dysfunction, proteinuria, or albuminuria. (21, 22)
- *inversion of the uterus* (see Fig. 58)—sometimes during the postdelivery stage, following delivery of the infant, the uterus begins to turn itself inside out. This usually starts in the area of the placental attachment of the fundus; the myometrium begins to prolapse downward through the remainder of the uterine cavity and can continue past the dilatated cervix into the vagina. This type of incident is reported to occur spontaneously about 40 percent of the time. (16)
- *involution of uterus*—postpartum return of uterus to its former shape and size. (31)
- *oligohydramnios*—deficient amount of amniotic fluid. (3)
- *phlegmasia alba dolens*—phlebitis of femoral vein; may occur postpartum.
- *placenta ablatio, placenta abruptio*—premature detachment of the placenta, generally causing severe hemorrhage. (1, 36)
- *placenta accreta*—adherent placenta; remains attached to uterus after delivery. (1, 8, 16)
- *placenta previa* (see Fig. 59)—displaced placenta, implanted in lower segment of uterine wall.
    - *—marginal insertion*—placenta comes up to the ostium uteri but does not cover it.
    - *—partial placenta previa*—placenta covers the ostium uteri incompletely.
    - *—complete or central placenta*—placenta entirely obstructs the ostium uteri.
- *polyhydramnios, hydramnios*—excessive amount of amniotic fluid. (3, 22)
- *puerperal hematoma*—escape of blood into the mucosa or subcutaneous tissues of the external genitalia, forming painful vaginal or vulvar hematomas (blood tumors). They may also form in broad ligaments. (31)
- *puerperal infection, puerpera fever, childbed fever, puerperal septicemia, puerperal sepsis*—infection of the genital tract occurring within the postpartum period. Fever is the dominant characteristic of puerperal infection; however, the puerpera may have fever from other causes, such as kidney, urinary tract, breast, or lung infections. Puerperal febrile morbidity is defined as a temperature elevation of 100.4°F. (38°C) or more occurring after the first 24 hours postpartum on two or more occasions that are not within the same 24 hours. (16, 31)
- *rupture of uterus, hysterorrhexis, metrorrhexis*—laceration of uterus; a torn uterus. (36)
- *subinvolution*—failure of the uterus to reduce to its normal size after delivery. (31, 39)
- *trophoblast*—layer of ectoderm that attaches the conceptus to the uterine wall, nourishes the embryo, and has invasive propensities and thus malignant potentials. (33)
- *trophoblastic disease (TRD)*—disease originating in trophoblast. (33)

Figure 57 Bimanual compression of uterus and massage with abdominal hand usually will effectively control hemorrhage from uterine atony.

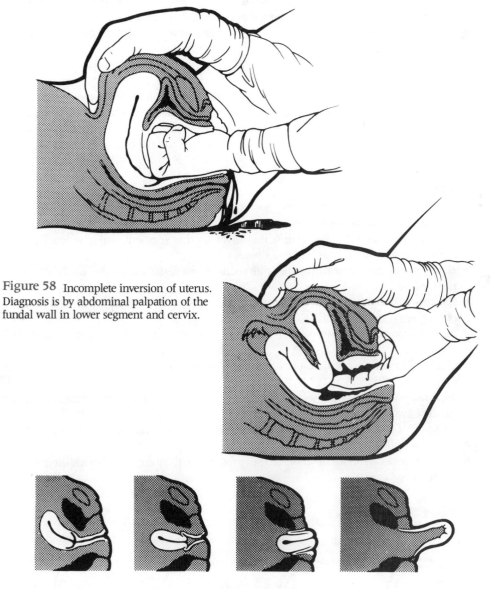

Figure 58 Incomplete inversion of uterus. Diagnosis is by abdominal palpation of the fundal wall in lower segment and cervix.

Progressive degrees of inversion.

—*chorioadenoma destruens*—malignant nonmetastasizing, invasive tumor that may penetrate the muscular coat and even the serosa of the uterus and neighboring structures, rendering its removal difficult. Trophoblastic proliferation tends to be excessive.

—*choriocarcinoma*—highly malignant, invasive tumor derived from fetal trophoblast. Neoplastic cells infiltrate the myometrium and readily metastasize to the liver, lungs, brain, and pelvic organs. Choriocarcinoma may be a complication of a hydatidiform mole.

*—hydatidiform mole—*developmental abnormality of the placenta characterized by the conversion of chorionic villi into a mass of vesicles that resemble hanging grapes. Embryonic growth is usually terminated, but if it continues to full term, the neonate will probably be stillborn. (22, 33)

- *uteroplacental apoplexy, Couvelaire uterus—*sudden, severe retroplacental bleeding into the myometrium. (1, 36)

Operative Terms

- *cesarean section—*removal of the fetus through an incision into the uterus. (34, 37)
- *episiotomy—*incision of perineum to facilitate delivery and prevent perineal laceration.
    *—median episiotomy—*midline incision of perineum.
    *—mediolateral episiotomy—*the incision is directed toward one side of the midline. (39)

Symptomatic Terms

- *attitude, obstetric—*the intrauterine position of the fetus. (9)
- *ballottement—*method of detecting pregnancy or testing for engagement of fetal head. The examiner sharply taps against the lower uterine segment with the forefinger in the vagina and tosses the embryo upward. (9)
- *Bandl's ring—*groove seen on the abdomen between the pubis and umbilicus after hard labor.
- *Braxton-Hicks sign—*painless contractions of the uterus throughout gestation. They occur periodically and last to term. (43)
- *bruit of placenta—*blowing sound heard on auscultation. It is caused by maternal circulation.
- *Chadwick's sign—*violet discoloration of the vaginal mucosa, presumptive evidence of pregnancy. (43)
- *colostrum—*yellowish fluid secreted by the mammary gland during pregnancy and for the first two or three days postdelivery. (31)
- *dilatation of cervix—*gradual opening of the cervix to permit passage of fetus. (39)
- *dystocia—*difficult birth. (40)
- *effacement—*obliteration of cervix; the process of thinning and shortening of the uterine cervix. (39)

Figure 59 Placenta types.

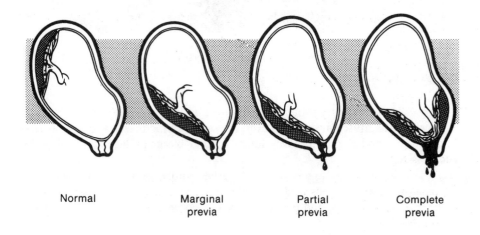

Normal   Marginal   Partial   Complete
              previa   previa   previa

- *engagement*—descent of the fetal head through the pelvic inlet. (22, 39)
- *engorgement*—excessive venous and lymph stasis of lactating breasts, usually referred to as caked breasts. (22, 39)
- *gestation*—pregnancy. (2, 43)
- *Goodell's sign*—softening of the uterine cervix, indicative of pregnancy. (43)
- *Hegar's sign*—softening of lower uterus; occurs in pregnancy. (43)
- *hemorrhage*—excessive blood loss.
    - —*antepartum*—before birth.
    - —*intrapartum*—during delivery.
    - —*postpartum*—after delivery. (8, 16, 36)
- *labor*—normal uterine contractions that result in the delivery of the fetus.
    - —*missed labor*—a few contractions at full-term, then cessation of labor and fetal retention, usually due to death of fetus in utero or extrauterine pregnancy.
    - —*precipitate labor*—hasty labor.
    - —*premature labor*—before full term.
    - —*protracted labor*—unduly prolonged. (15, 22, 35, 40)
- *labor*—three stages:
    - —*cervical dilatation*—first stage begins with uterine contractions and terminates with complete cervical dilatation.
    - —*expulsion*—second stage, from complete dilatation of the cervix to the birth of the baby.
    - —*placental separation and expulsion*—third stage, from delivery of neonate to expulsion of the placenta. (39)
- *lochia*—discharge from the birth canal following delivery. (31)
- *pica*—peculiar cravings of the pregnant woman for strange food or nonedibles. (43)
- *presentation or lie*—the relation which the long axis of the fetus bears to that of the mother. Accordingly, distinction is made between longitudinal and transverse presentations. Longitudinal presentation occurs in 99.5 percent of cases and includes the following varieties:
    - —*breech presentation*—presentation of the fetal buttock.
    - –*complete breech*—thighs flexed on abdomen and legs flexed on thighs.
    - –*footling*—the foot presents.
    - –*frank breech*—legs extended over ventral body surface.
    - –*knee*—the knee presents.
    - —*face presentation*—presentation of the fetal head.
    - –*brow*—the forehead presents.
    - –*sinciput*—the large fontanel presents.
    - –*vertex*—the upper and back part of the head presents. This is the most common variety.
    - Transverse presentation occurs in 0.5 percent of cases. (29, 39, 40)
- *quickening*—the pregnant woman's first perception of fetal life. (22, 43)
- *sterility*—total inability to conceive. (22, 23, 47)

The Fetal Period

Origin of Terms

amnion (G)—membrane around fetus	*fetus (L)*—offspring
anti- (G)—against	*terato- (G)*—monster
chorion (G)—membrane around fetus	*toxico- (G)*—poison

Anatomic Terms (20, 26, 27, 28)

- *amnion*—the innermost fetal membrane, which forms the bag of waters and encloses the fetus.
- *amniotic fluid*—fluid contained in the amniotic sac.
- *chorion*—outer envelope of the fetus.
- *embryo*—the product of conception, especially during the first three months of life.
- *fetus*—the unborn child after the first three months of development.

Diagnostic Terms

- *abortus (pl. abortuses)*—fetus that weighs about 500 grams (17 ounces) when expelled from the uterus and thus is unable to survive. (25, 43)
- *fetal anomaly, preventable*—malformed fetus caused by the mother taking teratogenic drugs during pregnancy; for example:
    - —anticarcinogens, such as aminopterin, cytoxin, methotrexate, and others.
    - —ovarian or testicular steroids, such as androgen, estrogen, progesterone.
    - —thalidomide, and others. (2, 32)
- *fetal anoxia, intrauterine asphyxia*—oxygen want of the fetus that may result from prolapse of the cord, placenta abruptio, compression of the umbilical vein, or other causes. Death is inevitable if fetus is not delivered promptly. (2)
- *fetal distress*—life-threatening condition caused by fetal anoxia, hemolytic disease, or other disorders. (2, 12, 13, 24)
- *fetal hemolytic disease*—blood disorder caused by antibody antigen reaction in ABO, Rh, or other blood group incompatibility. Maternal antibodies cross the placenta, agglutinate fetal blood cells, and destroy them. Fetal anemia develops. (2, 38)
- *fetotoxicity*—toxic effects of maternal medication on fetus and neonate. Some high risk agents are:

	Drugs	Toxicity
analgesics	acetylsalicylic acid (aspirin, excessive use) other salicylates	Bleeding of neonate Convulsions Encephalopathy
antianxiety drugs (ataractics, tranquilizers)	diazepam (Valium) meprobamate (Equanil)	Bleeding of neonate Retarded growth
anticoagulants (coumarin)	coumadin dicumarol warfarin	Bleeding of neonate Hypoprothrombinemia Fetal death
hypnotics, sedatives	barbiturates phenobarbital pentobarbital thiopental	Abstinence syndrome Retarded growth Bleeding of neonate Hyperbilirubinemia
narcotics	heroin meperidine (Demerol) methadone (Dolophine) morphine	Abstinence syndrome Convulsions Nerve damage Retarded growth Neonatal death

Among the many other hazards of fetotoxicity are maternal immunization (Sabin) for poliomyelitis, smallpox vaccination, and compulsive nicotine smoking. (2, 4, 19, 32, 43)

- *prolapse of cord*—premature descent of the umbilical cord, a cause of fetal death. (9, 19)

The Neonatal Period

Origin of Terms

chordo- (G)—cord

natus (L)—birth

neo- (G)—new, recent

neonate (L)—newborn

umbilicus (L)—naval

Anatomic Terms (14)

- *fontanel, fontanelle*—the junction point of cranial sutures that remains widely open in the newborn.
- *umbilical cord*—cord connecting placenta with fetal umbilicus. At birth it is chiefly composed of one umbilical vein and two umbilical arteries surrounded by gelatinous substance.

Diagnostic Terms

- *asphyxia neonatorum*—lack of oxygen in the blood of the newborn. (2, 14)
- *caput succedaneum*—tumorlike edema of presenting part of neonate's head. (2, 14)
- *cerebral hemorrhage*—brain hemorrhage due to birth injury or coagulation defects, resulting in anoxia, cyanosis, and convulsions. (2, 19)
- *congenital stridors*—breathing disorders associated with a crowing or stridulous noise from birth or first week of life caused by malformation or abnormal position of functioning of glottis, trachea, or vocal cords. (2)
- *cord hemorrhage*—bleeding from umbilical cord. (2, 19)
- *Down's syndrome, monogolism, trisomy G_{21}*—chromosome aberration characterized by mental retardation and many physical features, such as slanting eyes; flat facial profile; thick, fissured tongue protruding from open mouth; pudgy, broad neck; hypotonia; and absence of the Moro reflex in the newborn. (2, 45)
- *drug addiction in neonate*—withdrawal symptoms in the newborn appearing soon after birth. The infant is restless and has a shrill cry, tremors, twitching, and convulsions. Its manifestations may closely parallel those of adult withdrawal, such as yawning, sneezing, anorexia, and diarrhea. (2, 19, 32)
- *erythroblastosis fetalis*—hemolytic disease of the newborn.
    - —*anemic type*—damage to bone marrow, liver, and spleen; excessive hemolysis.
    - —*hydropic type*—extremely edematous, stillborn, or neonatal death.
    - —*icteric type*—marked jaundice; may be followed by kernicterus. (2, 38)
- *hydrocephalus*—abnormal fluid collection in the ventricles of the brain resulting in an enlargement of the head. (2)
- *hyperbilirubinemia, neonatal*—abnormally high bilirubin content of the circulating blood, predisposing the newborn to kernicterus due to unconjugated bilirubin concentration within brain tissue. (2, 19, 32)
- *hypoxia of the newborn*—reduction of oxygen supply to tissue below physiological levels despite adequate perfusion of the tissue by blood. After birth, the newborn's total bodily requirements of oxygen increase rapidly and if additional oxygen is not supplied immediately, permanent brain damage may result. It is important that the air passages be patent and not occluded by inhalation of amniotic fluid. It is essential that the inhaled oxygen reach the alveoli, so that adequate respiratory exchange can occur in the alveoli. (14, 19)

- *idiopathic respiratory distress syndrome, hyaline membrane disease*—serious breathing difficulty caused by hyaline material, a sticky exudate, filling the alveolar ducts and alveoli, thus obstructing the airway and preventing oxygenation. The condition, which occurs primarily in premature infants, may be fatal. (2, 5, 6, 12, 13, 24)
- *imperforate anus, atresia of anus*—rectum ending in a blind pouch. (2, 19)
- *infections of the newborn:*
  - —*congenital rubella syndrome*—neonate born with a rubella virus infection due to transplacental transmission, which is particularly serious when it occurs during the first trimester. The contagion lasts from 12 to 18 months after birth. The newborn may have cataracts, cardiovascular anomalies, microcephaly, mental retardation, deafness, and other defects.
  - —*epidemic diarrhea*—loose, yellow-green stools, dehydration, and acidosis.
  - —*impetigo contagiosa*—skin disease, with appearance of vesicles that change to pustules and later to crusts. It is caused by staphylococci.
  - —*neonatal chlamydial, cytomegaloviral, herpetic, and other infections.*
  - —*ophthalmia neonatorum*—purulent conjunctivitis. (2, 19, 32)
  - —*TORCH infections*—acronym for Toxoplasmosis, Other (e.g., syphilis), Rubella, Cytomegalovirus, and Herpes simplex. The effects of these viral infections may include abortion, fetal death, and growth retardation. Other complications that may surface are: microcephaly, congenital heart disease, eye damage, deafness, or hepatosplenomegaly with jaundice or purpura. (6, 11)
  - —*thrush*—fungus infection of oral mucous membrane forming white patches or aphthae.
- *kernicterus, nuclear jaundice, biliary encephalopathy*—irreparable brain damage complicating severe erythroblastosis. Excess serum bilirubin, liberated by destroyed erythrocytes and not converted into an excretable form, stains the brain nuclei and results in mental retardation, cerebral palsy, or deafness. The most severely affected infants die within a few days. Kernicterus can be prevented by exchange transfusions. (2)
- *meningocele*—meninges protruding through a defect in the spine or skull. (2)
- *phocomelia*—congenital deformities such as absence or stunting of extremities. Infants born of mothers who took thalidomide during the first trimester of pregnancy developed these malformations. (2)
- *retrolental fibroplasia*—disorder seen in premature infants who receive continuous oxygen therapy. The retina becomes edematous and detached. Partial or total blindness develops. (2, 32)
- *tongue-tie, ankyloglossia*—short frenulum linguae preventing neonate from taking feeding. (2)
- *umbilical hernia, omphalocele*—rupture of the umbilicus associated with protrusion of intestine. It occurs in the first weeks of life. (2, 32)

Operative Terms

- *clipping of frenulum linguae*—minor operation to relieve tongue-tie. (2)
- *repair of imperforate anus*—surgical creation of an opening. (2)

Symptomatic Terms

- *Apgar score*—assessing a neonate's physical condition by evaluating heart rate, respiratory effort, reflex irritability, and skin color according to a scoring system. (14, 32)
- *Chvostek's sign*—facial irritability in tetany evoked by a slight tap over the facial nerve. The spasm is unilateral.

- *congenital*—born with a certain condition.
- *eructation*—belching.
- *meconium*—black stools of the newborn. (32, 41)
- *Moro reflex, startle reflex*—reflex indicating an awareness of balance in the neonate. The reflex is stimulated by a sudden jarring of the crib or jerking of a blanket. The infant draws up the legs and throws the arms symmetrically forward. (14)
- *pylorospasm*—spasm of circular muscle of lower end of stomach. (2)
- *vernix caseosa*—fatty substance that covers the newborn. (14)

Special Procedures

Selected Procedures Pertaining to Delivery

- *bimanual compression of uterus*—massage of the posterior aspect of the uterus with abdominal hand massage and massage through the vagina of the anterior uterine aspect with the other fist, the knuckles of which contact the uterine wall.
- *breech extraction*—method of delivery when the presenting parts are the buttocks or feet. The fetus is pulled out. (39)
- *forceps application*—instrumental delivery of child.
    - *low forceps*—application of forceps when head is on perineum.
    - *midforceps*—application of forceps when head is at level of ischial spines.
    - *high forceps*—application of forceps before head has passed through the pelvic inlet. (10)
- *manual delivery of placenta* (Fig. 61)—this is performed by using one hand to grasp the placenta, which is held in the vagina or the lower uterine segment by gentle traction on the umbilical cord. When the placenta has been delivered to the introitus, its weight is supported, allowing more gradual delivery to avoid torn and retained fetal membranes. A clamp placed across the membrane to provide even tension during this portion of the delivery may prove to be helpful. (10, 38)
- *saline abortion*—intra-amniotic injection of hypertonic salt solution after 14 weeks of gestation to induce abortion. (42)
- *vacuum extraction*—instrumental delivery of infant with a vacuum extractor, indicated in:
    - fetal distress, malpresentation, or prolapse of arm.
    - maternal inertia, prolonged labor, heart-lung disease, shock, toxemia. (10, 39)
- *version*—the process of turning the fetus in the uterus.
    - *cephalic version*—the head is made the presenting part.
    - *podalic version*—the breech is made the presenting part. (9)

Selected Procedures Pertaining to Fetal Development

- *amniocentesis* (Fig. 60)—puncture of the amniotic cavity:
    - to aspirate fluid for amniotic fluid analysis
    - to inject radiopaque substance for amniography
    - to administer intrauterine transfusions to the fetus with severe hemolytic disease
    - to determine pressure changes of amniotic fluid, which permit the continuous monitoring of uterine contractibility
    - to monitor the fetal heart rate
    - to detect possible genetic disorders antenatally (18, 22, 27)
- *anti-D antibody injection*—preparation for passive immunization of Rh-negative mothers of D-positive babies, administered intramuscularly or intravenously within

Figure 60 Amniocentis late in pregnancy, performed suprapubically.

Figure 61 Manual removal of placenta. Fingers are alternately abducted, adducted, and advanced until placenta is detached.

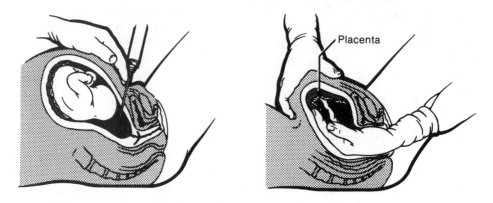

Placenta

72 hours after delivery. Its purpose is to prevent Rh isoimmunization and fetal hemolytic disease in future pregnancies. The individual sterile vaccine vials are prepared from plasma obtained from severely sensitized Rh-negative women who had stillborn hydropic fetuses or from gamma globulin from naturally or artificially sensitized donors. (6, 11)

- *fetal electrocardiography*—method of detecting and recording electric impulses of the fetal heart. In contradistinction to the larger, slower deflections of the maternal heart, the normal fetal heartbeat yields smaller and more rapid deflections. Fetal distress may be evidenced by a delay in the conduction time. (2, 42)
- *fetal monitoring*—continuous recording of fetal heart rate (FHR) patterns from a direct fetal electrocardiogram (FECG) electrode and uterine contractions using a transcervical catheter. Indications are clinical signs of fetal distress, FHR changes, suspected cephalopelvic disproportions, and high-risk pregnancies. (2, 3, 6, 42)
- *fetal phonocardiography*—the detection of fetal heart sounds by means of a phonocardiograph.
- *fetal telemetry*—wireless radio transmission that provides remote recordings of the fetal electrocardiography or other data. (42)
- *intrauterine transfusion*—the injection of red cell concentrate prepared from Rh-negative whole blood (packed erythrocytes) into the peritoneal cavity of the fetus to combat fetal hemolytic anemia and prevent fetal death. (2)
- *oxytocin challenge tests*—exercise tests estimate the ability of the fetus to withstand labor by the response of the fetal heart rate to induced uterine contractions. Late decelerations suggest that the placenta and fetus may be compromised. A negative stress test indicates fetal well-being for the next six to seven days. In the majority of cases, the test is negative. (15)

Selected Procedures Pertaining to the Neonate

- *extracorporeal membrane oxygenation (ECMO)*—medical technique that takes over the heart-lung functions for the neonate to allow the diseased organs to heal. It is a modification of the heart-lung machine and procedure used in open heart surgery. Although ECMO was developed initially for adults, currently its most common usage is in the treatment of newborns with severe respiratory and cardiopulmonary disorders. (13, 32, 38)

Figure 62 Right occipitoanterior (ROA) fetal position.

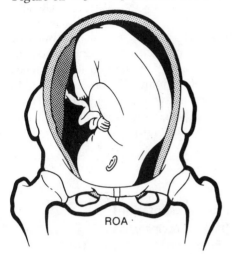

Figure 63 Left sacroposterior (LSP) fetal position.

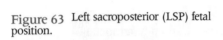

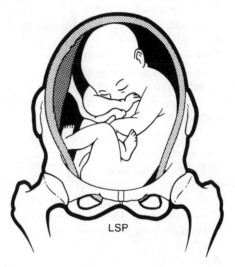

Figure 64 Right scapuloposterior (RScP) fetal position.

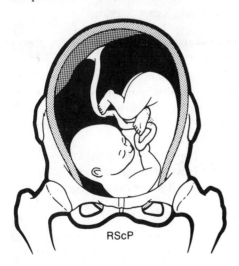

- *exchange transfusion*—replacing the blood of a neonate who has a severe antibody-antigen reaction caused by hemolytic disease with blood devoid of the offending antigen. (2, 38)
- *genetic fingerprinting, DNA fingerprinting*—molecular biologic technique displaying specific individual genetic makeup. DNA (deoxyribonucleic acid) carries an organism's genetic information. Each DNA molecule consists of four amino acids arranged in a code that is unique to each person. DNA fingerprinting has long been used in paternity cases. More recently, it has been applied to forensic biology in rape cases. Autoradiographs have displayed that the DNA patterns in the suspect's blood matched those in the semen found on the rape victim. (20)

Abbreviations

General

AFP—alpha (α) fetoprotein
BBT—basal body temperature
BPD—biparietal diameter
CDC—calculated day of confinement
CS—cesarean section
CWP—childbirth without pain
DNA—deoxyribonucleic acid
ECMO—extracorporeal membrane
      oxygenation
EDC—estimated day of confinement
FECG—fetal electrocardiogram
FHR—fetal heart rate
FHT—fetal heart tone
FTND—full-term normal delivery
HCG—human chorionic gonadotropin
HDN—hemolytic disease of newborn
HPL—human placental lactogen
HSG—hysterosalpingography
IUP—intrauterine pressure
LBW—low birth weight
LMP—last menstrual period
NB—newborn
OB—obstetrics
OGN—obstetric-gynecologic-neonatal
PPA pos—phenylpyruvic acid positive
      (phenylketonuria present)
PU—pregnancy urine
Rh neg—rhesus factor negative
Rh pos—rhesus factor positive
RML—right mediolateral (episiotomy)
UC—uterine contractions

Vertex Presentations

LOA—left occipitoanterior
LOP—left occipitoposterior
LOT—left occipitotransverse
ROA—right occipitoanterior (Fig. 62)
ROP—right occipitoposterior
ROT—right occipitotransverse

Face Presentations

LMA—left mentoanterior
LMP—left mentoposterior
LMT—left mentotransverse
RMA—right mentoanterior
RMP—right mentoposterior
RMT—right mentotransverse

Breech Presentations

LSA—left sacroanterior
LSP—left sacroposterior (Fig. 63)
RSA—right sacroanterior
RSP—right sacroposterior

Transverse Presentations

LScA—left scapuloanterior
LScP—left scapuloposterior
RScA—right scapuloanterior
RScP—right scapuloposterior (Fig. 64)

Size of Term Infant

AGA—appropriate for gestational age
LGA—large for gestational age
SGA—small for gestational age

Organizations

AAMIH—American Association for Maternal and Infant Health
ACNM—American College of Nurse Midwifery
ACOG—American College of Obstetricians and Gynecologists
FACOG—Fellow of American College of Obstetricians and Gynecologists
FCMC—Family-Centered Maternity Care
FSAA—Family Service Association of America
ICM—International Confederation of Midwives
NAACOG—Nurses' Association of the American College of Obstetricians and
　　　　　Gynecologists
USCB—United States Children's Bureau

Oral Reading Practice

Respiratory Distress Syndrome, Hyaline Membrane Disease

Respiratory distress syndrome **(RDS)** is the result of a complex disturbance of early neonatal adaptation in which several factors interact, such as **gestational age** (fetal maturity) and environmental influences **(asphyxia hypothermia),** along with probable genetic factors entering into this interaction. Unfavorable combinations of these factors present defects in **lung stability** and **cardiopulmonary functions,** which are classified as a syndrome. Studies in recent years have indicated that these problems arise from repeated cesarean sections performed without sufficient evaluation of fetal maturity. The death rate is highest in the first 24 hours, and 90 percent of the deaths occur by the fourth day.

The **hyaline membrane** lining of the **alveoli** gives the disease its alternate name. The hyaline material is the result of damage to the alveolar lining, and consists of **fibrin,** with additional transudates and secretions.

The main pathophysiological mechanism in RDS is a **surfactant** deficiency in the alveoli. The surfactant is a lipoprotein mainly composed of **dipalmitrol lecithin,** which begins to be secreted by the fetal lung about the twentieth to twenty-fifth week of pregnancy. An important function of this surfactant is to form a film at the interface between the **alveolar lining** and the oxygen in the **alveolus** per se. The result is an improvement in lung distensibility and lower alveolar surface tension. Without the surfactant, the alveoli collapse and greater **inspiratory pressure** is demanded on the next breath to expand the alveoli. Since **lung compliance** is extremely low, the neonate's work of breathing is increased. The pulmonary defects present right-to-left **cardiopulmonary shunting,** which is the central reason for the **arterial oxygen unsaturation.** This resistance may result from lung collapse and congestion of the capillary bed due to **hypoxia** and **acidosis,** which cause **arteriolar vasoconstriction.** Should **asphyxia** be acute and of short term, the main defect presenting may be **pulmonary vasoconstriction;** rapid resolution may follow when the asphyxia is corrected. When asphyxia persists and is longer term, the result is a gradual deterioration, resulting in full-blown respiratory distress syndrome. Recovery in these cases is much slower, and treatment must be aggressive.

Another lipoprotein, **sphingomyelin,** also is present in the amniotic fluid. Sphingomyelin concentrations do not increase as much as the lecithin concentrations. The high increase is noted around the thirty-second to the thirty-fourth week of gestation. The **L/S ratio** (ratio between lecithin and sphingomyelin concentrations) in the amniotic fluid provides an indication of the maturation of the fetal lung. An L/S ratio of two or more indicates that hyaline membrane disease is not likely to occur.

Recognition of respiratory distress syndrome is based on the respiratory effort, which may resemble **tachypnea** or may be slow; however, in all cases the neonate is laboring with **subcostal** retractions or retractions extending to the **sternum, intercostal** spaces, or **suprasternal** spaces. Grunting is often present with retractions and is indicative of serious disease; less grunting is usually a sign of improvement, unless it is associated with **apnea** or increasing **cyanosis** and **deterioration,** indications of failed respiratory effort.

Several pharmacologic agents or hormones may contribute to the acceleration of fetal pulmonary surfactant production. However, because of the potential maternal and fetal risk resulting from the usage of these drugs, it is essential that the drug of choice be individually justified and the risk-benefit ratio carefully evaluated prior to the administration of the drug.

Monitoring of the neonate with respiratory distress syndrome includes serial chest roentgenograms, periodic **blood gas analyses, acid-base evaluations, fluid** and **electrolyte balance, L/S ratio,** as well as maintenance of good **ventilation, oxygenation,** temperature control, and close observation of vital signs.

Approximately 70 to 90 percent of infants present with the disease in the moderately severe form. The remaining 10 to 30 percent of neonates are critically ill. Between 72 and 98 hours after birth, most infants will enter the recovery phase. The smaller the infant, the higher the mortality. The best site for care of **RDS** infants is in the neonatal intensive care unit where facilities and trained staff are available to monitor and provide treatment for these neonates on a continuous 24-hour basis. (2, 5, 6, 8, 12, 13, 24)

Table 15
Some Obstetric and Neonatal Conditions Amenable to Surgery

Organs Involved	Diagnosis	Type of Surgery	Operative Procedures
Cervix uteri Endometrium	Early incomplete abortion	Dilatation and curettage	Instrumental expansion of cervix and scraping of endometrium to remove blood clots and tissue
Cervix uteri	Dystocia Cervical stenosis Carcinoma of cervix in pregnancy; viable fetus	Cesarean section	Removal of fetus through incision into uterus
Uterine tube	Ruptured ectopic pregnancy with massive hemorrhage	Salpingectomy, unilateral	Removal of one fallopian tube

Organs Involved	Diagnosis	Type of Surgery	Operative Procedures
Perineum	Second stage of labor, tense perineum	Episiotomy, mediolateral or midline	Incision into perineum
Perineum	Obstetric laceration of the perineum	Perineorrhaphy	Suture of torn perineum
Pelvis	Inlet contraction of pelvis	Cesarean section	Abdominal delivery of fetus
Pelvis	Prolonged labor, dystocia	Elective forceps delivery	Fetus delivered by horizontal traction
Uterus	Total placenta previa antepartum or intrapartum hemorrhage	Cesarean section	Incision into corpus uteri and delivery of fetus through abdomen
Uterus	Rupture of uterus, fatal hemorrhage, maternal death	Postmortem cesarean section	Delivery of fetus by incision through abdominal wall and uterus after death of mother
Cervix uteri	Obstetric laceration of cervix	Trachelorrhaphy	Suture of torn cervix uteri
Blood of fetus	Fetal hemolytic disease, severe	Amniocentesis Intrauterine transfusion	Surgical puncture of amniotic cavity Injection of Rh-negative packed red cells into fetal peritoneal cavity
Blood of newborn	Erythroblastosis fetalis, Rh positive Hyperbilirubinemia	Exchange transfusions within 24 hours after birth	Replacing infant's red cells by transfusing with Rh-negative erythrocytes, which will remain unharmed by maternal antibodies
Intestine of newborn	Meconium ileus with intestinal obstruction due to mucoviscidosis	Intestinal resection	Surgical intervention to relieve intestinal obstruction

References and Bibliography

1. Anderson, Garland D. Abruptio placenta and placenta previa. In Phelan, Jeffrey P., and Clark, Steven L., eds., *Cesarean Delivery,* New York: Elsevier, 1988, pp. 99-114.

2. Behrman, Richard E., Vaughn, Victor C., and Nelson, Waldo E., eds. The fetus and the neonatal infant. In *Nelson Textbook of Pediatrics,* 13th ed. Philadelphia: W.B. Saunders

Co., 1987, pp. 358-435.

3. Bhatia, Rupinder, et al. Detection of high-risk pregnancy. In Pernoll, Martin L., and Benson, Ralph C., eds., *Current Obstetric & Gynecologic Diagnosis and Treatment—1987,* Norwalk, CT: Appleton & Lange, 1987, pp. 246-254.

4. Biswas, Mano, et al. Cardiac, hematologic, pulmonary, renal & urinary tract disorders. In Pernoll, Martin L., and Benson, Ralph C., eds., *Current Obstetric & Gynecologic Diagnosis & Treatment—1987,* Norwalk, CT: Appleton & Lange, 1987, pp. 353-385.

5. Carlo, Waldemar A., et al. Assisted ventilation and the complications of respiratory distress. In Fanaroff, Avroy A., and Martin, Richard J., *Neonatal-Perinatal Medicine,* 4th ed. St. Louis: The C.V. Mosby Co., 1987, pp. 591-603.

6. Catanzarite, V.A., et al. Assessment of fetal well-being. In Pernoll, Martin L., and Benson, Ralph C., eds., *Current Obstetric & Gynecologic Diagnosis & Treatment—1987,* Norwalk, CT: Appleton & Lange, 1987, pp. 278-302.

7. Chervenak, F.A., and Chervenak, J.L. Multiple gestations. In Phelan, Jeffrey P., and Clark, Steven L., eds., *Cesarean Delivery,* New York: Elsevier, 1988, pp. 54-69.

8. Clark, Steven L. Uterine hemorrhage. In Phelan, Jeffrey P., and Clark, Steven L., eds., *Cesarean Delivery,* New York: Elsevier, 1988, pp. 260-266.

9. Collea, Joseph V. Malpresentation & cord accidents. In Pernoll, Martin L., and Benson, Ralph C., eds., *Current Obstetric & Gynecologic Diagnosis & Treatment—1987,* Norwalk, CT: Appleton & Lange, 1987, pp. 424-440.

10. Danforth, David N. Operative delivery. In Pernoll, Martin L., and Benson, Ralph C., eds., *Current Obstetric & Gynecologic Diagnosis & Treatment—1987,* Norwalk, CT: Appleton & Lange, 1987, pp. 481-508.

11. Durfee R.B. Obstetric complications of pregnancy. In Pernoll, Martin L., and Benson, Ralph C., eds., *Current Obstetric & Gynecologic Diagnosis & Treatment—1987,* Norwalk, CT: Appleton & Lange, 1987, pp. 255-278.

12. Farrell, Philip M., and Perelman, Robert H. The developmental biology of the lung. In Fanaroff, Avroy A., and Martin, Richard J., eds., *Neonatal-Perinatal Medicine,* 4th ed. St. Louis: The C.V. Mosby Co., 1987, pp. 557-572.

13. Fox, William W., et al. Assessment of pulmonary function. In Fanaroff, Avroy A., and Martin, Richard J., eds., *Neonatal-Perinatal Medicine,* 4th ed. St. Louis: The C.V. Mosby Co., 1987, pp. 573-580.

14. Gill, William L. Essentials of normal newborn assessment & care. In Pernoll, Martin L., and Benson, Ralph C., eds., *Current Ob-stetric & Gynecologic Diagnosis and Treatment—1987,* Norwalk, CT: Appleton & Lange, 1987, pp. 205-215.

15. Herrera, Eduardo, and Pernoll, Martin L. Complications of labor & delivery. In Pernoll, Martin L., and Benson, Ralph C., eds., *Current Obstetric & Gynecologic Diagnosis & Treatment—1987,* Norwalk, CT: Appleton & Lange, 1987, pp. 450-455.

16. Kapernick, Peter S. Postpartum hemorrhage & the abnormal puerperium. In Pernoll, Martin L., and Benson, Ralph C., eds., *Current Obstetric & Gynecologic Diagnosis & Treatment—1987,* Norwalk, CT: Appleton & Lange, 1987, pp. 524-550.

17. Knuppel, Robert A., et al. Maternal-placental-fetal unit: Fetal & early neonatal physiology. In Pernoll, Martin L., and Benson, Ralph C., eds., *Current Obstetric & Gynecologic Diagnosis & Treatment—1987,* Norwalk, CT: Appleton & Lange, 1987, pp. 135-160.

18. Koontz, William L. Abnormal labor. In Phelan, Jeffrey P., and Clark, Steven L., eds., *Cesarean Delivery,* New York: Elsevier, 1988, pp. 21-35.

19. Koops, Beverly L., and Battaglia, Frederick C. The newborn infant. In Kempe, C. Henry, et al., eds., *Current Pediatric Diagnosis & Treatment—1987,* 9th ed. Norwalk, CT: Appleton & Lange, 1987, pp. 41-97.

20. Lewis, Ricki. DNA fingerprints: Witness for the prosecution. *Discover the World of Science,* 9:45-52, June 1988.

21. Marbie, Bill C., and Sibai, B.M. Hypertensive states of pregnancy. In Pernoll, Martin L., and Benson, Ralph C., eds., *Current Obstetric & Gynecologic Diagnosis & Treatment—1987,* Norwalk, CT: Appleton & Lange, 1987, pp. 340-352.

22. Margolis, Alan, J., and Greenwood, Sadja. Gynecology and obstetrics. In Schroeder, Steven A., Krupp, Marcus A., & Tierney, Lawrence M., Jr., eds., *Current Medical Diagnosis & Treatment—1988,* Norwalk, CT: Appleton & Lange, 1988, pp. 447-495.

23. Marshall, John R. Infertility. In Pernoll, Martin L., and Benson, Ralph C., eds., *Current Obstetric & Gynecologic Diagnosis & Treatment—1987,* Norwalk, CT: Appleton & Lange, 1987, pp. 919-937.

24. Martin, Richard J., and Fanaroff, Avroy A. The respiratory distress syndrome and its management. In Fanaroff, Avroy A., and Martin, Richard J., eds., *Neonatal-Perinatal Medicine,* 4th ed. St. Louis: The C.V. Mosby Co., 1987, pp. 580-590.

25. Moore, Keith L. Introduction to embryology. In *The Developing Human Clinically Oriented Embryology,* Philadelphia: W.B. Saunders Co., 1988, pp. 1-37.

26. ———. Formation of basic organs and sys-

tems: The fourth to the eighth weeks. Ibid., pp. 65-86.

27. ———. The fetal period: Ninth week to birth. Ibid., pp. 78-103.

28. ———. The placenta and fetal membranes. Ibid., pp. 104-130.

29. Moore, Thomas R. Malpresentation breech and transverse lie. In Phelan, Jeffrey P., and Clark, Steven L., eds., *Cesarean Delivery*, New York: Elsevier, 1988, pp. 36-53.

30. Morrison, John C., and Palmer, S.M. General medical disorders during pregnancy. In Pernoll, Martin L., and Benson, Ralph C., eds., *Current Obstetric & Gynecologic Diagnosis and Treatment—1987*, Norwalk, CT: Appleton & Lange, 1987, pp. 386-402.

31. Novy, Miles. The normal puerperium. In Pernoll, Martin L., and Benson, Ralph C., eds., *Current Obstetric & Gynecologic Diagnosis and Treatment—1987*, Norwalk, CT: Appleton & Lange, 1987, pp. 216-245.

32. Ogata, Edward S. Neonatal resuscitation and care of the newborn at risk. In Pernoll, Martin L., and Benson, Ralph C., eds., *Current Obstetric & Gynecologic Diagnosis and Treatment—1987*, Norwalk, CT: Appleton & Lange, 1987, pp. 509-523.

33. O'Quinn, A.G., and Barnard D.E. Gestational trophoblastic diseases. In Pernoll, Martin L., and Benson, Ralph C., eds., *Current Obstetric & Gynecologic Diagnosis and Treatment—1987*, Norwalk, CT: Appleton & Lange, 1987, pp. 891-900.

34. Perkins, Richard P. Cesarean delivery: The extraperitoneal approach. In Phelan, Jeffrey P., and Clark, Steven L., eds., *Cesarean Delivery*, New York: Elsevier, 1988, pp. 182-200.

35. Pernoll, Martin L. Untimely termination of pregnancy. In Pernoll, Martin L., and Benson, Ralph C., eds., *Current Obstetric & Gynecologic Diagnosis & Treatment—1987*, Norwalk, CT: Appleton & Lange, 1987, pp. 303-310.

36. ———. Third-trimester hemorrhage. Ibid., pp. 413-423.

37. Phelan, Jeffrey P., and Clark, Steven. Cesarean delivery: The transperitoneal approach. In Phelan, Jeffrey P., and Clark, Steven L., eds., *Cesarean Delivery*, New York: Elsevier, 1988, pp. 201-218.

38. Queenan, John T. Erythroblastosis fetalis. In Fanaroff, Avroy A., and Martin, Richard J., eds., *Neonatal-Perinatal Medicine*, 4th ed. St. Louis: The C.V. Mosby Co., 1987, pp. 153-163.

39. Russell, Keith P. The course and conduct of normal labor and delivery. In Pernoll, Martin L., and Benson, Ralph C., eds., *Current Obstetric & Gynecologic Diagnosis & Treatment—1987*. Norwalk, CT: Appleton & Lange, 1987, pp. 178-203.

40. Schlater, Sarah, and Pernoll, Martin L. Dystocia. In Pernoll, Martin L., and Benson, Ralph C., eds., *Current Obstetric & Gynecologic Diagnosis & Treatment—1987*, Norwalk, CT: Appleton & Lange, 1987, pp. 441-449.

41. Silverton, Arnold, and Roy, Claude C. Gastrointestinal tract. In Kempe, C. Henry, et al., eds., *Current Pediatric Diagnosis & Treatment—1987*, 9th ed. Norwalk, CT: Appleton & Lange, 1987, pp. 522-556.

42. Smith, Carl V. Fetal distress. In Phelan, Jeffrey P., and Clark, Steven L., eds., *Cesarean Delivery*, New York: Elsevier, 1988, pp. 70-90.

43. Taylor, C.M., and Pernoll, Martin L. Normal pregnancy & prenatal care. In Pernoll, Martin L., and Benson, Ralph C., eds., *Current Obstetric & Gynecologic Diagnosis & Treatment—1987*, Norwalk, CT: Appleton & Lange, 1987, pp. 161-177.

44. Tatum, Howard J. Contraception & family planning. In Pernoll, Martin L., and Benson, Ralph C., eds., *Current Obstetric & Gynecologic Diagnosis & Treatment—1987*, Norwalk, CT: Appleton & Lange, 1987, pp. 586-611.

45. Varner, Michael W. Disproportionate fetouterine growth. In Pernoll, Martin L., and Benson, Ralph C., eds., *Current Obstetric & Gynecologic Diagnosis & Treatment—1987*, Norwalk, CT: Appleton & Lange, 1987, pp. 311-320.

46. Wentz, Anne Colston. Contraception and family planning. In Jones, Howard W., III, Wentz, Anne Colston, and Burnett, Lonnie S., eds., *Novak's Textbook of Gynecology*, 11th ed. Baltimore: Williams & Wilkins, 1988, pp. 204-239.

47. ———. Infertility. Ibid., pp. 263-302.

Endocrine and Metabolic Disorders

Endocrine Glands

Origin of Terms

ad- (L)—near to, toward, in addition to
aden-, adeno- (G)—gland(s)
adreno- (L)—near kidney
end-, endo- (G)—within
ecto- (G)—outside
hormone (G)—to excite, to spur on

pituita (L)—phlegm
thalamus (G)—inner chamber
thymo- (G)—thymus
thyro- (G)—shield, thyroid
tropho- (G)—nourishment

Anatomic Terms (Refs. 55, 56, 57)

- *endocrine glands*—ductless glands producing internal secretions that are absorbed directly into the bloodstream and influence various body functions.
- *hormone*—active principle of an internal secretion.
- *hypophysis, pituitary gland*—small ovoid body situated in the hypophysial fossa of the sphenoid bone. It is composed of the adenohypophysis and neurohypophysis, each performing distinct functions. The adenohypophysis or anterior pituitary is known as the master endocrine gland because of its physiologic effect on the suprarenals, gonads, pancreas, and thyroid. Some important hormones of the adenohypophysis (see Fig. 65) are:
    - *adrenocorticotropic hormone (ACTH)*—affects the adrenal cortex and combats inflammatory processes. (ACTH is essential to maintain life.)
    - *follicle-stimulating and luteinizing hormones*—regulate the reproductive cycle.
    - *growth hormone*—promotes normal bone development.
    - *prolactin*—stimulates the secretion of milk.
    - *thyrotropic hormone*—evokes increased uptake of iodine by the thyroid.
  The neurohypophysis is thought to be not a true endocrine but a depot for neurosecretions known as antidiuretic hormone (ADH), which contain vasopressin and oxytocin.
- *pancreas*—abdominal gland extending from the concavity of the duodenum to the spleen. Its pancreatic islets, the islets of Langerhans, are approximately 20 percent A-cells, secreting glucagon; 75 percent B-cells, secreting insulin; and 5 percent D-cells, secreting somatostatin. A human pancreatic polypeptide has been recently

Figure 65 Hormones of adenohypophysis: direct and indirect effect on target organs.

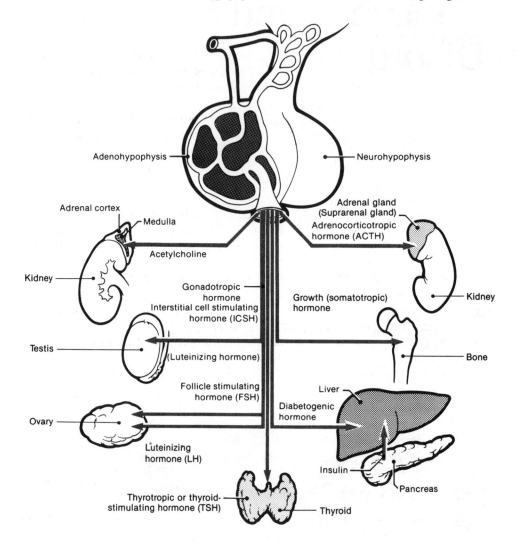

added as a fourth type of cell. The types of pancreatic cells differ chemically, functionally, and microscopically.

- *parathyroids*—two to four small glands, usually a pair attached to each thyroid lobe. They secrete a hormone that regulates the metabolism of calcium and phosphorus.
- *suprarenals, adrenals*—two glands, one on top of each kidney. They are composed of an inner medullary substance and an outer cortex. The medulla produces adrenalin and noradrenalin. The adrenal cortex forms the adrenocortical steroids, known as the corticosteroids or corticoids. They include the glucocorticoids and mineralocorticoids. C-19 derivatives yield androgens, and C-18 derivatives yield estrogens. Adrenocortical steroids help to regulate sodium, potassium, and chloride metabolism; water balance; and carbohydrate, protein, and fat metabolism.
- *thymus*—endocrine gland secreting thymin, a hormone that inhibits neuromuscular transmission.
- *thyroid*—gland that consists of two large lateral lobes and a central isthmus. It

produces the hormones, thyroxine and triiodothyronine, which have different physiologic properties.

Diagnostic Terms

- *acromegaly*—disease characterized by enlarged features, particularly of the face and hands. This is the result of oversecretion of the pituitary growth hormone. (9)
- *Addison's disease*—primary adrenal cortical insufficiency, a chronic syndrome. Pigmentation is a dominant trait. (9, 61)
- *adrenal crisis, Addisonian crisis*—acute adrenocortical insufficiency and a life-threatening event resulting from a lack of glucocorticoids, hyperkalemia, and depletion of extracellular fluid during acute stress. Clinical manifestations are lassitude, headache, mental confusion, gastric upset, circulatory collapse, coma, and death. (9, 40, 61)
- *adrenal neoplasms:*
    - *—adenomas and adenocarcinomas*—benign or malignant glandular tumors arising from the adrenal cortex. Oversecretion of androgen by the tumor may cause virilization in women and children; excess estrogen production by tumor may result in feminization in men.
    - *—neuroblastomas*—tumors arising from the adrenal medulla. They are generally associated with metastases to bones.
    - *—pheochromocytomas*—tumors usually arising from adrenal medulla and characterized by paroxysmal hypertension. (12)
- *Conn's syndrome, primary aldosteronism*—excessive secretion of aldosterone associated with pathology of adrenal cortex, resulting in potassium depletion, sodium retention, extreme exhaustion, paresthesias, cardiac enlargement, and increased carbon dioxide-combining power. (43, 59)
- *craniopharyngioma*—pituitary tumor of the intrasellar or suprasellar area that may compress the optic chiasm, causing blindness; and raise intracranial pressure, followed by severe headaches; and contain calcifications, cystic components, and cholesterol. (9)
- *Cushing's disease*—syndrome attributed to the hyperproduction of cortisone and hydrocortisone by the adrenal cortex. Obesity, weakness, and hypertension are typical manifestations. (30, 59)
- *dwarfism, pituitary*—congenital underdevelopment due to hyposecretion of the growth hormone. (9)
- *eunuchism*—total gonadal underdevelopment. (9, 21)
- *eunuchoidism*—partial gonadal underdevelopment. (9)
- *giantism*—abnormal growth, particularly of long bones before the closure of the epiphyseal lines. It is caused by overproduction of the growth hormone of the anterior pituitary. (9)
- *goiter*—an enlargement of the thyroid gland. It may be classified as:
    - *—nontoxic diffuse goiter*
    - *—toxic diffuse goiter*
    - *—nontoxic nodular goiter*
    - *—toxic nodular goiter (9, 14, 35)*
- *hypercalcemic syndrome*—abnormally high calcium levels of the blood seen in bone malignancies; endocrine and metabolic disorders such as multiple myeloma; acute adrenal insufficiency; hyperthyroidism; vitamin D intoxication; sarcoidosis; and milk-alkali syndrome. Prolonged bed rest may result in this hypercalcemic syndrome leading to the development of osteoporosis, Paget's disease, and other similar disorders. (4, 9)

- *hyperinsulinism due to islet cell tumor*—condition marked by hypoglycemic episodes with a blood sugar below 30 or 40 mg/dl (deciliter), convulsions increasing in frequency, and severity, and eventually coma. (9)
- *hyperparathyroidism, primary*—overproduction and overactivity of the parathyroid hormone present in hypercalcemia, osteitis fibrosa, and tissue calcification. (4, 9, 58)
- *hyperthyroidism, thyrotoxicosis, exophthalmic goiter, Graves' disease*—thyrotoxic state currently considered an immunologic disorder. The antigen, probably of thyroid origin, is still unknown. Excessive hormone secretion increases oxygen consumption and this accounts for the high metabolic rate. Clinical characteristics are goiter, protrusion of the eyeballs, tachycardia, tremors, emotional instability, sweating, and weight loss. (9, 16)
- *hypoparathyroidism*—abnormally decreased production of the parathyroid hormone causing hypocalcemia. It may be associated with reduced serum calcium and elevated serum phosphate levels. (9)
- *hypothyroidism*—condition resulting from insufficiency of thyroid hormones in the blood. (35, 49)
- *multiple endocrine neoplasia (MEN)*—endocrinopathies of tumors, genetically distinct and of autosomal dominant inheritance.
    - *—MEN, Type I, Wermer's syndrome*—familial disorder of pituitary, pancreatic, and parathyroid gland tumors exhibiting great variability in endocrine involvement and clinical manifestations.
    - *—MEN, Type II, Sipple's syndrome*—an inherited disorder, usually comprising medullary carcinoma associated with bilateral pheochromocytomas of the adrenal medulla.
    - *—MEN, Type III, mucosal neuroma syndrome*—sporadic syndrome similar to MEN, Type II, but with the following differences:
    (1) thyroid medullary carcinoma and pheochromocytomas that may be associated with disfiguring neuromas of the lips, buccal mucosal, and tongue. Café au lait spots may occur; ganglioneuromas of the gastrointestinal tract and the body habitus may resemble that seen in Marfan syndrome patients; (2) the presence of a severe degree of parathyroid hyperplasia that would cause frank hypercalcemia is rare; and (3) the mean survival time is shorter (30 versus 60 years) than in MEN, Type II; the history of family members being affected is present in about half of the cases. (37, 49)
- *myxedema*—hypothyroidism causing lethargy, nonpitting edema, and slow speech. (35)
- *pituitary apoplexy*—acute headache occurring with known pituitary lesions and usually resulting from infarction or hemorrhage into the tumor. Growth and metastasis of the tumor may involve the overlying optic chiasm or the laterally lying cavernous sinus, producing either visual loss or ocular palsies. Surgical drainage should be instituted for removal of the hemorrhagic or infarcted material. (46)
- *reactive hypoglycemia*—common hormonal disturbance initiated by an anxiety state that stimulates both increased consumption of carbohydrates and gastric emptying. This is followed by a high blood sugar, which in turn accelerates insulin production and causes reactive hypoglycemia. It is also known as postprandial reactive hypoglycemia. (17)
- *Simmond's disease, pituitary cachexia*—primary chronic pituitary insufficiency causing extreme weight loss and general debility.
- *tetany*—hypofunction of the parathyroids, resulting in intermittent, tonic spasms due to calcium deficiency. (9, 15)
- *thymic hypoplasia*—presents as congenital or acquired.

- *—congenital thymic hypoplasia*—consists of marked T-cell and variable B-cell immunodeficiency in neonates and infants.
- *—acquired hypoplasia*—thymic involution usually occurs with age or results from stress, malnutrition, pregnancy, x-rays, glucocorticoids, or cytotoxic drugs. Acquired immune deficiency syndrome (AIDS) and graft-versus host disease are common producers of severe thymic dysplasia. (53)
- *thymoma*—tumor of thymus that may be invasive and associated with myasthenia gravis or other syndromes. It tends to recur after removal. (53)
- *thyroid dysfunction*—malfunction of the thyroid hormones resulting in several thyrotoxic myopathies associated with muscle atrophy and weakness, depletion of energy, and other manifestations. (9, 15)
- *thyroiditis*—inflammation of the thyroid gland. (14, 15, 35)
  - *—acute thyroiditis*—sudden onset of inflammatory process with local tenderness of thyroid.
  - *—Hashimoto's thyroiditis, struma lymphomatosa*—lymphoid goiter or lymphocytic thyroiditis, thought to be an autoimmune hereditary disease and not an infectious or inflammatory disorder as the name suggests. It occurs almost exclusively in women. A medium-sized, rubbery, firm goiter, low metabolism, and hypothyroidism are common clinical findings.
  - *—Riedel's struma*—rare chronic type affecting the elderly and characterized by fibrotic changes and a wooden sensation in the neck.
  - *—subacute thyroiditis*—inflammation usually subsequent to viral infection in the respiratory tract, indicative of an immunologic response to the virus.
- *thyroid neoplasms:* (11, 14, 18)
  - *—adenomas*—benign glandular tumors.
  - *—follicular carcinoma*—malignant tumor more common in men than in women. It varies in appearance from well-differentiated types of tumors to nearly solid sheets of follicular epithelium with little evidence of follicle formation.
  - *—lymphomas*—malignant, nodular histiocytic tumor that usually arises in a gland affected by Hashimoto's thyroiditis.
  - *—medullary carcinoma*—malignant tumor originating from parafollicular or C-cells and producing large amounts of calcitonin. These tumors are characterized by sheets of tumor cells separated by a hyaline-amyloid containing stroma. Medullary carcinoma of the thyroid occurs in sporadic form (85%) and in familial form, which accounts for the remainder. Familial medullary carcinoma of the thyroid may be considered as part of a medullary thyroid carcinoma-pheochromocytoma syndrome, and it appears to be genetically determined as an autosomal dominant with a high degree of frequency.
  - *—papillary carcinoma*—most common malignant type of thyroid tumor seen in younger patients. This type of thyroid carcinoma is more common in women than in men.
  - *—extrathyroidal tumor*—extending through the thyroid capsule; involves surrounding tissue.
  - *—intrathyroidal tumors*—do not extend beyond the thyroid surface. Microscopically, these tumors consist of well-differentiated thyroid epithelium covering papillary fibrovascular stalks.

Operative Terms

- *adrenalectomy*—removal of adrenal gland or glands. (30)
- *cryohypophysectomy*—one of several procedures that uses the stereotaxic transsphenoi-

dal approach and achieves pituitary ablation (removal of hypophysis) by the application of a cryoprobe. (30)

- *hypophysectomy, total*—removal of hypophysis. Total hypophysectomy is required to correct hypercortisolism in approximately 10 percent of patients. Postoperative radiation may be required for unresectable tumors and persistent hypercortisolism. (30)
- *microneurosurgery of pituitary gland*—microdissection of tumor under magnification and with intense illumination using a binocular surgical microscope.
  Techniques are:
    - *Hardy's oronasal-transsphenoidal approach*—entering the sphenoid sinus via nasal septum for removal of intrasellar tumor.
    - *Rand's transfrontal-transsphenoidal approach*—opening the sphenoid sinus through a frontal craniotomy for removal of tumor attached to optic chiasm.
- *parathyroidectomy*—removal of parathyroid tissue to control hyperparathyroidism. (58)
- *thymectomy*—removal of thymus gland. (10)
- *thyroid surgery:* (14, 47)
    - *lobectomy of thyroid*—usually the removal of the isthmus and involved lobe for solitary thyroid nodule.
    - *partial thyroidectomy*—method of choice for removal of fibrous nodular thyroid.
    - *subtotal thyroidectomy*—the removal of most of the thyroid to relieve hyperthyroidism.

Symptomatic Terms

- *exophthalmos*—abnormal protrusion of the eyeballs. (9)
- *hirsutism*—excessive growth of hair. (9, 38)
- *malignant exophthalmos*—excessive protrusion of the eyeballs that fails to respond to treatment and leads to loss of sight. (35)
- *paroxysmal hypertension*—sudden recurrence of high blood pressure after a remission. It may be caused by conditions of the adrenal gland.
- *postural hypertension*—high blood pressure associated with changes in posture. (12)
- *pressor effect*—stimulating effect.
- *proptosis*—forward displacement of the globes in the orbit; exophthalmos. (35)
- *virilism*—masculinization in women. (9, 38)
- *vitiligo*—white patches on the skin of the hands and feet. They may be seen in hyperthyroidism. (44)

Metabolic Diseases

Origin of Terms

melano- (G)—black
meli- (G)—honey

meta- (G)—change, exchange, transformation
xantho- (G)—yellow

Diagnostic Terms

- *acid-base imbalance*—disturbance in acid-base balance of the blood concerned with carbon dioxide (carbonic acid) as the acid component and bicarbonate as the base component of the equation. As a result, abnormal changes develop in the carbon dioxide tension (Pco_2) and hydrogen ion concentration (pH). Lungs and kidneys play major roles in:

—*metabolic acidosis*—primary alkali deficit characterized by a low pH and Pco_2. It occurs in Addison's disease, starvation, diarrhea, renal and liver disease, overtreatment with acids, etc.

—*metabolic alkalosis*—primary alkali excess marked by increased pH and Pco_2. It is caused by excessive loss of acid, gastric suction, potassium deficit, Cushing's syndrome, overtreatment with alkaline salts, etc.

—*respiratory acidosis*—primary CO_2 excess, low pH, and high Pco_2 indicative of impaired gaseous exchange and hypoventilation resulting in carbon dioxide retention. It may develop in overdepression of respiratory center, lung disease, and heart failure.

—*respiratory alkalosis*—primary CO_2 deficit, high pH and low Pco_2 present in hyperventilation. It is seen in overstimulation of respiratory center, high altitudes, fever, hysteria, and anxiety. (2, 36)

- *alkalosis*—abnormal increase of alkalinity in the blood. (2, 36)
- *carcinoid syndrome, carcinoidosis*—peculiar metabolic disorder characterized by flushing, diarrhea, dyspnea, and valvular heart disease. The symptoms are related to an overproduction of serotonin by the malignant carcinoid tumor of the gastrointestinal tract, usually the terminal ileum. Metastases to the liver and adjacent lymph nodes may occur. (13, 41)
- *diabetes insipidus*—metabolic disorder caused by hyposecretion of the antidiuretic hormone of the pituitary gland. Its clinical manifestations are polydipsia and polyuria. (3)
- *diabetes mellitus*—chronic metabolic disease, thought to be genetically determined; in its advanced stage it is clinically manifested in a nonstressed patient by fasting hyperglycemia, glycosuria, ketoacidosis, atherosclerotic and microvascular changes, protein breakdown, and neuropathies. According to the National Diabetes Data Group and standards from the World Health Organization, diabetes mellitus can be separated into two general disease syndromes:

  —*Type I, insulin-dependent diabetes mellitus (IDDM), (formerly termed juvenile diabetes or juvenile-onset diabetes), ketosis-prone diabetes or brittle diabetes*—hyperglycemia caused by absent or insufficient secretion of insulin by B-cells of the pancreas in response to glucose. It is seen in the young and infrequently in adults, particularly thin or elderly adults.

  —*Type II, non-insulin-dependent diabetes mellitus (NIDDM), (formerly termed adult-onset or maturity-onset diabetes), ketosis-resistant or stable diabetes*—hyperglycemia related to varied amounts of pancreatic insulin; ketosis is limited to periods of stress or infection. This type of diabetes is prone to develop in obese individuals over 40 years of age. (31, 42)

- *secondary diabetic states*—exist when some other readily identifiable primary disorder or pathophysiologic state causes or is associated with the diabetic state. Any disorder that limits insulin secretion or impairs insulin action can cause secondary diabetes. Some examples of these disorders are chronic pancreatitis, cystic fibrosis, hemochromatosis, Cushing's disease, pheochromocytoma, and others. (31, 42)
- *diabetic ketoacidosis (DKA)*—due to insulin deficiency. Severe insulin deficiency leads to hyperglycemia and ketonemia and from these states all of the other pathophysiologic sequelae may occur. Acidosis and ketonuria are primarily caused by the buildup of the ketoacids beta-hydroxybutyrate and acetoacetate. Hyperglycemia and hyperketonemia cause an osmotic diuresis that produces intravascular volume depletion and dehydration and urinary electrolyte loss. DKA is a serious complication in diabetic persons of all ages that may be precipitated in the young by infection and in the elderly by acute stress, myocardial infarction, and infection. The onset is

gradual, with symptoms of polydipsia and polyuria, fever, nausea, vomiting, and extreme fatigue. It is followed by increasing mental stupor and rapid, deep respirations, with a fruity breath odor signaling ketoacetotic coma. This low blood pressure and rapid pulse reflect marked dehydration (5 to 10 liters) and salt depletion. (42)

- *galactosemia*—inborn error of carbohydrate metabolism resulting in an incapacity for metabolizing galactose. Consequently, galactose blood levels increase abnormally, and galactose may be present in the urine. The principal clinical manifestation in galactose deficiency is cataracts. Other manifestations that may develop include gastrointestinal disorders, ascites, cirrhosis, proteinuria, and mental retardation. The key treatment is the institution of a galactose-free diet. Untreated patients with galactose deficiency may not survive and those who do survive may be severely retarded mentally. (28, 51)

- *Gaucher's disease*—hereditary metabolic defect resulting in faulty lipid storage. Abnormal reticuloendothelial (Gaucher) cells proliferate and cause progressive splenomegaly, pigmentation of the skin, anemia, and frequently bone involvement. (29, 33)

- *glycogenoses*—glycogen storage diseases caused by an enzymatic defect in the buildup and breakdown of glycogen. (26)

- *gout, gouty arthritis*—disorder of purine metabolism and a recurrent form of arthritis manifested by an abnormal increase of uric acid in the blood, tophi, joint involvement, and, in severe cases, uric acid nephrolithiasis or renal failure. (32, 65)

- *hyperglucagonemia*—excess of glucagon in the circulating blood. It does not cause glucose intolerance in normal subjects or bring about deterioration of diabetic control. Glucagon in the insulin-deprived patient can worsen the condition. (22)

- *hypoglycemic states*—low blood sugar levels and neuroglycopenia (diminished glucose content of the brain) are essential characteristics of significant hypoglycemia. Nervousness, hunger, flushing or pallor, lethargy or somnolence, bizarre behavior, and syncopal attacks may be present in varying degrees. The most important cause of hypoglycemia is a pancreatic B-cell tumor, which may present as a solitary insulinoma and produce excessive amounts of insulin. Hypoglycemia may occur in the fasting state or postprandially. Some hypoglycemic disorders are presented.
  - *alcoholic hypoglycemia*—low plasma glucose production by the liver which has been damaged by excessive and prolonged alcohol ingestion.
    - *fasting hypoglycemia after alcoholic excess*—prolonged abstinence from food for 18 to 24 hours after ethanol ingestion tend to induce a profound hypoglycemia.
    - *postethanol-reactive hypoglycemia*—the use of soft drinks containing sugar to dilute alcoholic beverages seems to stimulate a marked insulin release, which is followed by a hypoglycemic reaction 3 or 4 hours later.
  - *fasting hypoglycemia related to some endocrine disorders*—low blood sugar episodes may occur in Addison's disease, hypopituitarism, and myxedema.
  - *fasting hypoglycemia caused by B-cell tumors of the pancreas:*
    - *adenomas of the islets of Langerhans may be associated with hypoglycemia.*
  - *Whipple's triad*—consists of: (1) the symptoms of hypoglycemia; (2) a low fasting flood sugar level of 40 mg/dl or less; and (3) a quick recovery after glucose administration. However, if insulinoma is the cause of hypoglycemia, the prognosis may be fatal. (31, 52)

- *lipid metabolism disorders*—there are four types of principal circulating lipids:
  - *cholesterol esters*
  - *free cholesterol*
  - *phospholipids*
  - *triglycerides*

Lipoproteins are classified according to specific differences into:
- —*HDL*—high-density lipoproteins
- —*LDL*—low-density lipoproteins
- —*VLDL*—very-low-density lipoproteins (7, 8)

- *lipidosis (pl. lipidoses)*—any disorder in which abnormal lipid concentrations are found in extracellular fluid and body tissues. Abnormally high plasma lipids and lipoproteins occurring in various metabolic disorders present problems of classification and treatment.
  These disorders include:
  - —*abnormal plasma lipoproteins:*
  - —*hyperlipoproteinemia, six types*
  - —*dyslipoproteinemia*
  - —*hypolipoproteinemia*
  - —*lipid storage diseases*—caused by functional deficiency of certain enzymes. Gaucher's disease and Wolman's disease belong in this category, as well as many other disorders.
  - —*granulomatous diseases with lipid storage, such as histiocytosis*
  - —*other xanthomatoses*
  - —*adipose tissue disorders:*
  - —*lipoatrophy, partial (lipodystrophy)*
  - —*lipoatrophy, complete*
  - —*other lipodoses* (7, 8, 29, 31)

- *obesity*—excess of adipose tissue that presents a potential risk to good health. The metabolic factor causing obesity may be the steroid excess of glucocorticoids in Cushing's syndrome. Since obese persons usually have hypertriglyceridemia and hypercholesterolemia, they are more prone to develop atherosclerosis, hypertension, and diabetes mellitus than thin persons. (45)

- *phenylketonuria*—hereditary metabolic disorder causing mental retardation. Phenylketone bodies are found in serum and urine. The disease is caused by an inborn error of amino acid metabolism. (48, 50, 54)

- *porphyria*—inborn faulty porphyrin metabolism resulting in porphyrinuria.
  - —*congenital, erythropoietic type*—porphyria characterized by skin lesions due to photosensitivity from porphyrin in subcutaneous tissue.
  - —*hepatic intermittent acute type*—porphyria noted for liver damage, brownish pigmentation of the skin, and neurologic symptoms. (6)

- *Wolman's disease*—rare familial xanthomatosis characterized by punctuate calcium deposits throughout the enlarged adrenal glands, hepatosplenomegaly, and visceral foam cells filled with triglyceride and cholesterol. The disease is lethal. (44)

- *xanthomatosis*—widespread eruption of xanthomas on the skin and tendons. The xanthomas are yellow, lipid-containing plaques usually associated with hyperlipoproteinemia. (24, 44)

Symptomatic Terms

- *exacerbation*—aggravation of symptoms. (60)
- *glycosuria*—the presence of sugar in the urine. (31, 42, 48)
- *hyperchloremia*—excessive chloride concentration in the circulating blood. (4)
- *hypercholesterolemia*—excessive cholesterol concentration in the circulating blood. (8, 31)
- *hyperchylomicronemia*—excessive chylomicron concentration in the blood. (8)
- *hyperglycemia*—excessive sugar concentration in the blood. (31, 42)
- *hyperkalemia*—excessive potassium concentration in the blood. (2, 61)
- *hypernatremia*—excessive sodium concentration in the blood. (61)

- *hypertriglyceridemia*—excessive triglyceride concentration in the blood. (8)
- *hyperuricemia*—excessive uric acid concentration in the blood. (65)
- *hyponatremia*—abnormally low serum sodium level due to a disturbed ratio of water to sodium. (2, 35, 59)
- *insulinopenia*—deficient insulin secretion by the pancreatic B-cells present in diabetes mellitus. (10)
- *ketosis*—excess ketone bodies in the body fluids and tissues due to incomplete combustion of fatty acids, which may result from a faulty or absent utilization of carbohydrates. Ketosis may produce severe acidosis. It develops in uncontrolled diabetes mellitus and starvation. (42)
- *Kussmaul breathing*—classic manifestations in diabetic acidosis marked by unusually deep respirations associated with dyspnea. This type of breathing is caused by abnormally increased acid content of the blood, resulting in continuous overstimulation of the respiratory center. (36, 42)
- *polydipsia*—excessive thirst. (9, 42)
- *polyphagia*—overeating.
- *remission*—symptoms decreased in severity. (60)
- *steatorrhea*—excess fecal fat due to malabsorption of lipids, an enzyme deficiency of the pancreas, or intestinal disease. (60)
- *tophi (sing. tophus)*—sodium biurate deposits near a joint. Condition is peculiar to gout. (65)

Hormonal Disorders and Cytogenetics

Origin of Terms

centre (G)—center
chromo- (G)—color
cyto- (G)—cell
gamete (G)—mature germ cell, sperm, ovum
-gen (G)—to produce
karyo- (G)—nucleus

mono- (G)—single
mutant (G)—to change
ovum (L)—egg
ovo- (L)—egg
spermato-, spermo- (G)—seed
syndrome (G)—running together

General Terms

- *acrocentric*—centromere located at one end. (60)
- *autosomal aberration*—abnormality of chromosomes.
  - *—acquired*—developed after birth, as in chronic myeloid leukemia.
  - *—congenital*—present at birth, as in mongolism. (34)
- *autosomal dominant inheritance*—one abnormal dominant gene of a pair is passed on to 50 percent of the offspring, although the affected parent has a normal mate. As a rule, autosomal dominant inheritance delineates the follow pattern:
  - *—equal distribution of the abnormal trait among males and females.*
  - *—direct transmission of the trait over two generations or more.*
  - *—abnormal trait affecting close to 50 percent of the members of the pedigree. (19, 60, 63)*
- *autosomal recessive inheritance*—abnormality is produced by paired defective genes, since both parents contribute one recessive abnormal gene. Criteria for establishing recessive inheritance are:

Figure 66 Chromosomes from a normal human male cell, grown in tissue culture and arrested at the metaphase.

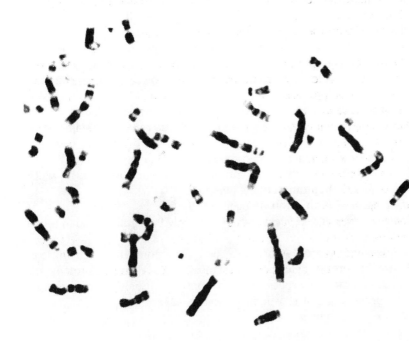

Figure 67 Human sex chromosomes, normal pattern and chromosomal aberrations.

Normal female

Normal male

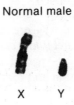

X X

X Y

Klinefelter's syndrome

Turner's syndrome

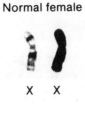

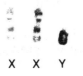

X X Y

X O

—consanguinity increases the chance that the affected gene is passed on by the two related parents.

—the same genetic disorder occurs in collateral family branches.

—the disease is present in 25 percent of the siblings. (19, 60, 63)

- *autosome, autosomal chromosome*—nonsex chromosome. (19, 60, 63)
- *banding*—banded or striped appearance of chromosomes when special staining is done to chromosomes at metaphase using the Giemsa method for karyotyping. (60)
- *centromere*—constriction in center of chromosome, dividing the chromosome into two lengths, or arms. (34)
- *chromatid*—one of the two halves of a chromosome. (34)
- *chromatin*—deoxyribonucleic acid (DNA) found in chromosomes and stainable by basic dyes. (23)
- *chromosomal aberration*—abnormality of chromosomes.

    —*acquired*—developed after birth, as in chronic granulocytic leukemia, in which the Philadelphia (Ph[1]) chromosome is present.

    —*congenital*—present at birth, as in mongolism. (5)
- *chromosomal breakage, chromosomal fragmentation*—anomaly frequently found in tumor cells. (23)
- *chromosome* (see Figs. 66 and 67)—threadlike body of chromatin in cell nucleus. Chromosomes are bearers of hereditary substances, called genes. Normally the number of chromosomes for each species remains constant. At present chromosomes have become the prime target of genetic investigation. (23)
- *chromosome analysis*—karyotyping. (60)
- *chromosome defects*—two types occur: (23, 60)

    —*aneuploidy*—abnormal chromosome number.

    —*aneuploid mosaics*—modal numbers differing in two or more distinct cell populations.

    —*heterosomal aneuploidy*—all cells possessing uniform aneuploidy, including:

    complex aneuploidy—two or more individual chromosomes in the same person show defects in numbers.

    monosomy—one member of a chromosome pair is absent.

    polysomy—the same chromosome is present four times or more.

    triploidy—each chromosome occurs in triplicate.

    trisomy—one chromosome occurs in triplicate.

    —*structural defects of chromosomes:* (23, 34, 60)

    —*deletion*—partial loss of a chromosome that is prone to occur during cell division and may be a long arm or short arm deletion. Usually there are two breaks in a chromosome, and the segment between fractures is lost.

    —*duplication*—condition in which a portion of a chromosome is represented more than once.

    —*isochromosome*—transverse division of the centromere during meiosis, which causes a chromosomal aberration.

    —*translocation*—chromosome segment that shifts to a different position. It is balanced if there is a full complement of genetic material, even if the arrangement happens to be unusual. It is unbalanced if there is too much or not enough genetic material.

    —*others*.
- *cytogenetics*—branch of science concerned with the origin and development of cells in heredity. (See Table 16 for cytogenetic studies). Examples of cytogenetic tests for chromosomal sex determination include:

  —*biopsy of human skin*—this is a microscopic examination of a small piece of epithelium to detect characteristic chromatin masses alongside the nuclear membrane in somatic cells. They are usually found only in females. (44)

  —*buccal or oral smear test, sex chromatin test, Barr test of nuclear sex*—a stained smear of epithelial cells, scraped from the mucosa of the cheek, is studied under the microscope for chromatin bodies. Normally males are chromatin negative and females chromatin positive. (34, 62)

  —*leukocyte cell smear for peripheral blood*—a cytologic test for chromosomal sex differentiation. A small number of circulating neutrophils poses a characteristic drumstick chromatin attachment distinguishable from the remaining nucleus. This drumstick formation on the cell nucleus has not been found in males. (60)

  —*tissue culture of human cells*—new method of culturing permits growth without chromosomal disorganization. Tissue is cultured in vitro to obtain sufficient mitoses. The culture is treated with colchicine to arrest mitosis in metaphase and with hypotonic saline to attain spreading of the chromosomes. Preparations are then squashed, stained, and photographed under a microscope. The photomicrograph is enlarged, and the chromosomes cut out and paired to make a karyotype. (60)

- *DNA, deoxyribonucleic acid*—chromosomal material thought to transmit hereditary characteristics, currently subject to intense research. (1, 5, 19)
- *dominant*—pertaining to a gene that exerts its effect even in the presence of a contrasting or opposite gene. (60)
- *equatorial plate*—same as metaphase plate. (60)
- *euploidy*—state pertaining to balanced sets of chromosomes in every number. (60)
- *fragment*—broken portion of a chromosome. In the acentric type no centromere is present. (60)
- *gamete*—mature germ cell, sperm, or ovum. (60)
- *gene*—basic unit of heredity found at a definite locus (place) on a particular chromosome. There may be thousands of genes to one DNA molecule. Genes, like chromosomes, come in pairs and are either:

  —*heterozygous*—each member of a gene pair carries a different instruction, or

  —*homozygous*—both members of the gene pair carry the same instruction. (19, 34)

- *genome*—a cell's or organism's entire genetic constitution. (60)
- *genotype*—genetic constitution, irrespective of external appearance. (60)
- *gonosome*—sex chromosome Y or X. (19, 23)
- *idiogram*—diagram representing the karyotype (chromosome pattern) of the cells of an individual. (60)
- *karyotype* (see Fig. 68)—group of characteristics (form, number, size) used to identify an individual's chromosomal pattern. A karyotype of a normal person has 46 chromosomes, including 22 autosomal pairs and two sex chromosomes. They are arranged and numbered according to the *1961 International Classification System of Denver, Colorado*. This is known as karyotyping. (19)
- *lagging*—anomaly resulting in the loss of material from chromosomes. These abnormal chromosomes are then located outside the mitotic spindle and are prone to develop micronuclei in the cytoplasm. (23)
- *mar*—symbol of unidentified chromosome of totally unknown origin, as defined by the 1966 Chicago Conference. (60)
- *marker chromosome*—an abnormal chromosome recognized by its unusual structure. (60)

- *meiosis*—special cell division that occurs in maturation of sex cells and causes each daughter nucleus to receive half of the number of chromosomes of the species' somatic cells. (19, 23)
- *metaphase*—chromosomes lying on the equatorial plate. (23)
- *mitosis*—process of cell division; longitudinal splitting of chromosomes into halves and migration of the halves. (19, 23)
- *mosaicism, chromosomal*—population of normal chromosomes together with a population of one or more abnormal types, varying in proportion. Mental and physical retardation are common clinical characteristics. (23, 62)
- *mutation*—change occurring in genes. (19, 64)
- *nondisjunction*—chromatid pair failing to separate in cell division.
- *phenotype*—apparent type with visible characteristics that may be independent of genotype (hereditary type). (62)
- *Philadelphia chromosome, Ph¹*—G group chromosome characterized by partial loss (deletion) of the long arm. It is present in typical CML (chronic myelocytic leukemia) and absent in atypical CML. (5)
- *recessive*—pertaining to a gene that is ineffective in the presence of contrasting or opposite genes. (63)
- *sex chromosomes*—those determining the sex of offspring; XX for female, XY for male. (19, 63)
- *stickiness*—chromosomal abnormality frequently present in tumor cells. It may cause clumping and abnormal distribution of chromosomes. (60)
- *X-chromosome*—sex chromosome, normally found in the male and female. (19, 23)
- *Y-chromosome*—sex chromosome present in the male. (19, 23)

Diagnostic Terms

- *Down's syndrome*—disorder with varying degrees of retardation and physical signs of mongolism, such as dwarfing of stature, slanting eyes, open mouth, and protruding tongue. The genetic basis may be a numerical chromosome abnormality (aneuploy), such as trisomy 21 with 47 chromosomes, or a structural chromosome abnormality, such as translocation with 46 chromosomes. (20, 25, 34, 49)
- *D-trisomy, trisomy 13-15*—common chromosome abnormality with 47 chromosomes; clinically characterized by hemangiomas, polydactylia, and microphthalmia. Less evident are cardiovascular and neurologic anomalies, which are detectable by chromosomal analysis. (23)
- *Edward's syndrome, trisomy E*—chromosome defect clinically manifested by a narrow long skull, prominent occiput, marked mental retardation, congenital cardiac disease, peculiar facies, and fingers with flexion deformities. (23)
- *hermaphrodite*—sex chromosome abnormality of variable phenotype and the presence of both ovarian and testicular tissue in gonads. (27, 62)
- *Klinefelter's syndrome, seminiferous tubule dysgenesis*—disorder in which chromosomal aberration results in sterility due to defective embryonic development of the seminiferous tubules. The symptom complex comprises various degrees of:
    - *aspermia or oligospermia*—lack or scanty secretion of semen.
    - *eunuchoidism*—sparsity of hair on face and body.
    - *gynecomastia*—overdevelopment of the mammary glands in the male.
    - *hypoplasia of testes, hypogonadism*—small, firm testes. Mental retardation and psychiatric disorders are common. (39, 62)
- *Noonan's syndrome, Bonnevie-Ullrich syndrome, male Turner's syndrome*—autosomal recessive disorder characterized by cryptorchism; insufficient spermatogenesis; webbed neck; short stature; cardiovascular defects; and other anomalies. Males with

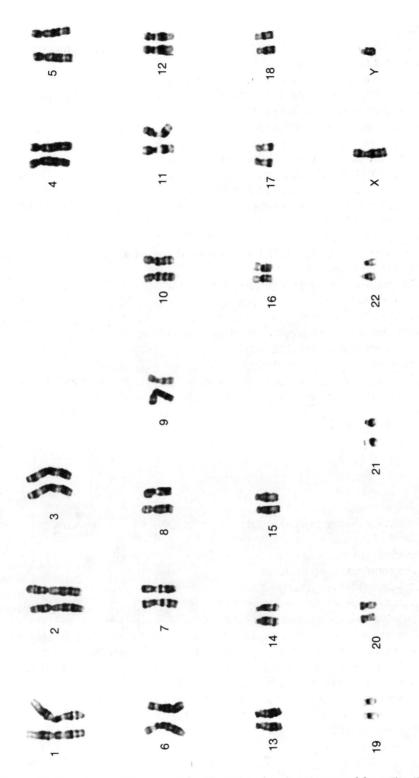

Figure 68 Karyotype or idiogram of a normal human male. Constructed from Fig. 67. Note banding of chromosomes.

Noonan's syndrome display primary testicular dysfunction with impairment of both sperm and androgen production, and elevated serum gonadotropin levels. It is not a chromosomal abnormality. (39, 62)

- *Turner's syndrome, gonadal dysgenesis, ovarian dysgenesis*—complex inherited disorder caused by chromosomal aberration. Constant clinical signs are rudimentary ovaries composed of a fibrotic streak in each broad ligament and infertility. The classic syndrome includes different degrees of:
  - *estrogen deficiency*—inadequate secretion of female hormones.
  - *hypomastia*—abnormally small breasts.
  - *malformations*—structural defects such as dwarfism, shieldlike chest, webbed neck, coarctation of the aorta, and others.
  - *true primary amenorrhea*—absence of menses. (27, 62) (See Table 16.)

Symptomatic Terms

- *arachnodactylia*—condition characterized by abnormal length and slenderness of the fingers and toes.
- *cylindruria*—presence of tube casts in the urine.
- *microphthalmia*—condition of abnormal smallness in all dimensions of one or both eyes.
- *polydactylia*—a developmental anomaly characterized by the presence of supernumerary digits on hands and feet.
- *xerostomia*—dryness of mouth.

Table 16
Cytogenetic Studies*

Chromosomal Findings	Normal Male	Normal Female	Klinefelter's Syndrome	Turner's Syndrome
Chromosome count	46	46	47	45
Chromosomal pattern	XY	XX	XXY	XO
Chromatin nuclear sex	Chromatin negative	Chromatin positive	Chromatin positive— genetic female	Chromatin negative— genetic male
Major clinical signs	Proper size and function	Proper size and function	Testicular hypoplasia Sterility	Ovarian hypoplasia Infertility

*(27, 39, 60, 62)

Abbreviations

Genetics and Cytogenetics

AD—autosomal dominant
AR—autosomal recessive
mar—marker chromosome

PH[1]—Philadelphia chromosome
XD—X (sex) linked dominant
XO—Turner's syndrome

XR—X (sex) linked recessive
XX—female sex chromosomes

XXY—Klinefelter's syndrome
XY—male sex chromosomes

Hormones and Miscellaneous

ACTH—adrenocorticotropic hormone
ADH—antidiuretic hormone
ATP—adenosine triphosphate
BMR—basal metabolic rate
CO_2—carbon dioxide
CRF—corticotropin-releasing factor
DKA—diabetic ketoacidosis
DOC—desoxycorticosterone
ECF—extracellular fluid
EFA—essential fatty acids
FBS—fasting blood sugar
FFA—free sugar acids
FSH—follicle-stimulating hormone
GTT—glucose tolerance test
HbA_{1c}—glycosylated hemoglobin
HDL—high-density lipoprotein
ICF—intracellular fluid
ICSH—interstitial cell-stimulating hormone
IDDM—insulin-dependent diabetes mellitus
IF—interstitial fluid

K—potassium
LATS—long-acting thyroid stimulator
LDL—low-density lipoprotein
LH—luteinizing hormone
MCT—medullary carcinoma of the thyroid
MSH—melanocyte-stimulating hormone
NaC1—sodium chloride
NIDDM—non-insulin-dependent diabetes mellitus
NPH—neutral protein Hagedorn (insulin)
P—phosphorus
PGH—pituitary growth hormone
PP—postprandial
PTH—parathyroid hormone, parathyrin
PZI—protamine zinc insulin
17-KS—17-ketosteroids
17-OH—17-hydroxycorticoids
TSH—thyroid-stimulating hormone
TTH—thyrotropic hormone
VLDL—very-low-density lipoprotein

Oral Reading Practice

Hypothyroidism

Hypothyroidism is a functional disorder caused by insufficiency of the circulating **thyroid** hormones. Any biologic, chemical, or physical factors that reduce the hormone supply may result in thyroid failure.

In primary hypothyroid states the condition may be congenital, such as in **cretinism,** or acquired, such as in **juvenile myxedema** or **adult myxedema.** Surgical excision, **atrophy,** or disease of the thyroid gland stop or lower hormone production, and a lack of **iodine** in food seriously hampers hormone synthesis.

In **secondary** hypothyroid states the pituitary gland elaborates an inadequate amount of **thyroid-stimulating hormone** (TSH), which drastically reduces thyroid function. This deficit of **thyrotropin** (TSH) occurs in **pituitary necrosis,** or Sheehan's disease, and **primary chronic hypopituitarism,** or Simmond's syndrome. A total absence of TSH is seen in **hypophysectomized** patients.

The judicious use of replacement therapy with **thyroxine** or **triiodothyronine** in thyroid failure and a thyrotropin preparation in pituitary failure is imperative to maintain relatively normal metabolic processes and overcome hypothyroidism. (9, 14, 15, 35)

Table 17
Some Endocrine Conditions Amenable to Surgery

Organs Involved	Diagnosis	Type of Surgery	Operative Procedures
Adrenal gland	Adenoma of adrenal cortex (unilateral) anterior to kidney	Unilateral adrenalectomy with excision of adenoma	Abdominal approach with preliminary exploration of ovaries in the female followed by removal of tumor
Adrenal gland	Cushing's syndrome secondary to adrenal neoplasm	Subtotal adrenalectomy Resection of tumor	Removal of one adrenal gland and tumor
Adrenal gland	Pheochromocytoma Paroxysmal hypertension	Adrenalectomy and tumor resection	Anterior transabdominal incision and removal of pheochromocytoma
Adrenal glands	Hypercortisonism	Bilateral adrenalectomy followed by autotransplantation	Both adrenals removed and healthy portion of gland implanted to maintain adrenal function
Pancreas	Insulinoma: hyperinsulinism and marked hypoglycemia	Resection of pancreas and excision of insulinoma	Removal of part of pancreas containing insulinoma to restore glycemia
Parathyroid	Parathyroid adenoma Hyperparathyroidism Nephrolithiasis	Excision of adenoma of parathyroid gland	Removal of parathyroid with adenoma to prevent recurrent renal calculi
Thyroid gland	Solitary thyroid nodule of unknown nature	Surgical exploration	Tissue from thyroid nodule removed; frozen section made
Thyroid gland	Graves' thyrotoxicosis	Subtotal thyroidectomy	Removal of part of thyroid gland
Thyroid gland	Papillary carcinoma with metastases to adjacent lymph nodes	Total thyroidectomy with neck dissection	Excision of entire thyroid gland with dissection of upper portion of neck
Thyroid gland	Postthyroidectomy hemorrhage	Thyroidotomy	Reopening of thyroid wound for removal of hematoma and control of hemorrhage
Thymus gland	Myasthenia gravis, nonthymomatous	Transcervical thymectomy	Incision across the suprasternal notch, removal of thymus

References and Bibliography

1. Anderson, W. French. Expectations from recombinant DNA research. In Wyngaarden, James B., and Smith, Lloyd H., Jr., eds., *Cecil's Textbook of Medicine*, 18th ed. vol. 1. Philadelphia: W.B. Saunders Co., 1988, pp. 158-161.

2. Andreoli, Thomas E. Disorders of fluid volume, electrolyte, and acid-base balance. In Wyngaarden, James B., and Smith, Lloyd H., Jr., eds., *Cecil's Textbook of Medicine*, 18th ed., vol. 1. Philadelphia: W.B. Saunders Co., 1988, pp. 528-558.

3. ———. The posterior pituitary. Ibid., vol. 2., pp. 1305-1313.

4. Arnaud, Claude D. The parathyroid glands, hypercalcemia and hypocalcemia. In Wyngaarden, James B., and Smith, Lloyd H., Jr., eds., *Cecil's Textbook of Medicine*, 18th ed., vol. 2. Philadelphia: W.B. Saunders Co., 1988, pp. 1486-1504.

5. Bishop, J. Michael. Oncogenes. In Wyngaarden, James B., and Smith, Lloyd H., Jr., eds., *Cecil's Textbook of Medicine*, 18th ed., vol. 1. Philadelphia: W.B. Saunders Co., 1988, pp. 1089-1092.

6. Bissell, D. Montgomery. Porphyria. In Wyngaarden, James B., and Smith, Lloyd H., Jr., eds., *Cecil's Textbook of Medicine*, 18th ed., vol. 1. Philadelphia: W.B. Saunders Co., 1988, pp. 1181-1188.

7. Brown, Michael S., and Goldstein, Joseph L. The hyperlipoproteinemias and other disorders of lipid metabolism. In Braunwald, Eugene, et al., eds., *Harrison's Principles of Internal Medicine*, 11th ed. New York: McGraw-Hill Book Co., 1987, pp. 1650-1661.

8. Brunzell, John D. The hyperlipoproteinemias. In Wyngaarden, James B., and Smith, Lloyd H., Jr., eds., *Cecil's Textbook of Medicine*, 18th ed., vol. 1. Philadelphia: W.B. Saunders Co., 1988, pp. 1137-1144.

9. Camargo, Carlos A., and Kolb, Felix O. Endocrine disorders. In Schroeder, Steven A., Krupp, Marcus A., and Tierney, Lawrence M., Jr., eds., *Current Medical Diagnosis & Treatment—1988*, Norwalk, CT: Appleton & Lange, 1988, pp. 676-748.

10. Chitwood, W. Randolph, Jr. The diagnosis and management of myasthenia gravis. In Sabiston, David C., Jr., ed., *Essentials of Surgery*, Philadelphia: W.B. Saunders Co., 1987, pp. 1036-1044.

11. Clarke, Susan E.M., et al. The role of technetium-99m pentavalent DMSA in the management of patients with medullary carcinoma of the thyroid. *The British Journal of Radiology* 60:1089-1092, Nov. 1987.

12. Cryer, Philip E. The adrenal medulla and the sympathetic nervous system. In Wyngaarden, James B., and Smith, Lloyd H., Jr., eds., *Cecil's Textbook of Medicine*, 18th ed. vol. 2. Philadelphia: W.B. Saunders Co., 1988, pp. 1461-1467.

13. ———. The carcinoid syndrome. Ibid., vol. 2, pp. 1467-1468.

14. Farndon, John R. The thyroid. In Sabiston, David C., Jr., ed., *Essentials of Surgery*, Philadelphia: W.B. Saunders Co., 1987, pp. 327-339.

15. Farid, Nadir R., and Balazs, C. Immunogenetics of thyroiditis and thyroid carcinoma. In Farid, Nadir R., ed., *Immunogenetics of Endocrine Disorders*, New York: Alan R. Liss, Inc., 1988, pp. 267-307.

16. Farid, Nadir R., and Stenszky, Valeria. Graves' disease. In Farid, Nadir R., ed., *Immunogenetics of Endocrine Disorders*, New York: Alan R. Liss, Inc., 1988, pp. 309-344.

17. Frohman, Lawrence A. The anterior pituitary. In Wyngaarden, James B., and Smith, Lloyd H., Jr., eds., *Cecil's Textbook of Medicine*, 18th ed., vol. 2. Philadelphia: W.B. Saunders Co., 1988, pp. 1290-1305.

18. Gogas, John, et al. Medullary carcinoma of the thyroid. *The American Surgeon* 53:347-349, June 1987.

19. Goldstein, Joseph L., and Brown, Michael S. Genetic aspects of disease. In Brunwald, Eugene, et al., eds., *Harrison's Principles of Internal Medicine*, 11th ed. New York: McGraw-Hill Book Co., 1987, pp. 285-296.

20. ———. Prevention and treatment of genetic disorders. Ibid., pp. 324-328.

21. Griffin, James E., and Wilson, Jean D. Disorders of the testis. In Braunwald, Eugene, et al., eds., *Harrison's Principles of Internal Medicine*, 11th ed. New York: McGraw-Hill Book Co., 1987, pp. 1807-1818.

22. Grunfeld, Carl. Pancreatic islet cell tumors. In Wyngaarden, James B., and Smith, Lloyd H., Jr., eds., *Cecil's Textbook of Medicine*, 18th ed., vol. 2. Philadelphia: W.B. Saunders Co., 1988, pp. 1387-1390.

23. Hamerton, John L. Chromosomes and their disorders. In Wyngaarden, James B., and Smith, Lloyd H., Jr., eds., *Cecil's Textbook of Medicine*, 18th ed., vol. 1. Philadelphia: W.B. Saunders Co., 1988, pp. 161-169.

24. Holmes, Edward W. Xanthuria. In Wyngaarden, James B., and Smith, Lloyd H., Jr., eds., *Cecil's Textbook of Medicine*, 18th ed., vol. 1. Philadelphia: W.B. Saunders Co., 1988, pp. 1170-1173.

25. Holmes, Lewis B. Congenital malformations. In Wyngaarden, James B., and Smith, Lloyd H., Jr., eds., *Cecil's Textbook of Medicine*, 18th ed., vol. 1. Philadelphia: W.B. Saunders Co., 1988, pp. 169-171.

26. Howell, R. Rodney. The glycogen storage diseases. In Wyngaarden, James B., and Smith, Lloyd H., Jr., eds., *Cecil's Textbook of Medicine*, 18th ed., vol. 1. Philadelphia: W.B. Saunders Co., 1988, pp. 1133-1135.

27. Imperato-McGinley, Julianne. Disorders of sexual differentiation. In Wyngaarden, James B., and Smith, Lloyd H., Jr., eds., *Cecil's Textbook of Medicine*, 18th ed., vol. 1. Philadelphia: W.B. Saunders Co., 1988, pp. 1380-1404.

28. Isselbacher, Kurt J. Galactosemia, galactokinase deficiency, and other rare disorders of carbohydrate metabolism. In Braunwald, Eugene, et al., eds., *Harrison's Principles of Internal Medicine*, 11th ed. New York: McGraw-Hill Book Co., 1987, pp. 1649-1650.

29. Isselbacher, Kurt J., and Podolsky, Daniel K. Infiltrative and metabolic diseases affecting the liver. In Braunwald, Eugene, et al., eds., *Harrison's Principles of Internal Medicine*, 11th ed. New York: McGraw-Hill Book Co., 1987, pp. 1353-1356.

30. Jeffrey, Stefanie S., and Clark, Orlo H. The pituitary and adrenal glands. In Sabiston, David C., Jr., ed., *Essentials of Surgery*, Philadelphia: W.B. Saunders Co., 1987, pp. 350-362.

31. Karam, John H. Diabetes mellitus, hypoglycemia, & lipoprotein disorders. In Schroeder, Steven A., Krupp, Marcus A., and Tierney, Lawrence M., Jr., eds., *Current Medical Diagnosis & Treatment—1988*, Norwalk, CT: Appleton & Lange, 1988, pp. 749-783.

32. Kelly, William N., and Patella, Thomas D. Gout and other disorders of purine metabolism. In Braunwald, Eugene, et al., eds., *Harrison's Principles of Internal Medicine*, 11th ed. New York: McGraw-Hill Book Co., 1987, pp. 1623-1632.

33. Klodny, Edwin H. Gaucher's disease. In Wyngaarden, James B., and Smith, Lloyd H., Jr., eds., *Cecil's Textbook of Medicine*, 18th ed., vol. 1. Philadelphia: W.B. Saunders Co., 1988, pp. 1145-1147.

34. Kosek, Margaret S. Medical genetics. In Schroeder, Steven A., Krupp, Marcus A., and Tierney, Lawrence M., Jr., eds., *Current Medical Diagnosis & Treatment—1988*, Norwalk, CT: Appleton & Lange, 1988, pp. 1035-1059.

35. Larsen, P. Reed. The thyroid. In Wyngaarden, James B., and Smith, Lloyd H., Jr., eds., *Cecil's Textbook of Medicine*, 18th ed., vol. 2. Philadelphia: W.B. Saunders Co., 1988, pp. 1315-1340.

36. Levinsky, Norman G. Acidosis and alkalosis. In Brunwald, Eugene, et al., eds., *Harrison's Principles of Internal Medicine*, 11th ed. New York: McGraw-Hill Book Co., 1987, pp. 208-214.

37. Loeb, John N. Polyglandular disorders. In Wyngaarden, James B., and Smith, Lloyd H., Jr., eds., *Cecil's Textbook of Medicine*, 18th ed., vol. 2. Philadelphia: W.B. Saunders Co., 1988, pp. 1458-1461.

38. Loriaux, D. Lynn. Hirsutism. In Wyngaarden, James B., and Smith, Lloyd H., Jr., eds., *Cecil's Textbook of Medicine*, 18th ed., vol. 2. Philadelphia: W.B. Saunders Co., 1988, pp. 1446-1448.

39. Matsumoto, Alvin M. The testis. In Wyngaarden, James B., and Smith, Lloyd H., Jr., eds., *Cecil's Textbook of Medicine*, 18th ed., vol. 2. Philadelphia: W.B. Saunders Co., 1988, pp. 1404-1421.

40. New, Maria L. HLA and adrenal disease. In Farid, Nadir, R., ed., *Immunogenetics of Endocrine Disorders*, New York: Alan R. Liss, Inc., 1988, pp. 309-344.

41. Oates, John A., and Roberts, L. Jackson, II. Carcinoid syndrome. In Braunwald, Eugene, et al., eds., *Harrison's Principles of Internal Medicine*, 11th ed. New York: McGraw-Hill Book Co., 1987, pp. 1585-1588.

42. Olefsky, Jerrold M. Diabetes mellitus. In Wyngaarden, James B., and Smith, Lloyd H., Jr., eds., *Cecil's Textbook of Medicine*, 18th ed., vol. 2. Philadelphia: W.B. Saunders Co., 1988, pp. 1360-1381.

43. Oparil, Suzanne. Arterial hypertension. In Wyngaarden, James B., and Smith, Lloyd H., Jr., eds., *Cecil's Textbook of Medicine*, 18th ed., vol. 1. Philadelphia: W.B. Saunders Co., 1988, pp. 276-293.

44. Parker, Frank. Skin diseases. In Wyngaarden, James B., and Smith, Lloyd H., Jr., eds., *Cecil's Textbook of Medicine*, 18th ed., vol. 2. Philadelphia: W.B. Saunders Co., 1988, pp. 2300-2353.

45. Pi-Sunyer, F. Xavier. Obesity. In Wyngaarden, James B., and Smith, Lloyd H., Jr., eds., *Cecil's Textbook of Medicine*, 18th ed., vol. 2. Philadelphia: W.B. Saunders Co., 1988, pp. 1219-1228.

46. Posner, Jerome B. Disorders of sensation. In Wyngaarden, James B., and Smith, Lloyd H., Jr., eds., *Cecil's Textbook of Medicine*, 18th ed., vol. 2. Philadelphia: W.B. Saunders Co., 1988, pp. 2128-2137.

47. Rieve, Thomas S. Surgery for hyperthyroidism. In Tompkins, Ronald K., ed.-in-chief, *Advances in Surgery*, vol. 21. Chicago: Year Book Medical Publishers, Inc., 1987, pp. 29-47.

48. Rosenberg, Leon E. Inherited disorders of amino acid metabolism. In Braunwald, Eugene, et al., eds., *Harrison's Principles of Internal Medicine*, 11th ed. New York: McGraw-Hill Book Co., 1987, pp. 1611-1616.

49. Schimke, R. Neal. Disorders affecting multiple endocrine systems. In Braunwald, Eu-

gene, et al., eds., *Harrison's Principles of Internal Medicine*, 11th ed. New York: McGraw-Hill Book Co., 1987, pp. 1853-1856.

50. Scriver, Charles R. Hyperaminoaciduria (with a classification of the inborn and developmental errors of amino acid metabolism). In Wyngaarden, James B., and Smith, Lloyd H., Jr., eds., *Cecil's Textbook of Medicine*, 18th ed., vol. 1. Philadelphia: W.B. Saunders Co., 1988, pp. 1149-1155.

51. Segal, Stanton. Galactosemia. In Wyngaarden, James B., and Smith, Lloyd H., Jr., eds., *Cecil's Textbook of Medicine*, 18th ed., vol. 1. Philadelphia: W.B. Saunders Co., 1988, pp. 1131-1133.

52. Service, F. John. Hypoglycemic disorders. In Wyngaarden, James B., and Smith, Lloyd H., Jr., eds., *Cecil's Textbook of Medicine*, 18th ed., vol. 2. Philadelphia: W.B. Saunders Co., 1988, pp. 1381-1387.

53. Sites, Daniel P. Diseases of the thymus. In Wyngaarden, James B., and Smith, Lloyd H., Jr., eds., *Cecil's Textbook of Medicine*, 18th ed., vol. 2. Philadelphia: W.B. Saunders Co., 1988, pp. 1974-1976.

54. Smith, Lloyd H., Jr. The hyperphenylalaninemias. In Wyngaarden, James B., and Smith, Lloyd H., Jr., eds., *Cecil's Textbook of Medicine*, 18th ed., vol. 2. Philadelphia: W.B. Saunders Co., 1988, pp. 1155-1157.

55. Spence, Alexander P., and Mason, Elliott B. The endocrine system. In *Human Anatomy and Physiology*, 3rd ed. Menlo Park, CA: The Benjamin/Cummings Publishing Co., 1987, pp. 473-504.

56. ———. The digestive system: anatomy and mechanical processes. Ibid., pp. 683-713.

57. ———. The digestive system: chemical digestion and absorption. Ibid., pp. 715-731.

58. Thompson, Norman W., and Gough, Ian R. The parathyroid glands. In Sabiston, David C., Jr., ed., *Essentials of Surgery*, Philadelphia: W.B. Saunders Co., 1987, pp. 340-349.

59. Tyrell, J. Blake, and Baxter, John D. Disorders of the adrenal cortex. In Wyngaarden, James B., and Smith, Lloyd H., Jr., eds., *Cecil's Textbook of Medicine*, 18th ed., vol. 2. Philadelphia: W.B. Saunders Co., 1988, pp. 1340-1360.

60. Volk, Sr. Leo Rita, M in Mt. Personal communications.

61. Williams, Gordon H., and Dluhy, Robert G. Diseases of the adrenal cortex. In Braunwald, Eugene, et al., eds., *Harrison's Principles of Internal Medicine*, 11th ed. New York: McGraw-Hill Book Co., 1987, pp. 1753-1774.

62. Wilson, Jean D., and Griffin, James E., III. Disorders of sexual differentiation. In Braunwald, Eugene, et al., eds., *Harrison's Principles of Internal Medicine*, 11th ed. New York: McGraw-Hill Book Co., 1987, pp. 1840-1853.

63. Wyngaarden, James B. Human heredity. In Wyngaarden, James B., and Smith, Lloyd H., Jr., eds., *Cecil's Textbook of Medicine*, 18th ed., vol. 1. Philadelphia: W.B. Saunders Co., 1988, pp. 146-152.

64. ———. Inborn errors of metabolism. Ibid., vol. 1. pp. 152-158.

65. ———. Gout. Ibid., vol. 1., pp. 1161-1170.

Disorders Pertaining to the Sense Organ of Vision

Eye

Origin of Terms

cornea (L)—horny
crystal (G)—clear ice
cyclo- (G)—circle
cysto- (G)—sac
enucleate (L)—to remove kernel
iris (G)—rainbow, halo
kerato- (G)—horny, cornea

nystagmus (G)—nod
oculo- (L)—eye
ophthalmo- (G)—eye
phaco-, phako- (G)—lens
pyo- (G)—pus
vitreous (L)—glassy
zonule (L)—tiny band

Anatomic Terms (Ref. 70)

- *bulb of the eye* (see Fig. 69)—the globe or eyeball.
- *chambers of the eye:*
  - *—anterior chamber*—space in front of the iris and back of the cornea.
  - *—posterior chamber*—space in back of the iris and in front of the lens.
- *coats of the eye:*
  - *—cornea*—anterior transparent part of the outer tunic of the eye. The sclera is the posterior opaque part of the outer tunic. It is composed of dense fibrous tissue that has a protective function.
  - *—retina*—innermost tunic that perceives and transmits the sensory impulses of light to the optic nerve.
  - *—uvea, uveal tract*—intermediate vascular tunic composed of the:
    - *–choroid*—contains a layer of blood vessels and provides nutrition for part of the retina, lens, and vitreous.
    - *–ciliary body*—thickened part of the vascular tunic of the eye. Its circularly arranged processes secrete aqueous humor. The ciliary muscle helps to regulate the shape of the lens.
    - *–iris*—anterior highly pigmented part of the uvea. The pupil is an opening in the center of the iris. Its size is controlled by a sphincter muscle and dilator muscle.
- *ciliary zonule*—suspensory ligament of the lens attaching the ciliary body and contiguous retina to the lens capsule.

Figure 69 Horizontal section of eyeball through optic nerve.

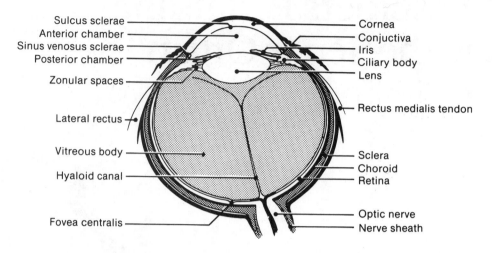

- *fovea*—small depression in the macula adapted for most acute vision.
- *fundus oculi*—inner posterior portion of the eye, which can be seen with an ophthalmoscope.
- *lens, crystalline lens*—transparent, biconvex body enclosed in a capsule and lying directly in back of the iris. It is a powerful refracting component of the visual system and focusing structure capable of changing its shape.
- *macula lutea*—small avascular area of the retina around the fovea.
- *orbit*—bony cavity of the skull in which lies the eyeball.
- *pars plana*—thin, flat layer of ciliary vessels and muscle covered by ciliary epithelium.
- *trabeculae (sing. trabecula)*—loosely arranged grayish white fibrous strands in the filtration angle of the anterior chamber through which the aqueous escapes.
- *vitreous body*—jellylike, transparent mass that occupies the space behind the lens and is normally in contact with the retina.

Diagnostic Terms

- *disorders of the cornea and sclera:*
  - —*arcus senilis*—degenerative change in the cornea commonly occurring in persons past age 50 and appearing as a grayish white ring about two millimeters wide. (48)
  - —*corneal dystrophy*—idiopathic degeneration of the cornea that may seriously interfere with vision. (48)
  - —*corneal injury*—damage to cornea by foreign body; chemical, thermal, or radiation burn; laceration; or penetrating wound, frequently accompanied by intraocular damage, such as traumatic cataract and iris prolapse. (48, 62)
  - —*corneal ulcer*—form of keratitis due to a pathogenic organism entering the corneal epithelium. The stroma may also break down. (48, 62)
  - —*dermoid*—skinlike tumor or cyst generally located at the limbus and involving both cornea and sclera. (12)
  - —*hypopyon*—pus in anterior chamber in back of cornea; sometimes associated with corneal ulcer. (12)
  - —*keratitis*—inflammation of the cornea. (48)
    - —*actinic keratitis, ultraviolet keratitis*—ultraviolet burns caused by strong sunlight

when skiing (snow blindness) or exposure to a welding arc resulting in extreme eye pain and photophobia 24 hours later. (48)

—*deep keratitis*—invasion of the deep layers of the cornea that may result in its perforation. Interstitial keratitis due to syphilis or tuberculosis may cause permanent opacification (loss of transparency) of the cornea. (48, 62)

—*herpes simplex keratitis*—corneal ulcer caused by herpes simplex virus (HSV). Primary infection by herpes simplex type I often causes undiagnosed localized ocular lesions in children, which may be accompanied by regional lymphadenopathy, infection, and fever. Herpes simplex type II often produces infection in the cornea and retina. When a high rate of recurrence at one site initiates secondary herpes infection, the condition is referred to as "reactivation disease." Reactivation disease presents as a severe inflammatory reaction and ulceration but fever and lymphadenopathy are not present. (20, 48, 62)

—*superficial keratitis*—inflammatory reaction of a loss of corneal epithelium and ulcer formation due to infection. (48, 62)

—*keratoconus*—conical bulging of the center of the cornea. (48, 62)

—*scars of cornea:*

—*leukoma*—white, opaque cornea.

—*macula*—opaque spot seen on cornea.

—*nebula*—grayish opacity of cornea. (48)

—*scleral injuries*—cause of scleral damage may include penetrating or blunt trauma, thermal burns, irradiation, chemical burns, and scleral lacerations. (63)

—*scleritis*—inflammation of the sclera. (12, 49, 63)

■ *disorders of the uveal tract:*

—*choroidal hemorrhage*—local bleeding of choroid that may be associated with vascular disorder, trauma, choroiditis, diabetes, or other diseases. (20)

—*iridocyclitis*—inflammation of the iris and ciliary body. (12)

—*iridodialysis*—detachment of outer margin of the iris from ciliary body. (51)

—*iritis*—inflammation of the iris.

—*sympathetic ophthalmia*—inflammation of uveal tract, following perforating wound of opposite eye, with incarceration or loss of uveal tissue. (20, 60)

—*synechia*—two kinds:

—*anterior synechia*—adhesion of the iris to the cornea.

—*posterior synechia*—adhesion of the iris to the lens. (20, 40)

—*tumors of the uveal tract*—intraocular tumors of the choroid, iris, or ciliary body.

—*nevi (sing. nevus), benign melanomas*—pigmental lesions that usually do not interfere with vision. (12, 20)

—*malignant melanomas*—pigmented cancerous lesions, usually unilateral, which lead to loss of vision and occur in the fifth or sixth decade of life. (12, 20)

—*uveitis*—inflammation of the uveal tract caused by:

—*allergy*

—organisms such as *Coccidioides immitis, Histoplasma capsulatum, Mycobacterium tuberculosis,* and *Toxoplasma gondii*

—*irritants and toxins*

—*connective tissue diseases* (12, 20, 60)

■ *disorders of the vitreous:*

—*vitreoretinal degeneration, Wagner's disease*—hereditary disorder of vitreous and retina characterized by marked liquefaction of central vitreous, reduced vision, vitreous floaters, and vitreous traction on retina, resulting in retinal tears and breaks leading to retinal detachment. (52)

—*vitreous detachment*—vitreous detached from retina in one or both eyes. It may lead to retinal tear. (20, 52)

—*vitreous hemorrhage*—rare but serious disorder, usually caused by rupture of a retinal vessel and followed by sudden loss of vision. (52)

—*vitreous infections*—bacterial, fungal, or parasitic infections resulting in liquefaction, opacification, and shrinkage of vitreous. (52)

- *disorders of the lens and intraocular pressure:*

  —*aphakia*—absence of the lens, congenital or acquired, due to surgical removal; binocular or monocular in both eyes or in one eye. (50)

  —*cataract*—an opacity in the lens, congenital or acquired. Lenticular opacity is usually linked with the process of aging. Insoluble proteins form in the lens and eventually lead to dehydration, lowered metabolism, and tissue necrosis. In the cataractous lens, sodium and calcium content tend to be increased, with potassium, protein, and ascorbic acid content decreased. Visual impairment is slowly progressive. (50)

  —*ectopia lentis*—displacement of the lens, seen primarily in Marfan's syndrome in its congenital form. It also may result from trauma. (50)

  —*glaucoma*—increased intraocular pressure; untreated, it leads to blindness. Some types of glaucoma are:

  —*acute glaucoma*—severe obstruction of aqueous humor drainage, sharp rise of intraocular tension, agonizing eye pain, dilated pupil, steamy cornea, and ciliary injection. (51)

  —*chronic glaucoma:*

    closed-angle glaucoma—intermittent attacks of angle closure of anterior chamber, formation of adhesions in angle with attacks, and gradual obliteration of angle, requiring peripheral iridectomy if unresponsive to medical therapy. (12, 50)

    open-angle glaucoma—interference with aqueous outflow, creating an elevated intraocular pressure. The open type is bilateral and, if untreated, leads slowly to visual impairment and cupping of optic disk. (12, 51, 60, 65)

  —*malignant glaucoma*—distinct type of angle closure with a forward movement of the lens and direct closure of the angle, occurring with or without glaucoma surgery. (34, 51, 65)

- *disorders of the retina:*

  —*atrophy and degeneration of retina*—a reduction of visual acuity due to degenerative processes seen in the elderly. (13)

  —*Coats' disease*—eye condition characterized by abnormalities of the retinal vasculature, retinal microaneurysms in areas of destruction of small vessels, retinal hemorrhage, and exudation. (13)

  —*edema of the retina*—condition due to active hyperemia, generally resulting from trauma. (13, 64)

  —*diabetic retinopathy*—condition characterized by pinpoint aneurysms, which may be caused by dilatation of the retinal capillaries in diabetes mellitus. (12, 13, 20, 64)

  —*hypertensive retinopathy*—retinal changes resulting from persistently high diastolic blood pressure. This condition may occur in essential hypertension, renal arteriolar sclerosis, glomerulonephritis, and toxemias of pregnancy. (13, 20, 60)

  —*macular degenerations*—group of degenerative disorders of the retina.

    —*circinate degeneration*—rather common macular retinopathy, seen in the elderly. It is usually bilateral and characterized by a girdle of yellow-white spots surrounding the macular area. The peripheral vision may be retained, but the central vision is lost. (13, 20)

—*cystic degeneration of macula*—sharply delineated red, round cystic defect in the macula. The wall of the fluid-filled cyst may rupture, and a macular hole may result. If the fovea is involved, central vision is blurred. (13)

—*disciform macular degeneration, Kuhnt-Junius disease*—dark, dome-shaped elevation in the macular area apparently containing extravasated blood from a retinal hemorrhage. Central vision is impaired or lost. (13)

—*retinoschisis*—separation of the sensory retina into two layers appearing as a shallow elevation of the peripheral retina. Defect may not be progressive, but vision in the involved area is affected. (13, 20)

—*occlusion of central retinal artery*—rare unilateral disorder due to thrombus, embolus, or atheromatous plaque suddenly causing total loss of sight in the affected eye. It may occur in advanced age or during oral contraceptive therapy. (12, 13, 20, 64)

—*occlusion of central retinal vein*—thrombosis of the central retinal vein leading to sudden, painless loss of sight. (12, 13, 20, 64)

—*retinal arteriolar sclerosis*—form of sclerosis due to hypertension characterized by copper-wire arterioles in the retina. In the advanced stage of sclerotic process the arterioles resemble silver wire. (13, 20)

—*retinal atherosclerosis*—obstructive changes in retinal vessels, which may cause a sudden vascular accident in the retina. (13, 20)

—*retinal detachment*—separation of the retina from the choroid. When the retina is torn, vitreous can pass through the tear and behind the sensory retina. The condition joined with vitreous traction and pull of gravity results in progressive detachment. This disorder may result in blindness, if not relieved.

Note: The term "*rhegmatogenous*" retinal detachment designates those detachments due to a retinal hole or tear. The Greek word, "*Rhegma,*" means a break in continuity. Two basic types of retinal detachment are termed "rhegmatogenous" and "nonrhegmatogenous." Nonrhegmatogenous retinal detachment (without tear or hole) presents in tumors of the choroid, retinal vascular lesions, vitreous traction from proliferative retinopathy. Rhegmatogenous retinal detachment may be further delineated as to location, e.g.:

—*equatorial*—near the equator or may occur behind the equator.

—*macular*—at the fovea.

—*oral*—within the vitreous base or may occur between the posterior border of the vitreous base and the equator. (13, 20, 60, 64)

—*retinal hemorrhage*—moderate or massive bleeding from the retina. (13)

—*retinal tears*—small holes or tears; unrepaired, they may enlarge and lead to retinal detachment and blindness. (13)

—*retinitis pigmentosa*—hereditary degenerative disease principally affecting the rod and cone layer of the retina. Ophthalmologic examination reveals spider-shaped pigment spots on the retina. Night blindness is the dominant feature. (13, 20, 64)

—*retrolental fibroplasia*—bilateral, retinal disease in premature infants associated with high oxygen concentration in the infant's environment. (13, 20, 64)

—*von Hippel-Lindau disease*—retinal angioma usually associated with cerebellar angioma and polycystic kidneys. (13)

■ *disorders of the optic nerve:*

—*optic atrophy*—destruction of the fibers of the optic nerve associated with loss of visual acuity. (12, 53)

—*optic coloboma*—congenital defect in the optic nerve resulting from imperfect closure of fetal cleft. Defects in the choroid and retina may coexist. Visual impairment is common. (53)

—*optic neuritis*—inflammation of the optic nerve; may involve the sheaths of the nerve (optic perineuritis) or its main body. (53)

—*papilledema, choked disk*—edema of the papilla or optic nerve head usually caused by increased intracranial pressure. (12, 20, 53)

—*papillitis*—inflammation of the papilla or head of the optic nerve. (53)

—*retrobulbar neuritis*—optic neuritis in which nerve involvement occurs behind the optic disk and cannot be seen ophthalmoscopically. Visual acuity is seriously affected or entirely lost. One of its most common causes is multiple sclerosis. (53)

- *ocular infections:*

—*endophthalmitis*—intraocular infection due to various etiologic agents. Early treatment may salvage the eye. (12)

—*panophthalmitis*—extensive ocular infection, usually resulting from eye injury and leading to corneal ulceration and total destruction of the eyeball.

- *ocular tumors:*

—*melanomas of choroid or iris*—malignant neoplasms derived from cells that form melanin, a black pigment. (12, 20)

—*optic nerve tumors:*

–*gliomas*—glial tumors, which may be derived from astrocytes of the optic nerve and are either solitary tumors or occur in von Recklinghausen's neurofibromatosis. (12, 53)

–*meningiomas*—usually orbital tumors arising in the sheath of the optic nerve. (12, 53)

—*retinoblastomas*—malignant tumors arising from the retina. They are hereditary, unilateral or bilateral, and readily metastasize to the optic nerve and brain. Other common tumors are hemangiomas and orbital lymphomas. (12, 20)

Operative Terms

- *cataract operations*—various procedures for the removal of an opaque lens.

—*anterior chamber lens implantation*—preparation of a 7.5 mm trephine opening followed by removal of cataract and insertion of anterior chamber lens through the trephine opening. Following an intraocular cataract extraction or as a secondary procedure, an anterior chamber type of lens is employed, while a posterior chamber type of lens is used after an extracapsular cataract extraction. (22, 44, 54)

—*posterior chamber lens implantation*—After an injection of sodium hyaluronate (Healon), an anterior capsulotomy is performed. The nucleus may be removed with an irrigating vectis technique followed by removal of the cortex. Additional Healon may be injected and the posterior lens implant inserted. Healon may be removed by aspiration. (2, 29, 44, 54, 56)

—*aspiration and irrigation procedure*—removal of a cataract by suction through a small limbal incision and simultaneous irrigation of the anterior chamber with normal saline solution through another limbal incision. The effective use of the operating microscope virtually permits aspiration of the entire opaque lens. Discission of the posterior capsule completes the procedure, which is used for patients under age 30. (8)

—*cryoextraction of cataract*—application of the tip of the cryoextractor to the anterior surface of the lens until the cataract firmly adheres to the instrument. When the freezing process has extended for two to three millimeters into the lens substance, the probe—with the lens frozen to it—is lifted out. (8)

—*enzymatic zonulysis, zonulolysis*—instillation of alpha-chymotrypsin, a fibrinolytic enzyme, into the anterior chamber to dissolve the ciliary zonules and thus facilitate the removal of the cataractous lens. The procedure is used in persons 20 to 50 years of age, who have tough zonules, making cataract extraction difficult. (8)

—*extracapsular cataract extraction*—incision into anterior capsule to express the opaque nucleus of the lens and some of the cortical material. (29, 44, 56)

—*intracapsular cataract extraction*—removal of entire lens in its capsule; a method of choice, especially for senescent (senile) cataracts. (44)

—*intraocular lens implantation*—removal of cataract and insertion of plastic lens, such as:

 —Binkhorst two-loop or four-loop lens

 —Choyce anterior chamber lens

 —Shearing posterior chamber lens

 —Sputnik or Fyodorow type II lens (1, 3, 16, 44)

—*pars plana lensectomy*—lens removal by:

 —irrigation with balanced salt solution.

 —ultrasonic fragmentation with Girard ultrasonic fragmentor.

 —aspiration through minute pars plana incisions. The technique is recommended for congenital and senescent (senile) cataracts, dislocated and traumatic cataracts, and other types. (8)

—*phacoemulsification, Kelman technique*—cataract removal by inserting a phacoemulsifier through a two- to three-millimeter incision and breaking up the sclerotic portion of the lens by ultrasonic vibration, followed by aspiration of the lens fragments and irrigation of the eye. (18, 44, 52)

—*phacoprosthesis*—usually referred to as intraocular lens, a less correct term, since the intraocular lens is either natural or artificial. (1, 3)

- *corneal operations:*

—*epikeratophakia*—form of corneal refractive surgery that alters the anterior surface of the patient's cornea by the addition of a precarved lenticule of donor corneal tissue. The procedure has been used to facilitate the treatment of amblyopia, aphakia, and keratoconus. Recently, epikeratophakia using commercially prepared tissue is another alternative technique that may be employed by the surgeon in this procedure. (5, 28, 62, 67)

—*keratocentesis*—puncture of the cornea.

—*keratoplasty, corneal graft, corneal transplant*—surgical replacement of a section of an opaque cornea with normal, transparent cornea to restore vision.

 —*lamellar keratoplasty*—using partial-thickness corneal transplant.

 —*penetrating keratoplasty*—using full-thickness corneal transplant. (42, 43, 45, 55)

—*radial keratotomy*—surgical procedure that aims at creating a given number of linear radial incisions at a prescribed depth through the corneal epithelium and stroma, while preserving an adequate clear central optical zone. (5, 11, 47)

—*thermokeratoplasty*—procedure based on proper application of heat to shrink corneal collagen and thus prevent corneal scarring. A well-controlled temperature probe flattens the keratoconus and makes the cornea more spherical. This operation is not indicated when scarring has already developed or when the cornea is very thin. (11)

- *enucleation*—removal of the eyeball, indicated in penetrating injuries, malignant tumors of the eye, and as an emergency measure in threatened sympathetic ophthalmia. (12, 58)

- *evisceration*—removal of contents of eyeball but leaving the sclera and cornea.

- *glaucoma operations*—surgical procedures for highly increased intraocular pressure, irreducible by miotics or other medical treatment.
  - *cyclocryosurgery*—direct application of the cryoprobe to the conjunctiva over different locations in back of the limbus. The intense vascular response reduces ciliary body function and aqueous production. No incision is necessary. (12, 64)
  - *cyclodialysis*—filtering procedure allowing aqueous to drain into the suprachoroidal space to lower intraocular tension. (8)
  - *iridencleisis*—filtering technique permitting aqueous to escape into the space below the conjunctiva, where it is reabsorbed by the circulating blood and diffused into the tear film. (65)
  - *goniotomy*—incision across the anterior chamber for establishing normal aqueous outflow through regular channels in congenital and infantile glaucoma. (64, 67)
  - *microsurgery in glaucoma*—use of the operating microscope to facilitate direct surgery on Schlemm's canal and trabecular meshwork in treating glaucoma. (65)
  - *Argon laser trabeculoplasty*—procedure whereby laser energy is directed through a goniolens to burn the trabecular meshwork. This produces blanching or fine bubble formation, thereby causing a purse-string type of contraction in the trabecular meshwork, and the outflow mechanism opens to facilitate the emergence of aqueous humor. This procedure achieves a clinically significant decrease in intraocular pressure. (21, 24, 37, 41, 65)
  - *trabeculectomy*—elevation of a conjunctival flap to expose the sclera at the limbus and excision of a scleral portion, including the trabecular meshwork. The appearance of a filtering bleb achieves ocular pressure control. Trabeculectomies have been successfully performed in adult phakic eyes with open-angle glaucoma. (8, 21, 40, 41, 65)
  - *trabeculotomy*—surgical fashioning of a scleral flap, meticulous dissection to locate Schlemm's canal, and insertion of a small probe into the canal and anterior chamber to relieve block to aqueous outflow, which is usually present in the trabecular meshwork. (21, 65)
  - *laser iridectomy*—application of the argon laser to penetrate the iris, producing thermal destruction with removal of a portion of the iris. Application of the neodymium YAG laser in this procedure produces mechanical disruption and explosion of tissue in contrast to the thermal lesion produced by the argon laser. (10)
  - *peripheral iridectomy*—raising a small conjunctival flap at the limbus and entering the anterior chamber through a four-millimeter incision to prevent pupillary block. This technique frees the filtration angle from the iris root and permits the aqueous to escape by the normal channel. (58)
  - *thermal sclerostomy, Scheie's operation*—filtering procedure for severe glaucoma. Anterior chamber is entered through limbal incision and posterior portion of incision is cauterized, resulting in tissue shrinkage. This is followed by a peripheral iridectomy, repositioning of conjunctival flap at the limbus, and wound closure. The use of the operating microscope is optional. (8)

Some types of laser tissue interaction are:
  - *photoablation*—tissue removal by a high-powered pulsed ultraviolet laser radiation. (54)
  - *photocoagulation*—use of light of appropriate intensity and wavelength at a given distance to cause coagulation of tissue. (59)

- *photodisruption*—application of high-powered laser pulse to achieve optical breakdown, plasma formation, and subsequent shock wave, which mechanically disrupts the tissue. (59)
- *argon laser beam*—blue-green light that is effectively absorbed by red hemoglobin choroid and pigment epithelium and that has been used with success in the treatment of diabetic retinopathy and tried in senescent (senile) macular degeneration. (24, 64)
- *xenon arc beam*—emission of a white light that includes all wavelengths in the visible spectrum and may be used in most ocular diseases and lesions for which argon laser is recommended. (8)
- *YAG laser*—yttrium, aluminum, and garnet (YAG) are the ingredients that form the crystal through which the laser's light is focused. It is absorbed by the body tissue, allowing for deep penetration of laser energy. Vessels up to four or five mm can be safely sealed. The YAG laser is particularly useful in cases following cataract extraction where the posterior membrane of the eye clouds over the pupil. Previously, this condition was treated by slitting the membrane with a scalpel. The YAG laser shatters the membrane with a shock wave effect and any subatomic debris caused by the YAG's shock wave is carried away through water in the eye. Unlike other lasers, which work by burning tiny pieces of tissue, the YAG laser tears tissue by delivering a great amount of energy in a very small amount of time. (10, 23, 44)
- *repair of retinal holes or tears and retinal detachment*—surgical reattachment of minor or major separations of the retina from the choroid. This can be accomplished by:
  - *cryopexy of sclera*—application of a supercooled probe to the sclera to produce a chorioretinal scar with minimal damage to the sclera.
  - *laser photocoagulation*—procedure for mending small retinal tears. A laser beam is directed through the dilated pupil to produce a chorioretinal inflammatory reaction that seals the small tear. (59, 64)
  - *retinopexy, pneumatic*—procedure whereby small superior retinal breaks or rents are treated with cryotherapy, intravitreal gas injection, and patient positioning. Pneumatic retinopexy provides an alternative technique to scleral buckling for the treatment of selected cases of retinal detachment. (8)
  - *scleral buckling operation*—removal of strip of sclera near the retinal separation, drainage of subretinal fluid, placement of implant, and tightening of sutures around the implant to buckle the sclera. (30, 36, 64)
- *vitrectomy, subtotal*—partial removal of the vitreous for vitreous opacity in severe retinopathy with vitreous hemorrhage or for the control of fibrotic overgrowth in severe intraocular trauma. Vitreous surgery is rare and preferably performed with the operating microscope and slit illumination. (7, 36, 46, 64)

Symptomatic Terms

- *amaurosis fugax*—fleeting blindness manifested by transient monocular blindness. It may result from transient embolization of retinal arterioles and suggest impending stroke. (4, 20, 61)
- *amblyopia*—dimness of vision in one eye that is normal on ophthalmoscopic examination. (4)
- *amblyopia ex anopsia*—diminished visual acuity in one eye not caused by organic eye disease. It is known as the "lazy eye."
- *ametropia*—optic defect or refractive error that does not permit parallel light rays to fall exactly on the retina. (69)
- *anisometropia*—inequality in refractive power of right and left eye. (9)

- *Argyll-Robertson pupil*—absence of light reflex without change in the contractile power of the pupil, a reliable sign of syphilis of the central nervous system. (4)
- *astigmatism*—images are warped and distorted because of irregular corneal curvature that prevents clear focusing of light. (69)
- *binocular blindness*—blindness in both eyes.
- *binocular vision*—ability to focus both eyes on one object and fuse the two images produced into one. (4)
- *color blindness*—reduced ability to distinguish between colors.
- *cystoid maculopathy, cystoid macular edema*—vascular abnormality that may develop after cataract extraction and reduces the vision at variable degrees (20/40 to 20/200). Fluorescein angiography reveals typical star-shaped staining of the macular area. (13)
- *diplopia*—double vision. (60)
- *Elschnig pearls*—clusters of transparent vacuoles, remnants of lenticular epithelium seen in the eye after incomplete cataract removal. (44)
- *emmetropia*—normal vision; no refractive error. (69)
- *enophthalmos*—recession of the eyeball into the orbit.
- *exophthalmos, exophthalmus*—protrusion of the eyeball in hyperthyroidism and orbital space-taking lesions. (60)
- *hypermetropia, hyperopia*—farsightedness; parallel rays of light from a distant object are focused behind the retina; a refractive error.
- *hyphemia*—blood in the anterior chamber in front of the iris.
- *iridodonesis*—a quivering of the iris when a person moves the eye is a common indication of lens dislocation and is caused by lack of lens support. This manifestation is characteristic of partially and completely dislocated lenses. (44)
- *leukokoria, white pupil*—white pupillary reflex referred to as amaurotic cat's eye, suggesting the presence of a sight-destroying condition such as a retinoblastoma, curable in its early phase. (12)
- *malignant exophthalmos, progressive proptosis*—increasing forward displacement of the eyeball in Graves' disease, causing severe ocular symptoms such as fullness of eyelids, lacrimation, epiphora, corneal ulcerations, chemosis, and edema of conjunctiva.
- *monocular blindness*—blindness in one eye. (4, 20, 60)
- *myopia*—nearsightedness; parallel rays from a distant object are focused in front of the retina; a refractive error. (13, 69)
- *nyctalopia*—night blindness. (13, 61)
- *nystagmus*—constant involuntary movement of the eyeballs. It may be caused by a disease of the central nervous system. (4)
- *photophobia*—marked intolerance to light. (60, 62)
- *presbyopia*—gradual loss of accommodation, a common condition in persons past middle age.
- *scotoma*—blind spot in the vision. (4, 61)
- *vitreous floaters*—dark opacities within the vitreous that are perceived as moving spots by the retina. (36, 52)
- *vitreous loss*—leakage of vitreous into the anterior chamber that disrupts the normal contact of the vitreous with the retina, exerts traction on the retina, and predisposes to the formation of retinal holes and tears. (36, 52)

Accessory Organs of Vision

Origin of Terms

blepharo- (G)—eyelid
canaliculus (L)—small canal
cantho- (G)—angle
dacryo- (G)—tear

dacryoaden- (G)—tear gland
dacryocyst- (G)—tear sac

oblique (L)—slanting
palpebra (L)—eyelid

Anatomic Terms (70)

- *canthus (pl. canthi)*—the lateral or medial angles at both ends of the palpebral fissures (slits between the eyelids).
- *cilia, eyelashes*—rows of hairs at the free margin of the eyelids.
- *conjunctiva (pl. conjunctivae)*—mucous membrane that lines the deep surface of the eyelid and is reflected over the front of the eyeball. It is divided into the:
  - *bulbar conjunctiva*—colorless, transparent portion covering the anterior part of the globe.
  - *palpebral conjunctiva*—lining of the posterior or deep surface of the lids.
- *fornix (pl. fornices) conjunctivae*—angle between the palpebral and bulbar conjunctivae.
- *lacrimal appartus:* (Fig. 70)
  - *lacrimal gland*—tear gland; its orbital part lies in the lacrimal fossa of the upper, outer part of the orbit; its palpebral part lies in the upper eyelid.
  - *lacrimal ducts*—tear ducts extending from the gland to superior conjunctival fornix.
  - *lacrimal canaliculi*—one canaliculus (canal) for each eyelid to conduct tears from lacrimal punctum to lacrimal sac.
  - *lacrimal puncta (sing. punctum)*—minute openings, the beginning of the canaliculi.
  - *lacrimal sac*—tear sac situated in lacrimal groove or medial wall of orbit.
  - *nasolacrimal duct*—duct-draining lacrimal sac and opening into inferior nasal meatus.
- *ocular muscles*—muscles controlling the movements of the eyeball.
  - *two oblique muscles (two obliqui).*
  - *four rectus muscles (four recti).*
- *palpebral fissure*—opening between the eyelids.
- *tarsal glands*—secretory follicles in the tarsal plate.
- *tarsal plate*—supporting connective tissue of the eyelid.

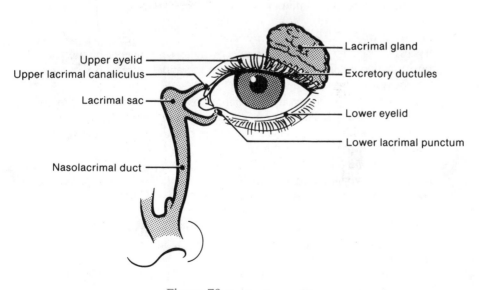

Figure 70 Lacrimal apparatus.

Diagnostic Terms

- *disorders of the eyelid:*
  - *blepharitis*—inflammation of the eyelid. (15, 57, 60)
  - *blepharoptosis*—drooping of the upper eyelid, congenital or acquired. (57)
  - *chalazion (pl. chalazia)*—true granuloma of the eye appearing as a painless swelling at the tarsus.
  - *distichiasis*—accessory row of lashes near or in the orifices of meibomian glands. (15)
  - *ectropion*—outward turning of the margin of the eyelid. (57, 60)
  - *entropion*—inward turning of the margin of the eyelid. (15, 57, 60)
  - *hordeolum (pl. hordeola)*
    - *external hordeolum*—pyogenic infection of a sebaceous gland at the margin of the lid.
    - *internal hordeolum*—purulent infection of a sebaceous gland embedded in the conjunctiva of the eyelid. (15, 57, 60)
  - *tumors of the lid*—congenital or acquired; dermoids, fibromas, hemangiomas, and carcinomas. (15, 60)
- *disorders of the conjunctiva:*
  - *allergic conjunctivitis*—chronic hypersensitivity reaction of the conjunctiva, frequently associated with hay fever. (12)
  - *bacterial conjunctivitis*—inflammation of the conjunctiva characterized by pain, edema, hyperemia, exudation, and infiltration. *Staphylococcus aureus, Streptococcus pneumoniae,* and Koch-Weeks and Morax-Axenfeld bacilli are common etiologic agents. (12, 60)
  - *chlamydial keratoconjunctivitis*—presents as:
    - *inclusion conjunctivitis*—venereal infection transmitted to the eyes by contact with genital secretions from a chlamydial urethritis in men or chlamydial cervicitis in women. (12, 60)
    - *neonatal inclusion conjunctivitis*—chlamydial infection of newborn contracted by passage through birth canal of infected mothers. Blenorrhea (inclusion conjunctivitis) develops within the first two weeks of life. (20)
    - *trachoma*—occurring endemically and a major cause of blindness, characterized by chronic inflammation of the follicular conjunctiva and followed by granulation, capillary infiltration of the cornea (pannus), and blindness. (20, 60)
  - *keratoconjunctivitis sicca (KCS), dry eye syndrome, Sjögren's syndrome*—ocular dryness caused by deficiency of one or more components of the tear film; mucin, aqueous, or liquid. This results in the appearance of dry spots on the conjunctival and corneal epithelium. (12, 57)
  - *ophthalmia neonatorum, gonococcal conjunctivitis of the newborn*—the conjunctival sac of the infant is filled with pus containing gonococci. (12, 20, 60)
  - *pterigium*—membrane of conjunctival tissue that extends like a wing from the limbus toward the center of the cornea. (20, 45, 60)
  - *viral conjunctivitis*—usually caused by adenovirus type 3 and marked by fever, malaise, pharyngitis, and glandular involvement. The palpebral conjunctiva looks red, and a copious watery discharge is present. (12, 20, 60)
- *disorders of the lacrimal apparatus:*
  - *acute dacryoadenitis*—unilateral or bilateral inflammation of the lacrimal gland. It is frequently seen in children as a complication of measles and parotitis (mumps). (57)
  - *chronic dacryoadenitis*—chronic, painless swelling of the lacrimal glands showing no signs of acute inflammation. (12, 57)

—*dacryocystitis*—acute or chronic inflammation of the lacrimal sac, usually due to nasolacrimal stenosis. (57, 60)

—*lacrimal abscess*—localized accumulation of pus in the lacrimal gland. (60)

■ *disorders of ocular motility:*

—*esotropia, convergent strabismus or squint*—common type of eye disorder, usually referred to as crossed eyes. The eyes are directed toward the medial line. (4, 9, 35)

—*exotropia, divergent strabismus or squint*—known as wall-eyes. The eyes are turned laterally (outward). (9)

—*hypertropia*—one eye deviated upward.

—*hypotropia*—one eye deviated downward. (9)

—*vergences*—disjunctive movements; the eyes move in opposite directions.

    –*convergence*—eyes turning inward.

    –*divergence*—eyes turning outward. (9, 35)

Operative Terms

■ *blepharectomy*—excision of an eyelid.

■ *blepharoplasty*—plastic repair of an eyelid. (15, 38, 39)

■ *blepharorrhaphy*—suture of a lacerated or injured eyelid.

■ *dacryoadenectomy*—removal of a lacrimal gland.

■ *dacryocystectomy*—removal of the lacrimal sac. (57)

■ *dacryocystorhinostomy*—surgical creation of an opening into the nose for the tears. (57, 66)

■ *Mohs' chemosurgery*—micrographic technique utilized to excise tumors of the skin. The tumor is fixed in place and a layer is removed. That portion is examined microscopically; this procedure is repeated until all of the tumor is removed. This technique gives the highest cure rate for both primary and recurrent eyelid tumors. (6)

■ *repair of strabismus:*

—*application of adjustable suture*—suture may be placed on the sclera at any point that will be accessible to the surgeon. The bow knot attached to the muscles may be adjusted as desired. i.e., tightened or loosened to change the eye position as necessary. However, eye alignment may not be permanent and further surgery may be necessary. (9)

—*Faden procedure*—technique whereby a new insertion site for the muscle is created far in the back of the eye by suturing the muscle to the sclera. This changes the functional insertion of a rectus muscle so that its vector force changes from a rotator to a retractor as the eye moves into the muscle's field of action. This procedure tends to weaken the muscle in its field of action. (9)

—*recession of ocular muscles*—technique to weaken muscles. The muscle is detached from the eye, separated from its facial attachments and allowed to retract. It is resewn to the eye a measured distance behind its original insertion site. (9)

—*resection of ocular muscles*—technique used to strengthen muscles. The muscle is detached from the eye and stretched longer by a measured amount and then resewn to the eye, usually at the original insertion site. Also, the muscle may be strengthened by tucking the tendon in graded amounts. (9)

—*tenotomy*—procedure of cutting through a tendon. For example, the superior oblique muscle weakening may be accomplished by cutting through the tendon.

—*transposition procedures*—techniques employed to move all or part of the extraocular muscles or tendons up or down or in any direction other than their natural line of action. The purpose of the procedure is to change the force generated by the muscle as well as the direction of that force. Transposition procedures are used to correct paresis and paralysis defects, torsional defects, and monocular concomitant hypertropia or hypotropia.

Examples of transposition procedures are:

–*Harda-Ito operation*—transfers the anterior half of the oblique tendon forward and laterally to increase the torsional effect of the superior oblique tendon.

–*Hummelsheim or Jensen procedure*—transfers a portion of the tendon or moves the tendon of the superior rectus and inferior rectus to the lateral rectus to correct paresis of the extraocular muscles in sixth cranial nerve palsy.* (14)

- *tarsorrhaphy*—surgical closure of an eyelid.

Symptomatic Terms

- *blepharedema*—puffy, swollen, edematous eyelids. (15)
- *chemosis*—conjunctival swelling near the cornea.
- *epiphora*—overflow of tears, often due to lacrimal duct obstruction. (57)
- *hyperemia*—congestion. (33)
- *lacrimation*—secretion of tears.
- *limbal damage*—injury at the corneoscleral junction that may be caused by the destruction of perilimbal blood supply, interfering with the nutrition of the cornea. (48)
- *pannus*—newly formed capillaries covering the cornea like a film. (48)
- *symblepharon*—adhesion between the palpebral and bulbar conjunctiva. (27)
- *xerophthalmia*—excessive dryness of the eye resulting from the destruction of mucin-producing goblet cells or lacrimal ducts and glands or from other causes. (12)

Special Procedures

Terms Related to Bacteriologic Studies

- *epithelial inclusion bodies*—bodies found in conjunctival disease, such as inclusion blennorrhea of the newborn, some adult forms of diffuse, follicular conjunctivitis, and in trachoma. Epithelial scrapings stained with Giemsa's or Wright's stain reveal the inclusion bodies. (60, 62)
- *epithelial scrapings from the cornea or conjunctiva*—procedure used for identifying the etiologic organism of bacterial conjunctivitis or keratitis. A thin layer of epithelial cells is removed with a spatula or scalpel. The scrapings are transferred to two or more slides and stained; one by Gram's method, the other with Giemsa's or Wright's stain. These methods permit the identification of the predominant organism, as well as eosinophils and epithelial inclusion bodies. Since pathogenic organisms are freely present in epithelial cells before they appear in secretions, the study of scrapings offers a valuable aid to early diagnosis. (60, 62)
- *etiologic organisms in conjunctival disease; those commonly seen include:*
    - *Diplococcus pneumoniae*
    - *Neisseria gonorrhoeae*
    - *Staphylococcus*
    - *Streptococcus*
    - *Chlamydia* (formerly virus of trachoma) (60, 62)

---

*Roger L. Hiatt. Transposition procedures in strabismus, *Annals of Ophthalmology,* 18:332-336, November, 1986. Reprinted with permission.

Terms Related Primarily to Functional Testing

- *accommodation*—ability to see at various distances due to the contraction and relaxation of the ciliary muscle. The focusing power is measurable. (44)
- *contact lenses*—small corneal lenses that fit directly on the eyeball under the eyelids, medically used to correct vision in keratoconus (cone-shaped cornea) and other eye conditions. (69)
- *corneal sensitivity*—the examiner touches the corneas with a cotton fiber to determine whether each cornea is normally sensitive.
- *dark adaptation*—ability of retina to adjust to low levels of illumination.
- *diopter*—unit of measurement of refractive power or strength of lenses. (69)
- *electroretinography*—the recording of retinal action currents. Procedure aids in the detection of degenerative disorders of the retina. (17, 19, 61)
- *"E" test, "E" game*—series of tests for the detection of visual acuity in preschool children and illiterate persons. (9)
- *fluorescein angiography*—intravenous injection of fluorescein followed by ophthalmoscopy or funduscopy and rapid serial photography. Fluorescence of the vasculature aids in the detection of normal and abnormal states of the retinal and choroidal vessels, including microaneurysms, neovascularization, atriovenous shunts, vascular leakage, retinal hemorrhage, and subtle vascular conditions of the macula. (13, 32, 61)
- *gonioscopy*—examination of the iris angle of the eye using an optical instrument. Obstruction of the filtration angle may occur in glaucoma. (61)
- *iris angiography*—procedure shows the blood supply to the iris and the permeability of the blood vessels of the iris in normal subject. (61)
- *keratometry*—measurement of the curves of the cornea with a keratometer.
- *major amblyoscopy*—test for evaluating the sensory status of the eyes; also used in orthoptic study before and after strabismus surgery. (9)
- *ophthalmodynamometry*—measurement of the pressure in the central retinal arteries for indirectly evaluating the blood flow in the carotid arteries. (61)
- *ophthalmoscopy*—examination of the eye grounds (fundi) with an ophthalmoscope. (61)
- *perimetry*—instrumental measurement of field of vision. Computerized automated perimetry utilizes test lights projected into a hollow bowl but with a static threshold testing method that is more precise and comprehensive. Two basic perimetry methods are:
  - *—kinetic (moving) perimetry*—test object is moved from a peripheral area toward the center and the patient indicates when the object is spotted.
  - *—static perimetry*—utilizes non-moving test object presented at a particular location and the patient indicates at what point he/she fails to see the object. (34, 61, 68)
- *probing of lacrimal drainage system*—establishing drainage of obstructed system after unsuccessful irrigation. A metal probe is passed through the upper or lower punctum and canaliculus and into the lacrimal (tear) sac, nasolacrimal duct, and nose.
- *retinoscopy*—light beam test for detecting refractive errors.
- *slit lamp biomicroscopy*—use of a combination of slit lamp and biomicroscope for intense illumination and high magnification of the eyeball or lids. Layers of cornea and lens are clearly visualized, and pathologic processes such as opacities are detected with accuracy. (32, 61)
- *tonometry*—determination of intraocular pressure by a tonometer, such as that of Schiotz. (61)
- *visual acuity*—determination of the minimum cognizable letter under standard

conditions of illumination using the Snellen chart or one of its modifications. (31, 60, 61, 69)

- *visual evoked potential (VEP), visual evoked response (VER)*—response to 50 to 100 flash stimuli recorded from over the right and left occipital poles. Since each eye is stimulated separately, it is possible to recognize lesions of the optic nerve by the reduced amplitude and delayed conduction. Different responses of each hemisphere suggest retrochiasmatic pathology. VER is of particular use in evaluating the vision pathways in nonresponsive patients and infants and recognizing subclinical lesions in certain neurologic disorders such as multiple sclerosis. (61)

Abbreviations

General

A, Acc—accommodation
$AgNO_3$—silver nitrate
anisometr.—anisometropia
C, Cyl—cylindric lens
C gl—with correction (with glasses)
CF—counting finger
CME—cystoid macular edema
cx—cylinder axis
D—diopter (lens strength)
EM—emmetropia
EOM—extraocular muscles
EPF—exophthalmos-producing factor
EPS—exophthalmos-producing substance
ET—esotropia
HM—hand motion
IOP—intraocular pressure
KW—Keith-Wagner (ophthalmoscopic findings)
LP, PL—light perception
L proj.—light projection
LR—light reaction

Myop.—myopia
NPC—near point of covergence
OD, RE—right eye (oculus dexter)
ODM—ophthalmodynamometry
Ophth., Oph.—ophthalmology
OS, LE—left eye (oculus sinister)
OU—each eye (oculus uterque)
PD—interpupillary distance
Pr—presbyopia
PRRE—pupils round, regular and equal
s gl—without correction (without glasses)
S, Sph—spherical lens
Tn, T—intraocular tension
VA—visual acuity
VE—visual efficiency
VEP—visual evoked potential
VER—visual evoked response
XT—exotropia

Organizations

NINDB—National Institute of Neurological Diseases and Blindness
NSPB—National Society for the Prevention of Blindness

Oral Reading Practice

Glaucoma

Glaucoma is a disease of the eye characterized by an elevated **intraocular pressure (IOP).** Normally, the internal pressure of the eye is about 18 to 22 mm Hg, a pressure higher than that of other organs. The maintenance of normal intraocular pressure depends primarily on the amount of **aqueous humor** present in the eye. The formation of aqueous humor and its elimination is a continuous process. If the production and absorption are in perfect balance, all is well, but if there is a disturbance of balance, the eye is seriously affected. (51)

The **ciliary** processes form the aqueous humor, which passes through the pupil space to the anterior chamber. It leaves through the **canal of Schlemm** and is picked up by the aqueous veins, which contain a mixture of blood and aqueous. In most cases of glaucoma the elevated intraocular pressure results from interference with the elimination of aqueous humor, although increased rate of production may be the source of imbalance. (51)

Primary open angle glaucoma presents spontaneously without the presence of related disorders and with no known origin other than **genetic** or **hereditary** predisposition. The disease is bilateral. The angle of the anterior chamber may be wide or narrow but it remains always open, whether the disease is in its initial stages or far advanced. The clinical picture is variable depending on the degree of elevation of intraocular pressure, which may vary from normal to significantly elevated pressures. Usually, there is a decreased facility of aqueous outflow, which tends to worsen over time with the progression of the disease. (20, 37, 51, 65)

Secondary open-angle glaucoma is characterized by partial or total blockage of the aqueous outflow to the tissues. This may result from the presence of **cells** and **particulate matter** carried into the **trabecular meshwork** along with aqueous or resulting from membrane or scar formation. Some types of **blunt trauma** to the anterior segment of the eye can produce blockage to aqueous outflow because of the simultaneous injury to the trabecular meshwork, the body of the **iris,** and the anterior aspect of the **ciliary** body, followed by scarring of the outflow channels. Some types of secondary open-angle glaucoma may be of short duration, lasting until the obstructing blockage has passed through the angle structures, while some types may be of longer duration, lasting long after the causative agent has been removed. (51)

Primary angle-closure glaucoma occurs in eyes with an anatomically narrow range. Abnormally small eyes **(nanophthalmus)** are more prone to angle closure. As the lens enlarges, the iris is held secure against the anterior lens surface, thus increasing the resistance to aqueous humor flow from the posterior chamber to the anterior chamber. In older adults, the anterior chamber loses depth and the lens enlarges with age, and thus this type of glaucoma is seen more often in that age category. (20)

Secondary angle-closure glaucoma represents antecedent pathologic factors responsible for causing closure of the angles. Some examples of these conditions are: **iritis, iridocyclitis, intraocular neoplasms, dislocations of the lens, central vein occlusion,** and **trauma.** (51, 65)

Preventing loss of visual function is the goal of treatment in glaucoma disorders. The treatment regimen is geared to lower the pressure, either by increasing the facility of outflow or suppressing formation of **aqueous humor** or both. Treatment consists of judicious use of drugs such as **miotics,** which sometimes constrict the pupil so effectively that the aqueous humor can escape. If no alleviation can be achieved, operative intervention becomes imperative. (51, 65)

Argon laser trabeculoplasty is usually considered before some of the more traditional surgical procedures are employed. Argon laser trabeculoplasty (ALT) is an operative procedure by which laser energy is directed through a goniolens to burn the trabecular meshwork producing blanching or a fine bubble formation, thereby causing a purse-string type of contraction in the trabecular meshwork, with resultant opening of the outflow mechanism to facilitate the emergence of aqueous humor. A series of 100 burns may be made in a 360 degree angle within the trabecular meshwork. Another approach is to perform this procedure in a two-step phase by having only an 180 degree angle of the trabecular meshwork treated with 50 burns. Then after a six week period, if the intraocular pressure is not adequately controlled, the other 180 degree angle can be treated with 50 more burns. Whatever the choice of approach, this procedure achieves a clinically significant decrease in intraocular pressure. (10, 37)

Various other forms of surgical drainage may be indicated, depending on the kind of glaucoma and the presence or absence of **anterior synechiae.** Other procedures of choice may include **peripheral iridectomy, laser iridectomy, sclerectomy, cyclodialysis** or **goniotomy.** Additional surgical procedures are combined **phacoemulsification, trabeculectomy** and **capsulocleisis.** (10, 65)

Table 18
Some Eye Conditions Amenable to Surgery

Organs Involved	Diagnosis	Type of Surgery	Operative Procedures
Eyeball	Penetrating wound of eyeball	Enucleation of eyeball	Removal of eyeball
Eyeball	Graves' disease with malignant exophthalmos and corneal ulceration	Orbital decompression of proptosed globe Krönlein orbitotomy	Lateral opening of orbit; Krönlein approach allowing orbital contents to overflow into temporal fossa
Retina Uvea Iris Conjunctiva	Retinoblastoma Malignant melanoma Epidermoid carcinoma	Enucleation of eyeball	Removal of eyeball and as much as possible of optic nerve in retinoblastoma
Retina Choroid Sclera	Detachment of retina	Scleral buckling operation	Diathermy to sclera and choroid; release of subretinal fluid Inward buckling of treated area and insertion of silicone implant; firm contact of choroid with retina reestablished
Retina Choroid Sclera	Detachment of retina	Cryopexy	Application of freezing probe to sclera to promote formation of chorioretinal scar and thus fusion
Cornea	Corneal scar Keratoconus	Keratoplasty; lamellar transplant or penetrating transplant	Replacement of opaque cornea with transparent cornea using partial-thickness or full-thickness corneal graft
Vitreous Cornea	Small foreign body in vitreous	Haab giant magnet technique Keratotomy	Foreign body dislodged by magnet and removed through corneal incision

Organs Involved	Diagnosis	Type of Surgery	Operative Procedures
Cornea Iris Vitreous	Glaucoma acute, primary	Keratocentesis Peripheral iridectomy Cyclodialysis	Paracentesis of cornea Surgical removal of part of iris Surgical communication between anterior chamber and suprachoroidal space
Cornea Sclera Trabeculum	Glaucoma open angle or narrow angle	Trabeculectomy	Positioning the operating microscope appropriately Raising a conjunctival flap to expose sclera Removing part of sclera together with trabecular meshwork
Sclera vitreous	Aphakic glaucoma or Open-angle glaucoma	Pars plana filter including sclerotomy vitrectomy	Sclera incised bilaterally Irrigation, fragmentation, and aspiration to remove formed vitreous Aqueous escaping through sclerotomy openings
Crystalline lens	Cataract congenital senescent (senile) traumatic	Pars plana lensectomy	Lens removed by irrigation, fragmentation, and aspiration through pars plana incisions
Crystalline lens	Cataract	Cryoextraction of cataract Anterior chamber lens implantation	Trephine opening to 7.5 mm Cataract frozen to cryoextractor and removed Insertion of intraocular lens through trephine opening
Crystalline lens Iris	Cataract congenital senescent (senile)	Discission Peripheral iridectomy Intracapsular extraction of cataract	Needling of lens Approach to cataract by removal of part of iris Excision of cataract within capsule
Crystalline lens	Cataract infantile juvenile young adult	Aspiration-irrigation method of cataract removal	Use of operating microscope Two limbal incisions, one for insertion of needle knife into lens to aspirate cataract, the other for insertion of hollow-bore needle to irrigate anterior chamber with saline

Organs Involved	Diagnosis	Type of Surgery	Operative Procedures
Crystalline lens	Cataract congenital infantile senescent	Microsurgical phacoemulsification Kelman technique	Operating microscope in position Tiny limbal incision followed by: Excision of small capsular portion of prolapse lens into anterior chamber Insertion of phacoemulsifier into lens using ultrasound for its emulsification Aspiration of lens fragments and irrigation of eye
Iris	Cyst of iris	Electrolysis	Insertion of an electrolysis needle in the center of cyst to induce shrinkage
Ocular muscle	Strabismus	Recession of ocular muscle	Correction of defect by drawing muscle backward
Canthus Eyelid Lacrimal sac	Basal cell carcinoma medial canthal region—eyelid	Surgical ablation of entire malignant lesion Reconstruction of canthal region and lid	Excision of tumor lacrimal sac canalicula medial half of lid Surgical creation of midline forehead flap covering the lid
Eyelid	Laceration of eyelid Hordeolum Blepharoptosis	Blepharorrhaphy Blepharotomy Repair of eyelid	Suture of eyelid Incision with drainage of meibomian gland Surgical correction of ptosis
Lacrimal sac	Abscess of lacrimal sac	Dacryocystotomy	Incision and drainage of tear duct
Lacrimal gland	Retention cyst of lacrimal gland	Dacryoadenectomy	Removal of tear gland
Lacrimonasal duct	Stenosis of lacrimonasal duct	Dacryocystorhinostomy	Fistulization of lacrimal sac into nasal cavity

References and Bibliography

1. Alpar, John J., and Fechner, Paul U. History of modern lens implantation. In *Fechner's Intraocular Lenses*, New York: Thieme Inc., 1987, pp. 6-23.
2. ———. Viscoelastic and other materials for cushioning the anterior chamber and coating the intraocular lens. Ibid., pp. 118-123.
3. ———. Survey of modern lenses. Ibid., pp. 178-205.
4. Baloh, Robert W. The special senses. In Wyngaarden, James B., and Smith, Lloyd H., Jr., eds., *Cecil's Textbook of Medicine,* 18th ed. Philadelphia: W.B. Saunders Co., 1988, pp. 2109-2124.

5. Biswell, Roderick. Refractive corneal surgery. In Vaughan, Daniel, and Asbury, Taylor, eds., *General Ophthalmology,* 11th ed. Los Altos, CA: Lange Medical Publications, 1986, pp. 125-127.

6. Callahan, Michael A., et al. Mohs' fresh tissue technique for periorbital skin cancer. In Hornblass, Albert, and Hanig, Carl J., eds., *Occuloplastic, Orbital, and Reconstructive Surgery,* vol. 1. Baltimore: Williams & Wilkins, 1988, pp. 643-650.

7. de Bustros, Serge, et al. Vitrectomy for macular pucker. *Archives of Ophthalmology* 106: 758-760, June 1988.

8. Drews, Robert C., MD. Personal communications.

9. Eggers, Howard M. Strabismus. In Vaughan, Daniel, and Asbury, Taylor, eds., *General Ophthalmology,* 11th ed. Los Altos, CA: Lange Medical Publications, 1986, pp. 200-222.

10. Epstein, David L. *Chandler and Grant's Glaucoma,* 3rd ed. Philadelphia: Lea & Febiger, 1986, pp. 104-125.

11. Fogle, Jerry. Radial keratotomy. In Schwab, Ivan R., ed., *Refractive Keratoplasty,* New York: Churchill Livingstone, Inc., 1987, pp. 125-144.

12. Gittinger, John W., Jr. Eye diseases. In Wyngaarden, James B., and Smith, Lloyd H., Jr., eds., *Cecil's Textbook of Medicine,* 18th ed. Philadelphia: W.B. Saunders Co., 1988, pp. 2289-2299.

13. Green, W. Richard. Retina. In Spencer, William H., ed., *Ophthalmic Pathology: An Atlas and Textbook,* 3rd ed., vol. 2. Philadelphia: W.B. Saunders Co., 1985, pp. 589-1291.

14. Hiatt, Roger L. Transposition procedures in strabismus. *Annals of Ophthalmology* 18:332-336, Nov. 1986.

15. Hornblass, Albert, and Gross, Neil D. Evaluation of the blepharoplasty patient. In Hornblass, Albert, and Hanig, Carol J., eds., *Occuloplastic, Orbital, and Reconstructive Surgery,* vol. 1. Baltimore: Williams & Wilkins, 1988, pp. 467-473.

16. Hu, Benjamin V., et al. Implantation of posterior chamber lens in the absence of capsular and zonular support. *Archives of Ophthalmology* 106:416-420, March 1988.

17. Johnson, Mary A., et al. Neovascularization in central retinal vein occlusion: Electroretinographic findings. *Archives of Ophthalmology* 106:346-352, March 1988.

18. Johnson, Stephen H., et al. Emulsification of the nucleus: The bimanual technique. In Abrahamson, Ira A., ed., *Cataract Surgery,* New York: McGraw-Hill Book Co., 1986, pp. 55-73.

19. Kaye, Stephen B., et al. Early electroretinography in unilateral central retinal vein occlusion as a predictor of rubeosis iridis. *Archives of Ophthalmology* 106:353-359, March 1988.

20. Klintworth, Gordon K. The eye. In Rubin, Emanuel, and Farber, John L., eds., *Pathology,* Philadelphia: J.B. Lippincott Co., 1988, pp. 1500-1531.

21. Layden, William E. Trabecular surgery. In Weinstein, George W., ed., *Open Angle Glaucoma,* New York: Churchill Livingstone, Inc., 1986, pp. 155-181.

22. Leiske, Larry G., and Shepard, Dennis. Anterior chamber lenses. In Abrahamson, Ira A., ed., *Cataract Surgery,* New York: McGraw-Hill Book Co., 1986, pp. 80-90.

23. Lin, T.Y., et al. The effect of YAG laser anterior capsulotomy of prostaglandin concentration in aqueous humor. *Annals of Ophthalmology* 20:95-99, March 1988.

24. Lisman, Richard D., et al. Use of cutaneous argon laser in ophthalmic plastic surgery. In Hornblass, Albert, and Hanig, Carl J., eds., *Occuloplastic, Orbital, and Reconstructive Surgery,* vol. 1. Baltimore: Williams & Wilkins, 1988, pp. 680-692.

25. Marrone, Alfred. Thermal eyelid burns. In Hornblass, Albert, and Hanig, Carl J., eds., *Occuloplastic, Orbital, and Reconstructive Surgery,* vol. 1. Baltimore: Williams & Wilkins, 1988, pp. 433-447.

26. Maxwell, W. Andrew, and Nordan, Lee T. Optical and wound complications of keratomileusis: Incidence and treatment. In Cavanagh, H. Dwight, ed., *The Cornea: Transactions of the World Congress on Cornea III,* New York: Raven Press, 1987, pp. 597-601.

27. McCarthy, Rodney W. Symblepharon. In Hornblass, Albert, and Hanig, Carl J., eds., *Occuloplastic, Orbital, and Reconstructive Surgery,* vol. 1. Baltimore: Williams & Wilkins, 1988, pp. 659-667.

28. McDonald, Marguerite B., and Dingeldein, Steven A. Complications of epikeratophakia. In Cavanagh, H. Dwight, ed., *The Cornea: Transactions of the World Congress on Cornea III,* New York: Raven Press, 1987, pp. 603-608.

29. McGuigan, Lorraine J.B., et al. Extracapsular cataract extraction and posterior chamber lens implantation in eyes with preexisting glaucoma. *Archives of Ophthalmology* 104: 1301-1308, Sept. 1986.

30. Morse, Peter H. Scleral buckling for retinal separation: with and without encirclement. *Annals of Ophthalmology* 20:92-94, March 1988.

31. Newell, Frank. Functional examination of the eyes. In *Ophthalmology: Principles and Concepts,* 6th ed. St. Louis: The C.V. Mosby Co., 1986, pp. 154-164.

32. ———. Physical examination of the eyes. Ibid., pp. 165-179.

33. ———. Injuries of the eye. Ibid., pp. 183-194.

34. ———. The glaucomas. Ibid., pp. 378-398.

35. ———. Ocular motility. Ibid., pp. 399-414.

36. O'Malley, Conor. Vitreous. In Vaughan, Daniel, and Asbury, Taylor, eds., *General Ophthalmology,* 11th ed. Los Altos, CA: Lange Medical Publications, 1986, pp. 151-162.

37. Pollack, Irvin P., et al. Laser surgery for open-angle glaucoma. In Weinstein, George W., ed., *Open Angle Glaucoma,* New York: Churchill Livingstone, Inc., 1986, pp. 227-249.

38. Putterman, Allen M. Upper eyelid blepharoplasty. In Hornblass, Albert, and Hanig, Carl J., eds., *Occuloplastic, Orbital, and Reconstructive Surgery,* vol. 1. Baltimore: Williams & Wilkins, 1988, pp. 467-473.

39. Rees, Thomas D., and Nolan, William B. Lower eyelid blepharoplasty: The cutaneous approach. In Hornblass, Albert, and Hanig, Carl J., eds., *Occuloplastic, Orbital, and Reconstructive Surgery,* vol. 1. Baltimore: Williams & Wilkins, 1988, pp. 485-499.

40. Rouhiainen, Harri J. Peripheral anterior synechiae formation after trabeculoplasty. *Archives of Ophthalmology* 106:189-191, Feb. 1988.

41. Rouhiainen, Harri J., et al. The effect of some treatment variables on the results of trabeculoplasty. *Archives of Ophthalmology* 106:611-613, May 1988.

42. Schwab, Ivan R. Perspectives of refractive surgery. In Schwab, Ivan R., ed., *Refractive Keratoplasty,* New York: Churchill Livingstone, Inc., 1987, pp. 1-16.

43. ———. The refractive aspects of corneal transplantation. Ibid., pp. 171-195.

44. Shock, John P. Lens. In Vaughan, Daniel, and Asbury, Taylor, eds., *General Ophthalmology,* 11th ed. Los Altos, CA: Lange Medical Publications, 1986, pp. 142-150.

45. Small, Robert G. Pterygium. In Hornblass, Albert, and Hanig, Carl J., eds., *Occuloplastic, Orbital, and Reconstructive Surgery,* vol. 1. Baltimore: Williams & Wilkins, 1988, pp. 693-701.

46. Smiddy, William E., et al. Vitrectomy for macular traction caused by incomplete vitreous separation. *Archives of Ophthalmology* 106:624-628, May 1988.

47. Smith, Randolph. Eyes right? In *St. Louis Post-Dispatch.* Saturday, May 21, 1988, pp. D1 & D8.

48. Spencer, William H. Cornea. In Spencer, William H., ed., *Ophthalmic Pathology: An Atlas and Textbook,* 3rd ed., vol. 1. Philadelphia: W.B. Saunders Co., 1985, pp. 229-338.

49. ———. Sclera. Ibid., pp. 389-422.

50. ———. Lens. Ibid., pp. 423-479.

51. ———. Glaucoma. Ibid., pp. 480-547.

52. ———. Vitreous. Ibid., vol. 2., 1985, pp. 548-588.

53. ———. Optic nerve. Ibid., vol. 3., 1986, pp. 2337-2458.

54. Steedle, Thomas O., et al. Cortex removal in extracapsular cataract extraction. In Abrahamson, Ira A., ed., *Cataract Surgery,* New York: McGraw-Hill Book Co., 1986, pp. 74-79.

55. Steinert, Roger F., and Wagoner, Michael D. Long term comparison of epikeratoplasty and penetrating keratoplasty for keratoconus. *Archives of Ophthalmology* 106:493-496, April 1988.

56. Stone, Lawrence S., and Kline, Oram R., Jr. Extracapsular cataract surgery and posterior chamber intraocular lenses. In Reinecke, Robert D., ed., *1985 Ophthalmology Annual,* vol. 1. Norwalk, CT: Appleton-Century-Crofts, 1985, pp. 1-27.

57. Sullivan, John H. Lids & lacrimal apparatus. In Vaughan, Daniel, and Asbury, Taylor, eds., *General Ophthalmology,* 11th ed. Los Altos, CA: Lange Medical Publications, 1986, pp. 63-71.

58. Thawley, Stanley E., and Panje, William R. Treatment of tumors of the eye, orbit and lacrimal apparatus. In Thawley, Stanley E., and Panje, William R., eds., *Comprehensive Management of Head and Neck Tumors,* Philadelphia: W.B. Saunders Co., 1987, pp. 1767-1839.

59. Trokel, Stephen. Laser surgery of the cornea. In Schwab, Ivan R., ed., *Refractive Keratoplasty,* New York: Churchill Livingstone, Inc., 1987, pp. 273-297.

60. Vaughan, Daniel. Eye. In Schroeder, Steven A., Krupp, Marcus A., and Tierney, Lawrence M., Jr., eds., *Current Medical Diagnosis and Treatment—1988,* Norwalk, CT: Appleton & Lange, 1988, pp. 94-109.

61. Vaughan, Daniel, and Asbury, Taylor, eds. Examination. In *General Ophthalmology,* 11th ed. Los Altos, CA: Lange Medical Publications, 1986, pp. 14-32.

62. ———. Cornea. Ibid., pp. 106-127.

63. ———. Sclera. Ibid., pp. 128-131.

64. ———. Retina. Ibid., pp. 163-183.

65. ———. Glaucoma. Ibid., pp. 184-199.

66. Vila-Coro, A.A., et al. Inflatable catheter for dacryocystorhinostomy. *Archives of Ophthalmology* 106:692-694, May 1988.

67. Werblin, Theodore P. Epikeratophakia. In Schwab, Ivan R., ed., *Refractive Keratoplasty,* New York: Churchill Livingstone, Inc., 1987, pp. 17-39.

68. Werner, Elliot B., et al. A comparison of experienced observers and statistical tests in detection of progressive visual field loss in glaucoma using automated perimetry. *Ar-*

chives of Ophthalmology 106:619-623, May 1988.

69. White, Orson W. Optics and refraction. In Vaughan, Daniel, and Asbury, Taylor, eds., *General Ophthalmology,* 11th ed. Los Altos, CA: Lange Medical Publications, 1986, pp. 345-361.

70. Woodburne, Russell T., and Burkel, William E. The head and neck. In *Essentials of Anatomy,* New York: Oxford University Press, 1988, pp. 179-323.

Disorders Pertaining to the Sense Organ of Hearing

Ear

Origin of Terms

acoustic (G)—sound
auricle (L)—little ear
cochlea (G)—snail, shell, spiral form
myringo- (L)—eardrum

ossicle (L)—small bone
ot-, oto- (G)—ear
salpingo- (G)—tube, trumpet
vestibule (L)—antechamber

Anatomic Terms (Refs. 7, 30, 46)

- *external ear*—division of ear consisting of the auricle and the external auditory canal or meatus.
    - —*auricle, pinna*—the external ear, made up chiefly of elastic fibrocartilage that is shaped to catch the sound waves.
    - —*cerumen*—ear wax, formed by the ceruminous glands of the skin lining the meatus.
    - —*external auditory meatus*—ear passage, composed of a cartilaginous and a bony part.
    - —*helix*—outer folded margin of the auricle.
- *middle ear, tympanic cavity* (see Fig. 71)—division of ear containing the ossicles for the conduction of airborne sound waves.
    - —*auditory tube, eustachian tube, pharyngotympanic tube*—channel of communication between pharynx and middle ear.
    - —*orifices of the tympanic cavity:*
    - –*aditus and antrum*—opening to the mastoid antrum.
    - –*fenestra cochleae, fenestra rotunda*—round window facing the internal ear.
    - –*fenestra vestibuli, fenestra ovalis*—oval window in which the stapes lodges.
    - –orifice from the external auditory meatus into the middle ear. It is closed by the tympanic membrane of eardrum.
    - –opening into auditory tube.
    - —*ossicles of the tympanic cavity*—three tiny bones: malleus (hammer), incus (anvil), and stapes (stirrup). They transmit vibrations to the internal ear.
- *inner ear* (see Fig. 71)—division of ear composed of a number of fluid-filled spaces and the membranous labyrinth, which lies within the bony (osseous) labyrinth. The

Figure 71 Schematic section through middle and inner ear.

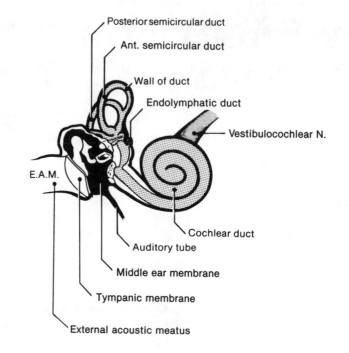

Figure 72 Distribution of vestibulocochlear nerve to inner ear.

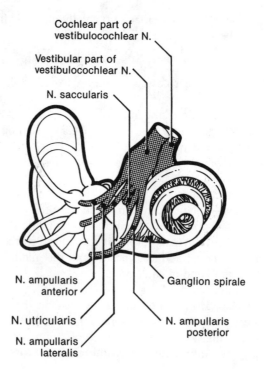

perilymphatic space of the bony labyrinth contains the cochlea, vestibule, and semicircular canals. Because of the complexity of the structures, only a few basic facts are given here.

—*cochlea*—spiral tube possessing a bony core, the modiolus, which contains the spiral ganglion and transmits the cochlear nerve. It is the essential organ of hearing.

—*vestibular apparatus*—the utricle and semicircular ducts, which are concerned with the maintenance of the equilibrium.

—*vestibulocochlear nerve, eighth cranial nerve, formerly acoustic or auditory nerve*— nerve comprising two distinct fiber sets. (see Fig. 72)

—*cochlear branch*—fibers distributed to the hair cells of the spiral organ. They are concerned with hearing.

—*vestibular branch*—fibers distributed to portions of the utricle, saccule, and semicircular ducts. They aid in maintaining body balance.

Diagnostic Terms

■ *conditions of the external ear:*

—*abscess of auricle or of external auditory meatus*—localized collection of pus of auricle or meatus. (29, 37)

—*congenital or acquired defects:*

—*atresia of external auditory meatus*—absence of the normal opening of the ear or closure of the external auditory meatus. (29)

—*congenital microtia*—usually a deformed or misplaced, small aural tag associated with absence of meatus and tragus. (3)

—*traumatic avulsion of auricle*—loss of pinna due to injury. (29)

—*dermatitis of external ear*—inflammation of skin of auricle and external auditory meatus. Types encountered: dry, moist, exfoliative, contact, eczematous, allergic, and seborrheic. (29)

—*frostbite of auricle*—exposure to extreme cold resulting in hyperemia, blanching, and in severe cases ulceration and gangrene. (10, 29)

—*furuncle of the external auditory canal*—painful nodule of the skin formed by circumscribed inflammation of the skin and subcutaneous tissue: usually may resemble a mild infection of the sebaceous glands and hair follicles. Staphylococci enter through the hair follicles. (9, 29)

—*tumors of external auditory canal:*

—*adenocarcinoma of cerumen gland*—malignant tumor originating in ceruminous glands characterized by a tendency to invade soft tissues and bones and to recur after surgical removal. (10, 29)

—*aural polyp*—benign tumor on a pedicle that may occlude the external auditory canal and thus interfere with sound conduction. (10, 29)

—*cerumen gland adenoma*—benign tumor originating in ceruminous glands. (9, 10, 29)

■ *conditions of the tympanic membrane:*

—*myringitis, tympanitis*—inflammation of the eardrum. (9)

—*perforation of tympanic membrane*—hole in eardrum; if small it will heal without treatment; if large it may require tympanoplasty. (9)

—*rupture of tympanic membrane*—condition usually due to trauma, such as direct injury to ear.

—*tumors*—rare disorders that may be endotheliomatous, fibromatous, or angiomatous or show other histologic patterns.

—*tympanosclerosis*—involvement of the mucous membrane of the middle ear or drum by sclerosis of exudate, with fixation of the ossicles and drum, diffuse calcification, and thickening of the mucosal lining of the cavity. (9)

- *conditions of the middle ear:*
  - —*aerotitis media, barotitis media, aural barotrauma*—painful condition caused by atmospheric pressure changes in middle ear, chiefly during ascent and descent of air travel or experienced on descent by divers. (10)
  - —*cholesteatoma*—globular pearly mass covered with a thin shell of epidermis and connective tissue. It usually forms following middle ear infection and is the body's way of arresting suppuration. Pseudocholesteatomas are common. (2, 9, 32, 37)
  - —*glomus tumors, chemodectomas*—common neoplasm of the head and neck.
    - –*glomus tympanicum*—tumor originates in the middle ear and can usually be surgically removed.
    - –*glomus jugulare*—tumor containing chemoceptor cells arises from the jugular bulb in the middle ear. It may cause episodes of dizziness, nystagmus, blackouts, and facial paralysis. Labyrinthine and cochlear invasion by the glomus leads to deafness. Complete surgical excision depends on the location and size of the tumor.
    - –*glomus vagale*—tumor arises along the course of the vagus nerve and is relatively uncommon. (2, 9, 32, 37, 41)
  - —*mastoiditis*—infection of the middle ear that has extended to the antrum and mastoid cells. Mastoiditis may be acute, subacute, chronic, and recurrent. (9, 44)
  - —*middle ear effusion*—acute or chronic presence of fluid in middle ear, generally without infection. (4)
    - –*secretory otitis media, mucoid otitis media, glucotitis*—thick, cloudy, viscous exudate in middle ear containing cells and mucous strands. (4, 9)
    - –*serous otitis media*—thin, clear amber fluid in middle ear. (4)
    - –*serous otitis media with hemotympanum*—serum and blood in middle ear space resulting from temporal bone fracture, tumor, or blood disorder. (4, 9)
  - —*otitis media*—inflammation of the middle ear. Common types encountered are:
    - –*acute suppurative otitis media*—marked by intense congestion of mucosa of middle ear, blockage of eustachian tube, serous exudate that becomes infected, and rupture of the eardrum. Bacterial invaders are *Staphylococcus aureus, Diplococcus pneumoniae, Streptococcus pyogenes, Hemophilus influenzae,* and others. (4, 9)
    - –*chronic suppurative otitis media*—characterized by continuation of middle ear infection resulting in protracted suppuration. (4, 9)
  - —*salpingitis of eustachian tube*—inflammation of the auditory tube. It may be acute or chronic. (9)
- *conditions of the inner ear:*
  - —*acoustic neuroma*—benign tumor of the eighth cranial nerve affecting the vestibular branch more than the cochlear branch of the nerve and causing vertigo, tinnitus, and hearing impairment. (10)
  - —*labyrinthitis*—inflammation of the labyrinth, usually secondary to acute or chronic suppurative otitis media with or without cholesteatoma or to acute upper respiratory infection. (14, 20)
  - —*Menière's disease, endolymphatic hydrops*—neurologic disorder exhibiting a triad symptom complex in its classic form:
    - –explosive attacks of true vertigo
    - –fluctuating hearing loss of the sensorineural type

−tinnitus

Dizziness, ataxia, and a feeling of fullness in the ear are usually present. Remissions may last years. (12)

—*otosclerosis, otospongiosis*—newly formed spongy bone replacing the hard bone of the labyrinth. It may result in conduction deafness with fixation of the stapes and stapedial footplate, followed later by nerve degeneration resulting in mixed deafness. (21)

—*tinnitus*—auditory perception of internal origin (noise), usually localized as presenting from within and rarely heard by others. It affects both men and women and generally occurs between the ages of 40 and 80.

−*vibratory tinnitus*—real sounds, mechanical in origin, arising within or near the ear.

−*nonvibratory tinnitus*—neural excitation and conduction from anywhere within the auditory system to the auditory cortex, without a mechanical basis. Nonvibratory tinnitus appears to be more common than vibratory tinnitus. (13, 23)

- *hearing loss:*
  - *Two basic types are recognized:*
    - *conductive hearing loss*—impairment of hearing resulting from obstruction of sound waves that do not reach the inner ear. The interference may be caused by impacted cerumen, exudate, blockage of external auditory canal or eustachian tube, otosclerosis, or other causes. Otitis media of some type is the most common cause of conductive hearing loss. (8, 12, 25)
    - *sensorineural hearing loss*—inability of the cochlear division of the eighth cranial nerve to transmit electric impulses to the brain or the hair cells of the organ of Corti to change sound to electric energy. Dysfunction may result from neural degeneration of the organ of Corti, alterations in endolymph, cochlear conductive disorder, or other causes. (8, 12, 25)
  - Conductive or sensorineural hearing loss or both may be found in the following types.
    - *congenital deafness*—loss of hearing from birth. (12)
    - *hysteric deafness*—simulated hearing loss associated with neurotic behavior and emotional instability, thus psychogenic in nature. (12)
    - *Mondini's deafness*—genetic deafness caused by aplastic changes in the osseous and membranous labyrinth. (5)
    - *noise deafness, industrial hearing loss, occupational hearing loss*—impairment or loss of hearing induced by constant noise, explosions, or blows to the head. It disappears in a quiet environment if neural damage is in its early phase. (12)
    - *sudden hearing loss, spontaneous hearing loss*—usually an abrupt onset of sensorineural loss of hearing in one ear due to viral infection, vascular accident, trauma, shrinkage of organ of Corti, or other causes. Bilateral sudden hearing loss is uncommon. (12, 36)

Operative Terms

- *microsurgery*—the use of a high-power binocular dissecting microscope with built-in illumination for ear surgery.
- *external ear:*
  - *otoplasty*—correction of deformed pinna. (11)
  - *pedicle tube insertion*—technique useful in repairing a large defect in the auricular area, such as results from trauma or from total excision of the auricle for extensive carcinomas. A skin incision is made over the defective area, the

skin flap is raised, and a tube is inserted and closed with continuous or interrupted sutures. By sliding and undermining, the donor site can be closed beneath the tube, then defects at the end of the tube are closed. (12)

—*repair of auricular deformity (microtia), excision of microtia*—proper surgical revision of existing malformation as a foundation for prosthesis and prosthetic reconstruction of auricle.

—*sebaceous cyst and keloid excision*—complete removal of entire sebaceous cyst and keloid from its site. (11)

■ *middle ear:*

—*fenestration operation (Lempert)*—a one-stage surgical procedure to create a new opening in the labyrinth of the ear for the restoration of hearing in cases of otosclerosis. (12)

—*insertion of plastic tubes*—the process whereby plastic tubes may be introduced into the middle ear area; the tubes act temporarily or permanently as an artificial eustachian tube.

—*mastoid antrotomy*—surgical opening of mastoid antrum, usually done for children with middle ear infection. (26)

—*mastoidectomy, complete, Schwartze operation*—mastoid air cells completely exenterated, antrum drained, and myringotomy performed to promote escape of drainage in the presence of a subperiosteal abscess. (9, 26)

—*mastoidectomy, radical*—removal of all diseased tissue in mastoid antrum and tympanic cavity and conversion of both into one dry cavity that communicates with the external ear. An operating microscope is used. (9, 26)

—*mastoidectomy, simple*—postaural or endaural incision and removal of mastoid cells. In the presence of fluid in the middle ear, a myringotomy is performed to establish drainage. (9, 26)

—*myringotomy, tympanotomy*—opening of the eardrum in an area that tends to heal readily, to avoid spontaneous rupture at a site that rarely closes. (9)

—*myringoplasty*—surgical repair of tympanic membrane by tissue grafts. (12)

—*paracentesis tympani*—surgical puncture of the eardrum for evacuation of fluid from middle ear. (4)

—*stapedectomy*—removal of stapes, reestablishing connection between incus and oval window by interposition of prosthesis and tissue or inert cover over oval window. (12, 16, 40)

—*tympanoplasty*—repair of perforated tympanic membrane with erosion of malleus by closing tympanum with graft against incus or remnant of malleus. Several tympanoplastic procedures have been devised. (2, 9, 26, 41)

—*tympanotomy, exploratory*—exploration of middle ear through tympanomeatal approach. (2, 9, 26, 41)

■ *inner ear:*

—*cochlear implant, cochlear prosthesis*—electronic device assigned to initiate motion in the ossicular chain and cochlear fluid and depolarize peripheral neurons, thus producing auditory sensations. By generating electric stimulation of various segments of the cochlear branch of the eighth cranial nerve, the cochlear prosthesis promises to become a functional implantable hearing aid enhancing the speech rehabilitation of the totally deaf. (16, 31)

—*cochleosacculotomy*—creation of a fistula between the perilymphatic and dilatated endolymphatic compartments by inserting a hook through the round window membrane and the osseous spiral lamina of the basal end of the cochlea. Penetration of the tip of the hook can be monitored by movement of the stapes footplate. The defect in the round window is obliterated with Gelfoam. (43)

—*decompression of endolymphatic sac*—removal of bone around the sac for improvement of vascularization so that endolymph can escape to cerebrospinal fluid system. (19)

—*labyrinthectomy*—total destruction of labyrinth with or without removal of Scarpa's ganglion for intractable vertigo. (19, 43) (see Fig. 73)

—*labyrinthectomy, transmeatal with cochleovestibular neurectomy*—the transcanal labyrinthectomy can be extended, the internal auditory canal opened, and the cochlear and vestibular nerves sectioned. This procedure has the advantage of ruling out an acoustic neuroma and also may give better results in relieving tinnitus. (43)

—*ligation of internal jugular vein*—tying of the internal jugular vein to relieve objective venous tinnitus, formerly known as cephalic bruit. (43)

—*surgery of internal auditory canal*—transvestibular approach to canal:

    –for relief of disabling vertigo and tinnitus by section of the vestibular nerve or excision of acoustic neuroma.

    –for facial paralysis by decompression of the facial nerve and facial nerve grafting. (43)

Symptomatic Terms

- *anacusis*—sound perception completely lost.
- *impacted cerumen*—dried ear wax. (9)
- *nystagmus*—involuntary rhythmic movements in one eye or both that may be horizontal, rotary, vertical, circulatory, oblique, or mixed type. They commonly occur in vestibular disease.
- *otalgia*—pains in ear; severe earache. (43)
- *paracusis of Willis*—ability of person with conductive hearing loss to hear better in the presence of noise.

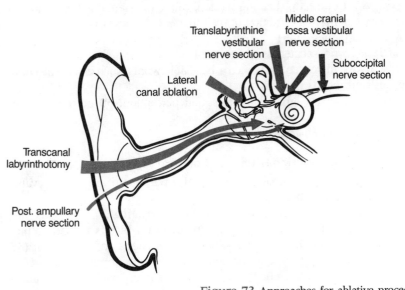

Figure 73 Approaches for ablative procedures for treatment of vertigo.

- *presbycusis*—impaired hearing that is part of the aging process. (12)
- *tinnitus*—ringing in the ears. (13, 23, 25)
- *vertigo* (see Fig. 73)—illusion of movement of a person in relation to the environment. The patient feels that he himself is spinning (subjective type) or the objects are whirling about him (objective type).
  - —*central vertigo*—present in disorders of vestibular nuclei, cerebellum, or brainstem, characterized by slow onset, prolonged duration, and absence of hearing impairment or tinnitus.
  - —*peripheral vertigo*—present in disorders of vestibular nerve and semicircular canals. It is episodic and explosive; marked by sudden, violent attack, lasting minutes to hours; and usually accompanied by tinnitus and impaired hearing. (43)

Special Procedures

Basic Terms Related to Audiology

- *air conduction*—aerotympanic route or aerial transmission of sound waves across the tympanic cavity (middle ear) and through the round window into the inner ear. (27)
- *bone conduction*—ossicular route or transmission of sound waves across the ossicles and through the oval window into the inner ear. The mechanical force of air and bone conduction is transformed in the inner ear into electric energy, which travels along the cochlear branch of the eighth cranial nerve to the brain, where it is perceived as speech. (27)
- *decibel*—unit expressing intensity of sound. (1)
- *discrimination*—ability to distinguish accurately between similarly sounding words. (27)
- *frequency*—the number of regularly recurrent sound vibrations emanating from a source and expressed in cycles per second. (1, 27)
- *intensity of sound*—pressure exerted by sound and measured in decibels.
- *loudness*—sound heard by person with normal hearing differing from that perceived by person with defective hearing while the intensity remains the same. (1)
- *recruitment*—abnormal condition of the inner ear characterized by an extremely rapid increase in loudness. (45)
- *sensitivity to sound*—acuteness of hearing.
- *spondee words*—in speech audiometry, bisyllabic words, such as nosebleed, headache, and eardrum. (27)
- *threshold*—the lowest limit of initial sound perception; 50 percent of words heard correctly. (20, 27)
- *tone decay*—the tone becomes inaudible.

Terms Related to Functional Tests of Cochlear Apparatus (see Fig. 74)

- *audiometry*—measurement of hearing for the purpose of accurately evaluating the extent and nature of hearing impairment. (8)
- *audiometric test*—quantitative measurement of hearing loss. Results are plotted according to an established norm on an audiogram, which is a graphic representation of patient's threshold of hearing at different frequencies and intensities. (35)
- *Békésy audiometric test*—test automatically presenting continuous pure tones and interrupted tones at different frequencies. The subject controls the intensity of the testing signal, and a needle plots the audiogram on a record form. (27)
- *electrocochleography*—new method of testing hearing, particularly in infants one to six

Figure 74 Different frequencies creating different wave patterns in basilar membrane within the cochlea. High-frequency sound vibrates basilar membrane at base of cochlea. Medium-frequency sound vibrates middle area of cochlea. Low-frequency sound vibrates apex of cochlea. Hearing depends on sound waves entering the inner ear.

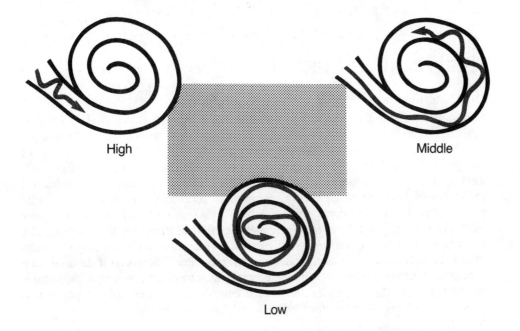

High   Middle

Low

months old. Electrodes are positioned on or near the cochlea, and a computer records low-voltage electric potentials obtained from the inner ear. (24)

- *pure tone audiometry*—use of an electric instrument for quantitatively measuring pure tones both by air conduction and bone conduction at threshold levels. Test detects the type of hearing loss. (27)
- *short-increment sensitivity index*—test presenting continuous pure tone to subject and superimposing short pips of one decibel increments on constant pure tone. Subjects with cochlear impairment experience no difficulty in perceiving the pips, whereas those with normal hearing do. (8)
- *speech audiometry*—valuable aid in clinical audiology. The patient's functioning in the environment is estimated by a speech discrimination score. (8, 27)
- *tone decay test*—valuable special auditory test that demonstrates the phenomenon of a tone becoming inaudible.
- *tuning fork tests*—means for determining the type of hearing impairment in relation to sound conduction and sound perception. The Rinne, Bing, and Weber tests are commonly used. (6, 8, 16, 25)

Terms Related to Functional Tests of the Vestibular Apparatus

- *caloric test*—procedure that conveys information of the functional capacity of each labyrinth and the presence of horizontal and rotary nystagmus. (20, 34)
- *electronystagmogram*—record of eye movements by electric tracing induced by caloric or positional stimulation. (20)
- *Romberg test*—procedure that tests body balance when eyes are closed and feet are together side by side. (20)

Abbreviations

AC—air conduction
BC—bone conduction
ENT—ear, nose, and throat
ETF—eustachian tubal function

PTS—permanent threshold shift
SISI—short-increment sensitivity index
TDT—tone decay test
TTS—temporary threshold shift

Oral Reading Practice

Otitic Meningitis

Meningitis is one of the most serious **sequelae** of ear infections. Its incidence is higher in small children than in adults because of the intimate relation of the middle ear to the **middle cranial fossa** in early life. Symptoms may develop slowly, or there may be an abrupt onset of the disease with **prodromal** manifestations. A chill occasionally signals the beginning of the acute phase. With the cerebral invasion of pathogenic organisms, the cardinal symptoms make their appearance: a constantly high fever, a headache progressively becoming worse to the point of being excruciating, and **vertigo,** particularly in the presence of **labyrinthine** involvement. **Purulent labyrinthitis** can occur as the infarction spreads from the **subarachnoid space** into the **cochlea** through the **cochlear aqueduct** or along the **vascular** and **nerve channels** of the **auditory canal.** As the disease progresses, prostration increases, **convulsions** occur, particularly in children, and the patient becomes very irritable, exhibiting marked personality changes. In infants, the large **fontanelle** is bulging, but there is no pulsation.

Bacterial meningitis is a common cause of unilateral or bilateral **sensorineural hearing impairment.** In children, the most common cause of **conductive hearing impairment** is otitis media with effusion, and a persistent effusion may cause a conductive hearing loss. Chronic **suppurative otitis media** causes meningitis by direct extension through bone and dura or through the inner ear via a **labyrinthine fistula** caused by a **cholesteatoma,** or through the bloodstream: e.g., **bacteremia** is thought to be responsible for the majority of **bacterial meningitis** (otitic and nonotitic). Acute or chronic suppurative otitis media may be followed by **intracranial** complications such as **thrombophlebitis** of the **lateral sinus, extradural** or **intradural** abscess, facial paralysis, and other disorders.

The **Kernig's sign** is positive, as evidenced by pain and reflex contraction in the hamstring muscles when the examiner attempts to extend the leg after flexing the thigh upon the abdomen. Muscular rigidity of back and neck and retraction of the head are characteristic manifestations. In addition, the patient suffers from **photophobia, hyperesthesia** at touch, and **opisthotonos.** If treatment remains ineffectual, progressive drowsiness and coma develop, the deep reflexes disappear, and the prognosis is poor.

Spinal fluid findings confirm the diagnosis. The fluid appears cloudy and purulent, and the pressure is increased. The cell count is high in **lymphocytes** and **polymorphonuclear leukocytes.** The protein content of the spinal fluid markedly rises, whereas the sugar drops. An excessively high protein content is usually associated with **ventricular blockage** and signals a fatal outcome.

Smear and culture findings generally indicate that the bacterial invaders causing the ear infection are the same as those of the otogenic complication in the brain.

Streptococcus pyogenes and *Diplococcus pneumoniae* are the common etiologic agents of diffuse purulent meningitis, whereas *Neisseria meningitidis,* a very pyogenic diplococcus, provokes epidemic cerebrospinal meningitis.

The treatment of meningitis consists of intravenous antibiotic therapy and adequate drainage of the suppurative focus in the ear. Monitoring the cerebral spinal fluid is important to ensure the adequacy of the antibiotic therapy. Progress may be monitored by periodic lumbar puncture. Once the disease has developed, vigorous treatment must be instituted to combat the infection, prevent ventricular blocking, and maintain electrolyte balance and nutrition. Surgical intervention is limited to the rapid eradication of the ear infection and any additional intracranial complications requiring surgery. (9, 17, 18, 22, 28, 33, 39, 42)

Table 19
Some Ear Conditions Amenable to Surgery

Organs Involved	Diagnosis	Type of Surgery	Operative Procedures
Ear	Carcinoma of ear	Amputation of ear Otoplasty	Removal of ear Plastic repair of ear
External auditory meatus	Foreign body in external auditory meatus Papilloma	Otoscopy with removal of foreign body Excision of papilloma	Endoscopic examination of external auditory meatus for removal of foreign body or lesion
Middle ear	Otitis media, acute serous	Paracentesis tympani Myringotomy	Puncture of eardrum and evacuation of fluid from middle ear Incision of eardrum and drainage of middle ear
Middle ear	Perforation of eardrum, chronic	Myringoplasty	Reconstruction of eardrum
Middle ear Mastoid	Otitis media, acute Mastoiditis, acute	Complete mastoidectomy	Scooping out and obliterating infected air cells Removal of diseased mastoid process
Middle ear Mastoid	Otitis media, chronic suppurative Mastoiditis, chronic suppurative or recurrent	Radical mastoidectomy or modified radical mastoidectomy Repair of middle ear Tympanoplasty	Endaural approach to temporal bone and thorough removal of diseased tissues Surgical creation of new cavity composed of healthy mastoid tissue, tympanum, and external auditory canal
Mastoid	Mastoiditis, chronic perforation of pars tensa	Tympanoplasty with or without mastoidectomy	Closure of perforation by skin graft or vein or fascia or perichondrium

Organs Involved	Diagnosis	Type of Surgery	Operative Procedures
Middle ear	Otosclerosis, conductive deafness with fixation of stapes	Stapedectomy Stapedioplasty	Removal of stapes Insertion of delicate prosthesis to replace stapes
Middle ear Tympanum Mastoid	Tympano-mastoiditis Cholesteatoma	Tympano-mastoidectomy Tympanoplasty	Postauricular incison Removal of necrotic incus Malleus and stapes freed by dissection, tympano-sclerosis removed Complete enucleation of diseased mastoid Fascial graft placed on canal wall Tympanomeatal flap positioned and secured with Gelfoam and Silastic sponge
Internal ear	Menière's disease unilateral bilateral	Labyrinthectomy Exenteration of air cells Avulsion of endolymphatic labyrinth Ultrasonic surgery	Endaural or postaural approach to inner ear Removal of air cells Destruction of membranous labyrinth Selective destruction of osseous vestibular labyrinth by ultrasonic waves, avoiding bombardment of cochlea
Vestibulo-cochlear nerve	Acoustic neuroma	Excision of neoplasm	Removal of neoplasm that involved some area of neural passageway of hearing

References and Bibliography

1. Abel, Sharon M. Acoustics and psycho-acoustics. In Alberti, P.W., and Ruben, R.J., eds., *Otologic Medicine and Surgery,* vol. 1. New York: Churchill Livingstone, Inc., 1988, pp. 201-221.

2. Abramson, Maxwell, et al. The natural history of cholesteatoma. In Alberti, P.W., and Ruben, R.J., eds., *Otologic Medicine and Surgery,* vol. 1. New York: Churchill Livingstone, Inc., 1988, pp. 803-811.

3. Bauer, Bruce S. Management and therapy of congenital malformations and traumatic deformities of the pinna. In Alberti, P.W., and Ruben, R.J., eds., *Otologic Medicine and Surgery,* vol. 2. New York: Churchill Livingstone, Inc., 1988, pp. 1025-1072.

4. Bluestone, Charles D. Management and therapy of otitis media. In Alberti, P.W., and Ruben, R.J., eds., *Otologic Medicine and Surgery,* vol. 2. New York: Churchill Livingstone, Inc., 1988, pp. 1173-1201.

5. Bodurtha, Joann, and Nance, Walter E. Genetics of hearing loss. In Alberti, P.W., and Ruben, R.J., eds., *Otologic Medicine and Surgery,* vol. 1. New York: Churchill Livingstone, Inc., 1988, pp. 831-853.

6. Chole, Richard A., et al. Rinne test for conductive deafness. *Archives of Otolaryngology—Head & Neck Surgery* 114:399-403, April 1988.

7. DeWeese, David D., et al. Anatomy and physiology. In *Otolaryngology—Head and Neck Surgery,* 7th ed. St. Louis: The C.V. Mosby Co., 1988, pp. 347-369.

8. ———. Special diagnostic procedures in treating for hearing. Ibid., pp. 371-390.

9. ———. Infection and inflammation of the ear. Ibid., pp. 395-425.

10. ———. Trauma to the external ear. Ibid., pp. 427-432.

11. ———. Tumors. Ibid., pp. 433-444.

12. ———. Hearing loss. Ibid., pp. 445-477.

13. ———. Tinnitus. Ibid., pp. 479-482.

14. ———. Dizziness and vertigo. Ibid., pp. 483-501.

15. ———. The facial nerve. Ibid., pp. 503-517.

16. Eviatar, Abraham. Stapes surgery. In Alberti, P.W., and Ruben, R.J., eds., *Otologic Medicine and Surgery,* vol. 2. New York: Churchill Livingstone, Inc., 1988, pp. 1261-1275.

17. Ford, Regina Daley, ed. Additional body fluid testing. In *Diagnostic Tests Handbook,* Springhouse, PA: Springhouse Corporation, 1987, pp. 279-312.

18. ———. Diagnostic tests profiles for common disorders. Ibid., pp. 321-385.

19. Friberg, Ulla, et al. Variations in surgical anatomy of the endolymphatic sac. *Archives of Otolaryngology—Head & Neck Surgery* 114:389-394, April 1988.

20. Gibson, W.P.R. Vestibular diagnostic tests. In Alberti, P.W., and Ruben, R.J., eds., *Otologic Medicine and Surgery,* vol. 1. New York: Churchill Livingstone, Inc., 1988, pp. 487-505.

21. Gristwood, Ronald E. Otosclerosis (otospongiosis): General considerations. In Alberti, P.W., and Ruben, R.J., eds., *Otologic Medicine and Surgery,* vol. 1. New York: Churchill Livingstone, Inc., 1988, pp. 911-941.

22. Harter, Donald H., and Petersdorf, Robert G. Pyogenic infections of the central nervous system. In Braunwald, Eugene, et al., eds., *Harrison's Principles of Internal Medicine,* 11th ed. New York: McGraw-Hill Book Co., 1987, pp. 1980-1987.

23. Hazell, Jonathan W.P. Tinnitus. In Alberti, P.W., and Ruben, R.J., eds., *Otologic Medicine and Surgery,* vol. 2. New York: Churchill Livingstone, Inc., 1988, pp. 1605-1622.

24. Hyde, Martyn L. Auditory evoked potentials. In Alberti, P.W., and Ruben, R.J., eds., *Otologic Medicine and Surgery,* vol. 1. New York: Churchill Livingstone, Inc., 1988, pp. 443-485.

25. Jackler, Robert K., and Kaplan, Michael J. Ear, nose & throat. In Schroeder, Steven A.,

Krupp, Marcus A., and Tierney, Lawrence M., Jr. eds., *Current Medical Diagnosis & Treatment—1988,* Norwalk, CT: Appleton & Lange, 1988, pp. 110-131.

26. Kinney, Sam E. Surgical techniques for mastoidectomy. In Alberti, P.W., and Ruben, R.J., eds., *Otologic Medicine and Surgery,* vol. 2. New York: Churchill Livingstone, Inc., 1988, pp. 1319-1340.

27. Kruger, Barbara. Basic audiologic evaluation. In Alberti, P.W., and Ruben, R.J., eds., *Otologic Medicine and Surgery,* vol. 1. New York: Churchill Livingstone, Inc., 1988, pp. 365-395.

28. Lambert, Paul R. Meningitis and facial paresis. *Archives of Otolaryngology—Head & Neck Surgery* 113:1101-1103, Oct. 1987.

29. Lucente, Frank, et al. Diseases of the external ear. In Alberti, P.W., and Ruben, R.J., eds., *Otologic Medicine and Surgery,* vol. 2. New York: Churchill Livingstone, Inc., 1988, pp. 1073-1092.

30. Magnuson, Bengt, and Falk, Bernt. Eustachian tube malfunction in middle ear disease. In Alberti, P.W., and Ruben, R.J., eds., *Otologic Medicine and Surgery,* vol. 2. New York: Churchill Livingstone, Inc., 1988, pp. 1153-1171.

31. Michelson, Robin P. Cochlear implants. In Alberti, P.W., and Ruben, R.J., eds., *Otologic Medicine and Surgery,* vol. 2. New York: Churchill Livingstone, Inc., 1988, pp. 1719-1737.

32. Morrison, W.V., and Anand, V.K. Ear, nose, paranasal sinuses, pharynx, and larynx. Hardy, James D., ed., *Hardy's Textbook of Surgery,* 2d ed. Philadelphia: J.B. Lippincott Co., 1988, pp. 283-312.

33. Neely, J. Gail. Complications of temporal bone infection. In Harker, Lee A., ed., *Otolaryngology—Head and Neck Surgery,* vol. 4. St. Louis: The C.V. Mosby Co., 1986, pp. 2998-3015.

34. O'Leary, Dennis P. Physiology of the vestibular system. In Alberti, P.W., and Ruben, R.J., eds., *Otologic Medicine and Surgery,* vol. 1. New York: Churchill Livingstone, Inc., 1988, pp. 223-251.

35. Parving, Agnete, and Salomon, Gerhard. Detection of the hearing-impaired infant and child. In Alberti, P.W., and Ruben, R.J., eds., *Otologic Medicine and Surgery,* vol. 2. New York: Churchill Livingstone, Inc., 1988, pp. 1653-1663.

36. Pfaltz, C.R. Sudden and fluctuant hearing loss. In Alberti, P.W., and Ruben, R.J., eds., *Otologic Medicine and Surgery,* vol. 2. New York: Churchill Livingstone, Inc., 1988, pp. 1577-1603.

37. Ruben, Robert J. Management and therapy of congenital malformations of the external and middle ears. In Alberti, P.W., and

Ruben, R.J., eds., *Otologic Medicine and Surgery,* vol. 2. New York: Churchill Livingstone, Inc., 1988, pp. 1135-1151.

38. Sheehy, James L. Cholesteatoma surgery: Canal wall down procedures. *Annals of Otology, Rhinology & Laryngology* 97:30-35, Jan.-Feb. 1988.

39. Smith, Richard J.H. Medical diagnosis and treatment of hearing loss in children. In Harker, Lee A., ed., *Otolaryngology—Head and Neck Surgery,* vol. 4. St. Louis: The C.V. Mosby Co., 1986, pp. 3225-3246.

40. Smyth, Gordon D.L. Surgical techniques of tympanoplasty. In Alberti, P.W., and Ruben, R.J., eds., *Otologic Medicine and Surgery,* vol. 2. New York: Churchill Livingstone, Inc., 1988, pp. 1277-1297.

41. ———. The management of cholesteatoma. Ibid., pp. 1341-1362.

42. Swartz, Morton N. Bacterial meningitis—meningococcal disease—infections caused by hemophilus species. In Wyngaarden, James B., and Smith, Lloyd H., eds., *Cecil's Textbook of Medicine,* 18th ed. Philadelphia: W.B. Saunders Co., 1988, pp. 1604-1621.

43. Thomsen, Jens. Surgical management of vestibular disorders. In Alberti, P.W., and Ruben, R.J., eds., *Otologic Medicine and Surgery,* vol. 2. New York: Churchill Livingstone, Inc., 1988, pp. 1535-1559.

44. Tos, Mirko. Tympanomastoiditis: Management and treatment. In Alberti, P.W., and Ruben, R.J., eds., *Otologic Medicine and Surgery,* vol. 2. New York: Churchill Livingstone, Inc., 1988, pp. 1203-1239.

45. Wilber, Laura Ann. Acoustic impedance and auditory reflexes. In Alberti, P.W., and Ruben, R.J., eds., *Otologic Medicine and Surgery,* vol. 1. New York: Churchill Livingstone, Inc., 1988, pp. 347-413.

46. Woodburne, Russell T., and Burkel, William E. The head and neck. In *Essentials of Human Anatomy,* 8th ed. New York: Oxford University Press, 1988, pp. 179-323.

Multisystem Disorders

Infectious Diseases

Origin of Terms

ameba- (G) — change
bacillus (L) — rod
coccus (G) — berry
gono- (G) — seed
helminth (G) — worm
lympho- (L) — lymph, lymphoid tissue
myco- (G) — fungus
proto- (G) — first

pseudopod (G) — false foot
sapro- (G) — rotten
strepto- (G) — curved, twisted
tricho- (G) — hair
vector (L) — carrier
virus (L) — poison
zoster (G) — girdle

General Terms

- *acid-fast bacilli* — organisms that resist acid-alcohol decolorization after they have been stained with a special dye (carbofuchsin). (Ref. 81)
- *aerobes* — organisms requiring oxygen for growth. (68)
- *agglutination* — clumping of bacteria (or blood cells) following mixture with antisera. (42)
- *allergen* — substance capable of bringing about a hypersensitive state when introduced into the body.
- *allergy* — state of hypersensitivity in which a person experiences certain symptoms when coming in contact with an allergen.
- *anaerobes* — organisms capable of growing in the absence of atmospheric oxygen. (50, 68)
- *antiseptic* — substance that prevents bacterial growth.
- *antitoxin* — immune serum that prevents the deleterious action of a toxin.
- *bacterium (pl. bacteria)* — "little rod"; in general, any of the unicellular prokaryotic microorganisms that commonly multiply by cell division (fission) and whose cell is typically contained within a cell wall. The bacteria may be aerobic, anaerobic, phytic, parasitic, or pathogenic. (68)
- *contagious* — communicable.
- *culture medium* — a milieu that promotes the growth of bacteria. (81)
- *direct contact* — spread of disease from person to person.

- *exudate*—fluid or blood elements that have escaped into body cavities or tissues.
- *fungus (pl. fungi)*—a vegetable, unicellular organism that feeds on organic matter. (56)
- *gram-negative*—pertaining to bacteria that do not retain Gram's stain (an iodine-crystal violet complex). (81, 104)
- *gram-positive*—pertaining to bacteria that retain Gram's stain after suitable decolorization. (81)
- *immunity*—resistance to disease, either natural or acquired. (13)
- *inoculation*—the process of introducing pathogenic organisms.
- *microorganism*—plant or animal only recognized under microscopic vision.
- *molds*—plants belonging to a division of organisms known as fungi.
- *multisystem disorder*—any disease with involvement of many systems; it need not have an immunologic basis. Examples are infections, connective tissue disorders, or metabolic diseases.
- *mycology*—the study or science of fungi. (19, 22)
- *neutralization*—process by which antibody or antibody complement neutralizes the infectivity of microorganisms. (22)
- *nosocomial infections*—hospital-acquired infections usually occurring in patients with defective host resistance or in recipients of cytotoxic drugs for malignancies or of organ transplants treated with immunosuppressive therapy. Infective agents may be *Aspergillus, Candida, Nocardia, Pneumocystis carinii,* cytomegalovirus, and other pathogenic or opportunistic microorganisms. (22, 27, 41)
- *nosology*—the science or study of disease classification.
- *nucleus*—functional center of a cell.
- *opportunistic infection*—refers to those pathogens that produce disease through some defect or group of defects in the ability of the host to defend against and destroy the potential invader. A member of the normal flora, usually regarded as harmless in a specific location, may produce disease if introduced to another part of the body or if predisposing factors such as neoplasm, trauma, or immunosuppressive antibiotic therapy are present. *Candida* is an example of an opportunistic pathogen. While part of the normal flora of the mouth, skin, vagina, and pharynx, when *Candida* is exposed to broad-spectrum antibiotic therapy or corticosteroid or other immunosuppressive chemotherapy, it may cause clinically significant local infection involving the mouth, skin, vagina, pharynx, or esophagus. In the setting of an infected intravascular catheter, marked granulocytopenia, or certain postoperative states, it may invade the bloodstream and produce disseminated systemic disease. (21, 22, 23)
- *parasite*—plant or animal that lives within or on another and derives nourishment from its host. Medical parasitology studies parasites in human beings, their life cycle in their hosts, pathogenic effect, prevention, and control. It deals with two major phyla:
  - *Metazoa*—multicellular parasites, for example:
    - *helminthic infection*—infestation by worms.
    - *platyhelminthic infection*—infestation by flatworms: tapeworms or flukes.
    - *polyhelminthism*—infestation by several species of worms. (90, 91, 92)
  - *Protozoa*—unicellular parasites, for example:
    - *Leishmania donovani*—etiologic agent of visceral leishmaniasis or kala-azar, causing splenomegaly, bleeding, edema, and emaciation. (25, 73)
    - *Trypanosoma*—protozoal parasites causing sleeping sickness in Africa and Chagas' disease in America. The latter, affecting primarily children, is characterized by intermittent parasitemia, fever, acute lymphadenitis, and eyelid edema. (25, 82, 84)

- *pathogenic*—disease producing.
- *putrefaction*—decomposition of organic material.
- *pyogenic*—pus forming.
- *saprophyte*—an organism that grows on dead matter.
- *sensitivity (drug related)*—ability of infective organism to respond to the bacteriostatic or bacteriocidal action of an antibiotic or other agent.
- *susceptibility*—ability to acquire an infection following exposure to pathogenic organisms.
- *taxonomy*—the classification of organisms of the plant or animal kingdom, including the following categories: phyla, classes, orders, families, genera, species, and varieties. The scientific names of organisms are binomial, composed of a genus, which is capitalized, and a species, which is given in small letters.
    - —*genus (pl. genera)*—the division between family and species.
    - —*species*—the division between genus and variety. (103)
- *virus (pl. viruses)*—infectious agent of protein-coated nucleic acid, either ribonucleic acid (RNA) or deoxyribonucleic acid (DNA), and submicroscopic size, depending completely on the cells of its host and insusceptible to common antibiotics. (58)
- *yeast*—unicellular organism that usually reproduces by budding. (56)

Terms Pertaining to Infections Caused by Viruses

- *adenoviral infections*—31 serotypes of DNA-bearing adenovirus, transmitted by person-to-person contact and capable of latency in lymphoid tissue. (60) Adenoviruses may cause epidemic outbreaks of
    - —*febrile pharyngitis*—inflammation of pharynx with exudate, enlarged cervical lymph nodes, and fever. (39, 115)
    - —*keratoconjunctivitis, epidemic*—serious eye infection with corneal infiltrates and follicular conjunctival lesions. Associated symptoms that may be present include headache and/or swelling of regional lymph nodes. (108)
    - —*pharyngoconjunctival fever*—severe type of pharyngitis associated with acute follicular conjunctivitis, usually lasting five days. (6)
    - —*pneumonia, adenoviral*—highly fatal bronchopneumonia in infants, with sore throat, cough, prostration, and high fever. (36)
- *arboviral infections*—arthropod-borne viral infections that are usually transmitted to human beings by the bite of a blood-sucking (hemaphagous) insect. The viruses multiply in susceptible arthropods without producing the disease. The arthropod vector acquires a lifelong infection by ingesting vertebrate blood from a viremic host and maintains a complex vertebrate-arthropod-vertebrate cycle. (103)
- *arbovirus encephalitides*—various types of encephalitis, each having a specific host and viral vector according to its geographic distribution. Those prevalent in the Americas are:
    - —*eastern equine encephalitis (EEE)*—in eastern and southern United States.
    - —*St. Louis encephalitis (SLE)*—in nearly all the United States.
    - —*Venezuelan equine encephalitis (VEE)*—in Central and South America and southern United States.
    - —*western equine encephalitis (WEE)*—chiefly in Canada and western United States. The encephalitogenic arbovirus attacks the neural tissues of the central nervous system, especially those of the brain, the cerebral cortex, meninges, cerebellum, neurons, and supportive structures. (103)
- *chickenpox, varicella*—acute varicella-zoster virus infection, characterized by sudden onset, fever, and skin eruption. It is highly infectious. The prognosis is good. (66, 116)

- *cytomegalovirus infections (CMV)*—common viral infection occurring congenitally or in acquired forms in the newborn, child, or adult, with or without symptoms, as local or systemic disorders. Infected cells are oversized and contain intranuclear and cytoplasmic inclusion bodies. Diagnosis is made serologically or by culturing white blood cells or urine.

    —*acute acquired cytomegalovirus disease (CMV infectious mononucleosis)*—similar clinical picture as that of infectious (Epstein-Barr virus) mononucleosis. There is fever, malaise, muscle and joint pains, enlarged liver, and generalized lymphadenopathy. This disorder can occur spontaneously or after transfusions of fresh blood during surgery (postperfusion syndrome).

    —*congenital cytomegalic inclusion disease*—infection developing in utero and primarily affecting premature infants. Lungs, kidneys, liver, spleen, pancreas, thymus, adenoids, parotid glands, and other organs are infiltrated by viral foci in the fatal form of the disease in the neonate.

    —*cytomegalic inclusion disease in the immunosuppressed host*—system disorder in immunocompromised persons whereby the cytomegalovirus can cause a severe opportunistic pneumonia. Individuals with acquired immune deficiency syndrome (AIDS) often are susceptible to severe infections with cytomegalovirus, including retinitis, enterocolitis, and pneumonitis. Other persons who may develop cytomegalovirus pneumonitis or hepatitis and occasionally generalized disease include those with malignancies or immunologic defects or those receiving immunosuppressive therapy for organ transplantation. (22, 34, 66, 105)

- *German measles, rubella*—mildly contagious disease with catarrhal symptoms and a rash resembling measles. (64, 98)

- *herpes simplex, herpes febrilis, fever blisters*—acute infectious condition of the skin or oral or genital mucous membranes, marked by vesicular lesions that may become secondarily infected. After a primary infection, latency usually is established and may lead to recurrences. (11, 22, 66)

- *herpes zoster*—recurrent varicella-zoster virus infection affecting primarily one or more dorsal root ganglia or extramedullary cranial nerve ganglia. It is characterized by a vesicular eruption in the affected ganglia. Contact with vesicular fluid can cause chickenpox in a nonimmune person. (66, 116)

- *infectious mononucleosis*—usually a benign infection caused by Epstein-Barr virus. It exhibits a characteristic lymphocytosis and irregular clinical pattern. Glandular swelling (lymph node enlargement), throat symptoms, fever, and splenomegaly are common manifestations. The disease occurs chiefly in adolescents and young adults. (5, 7, 59, 105)

- *influenza*—acute febrile disease caused by influenza virus A, B, or C. It is generally characterized by prostration, muscle ache, joint pains, and respiratory symptoms. It may occur in epidemic or even pandemic form. (18, 63)

- *measles, rubeola*—highly communicable disease; clinically manifested by Koplik's spots of the buccal mucosa (small, irregular, bright red spots on the buccal and lingual mucosa, with a very small, bluish white speck in the center of each); a rash; and catarrhal symptoms. (64, 97)

- *mumps, infectious parotitis*—virus disease of the salivary glands, which tend to involve other organs, especially the testes and ovaries. (64, 101)

- *rabies, hydrophobia*—acute encephalitis that causes paralysis, delirium, convulsions, and death. (12)

- *Reye's syndrome*—neurologic disease that develops subsequent to mild or acute viral illness and is often related to an epidemic of influenza B or chickenpox.

Manifestations include pernicious vomiting, agitated delirium, and in fatal cases cytotoxic (intracellular) cerebral edema and decerebrate coma. Highly increased serum enzyme and ammonia levels reflect liver damage and impending death. (22, 40)

- *smallpox, variola*—communicable disease characterized by a rash that changes from macules, papules, vesicles, and pustules to scabs. Vigorous control efforts by the World Health Organization appear to have eradicated this disease. (22, 90)
- *viral hepatitis, acute*—disease associated with jaundice, liver damage resulting from hepatic cell necrosis, followed by hepatomegaly, splenomegaly, and virema. Several forms, immunologically distinct but clinically similar, are recognized:
  - *hepatitis A*—incubation period 15 to 20 days, infective agent is hepatitis A virus (HAV), transmitted orally or parenterally. Virus present in feces. Early symptoms are cough, pharyngitis, and muscle pains.
  - *hepatitis B*—incubation period 50 to 80 days, infective agent is hepatitis B virus (HBV), transmitted parenterally. Virus rarely found in feces. A circulating antigen, HBsAg, is present in the early phase of hepatitis B and in chronic carriers.
  - *hepatitis D* (delta-agent)—the delta agent hepatitis D virus (HDV) is a defective RNA virus which coinfects and requires the presence and helper function of HBV for its infection of the host cell. Because the delta agent relies on HBV for its expression and replication, the duration of the delta infection is determined by the duration of and cannot outlast the HBV infection.
  - *hepatitis non-A, and non-B* (NANBH)—clinically similar to hepatitis B. This entity represents the majority of transfusion-associated hepatitis cases in the United States. NANBH is a term to describe viral hepatitis not due to either HAV or HBV. Two identified forms of NANBH are:
    - epidemic type transmitted enterically
    - parenterally transmitted form caused by hepatitis C virus (HCV)
  - *hepatitis C*—a cloned genome of NANBH agent, designated the hepatitis C virus (HCV). HCV appears to be the major cause of chronic NANBH throughout the world. Research keys such as the recombinant-based assay for detection of HCV antibodies combined with the availability of HCV hybridization probes will unlock opportunities for future research of the issue of whether other parenteral NANBH agents exist. (17, 22, 62, 72, 114)
- *viral hepatitis, chronic active*—long-term infection characterized by progressive destruction of liver cells and fibrotic changes followed by terminal cirrhosis. (113)

Terms Pertaining to Infections Caused by Chlamydiae

- *chlamydiae (sing. chlamydia)*—nonmotile, gram-negative bacteria, restricted to an intracellular parasitic existence. Two species are:
  - *C. psittaci*—species that produces diffuse intracytoplasmic inclusions that lack glycogen. It is inhibited by sulfonamides.
  - *C. trachomatis*—species that produces compact intracytoplasmic inclusions that contain glycogen. It is inhibited by sulfonamides. (22, 55, 109)
- *psittacosis, ornithosis, parrot fever*—infectious disease characterized by variable symptoms, mild to acute fever, headache, lung involvement, cough, delirium, prostration, and even death. Psittacosis is a disease of birds that may be transmitted to humans. In humans, the agent *C. psittaci* produces a wide range of clinical manifestations ranging from severe pneumonia and sepsis with a high mortality to that of a very mild infection. Tetracyclines are the drug of choice to inhibit growth or extension of the disease. (22, 29, 109)

- *trachoma and inclusion conjunctivitis (TRIC)*—chronic infectious diseases of the conjunctiva that may be associated with infections of the urogenital tract. The etiologic agents, chlamydiae, are transmitted by human contact or flies. If left untreated, TRIC infections persist for years and produce corneal scarring and blindness. (29, 37, 109)

Terms Pertaining to Infections Caused by Sexually Transmitted Diseases

- *acquired immunodeficiency syndrome (AIDS)*—probably the most dramatic occurrence of an infectious sexually transmitted disease in this century. The causative agent is a retrovirus called human immunodeficiency virus (HIV). The virus is transmitted through intimate sexual contact. The HIV infection appears to ultimately result in the almost total collapse of the body's cell-mediated immune system, leaving the person susceptible to malignancies (Kaposi's sarcoma) and opportunistic infections (*Pneumocystis carinii* pneumonia), against which the body is unable to defend itself. See the AIDS definition, p. 357 for further information regarding this disease. (10, 21, 22, 27, 41, 67, 107)

- *gonorrhea*—sexually transmitted infection that usually begins in the urethra and attacks the genital mucosa membrane. The infection also may affect the conjunctiva and joints. The etiologic agent is *Neisseria gonorrhoeae* (gonococcus). The primary symptoms in males during acute infection include dysuria, urethritis, and a purulent discharge. Symptoms in females include endocervical infection, which extends to the urethra and vagina. Mucopurulent discharge is present and the infection may progress to the uterine tubes. A serious complication of gonorrhea is pelvic inflammatory disease (PID). (22, 49, 107)

- *granuloma inguinale*—a progressive granulomatous disease of the skin and mucosa. The causative agent is an intracellular gram-negative bacillus. *Calymmatobacterium granulomatis* (also called Donovan bodies, when identified within the histiocytes of a typical lesion). It is transmitted mainly through sexual contact. The primary lesion of granuloma inguinale presents as a red granulated ulcer tissue, which readily bleeds on contact. The primary lesion involves the genital and/or perianal areas and may occur as single or multiple lesions. (50, 107)

- *herpes simplex genital infection*—Type II herpes simplex virus (HSV II) is the causative agent of herpes simplex. It infects the genital area in both men and women. Infection is contracted from a person who is shedding viral particles at the time of intercourse. Pain, vaginal, penile, or urethral lesions occur in most cases. (11, 22, 66, 116)

- *lymphogranuloma venereum (LGV)*—*Chlamydia trachomatis* serotypes L-1, L-2, and L-3 can cause this sexually transmitted disease. The primary lesion of LGV may appear as either a papule, small ulcer, or as a herpes-type lesion. The most frequent symptom is progressive lymphadenopathy. In its advanced course, the disease exhibits systemic manifestations such as fever, skin rashes, gastric upset, back pain, headache, and meningeal irritation. (22, 29, 55, 107, 109)

- *syphilis*—*Treponema pallidum* is the causative agent of syphilis. Sexual contact accounts for almost all syphilitic infections. Syphilis is an infectious, relapsing disease characterized by primary lesion or hard chancre. It is followed by a secondary skin eruption with typical reddish brown, coppery spots; periods of latency; and later lesions in the central nervous system and cardiovascular systems. A transient nephrotic syndrome also may occur in some cases. (22, 30, 38, 53, 107)

- *trichomoniasis*—venereal infection caused by a flagellate protozoan, *Trichomonas vaginalis*. In the female, trichomoniasis usually is manifested by a persistent vaginitis. The characteristic finding on vaginal examination is the strawberry appearance of the vaginal mucosa and the portio vaginalis of the cervix due to the marked congestion and petechial hemorrhages present. Patients may experience vulvovaginitis, urethritis, cystitis, cervicitis, and infections in the Skene's ducts and the Bartholin's gland. (22, 88, 109)

- *urethritis, salpingitis, and pelvic inflammatory diseases*—these diseases represent common sexually transmitted diseases, which may be caused by *Chlamydia trachomatis.* (29, 37, 107, 109)
- *vulvovaginitis candidiasis*—the causative agents of this vulvovaginal infection can be either *Candida albicans* or *Candida glabrata.* The most frequent clinical finding is vulvar pruritus. Vaginal discharge is usually minimal and may resemble cottage cheese or have a watery consistency. Also present may be vaginal soreness, dyspareunia, dysuria, and erythema and swelling of the labia and vulva. (22, 29, 37, 107, 109)

Terms Pertaining to Infections Caused by Pathogens of the Family Legionellaceae

- *legionnaires' disease*—respiratory disease occurring in sporadic and epidemic outbreaks and in mild and fulminant form. Its etiologic agent is *Legionella pneumophila,* the legionnaires' disease bacterium (LDB), and other related bacteria, probably inhaled in droplets from contaminated water-cooled air-conditioning towers or dust. In mild cases malaise, chills, fever, cough, sputum, diarrhea, and joint and muscle pains gradually subside. In the fulminant type these symptoms rapidly increase in severity. A widespread pneumonia develops and is associated with shaking, chills, hypoxia, pleuritic pain, delirium, a deepening coma, and death. Nosocomial outbreaks in immunosuppressed patients have been reported. Other bacteria of the *Legionella* family may include:
    - *flurobacter species*—three *Legionella*-like pathogens showing blue-white fluorescence in the presence of long-wave ultraviolet light.
    - *Tatlockia micdadei*—blue-gray organisms causing legionnaires' disease.
    - *Pittsburgh pneumonia*—condition initiated by Pittsburgh pneumonia agent (PPA) and prevalent in patients on immunosuppressive therapy. The Pittsburgh pneumonia agent is a bacterium phenotypically similar to *Legionella pneumophila* and identical to tatlock bacteria. (3, 22, 36, 50)

Terms Pertaining to Infections Caused by Mycoplasmas

- *mycoplasmas*—pathogenic bacteria without cell walls that may cause infections of the respiratory and urogenital tract. They were formerly known as pleuropneumonia-like organisms (PPLO).
- *mycoplasma pneumonia, primary atypical pneumonia*—a pneumonitis that may range from asymptomatic to serious lung disease. It is clinically manifested by an insidious onset, headache, malaise, fever, severe cough, and sore throat. (9, 22, 36, 51)

Terms Pertaining to Infections Caused by Rickettsiae

- *spotted fever group:*
    - *rickettsialpox*—benign, self-limited disease that develops from *Rickettsia akari* and is transmitted from the house mouse to human beings by mites. Its clinical manifestations are a papulovesicular skin eruption, chills, fever, headache, and aching muscles.
    - *Rocky Mountain spotted fever*—acute febrile disease from *Rickettsia rickettsii* infection, usually transmitted to human beings by infected ticks and clinically manifested by an abrupt onset with chills, high fever, delirium, excruciating headache, and atypical rash on extremities and trunk and progressing to shock, kidney failure, and frequently death. (28, 54, 117)

- *typhus group:*
  —*endemic murine typhus*—acute fever caused by *Rickettsia typhi (R. mooseri)* infection, transmitted to human beings by fleas and clinically manifested by fever lasting about two weeks, a rash, and muscle pain.
  —*epidemic louse-borne typhus*—acute febrile illness due to *Rickettsia prowazekii*, transmitted to human beings by body lice *(Pediculus humanus corporis).*
  —*recrudescent typhus, Brill-Zinsser disease*—recurrent epidemic typhus that develops years after recovery from epidemic typhus, has a similar rash, similar liver, kidney, and neural manifestations, and the same etiologic agent, *Rickettsia prowazekii.* (28, 54, 117)
- *other rickettsial groups:*
  —*Q fever ("Q" for query)*—severe febrile illness caused by *Coxiella burnetii* living in ticks. They infect cattle, sheep, and goats and are transmitted to human beings by the inhalation, ingestion, or rarely by the transfusion of contaminated air, milk, meat, or blood. Headache, fever, chills, malaise, anorexia, and aching muscles are common symptoms. There is no transmission of the infection between human beings. (28, 54, 115)
  —*trench fever, quintan fever, shin bone fever, His-Werner disease, Volhynia fever*—illness caused by *Rickettsia quintana* found extracellularly in the gut of lice and transmitted to human beings by infected feces rubbed on broken skin or conjunctiva. The clinical course of trench fever ranges from afebrile to severely debilitating disease, manifesting in its acute form headache, fever, malaise, bone pain, muscle soreness, and macular skin eruption. Relapses are common. (28, 54, 117)

Terms Relating to Infections Caused by Cocci

- *erysipelas*—acute febrile, inflammatory disease marked by localized skin lesions that tend to migrate. The infection is caused by the *Streptococcus pyogenes.* (6, 50)
- *furunculosis*—condition resulting from boils, generally caused by *Staphylococcus aureus.* (73)
- *gonorrhea*—sexually transmitted infection that usually begins in the urethra and attacks the genital mucous membrane. The infection may also affect the conjunctiva and joints. The etiologic agent is *Neisseria gonorrhoeae* (gonococcus). (22, 49, 107)
- *meningitis*—inflammation of meninges. The epidemic form is caused by *Neisseria meningitidis.* (29)
- *staphylococcal food intoxication*—food poisoning caused by staphylococci and associated with more or less violent and abrupt onset of nausea, vomiting, and prostration. Severe diarrhea may occur. (8)
- *toxic shock syndrome (TSS)*—severe multisystem illness with sudden onset of high fever, vomiting, diarrhea, and myalgia. An erythematous (sunburnlike) rash is noted during the acute phase of the illness. Hypotension with cardiac and renal failure occur in the most severe cases. TSS frequently occurs within four to five days of the onset of menses in young women who use tampons. Toxic shock syndrome-associated *Staphylococcus aureus* has been found in the vagina and on tampons. Most *Staphylococcus aureus* strains isolated from individuals with toxic shock syndrome produce a toxin called toxic shock syndrome toxin 1 (TSST-1). This toxin is associated with fever, shock, and multisystem involvement. Prolonged use of certain brands of hyperabsorbent tampons linked with the capacity of these materials to bind magnesium have increased the growth of intravaginal *S. aureus* and TSST-1 production. Removal of the hyperabsorbent tampons from the market and public

education concerning this disorder have decreased the number of TSS cases reported in the United States. (29, 46, 73)

Terms Pertaining to Infections Caused by Bacilli

- *bacillary dysentery, shigellosis*—acute infection marked by diarrhea, tenesmus, fever, and in severe cases mucus and blood in the stool. Prognosis tends to be serious in infants and debilitated elderly persons. The disease is caused by various species of *Shigella*. (48, 79)
- *diphtheria*—acute infection, generally associated with fever and the formation of a grayish membrane in the throat, from which the Klebs-Loeffler bacillus *(Corynebacterium diphtheriae)* can be cultured. (29)
- *food poisoning*—disease characterized by an abrupt onset of gastrointestinal symptoms caused by food intoxication or infection.
    - *—botulism*—afebrile condition, marked by weakness, constipation, headache, and forms of paralysis, may be fatal. The intoxication results from the botulinus bacillus *(Clostridium botulinum)* toxin. (2)
    - *—Salmonella infection, salmonellosis*—condition causing typhoid and paratyphoid fevers. (31)
- *septic shock*—manifested by inadequate tissue perfusion, following bacteremia most often with gram-negative enteric bacilli. Septic shock also may be associated with gram-positive infections. Usually these result from *Staphylococcus*, *Pneumococcus*, and *Streptococcus*. Other frequent etiologic organisms include *Escherichia coli*, *Klebsiella-Enterobacter*, *Proteus*, *Pseudomonas*, and *Serratia*. The circulatory insufficiency is caused by diffuse cell and tissue injury and the pooling of blood in microcirculation. Hypotension, oliguria, tachycardia, and tachypnea occur in most cases. Respiratory failure is the primary cause of death in patients with septic shock. (15)
- *undulant fever, brucellosis*—general infection characterized by intermittent or continuous fever, headache, chills, and profuse perspiration. The etiologic agents are three species of *Brucella*. (29, 70)

Terms Pertaining to Infections Caused by Actinomycetes

- *actinomycetes*—a heterogeneous group of filamentous bacteria related to the corynebacteria and mycobacteria. Actinomycetes superficially resemble fungi. They usually grow as gram-positive, branching organisms that fragment into bacteria-like pieces. Most are free living in soil; however some are acid-fast. The anaerobic species are part of the mouth's normal flora. (22, 56)
- *actinomycosis*—chronic disease characterized by multiple abscesses that form draining sinuses. It is caused by *Actinomyces israelii* and related anaerobic filamentous bacteria. Lesions occur on the face, neck, lungs, and abdomen. Pelvic actinomycosis has occurred in women wearing intrauterine contraceptive devices (IUDs). (5, 22, 56)
- *nocardiosis*—infection chiefly caused by *Nocardia asteroides* and *Nocardia brasiliensis*, either localized in the lungs or disseminated through multiple systems: skin, subcutaneous tissue, brain, and other organs. Disorders caused by these organisms may be seen in patients immunosuppressed by such disorders as leukemia, lymphoma, AIDS, and drugs. (5, 22, 56)

Terms Pertaining to Infections Caused by Fungi and Yeasts

- *aspergillosis*—infection with *Aspergillus* that attacks the lungs, skin, external ear, nasal sinuses, meninges, and bones. Severe infection is found in immunosuppressed patients. (19)

- *blastomycosis*—mycotic infection that follows inhalation of the conidia of *Blastomyces dermatitidis*. The infection may be limited to either subcutaneous tissue or disseminated throughout the lungs or multiple body systems. The most commonly affected organs are the lungs, skin, bones, and male genitourinary system. It is prevalent in the southeastern United States and in areas surrounding the Great Lakes. The disease also is found in Africa, Mexico, and in Central and South America. (4, 19)
- *candidiasis*—represents a general term for diseases produced by *Candida* species. It may be an acute or subacute fungus infection that causes thrush, glossitis, vaginitis, onychia, and pneumonitis. *Candidiasis* occurs worldwide. (4, 19, 56)
- *coccidioidomycosis*—caused by *Coccidioides immitis*, a dimorphic fungus. It may occur as either a primary, acute infection of the lungs, lymph nodes, or skin with a favorable prognosis or a generalized infection that includes invasion of the meninges, which can be fatal. Patients with AIDS are at increased risk of coccidioidal dissemination. It is prevalent in the southwestern United States. (4, 19, 106)
- *cryptococcosis*—often presents as a noncontagious opportunistic mycosis characterized by acute or chronic pulmonary infection, or hematogenous dissemination, usually with meningitis. The mycotic infection forms multiple abscesses and lesions of skin, subcutaneous tissue, lungs, and meninges. The etiologic agent is *Cryptococcus neoformans*. The disease occurs worldwide. (4, 19, 56)
- *histoplasmosis*—mycotic disease caused by *Histoplasma capsulatum* that produces benign pulmonary lesions. Histoplasmosis occurs worldwide and is presently considered the most common endemic respiratory mycosis in the United States. (4, 19, 56)
- *mycosis (pl. mycoses)*—any fungus disease. (19)

Terms Pertaining to Infections Caused by Spirochetes

- *leptospirosis*—acute infection by one of the *Leptospira* species, transmitted to human beings by the ingestion of food that has been contaminated by the excretions of a reservoir animal: dog, rat, cattle, or swine. Clinical manifestations include sudden onset of fever, chills, abdominal and muscular pains, intense headache, a palpable liver, jaundice, conjunctival redness, purpura, erythema of skin, and, in severe cases, meningeal irritation. (53, 103)
- *Lyme disease*—an inflammatory arthropathy disorder transmitted by small ixodid ticks, often *Ixodes dammini*, which carry the infectious spirochete organism called *Borrelia burgdorferi*. The first cluster of this disease was reported in Lyme, Connecticut, the town that gave the disease its name. Most of the cases of Lyme disease occur on the northeastern seaboard of the United States. The symptoms include headache, stiff neck, fever, myalgia, arthralgia, lymphadenopathy, and also an expanding red skin rash with a pale center that appears and then vanishes. The worst consequences of the disorder are the secondary symptoms that can develop after the initial infection, such as arthritis, meningitis, and occasional cardiac problems. Early treatment with penicillin or tetracycline usually results in prompt recovery and prevents developing complications. (22, 53, 86)
- *Weil's disease*—severe leptospirosis with hepatic or renal involvement or both, hemorrhages, fever, and muscle pain. (102)
- *rat-bite fever*—two kinds, according to etiologic agent:
  —*Streptobacillus moniliformis*—bite causing high fever, chills, headache, vomiting, joint pains, and rash; present in the United States.
  —*Spirillus minus*—wound healing of bite followed by fever, local lymphadenitis, and sometimes rash. (35)

■ *relapsing fever*—acute spirochetal infection by *Borrelia recurrentis*, transmitted to human beings by insect vectors (lice) or infected insects (tics). Relapses of fever occur abruptly every week or two and gradually decrease in severity. They are accompanied by nausea and vomiting, joint and muscle pains, tachycardia, and psychic, neurologic, and hemorrhagic manifestations. Relapsing fever is endemic in western United States and many other countries. (80)

Terms Pertaining to Infections Caused by Protozoa

■ *African trypanosomiasis, sleeping sickness*—protozoal disease transmitted to human beings by the bite of infected tsetse flies. Its clinical manifestations are irregular fever, enlarged spleen and lymph glands, rapid pulse, and damage to the myocardium and central nervous system. (25, 85)

■ *American trypanosomiasis, Chagas' disease*—infection by *Trypanosoma cruzi* spread to the human host by blood-sucking insects. Usual clinical signs are unilateral eyelid and facial edema; intermittent fever, a chagoma (small painful, hard skin nodule); Romaña's sign (conjunctivitis); an enlarged liver; and myocardial and cerebral involvement. (25, 85)

■ *amebic dysentery, amebiasis*—parasitic infection marked by diarrhea, pain, and fever. It is caused by the protozoan *Entamoeba histolytica*. (25, 84)

■ *giardiasis*—infectious disease caused by the intestinal parasite *Giardia lamblia* that produces a wide range of clinical symptoms, from gastrointestinal discomfort to acute or chronic diarrhea, sometimes progressing to steatorrhea and malabsorption syndromes. Endemics of giardiasis occur in many countries of the world. (25, 87)

■ *leishmaniasis*—infection by genus *Leishmania* and several species related to their geographic distribution. Transmission may result from bites by infected sandflies. Three forms are recognized:
  —*cutaneous leishmaniasis*—lesions may be ulcerating, moist or dry, or diffuse.
  —*visceral leishmaniasis, kala-azar*—fever is irregular and chronic, enlargement of liver and spleen is progressive and complicated by anemia, leukopenia, stomatitis, and dysentery.
  —*mucocutaneous leishmaniasis*—manifests naso-oral lesions and erosions affecting the nasal septum. (25, 74)

■ *malaria*—disease caused by protozoa of the genus *Plasmodium*, which are parasitic in the red blood cells. It is manifested by fever, chills, splenomegaly, and anemia, and is transmitted to human beings by the bites of infected mosquitoes of the genus *Anopheles*. Some types of malaria include:
  —*vivax malaria*—caused by *Plasmodium vivax*.
  —*ovale malaria*—caused by *Plasmodium ovale*.
  —*falciparum malaria*—caused by *Plasmodium falciparum*. (25, 94)

■ *pneumocystis pneumonia*—lung infection caused by *Pneumocystis carinii* that produces an interstitial plasma cell pneumonitis. Outbreaks may occur in nurseries, particularly among premature and marasmic infants. Adults receiving cytotoxic or corticosteroid therapy over a prolonged period are likely to develop this disease. This disease is the most common opportunistic infection in AIDS patients. (22, 25, 27, 112)

■ *toxoplasmosis*—protozoal infection by *Toxoplasma gondii* that may be:
  —*congenital*—the prenatal infection from the mother; if active after birth, it may be manifested in the neonate by fever, convulsions, enlarged liver and spleen, lymphocytosis, muscle and nerve involvement, microcephaly, and mental retardation.

*—acquired—*this infection is usually mild, with lymphadenopathy, malaise, fever, and rash present; if severe, encephalitis, pneumonia, retinochoroiditis, and myocarditis may develop, especially in the immunologically incompetent host. CNS toxoplasmosis is seen often in AIDS patients. (22, 25, 76)

Terms Pertaining to Infections Caused by Helminthic Parasites

■ *cestodes—*tapeworms. (26, 96)

—*cestodiasis—*infestation of the intestinal tract with a tapeworm.

—*echinococcosis, hydatid disease—*hydatid cyst of liver or lung caused by larvae of *Echinococcus granulosa*, a small tapeworm that has been sporadically endemic in Alaska, Canada, California, and Utah. Human beings are usually infected hand-to-mouth by a host dog that harbors eggs in its fur. Ingested eggs deliver larvae that penetrate the intestinal wall and are carried by the circulating blood to the liver and sometimes to the lungs, where they form a hydatid cyst. The cysts are asymptomatic unless rupture occurs.

—*taenia, tapeworm infection—*human parasitic infestation by the beef or pork or fish tapeworm caused by the ingestion of poorly cooked, infected meat or fish. A tapeworm has three distinct parts: the head or scolex, the neck, and the segments or proglottids. Its length may exceed 10 feet. Single segments are prone to detach themselves from the entire chain and to be eliminated in the feces. A rupture of a gravid (pregnant) segment delivers a huge number of eggs, which may be eaten by cattle, develop into embryos in their animal host, and lodge in muscles as cysticerci. When infected meat is consumed by human beings, a cysticercus grows into an adult tapeworm. Larvae of the pork tapeworm are disseminated to all organs of the body.

—*cerebral cysticercosis—*larval invasion of the brain results in epilepsy, mental decline, internal hydrocephalus, headache, nerve palsies, and personality disorders.

—*muscle cysticercosis—*larval invasion of muscles is followed by calcification of cysticerci after prolonged infestation, as confirmed by radiographic studies.

■ *nematodes—*roundworms. (26, 89, 90, 92)

—*ascariasis—*human infestation with the giant intestinal roundworm, *Ascaris lumbricoides*, and in the past endemic in the southern United States. Larvae of the roundworm may severely damage the lungs, causing an *Ascaris* pneumonitis prevalent in children. Adult ascarids may be expelled in vomitus or feces.

—*enterobiasis—*pinworm infection usually found in children, dormitory groups, and in mental hospitals. The gravid (pregnant) female migrates from the lower intestine to lay her eggs on the perianal skin, where they cause intense itching.

—*filariasis—*filarial roundworm infection transmitted to human beings by the bite of certain mosquitoes that are the hosts of infective larvae. These larvae grow into adult worms near or in lymph nodes of the human host. The adults release numerous motile larvae, the microfilariae, which usually circulate in the blood during the night. In advanced filariasis obstruction of the lymph flow leads to elephantiasis, lymphedema, hydrocele, and skin and other problems.

—*hookworm disease—*infection by *Necator americanus*, the American hookworm of the southern states, one centimeter in length, its head curved backward and attached to the intestinal mucosa. Tarry, viscous stools associated with poor digestion, malnutrition, anemia, and moderate heart failure suggest heavy intestinal infection. The initial reaction to larval invasion is ground itch. There may be a creeping eruption, tortuous and raised, caused by the larvae's subcutaneous tunnels.

—*onchocerciasis*—disease caused by microfilariae, infective larvae of a roundworm, which are transmitted to human beings by the bite of a black fly. Intense pruritus and skin eruptions are early symptoms. Painful nodules that form around dead and living worms and serious ocular lesions occur late in the disease.

—*strongyloidiasis*—threadworm infection, prevalent in southern United States. It is characterized by a high degree of toxemia, urticaria, and prolonged mucous diarrhea indicative of intestinal invasion.

—*trichiniasis, trichinosis*—infection acquired by the ingestion of encysted larvae of *Trichinella spiralis* in poorly cooked pork.

—*trichuriasis*—whipworm infection producing serious toxic reactions in the host, such as marked emaciation, anemia, diarrhea, and bloody stools.

- *trematodes*—flukes. (27, 78, 93)

—*fasciolopsiasis*—infection with large intestinal fluke by eating uncooked infected water plants. The flukes may cause severe cramping pain, nausea, anorexia, diarrhea, and finally edema, ascites, cachexia, and death.

—*schistosomiasis, bilharziasis*—*Schistosoma* infection by fluke invasion causing several trematode diseases in Asia, Africa, and South America.

—*intestinal schistosomiasis*—cercariae, infective larvae, pierce the human skin or mucous membranes, where they are in contact with water. Maturation, mating, and delivery of eggs takes place in the veins of the intestinal wall. Eggs may be eliminated in feces or reach the liver, provoking cirrhosis, portal hypertension, and ascites in the advanced stage.

—*vesical or urinary schistosomiasis*—maturation of the fluke occurs in the venous networks of the prostate, bladder, and uterus, leading to cystitis, pyelonephritis, and later terminal hematuria, uremia, and death.

Terms Pertaining to Conditions of Undetermined Cause

- *cystic fibrosis*—systemic hereditary disease of unknown etiology seen in children and adolescents. It is characterized by a more or less extensive involvement of the exocrine glands, especially those secreting mucus and sweat. It may include a variety of clinical conditions:

—*meconium ileus*—causing intestinal obstruction in the newborn.

—*chronic pulmonary disease*—often leading to fatal complications.

—*pancreatic insufficiency*—resulting in malnutrition.

—*abnormally raised levels of sweat electrolytes*—causing salt depletion and cardiac collapse in hot weather. (71)

- *fever of unknown origin*—persistent elevated body temperature, unexplained by serologic and bacteriologic studies or other diagnostic measures. (41, 81)

- *Kawasaki syndrome, mucocutaneous lymph node syndrome*—febrile disorder of undetermined cause. It is clinically manifested by prolonged fever; cracked lips; conjunctivitis; pharyngitis; strawberry tongue; red rash and edema of extremities with desquamation of hands and feet; lymphadenopathy; and in some cases angiitis of the coronary arteries occurs. Most frequently, the disorder occurs in children under five years of age. (41)

- *sarcoidosis*—systemic granulomatous disease of undetermined etiology and pathogenesis. Mediastinal and peripheral lymph nodes, lungs, liver, spleen, skin, eyes, phalangeal bones, and parotid glands are most often involved, but other organs and tissues may be affected. (14)

See Fig. 75 for examples of selected microscopic organisms.

Figure 75 Some selected organisms

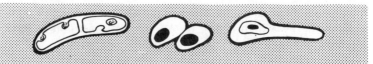

Bacilli. Rod-shaped or club-shaped organisms.

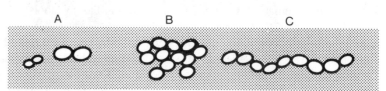

Cocci. Spherical or oval organisms. A. Diplococci (in pairs). B. Staphylococci (in cluster). C. Streptococci (in chains).

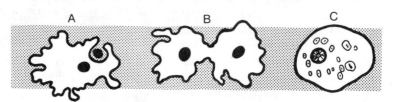

Amebae. Unicellular animal-organisms, capable of changing form by throwing out footlike processes (pseudopodia), which help them to move about and obtain nourishment. A. Ameba. B. Ameba dividing. C. Cyst of Entamoeba histolytica.

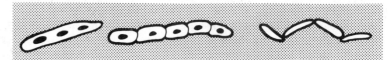

Salmonella or shigella. Simple, non-spore-forming rods, often joined end-to-end.

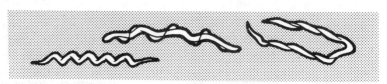

Treponema pallidum. Coiled, virulent organisms containing 8 to 14 spirals.

Table 20
Laboratory Tests for Major Infectious Diseases

Major Viral Diseases

Diseases	Etiologic Agent	Tests for Diagnosis
Acute respiratory disease Conjunctivitis	Adenovirus (65) type 4, 7, and others	Virus isolation from throat and conjunctival swabs or washings
Keratoconjunctivitis	type 3, and others	Complement fixation Neutralization
Pharyngitis	type 8, 3, and 7	Hemagglutination inhibition (110)
Classic influenza	Orthomyxovirus (63) influenza A, B, C	Virus isolation from nasal swabs and throat washings Complement fixation Neutralization (110) Hemagglutination inhibition
Laryngotracheitis Bronchitis Bronchiolitis Pneumonitis Croup	Paramyxovirus Parainfluenza 1, 2, 3, 4 (64)	Virus isolation from throat or nasopharyngeal swab, wash, or aspirate Hemagglutination inhibition Complement fixation Neutralization (110)
Bronchitis Bronchiolitis Pneumonia Coryza	Respiratory syncytial virus (RSV) (57, 59)	Virus isolation from naso-pharyngeal swab, aspirate, or wash Direct immunofluorescence with RSV antiserum can be applied to nasopharyn-geal smears containing exfoliated cells (110)
Measles (rubeola)	Measles virus (64, 97)	Virus isolation from blood and nasopharynx Hemagglutination inhibition Complement fixation Neutralization (110)
German measles (rubella)	Rubella virus (64, 98)	Virus isolation from cell culture Enzyme linked immunosor-bent assay (ELISA) Hemagglutination inhibition Indirect immunofluorescence
Congenital rubella syndrome		Virus isolation from throat, nasopharynx, urine, and blood (110)
Mumps (epidemic parotitis)	Mumps virus (64, 101)	Virus isolation from saliva, urine, and cerebrospinal fluid Complement fixation Hemagglutination inhibition Skin test antigen Hemadsorption (110)

Diseases	Etiologic Agent	Tests for Diagnosis
Common cold (Coryza)	Picornavirus Rhinovirus (61)	Virus isolation from nose and throat
Herpangina Pleurodynia Aseptic meningitis Myocardiopathy Neonatal disease	Coxsackie virus A Coxsackie virus B	Virus isolation from lesion Virus isolation from cerebro-spinal fluid, rectal swabs, or throat swabs Neutralization Complement fixation (110)
Febrile illnesses with or without rash	Echoviruses (30 serotypes) (61, 100)	Virus isolation from body flu-ids or from lesions, and virus isolation from feces, throat, or cerebrospinal fluid
Aseptic meningitis		Complement fixation Hemagglutination inhibition (110)
Poliomyelitis abortive nonparalytics paralytic	Poliovirus (61, 100)	Cytology of cerebrospinal fluid Virus isolation from throat and feces, rarely from cere-brospinal fluid, Comple-ment fixation Neutralization test (110)
Acute hemorrhagic conjunc-tivitis (AHC)	Enterovirus 70 (61, 100)	Virus isolation in human cell culture (110)
Meningitis Encephalitis	Enterovirus 71 (61, 100)	Virus isolation from brain (postmortem) (110)
Viral hepatitis A	Hepatitis A virus (virus HAV) (17, 62)	Enzyme linked immunosor-bent assay (ELISA) for IgM to HAV Radioimmunoassay (RIA) for IgM to HAV Immune adherence hemag-glutination Tissue from liver biopsy Liver function tests Serum alaine aminotrans-ferase Serum aspartate trans-aminase (110)
Viral hepatitis B	Hepatitis B virus (virus HBV) (17, 62)	ELISA and RIA for HBsAg, HBsAb, HBcAb Serum alanine aminotrans-ferase Serum aspartate trans-aminase Complement fixation Counterelectrophoresis Red cell agglutination (RCA) (110)

Diseases	Etiologic Agent	Tests for Diagnosis
(Continued) Viral hepatitis Non-A, Non-B Post-transfusion hepatitis	Hepatitis C virus (virus HCV) (17, 72, 114)	Serum alanine aminotransferase Serum aspartate transaminase Radioimmunoassay for antibodies to HCV (110)
Herpes simplex Aphthous stomatitis Keratoconjunctivitis Meningoencephalitis	Herpesvirus Herpesvirus type 1	Virus isolation from herpetic lesions of skin, cornea, brain, throat, saliva, and feces
Genital herpes Neonatal herpes	Herpesvirus type 2 (11, 66)	Antibodies measured by: neutralization, complement fixation, ELISA, RIA, or immunofluorescence tests (110)
Varicella (chickenpox)	Varicella-zoster virus (VZV) (66)	Virus isolation from vesicular fluid of skin lesion Antibodies to varcella-zoster virus measured by: complement fixation, neutralization, gell precipitation, tests Indirect immunofluorescence to virus-induced membrane antigens tests (110)
Cytomegalic inclusion disease	Cytomegalovirus (CMV) (34, 66)	Virus isolation from mouth, adenoids, urine, kidneys, liver, and peripheral leukocytes Detection of antibodies in human sera by: ELISA, RIA, immunofluorescence, complement fixation, and neutralization tests DNA hybridization quantitative method to identify virus in urine (110)
Infectious mononucleosis (glandular fever) Burkitt's lymphoma Nasopharyngeal carcinoma	Epstein-Barr virus (EBV) or EB herpesvirus (66, 105)	Heterophil agglutination test Commercial mononucleosis spot tests Antibodies against EBV immunofluorescence with virus-containing cells (110)

Diseases	Etiologic Agent	Tests for Diagnosis
Acquired immunodeficiency syndrome (AIDS)	Human immunodeficiency virus (HIV) (10, 21, 27, 67)	Antibodies detected by: ELISA, RIA, and immuno-fluorescence assay or by Western blot analysis and radio-immunoprecipitation (RIP) T4-T8 ratio (110)

Major Rickettsial Diseases

Diseases	Etiologic Agent	Tests for Diagnosis
Rickettsialpox	*Rickettsia akari* (28, 54)	Serologic Weil-Felix reaction Complement fixation Microimmunofluorescence Microagglutination (110)
Rocky Mountain spotted fever	*Rickettsia rickettsii (Rickettsia mooseri)*	Serologic Same as for Rickettsialpox (110)
Endemic murine typhus	*Rickettsia typhi*	Serologic Same as for Rickettsialpox (110)
Epidemic louse-borne typhus	*Rickettsia prowazekii*	Serologic Same as for Rickettsialpox (110)
Brill-Zinsser disease	*Rickettsia prowazekii*	Serologic Same as for Rickettsialpox (110)
Scrub typhus	*Rickettsia tsutsugamushi* (28, 54, 117)	Serologic Same as for Rickettsialpox (110)
Q fever	*Coxiella burnetii* (28, 54, 117)	Serologic Complement fixation Microagglutination Immunofluorescent antibody (110)
Trench fever (quintan fever, shin-bone fever, Volhynia fever, and His-Werner disease)	*Rochalimaea quintana* (28, 54, 117)	Serologic Enzyme-linked immuno-sorbent assay (ELISA) Passive hemagglutination (110)

Major Bacterial Diseases

Diseases	Etiologic Agent	Tests for Diagnosis
Abscesses	*Staphylococcus aureus* (46, 73)	Microscopic Smears and cultures from infected lesions
Bacterial endocarditis	*Streptococcus:* various kinds (6, 47)	Microscopic Blood culture (110)

Diseases	Etiologic Agent	Tests for Diagnosis

Erysipelas
Puerperal fever
Sepsis
	Streptococcus pyogenes (6, 47)	Microscopic
		    Smears and cultures
		        obtained from lesions

Scarlet fever	*Streptococcus pyogenes (beta-
	    hemolytic streptococci)* (6, 47)
		Skin tests
		Dick test: intradermal injec-
		    tion of dilute scarlet fever
		    streptococcus toxin
		Schultz-Charlton test, Rash
		    extinction test for scarlet
		    fever: intradermal injection
		    of convalescent scarlet fever
		    serum (110)

Pneumonia	*Streptococcus pneumoniae*
	    (6, 47)
		Microscopic
		    Capsule swelling test
		        (Quellung reaction)
		    Blood culture
		    Sputum smears (110)

Enteric infections
Genitourinary infections
	Enterobacteriaceae
	
	Escherichia (E. coli)
	Klebsiella-Enterobacter-Serratia
	    group
	Proteus-Morganella-Providencia
	    group
	Citrobacter
	Salmonellae
	Shigellae (48, 104)
		Microscopic
		    Smears and cultures (110)

Gonococcal infections	*Neisseria gonorrhoeae*
	    (gonococcus) (49)
		Microscopic
		    Smears and cultures
		    (Thayer-Martin medium)
		    from lesions (110)

Meningitis	*Neisseria meningitidis*
	Haemophilus influenzae
	Streptococcus pneumoniae (18,
	    47, 49)
		Microscopic
		    Culture of cerebrospinal
		        fluid
		    Quellung reaction with type-
		        specific serum helps in
		        identification (110)

Undulant fever (brucellosis)	*Brucella melitensis*
	    B. abortus suis (29, 69)
		Serologic: Agglutination test
		    for undulant fever (110)

Whooping cough	*Bordetella pertussis* (29)	Microscopic: Culture on
		    cough plate from speci-
		    mens from nasopharyngeal
		    swabs or cough droplets
		Direct fluorescent antibody
		    (FA) test is quite useful in
		    detecting *B pertussis* after
		    culture on solid media (110)

Diseases	Etiologic Agent	Tests for Diagnosis
Diphtheria	*Corynebacterium diphtheriae* (Klebs-Loeffler bacillus) (28, 45)	Microscopic: Culture from throat or larynx Shick test: intradermal injection of diluted diphtheria toxin (110)
Food poisoning (botulism)	*Clostridium botulinum* (2, 44)	Animal inoculation for toxin in suspected food (110)
Gas gangrene	*Clostridium perfringens* (Welchii) (29, 44)	Microscopic: Anaerobic culture from lesion (110)
Legionnaires' disease	*Legionella pneumophilia* (3, 50)	Serologic: Indirect fluorescent antibody (IFA) Microagglutination (MA) Direct fluorescent antibody Enzyme-linked immunosorbent assay (ELISA) Culture: Isolation of organism (110)
Leprosy (Hansen's disease)	*Mycobacterium leprae* (Leprosy of Hansen's bacillus) (29, 52, 77)	Microscopic: smear and culture from cutaneous skin lesions, nodules, plaques, and ulcers Animal inoculation Lepromin test: skin reaction to extracts of M. leprae (110)
Tuberculosis, pulmonary and extrapulmonary	*Mycobacterium tuberculosis* (tubercle bacillus) (16, 52)	Microscopic: smears and cultures from acid-fast bacilli from sputum, gastric and bronchial washings, drainage, and tuberculous lesions from organs Animal inoculation Tuberculin tests: Mantoux, Tine, and others Detection of antibodies by precipitation, complement fixation, passive hemagglutination and enzyme-linked immunosorbent assay (ELISA) (110)
Tularemia	*Francisella tularensis* (69)	Serologic: Agglutination test Animal inoculation Skin test for tularemia (110)
Typhoid fever Parathyroid fever Food infection	*Salmonella typhi* *Salmonella paratyphi*—*A, B,* or *C* (29, 31, 48)	Microscopic: Culture from stool, urine, and blood Serologic: Widal reaction agglutination of bacilli (110)

Major Mycotic Diseases

Diseases	Etiologic Agent	Tests for Diagnosis
Actinomycosis	Actinomyces (*Actinomyces israelii*) (5, 56)	Microscopic: direct smears or cultures from sinuses and sputum Animal inoculation Gel diffusion methods or immunofluorescence can differentiate *A. israelii* from other *Actinomycete* species (110)
Blastomycosis	Blastomyces (*Blastomyces dermatitidis*) (4, 56)	Microscopic: direct smears and cultures from sputum, pus, exudates, urine, and biopsies from lesions Animal inoculation Complement fixation Immunodiffusion test (110)
Candidiasis	*Candida albicans* (Monilia) (4, 56)	Microscopic: direct smears and cultures from skin, and nail scrapings, sputum and material from vagina Antigen detection by immunodiffusion, precipitation, counterimmunoelectrophoresis, latex agglutination tests, and others (110)
Coccidioidomycosis	*Coccidioides immitis* (4, 56)	Microscopic: direct smears or culture from sputum, gastric content, pleural fluid and abscesses Animal inoculation Serologic: immunodiffusion and latex agglutination tests Skin test (110)
Histoplasmosis	*Histoplasma capsulatum* (4, 56)	Microscopic: direct smears or cultures of bone marrow and lymph nodes Animal inoculation Serologic: latex agglutination, immunodiffusion, and complement fixation Skin tests: Tine and intradermal (110)
Nocardiosis	*Nocardia asteroides* (and related species) (5, 56)	Microscopic: Cultures from sputum, lung abscesses, brain abscesses, and skin or other lesions (110)

Major Spirochetal and Protozoal Diseases

Diseases	Etiologic Agent	Tests for Diagnosis
Leptospirosis	*Leptospira* species: *Leptospira canicola* (of dogs) *Leptospira icterohaemor-rhagiae* (of rats) *Leptospira pomona* (of cattle and swine) (30, 102)	Urine culture Dark-field examination of patient's blood Culture on Korthof's medium Specific agglutination titer Specific serologic tests of anicteric form of leptospi-rosis (110)
Lyme disease	*Borrelia burgdorferi* (transmit-ted by ixodid ticks, often by *Ixodes dammini*) (30, 53)	Specific immunoglobulin antibody titers Culture of *B burgdorferi* (not often successful) Other elevated test values are reflected in serum glutamic-oxaloacetic trans-aminase (SGOT) and erythrocyte sedimentation rate (110)
Syphilis	*Treponema pallidum* (30, 38)	Dark-field examination of scraping or fluid exudate from chancre Immunofluorescence micros-copy for fluorescent spirochetes Nontreponemal antigen tests: Flocculation tests Venereal Disease Research Laboratories (VDRL) Rapid plasma reagin (RPR) Complement fixation (CF) tests (Wasserman, Kolmer) Treponemal antibody tests: Fluorescent treponemal antibody test T *pallidum* immobilization test T *pallidum* complement fixation test T *pallidum* hemagglutina-tion test (110)
Amebic dysentery	*Entamoeba histolytica* (28, 84)	Microscopic: examination of fresh stools (110)
Giardiasis	*Giardia lamblia* (25, 87)	Microscopic: identification of trophozoites and/or cysts in stool specimen Serologic: indirect immuno-fluorescence (110)

Diseases	Etiologic Agent	Tests for Diagnosis
Malaria	*Plasmodium vivax malariae falciparum* (25, 94)	Microscopic: examination of blood smears (110)
Pneumocystis pneumonia	*Pneumocystis carinii* (25)	Lung puncture biopsy (110)

Toxoplasmosis	*Toxoplasma gondii* (25, 76)	Microscopic: smears and sections stained with Giemsa's stain may detect organism
		Animal inoculation
		Serologic:
		  Sabin-Feldman dye test,
		  Enzyme-linked immunosorbent assay (ELISA),
		  Indirect fluorescent antibody test
		  Complement fixation test
		  Indirect hemagglutination test
		Skin test (110)

Major Helminthic Diseases

Diseases	Etiologic Agent	Tests for Diagnosis
Ascariasis	Nematodes *Ascaris lumbricoides* (large intestinal roundworm) (26, 92)	Stool specimen containing characteristic ova (eggs) Sputum occasionally containing larvae (110)
Enterobiasis	*Enterobius vermicularis* (pinworm) (26, 92)	Stool specimen containing adult worms Microscopic: pinworm ova smears identified with cellophane tape test; gummed side of the cellophane pressed on the perianal area followed by sticking the tape to the slide (110)
Filariasis in advanced stage: elephantiasis	*Brugia malayi, Brugia timori, Wuchereria bancrofti* (and other infective larvae) (26, 90)	Day and night blood specimens for identification of microfilariae (motile larvae) Complement fixation Skin test for microfilaria (110)
Hookworm disease	*Ancylostoma duodenale* (European hookworm) *Necator americanus* (American hookworm) (26, 92)	Stool specimen containing characteristic eggs, guaiac positive Microscopic: fecal smears for egg and larvae detection (110)

Diseases	Etiologic Agent	Tests for Diagnosis
Onchocerciasis	*Onchocera volvulus* (filiarial roundworm) (26, 90)	Aspiration of nodules for detection of eggs Excision of nodules for demonstrating larvae and adult worms Microscopic: skin shavings and conjunctival snips Slit-lamp examination for ocular onchocerciasis (110)
Strongyloidiasis	*Strongyloides stercoralis* (threadworm) (26, 92)	Stool specimen containing larvae or adult worms Duodenal aspiration if not found in stool (110)
Trichinelliasis Trichiniasis Trichinosis	*Trichinella spiralis* (Pork roundworm) (26, 89)	Skin test Precipitation and complement fixation tests Muscle biopsy for encysted larvae (110)
Trichuriasis Trichocephaliasis	*Trichuris trichiura* (whipworm) (26, 92)	Stool specimen containing ova of whipworm Concentration by centrifugation if eggs not found in direct fecal smear (110)
Echinococcosis Cystic hydatid disease Alveolar hydatid disease	Cestodes *Echinococcus granulosus* *Echinococcus multilocularis* (tapeworm) (26, 96)	Microscopic: examination of cyst contents of hydatid tumor in liver or other organs Serologic: indirect hemagglutination test, complement fixation test, and immunoelectrophoresis test (110)
Taenia infestation	*Taenia lata* *Diphyllobothrium latum* (fish tapeworm) *Taenia saginata* (beef tapeworm) *Taenia solium* (pork tapeworm) (26, 96)	Stool specimens containing eggs and segments Microscopic: Examination of segment Serologic: indirect hemagglutination test, complement fixation test, and ELISA if cerebral cysticercosis is suspected (110)
Fasciolopsiasis	Trematodes *Fasciolopsis buski* (large intestinal fluke)	Stool specimen containing eggs and occasionally flukes Urine specimen containing eggs

Diseases	Etiologic Agent	Tests for Diagnosis
Schistosomiasis (Bilharziasis)	*Schistosoma haematobium* (vesical or urinary fluke) *Schistosoma japonicum* (intestinal fluke) *Schistosoma mansoni* (intestinal fluke) (26, 93)	Cystoscopic biopsy Stool specimen containing eggs Serologic: positive Stool specimen containing eggs Rectal biopsy (110)

Immunologic Diseases

Origin of Terms

auto- (G)—self
cyt- cyto- (G)—cell
histio-, histo- (G)—tissue, web

-lysis (G)—dissolution, breaking down
phylaxis (G)—protection
-phoresis (G)—transmission, breaking down

General Terms

- *anaphylaxis*—excessive hypersensitivity to foreign protein or other substance, clinically manifested by edema of the larynx, hypoxia, respiratory distress, hypotension, and vascular collapse. (1, 43)
- *antibodies*—specialized proteins or immunoglobulins, formed in response to an antigen. (42)
- *antigens*—substances that will cause the body to form antibodies. (42)
- *autoantibodies*—antibodies elicited by a person's own antigens.
- *autohemolysins*—antibodies acting on the corpuscles of a person's own blood.
- *autoimmunization*—the production of antibodies or other immunologic responses to antigens in a person without any artificial intervention.
- *cytopathic effect (of viruses)*—biologic changes produced by the multiplication of viruses in cell culture. (17)
- *cytotoxicity*—the destruction of cells of autoantibodies, as seen in acquired hemolytic anemia and other diseases. (42, 83)
- *fluorescein*—fluorescent dye used for diagnostic purposes. (42)
- *fluorescence*—luminescence of a substance when exposed to short-wave rays. (42)
- *histocompatibility*—tissue compatibility between a recipient and donor based on immunologic identity or similarity of tissues; necessary for successful transplantation. (43)
- *hypersensitivity*—exaggerated sensitivity to an infective, chemical, or other agent, such as an extreme allergic reaction to a foreign protein. Hypersensitivity may be of the:
  - *immediate type*—occurring within 1 to 30 minutes, such as anaphylactic shock.
  - *cell-mediated, delayed type*—developing gradually within 24 to 48 hours or longer, such as a tuberculin reaction.
  - *subacute delayed type, Arthus reaction*—developing within 4 to 10 hours and characterized by a marked infiltration of small vessels, with polymorphonuclear leukocytes, local edema, and bleeding without thrombus formation. (1, 42)
- *immune response*—formation of antibodies due to a specific stimulus. (1, 42, 108)

- *immunohematology*—branch of hematology dealing with antigen-antibody reactions and their effects on the blood.
- *immunoelectrophoresis*—procedure employed to separate and identify multiple protein components. In the test, use is made of physiochemical and immunologic specificity. (42, 108)
- *immunogen*—one of a group of substances capable of stimulating an immune response or initiating a certain degree of active immunity under favorable conditions. Its effects may be detrimental or beneficial.
- *immunogenicity*—the ability of an immunogen to evoke an immune response, or the ability of an antigen to stimulate antibody formation. Immunogenicity is the same as antigenicity. (117)
- *immunoglobulins (Igs)*—antibodies capable of reacting specifically with the antigen that caused their formation. They are similar in structure but diverse antigenically. Molecules of immunoglobulins are composed of:
  - *heavy (H) chains*—large polypeptide chains. Each of the five classes of immunoglobulins are antigenetically distinct:
    - γ *in IgG*—immunoglobulin G
    - α *in IgA*—immunoglobulin A
    - μ *in IgM*—immunoglobulin M
    - δ *in IgD*—immunoglobulin D
    - ϵ *in IgE*—immunoglobulin E
    Molecular weights are 50,000 to 70,000 daltons. (42, 108)
  - *light (L) chains*—small polypeptide chains, either of the kappa (κ) or lambda (λ) type.
    Molecular weight is 25,000 daltons. (42, 108)
- *immunoglobulin concentration*—the amount of serum protein components determined by immunoelectrophoresis for establishing the presence or absence of elevated or depressed immunoglobulin levels. Thus an exaggerated susceptibility to infection or antibody deficiency may be detected. (1)
- *immunology*—the medical science concerned primarily with immunity or resistance to disease in the human being. In its practical aspects it deals with methods of diagnosing or preventing disease or influencing its course by serotherapy and vaccination. (1)
- *immunopathology*—the study of disorders or diseases resulting from antigen-antibody reactions or alterations produced by immunologic responses. (22, 83)
- *immunosuppressive therapy*—treatment instituted to suppress all immune responses and thus prevent the rejection of the graft. (43)
- *lymphocytes*—white blood cells originating in lymphoid tissue and capable of responding to immunologic stimulation. There are two types of cells:
  - *B-lymphocytes*—about 20 percent of lymphocytes in the circulating blood. They are short-lived, capable of proliferating, differentiating, and maturing into plasma cells; functioning independently of the thymus; and are responsible for a specific immunoglobulin or serum antibodies.
  - *T-lymphocytes*—about 65 to 80 percent of lymphocytes in the circulating blood. They are long-lived; have few immunoglobulin molecules; depend on a functioning thymus; and are cytotoxic to grafted cells, thus causing graft rejection, a graft-versus-host reaction. (33, 42)
- *rejection phenomenon*—reaction to graft based on the formation of antibodies directed against the donated tissue or organ. (43)

■ *transplantation immunity*—immune responses to transplanting organs, depending on the histocompatibility of the type of graft.

— *allograft, homograft*—tissue or organ from one individual is transferred to another individual of the same species.

— *autograft*—tissue or organ is transplanted from one part of the body to another in the same person.

— *isograft*—tissue or organ is transplanted from one identical twin to another. Histocompatibility exists in its most complete form.

— *xenograft, heterograft*—tissue or organ from donor from one species is implanted in recipient from another species. Grafts between species are subject to intense medical research. (22, 43)

Diagnostic Terms

■ *acquired immune deficiency syndrome (AIDS)*—an ultimately fatal disease first described in promiscuous homosexual men in 1980. Also, it has been reported in such groups as Haitian men and women, intravenous drug users, female partners of these drug users, infants, and children, as well as patients who receive infected blood transfusions. The etiologic agent of AIDS is a retrovirus called human immunodeficiency virus (HIV). Formerly, the AIDS causative agent was termed human T lymphotropic virus type III (HTLV III) or lymphadenopathy-associated virus (LAV), as well as AIDS-associated retrovirus (ARV). The human immunodeficiency virus (HIV) attacks T lymphocytes and severely damages the immune system. The virus is transmitted through intimate sexual contact and through contaminated blood and blood products. The HLV infection appears to ultimately result in the almost total collapse of the body's cell-mediated immune system, leaving the patient susceptible to malignancies (e.g., Kaposi's sarcoma) and opportunistic infections (e.g., *Pneumocystis carinii* pneumonia), against which the body is unable to defend itself. The presence of antibodies to AIDS retrovirus is helpful for screening blood donors but is not diagnostic of AIDS. Antibodies may be detected by enzyme-linked immunosorbent assay (ELISA). Other alternative tests include immunofluorescence assay, radioimmunoprecipitation assay, and the Western blot analysis. (10, 21, 22, 27, 41, 67, 107)

■ *AIDS-related complex (ARC)*—presence of such conditions as generalized lymphadenopathy; unexplained fever; weight loss; hematologic abnormalities (thrombocytopenia, anemia, and neutropenia), and neurologic abnormalities in a person with HIV infection but without the clinical picture of full-blown AIDS. (10, 21, 22, 27, 41, 107)

■ *angioimmunoblastic lymphadenopathy (AIL)*—newly recognized systemic disorder with widespread involvement of peripheral and deep lymph nodes by movable and soft lesions that are two or three centimeters in diameter. The syndrome is clinically marked by an acute onset of chills, fever, diaphoresis, polyarthralgia, anorexia, edema, ascites, and vasculitis and occurs primarily in the elderly. The fatal prognosis is about 60 percent of victims may result from severe infection and immunologic incompetence. (32)

■ *autoimmune diseases*—immunologic disorders in which the patient's own tissues produce antigenic stimuli. By using fluorescein antibody technique, the presence of autoimmunity has been detected in certain cases of chronic thyroiditis, disseminated lupus erythematosus, rheumatoid arthritis, viral hepatitis, and other diseases. (22, 43)

—*autoimmune hemolytic anemia*—clinical syndrome of uncompensated hemolytic anemia caused by aberrant immune response initiated by a host and directed against the host's normal red cell antigens.

—*secondary autoimmune hemolytic anemia*—hemolytic anemia characterized by the presence of autoantibodies and a coexisting disease that constitutes the basic ailment; for example, anemia caused by chronic infection or neoplasm. (43, 108)

■ *heavy-chain diseases*—disorders demonstrating a typical heavy-chain immunoglobulin fragment in urine, serum, or both.

—*alpha (α)heavy-chain disease*—lymphocyte dyscrasia usually associated with malignant lymphoma of intestine resulting in nutritional malabsorption. The diagnosis is based on the detection of an abnormal protein in the urine and serum that reacts with antiserums to alpha chains. (42, 75, 108)

—*gamma (γ)heavy-chain disease*—disorder primarily seen in the elderly, clinically manifested by weight loss, weakness, enlarged liver, recurrent infections, involvement of lymph glands, lymphocytosis, anemia, and platelet deficiency. (42, 75, 108)

■ *immunologic deficiency states*—disorders reflecting defective cellular immunity, decreased antibody production, or both, resulting in increased susceptibility to infection. (108)

—*Bruton's agammaglobulinemia*—severe familial X-linked deficiency of all classes of immunoglobulins and absence of plasma cells. (10, 108)

—*DiGeorge's syndrome*—occurs because of failure of embryogenesis of the third and fourth pharyngeal pouches, resulting in aplasia of the parathyroid and thymus glands. The syndrome is an example of pure T-cell functional deficiency with intact B-cell function. (10, 108)

—*severe combined immunodeficiency (SCID)*—syndrome caused by marked lymphopenia of both T-cells and C-cells. This immunologic defect is related to deficiency of adenosine deaminase (ADA), an enzyme active in purine metabolism. (10, 108)

—*Wiskott-Aldrich syndrome*—severe immunodeficiency disease of a familial type, characterized by eczema, low platelet count, and frequent infections and associated with abnormal immunoglobulins, lymphopenia, delayed hypersensitivity, and impaired immune response. (108)

■ *plasma cell and lymphocyte dyscrasias*—disorders manifesting uncontrolled proliferation of cells usually active in antibody synthesis and homogenous immunoglobulin synthesis. Typical protein abnormalities in serum and urine confirm the diagnosis. (75)

—*macroglobulinemia, Waldenström's macroglobulinemia*—dyscrasia, including several clinical disorders, in which the common denominator is the presence of monoclonal macroglobulin formed by cells involved in immunoglobulin M (IgM) synthesis. Clinical features are anemia, bleeding, lymph gland involvement, and enlarged spleen and liver. (75)

—*multiple myeloma*—severe plasma cell dyscrasia associated with decreased antibody synthesis and low immunoglobulin levels resulting in recurrent infections. There is considerable infiltration of the bone marrow by neoplastic plasma cells, which proliferate in advanced disease, causing osteoporosis, typical punched-out skeletal lesions, and pathologic fractures, especially of the ribs and vertebrae. Renal disease and anemia are usually present. Multiple myeloma runs a progressive course, extending over one or more decades. (75)

Diseases of Connective Tissue

Origin of Terms

colla (G)—glue

erythema (G)—redness

lupus (L)—wolf, meaning destructive

sclero- (G)—hard

Anatomic Terms (95)

- *collagen*—a substance present between the fibers of connective tissue throughout the body.
- *collagen diseases*—group of diseases in which the connective tissues have undergone pathologic changes. The prognosis is usually fatal.
- *connective tissue*—a variety of tissues composed of widely spaced cells between which intercellular material is deposited. This intercellular substance offers the distinguishing mark of the specific connective tissue; for example, mineral salts are located in the interspaces of bone and are responsible for its hardness, whereas for blood the intercellular substance is liquid. Other variations of connective tissue are areolar, adipose, fibrous, cartilage, and lymphoid tissues.

Diagnostic Terms

- *CREST syndrome*—presence and coexistence of calcinosis, Raynaud's phenomenon, esophageal hypomotility, sclerodactyly, and telangiectasia. Initially, this disorder was considered a benign form of progressive systemic sclerosis. Pulmonary hypertension may occur during any phase of the syndrome's course. (24)
- *dermatomyositis*—disease of unknown etiology. It is characterized by an insidious onset and subsequent dermatitis and widespread degeneration of the skeletal muscles. (7)
- *Marfan's syndrome, arachnodactyly*—hereditary disorder of a connective tissue element resulting in skeletal, ocular, and cardiovascular abnormalities. Clinical features are spidery fingers; disproportionately long limbs; funnel chest; lax, redundant ligaments; and ectopia lentis (displaced lens) with impaired vision. Hemodynamic stress on the media of the aorta may lead to dissecting aortic aneurysm. Other disorders may be present. (95)
- *mixed connective tissue disease (MCTD)*—clinical syndrome with overlapping features of systemic lupus erythematosus, scleroderma, and myositis are present along with high titers of extractable nuclear antigen (ENA). Patients with this disorder may have nondeforming arthritis, swollen hands, Raynaud's phenomenon, and myositis. (106)
- *polyarteritis, periarteritis nodosa*—systemic disease characterized by nodules along the course of the muscular arteries. (20, 106)
- *scleroderma, progressive systemic sclerosis*—chronic disease causing a leathery induration of the skin, progressive atrophy, and pigmentation. Systemic involvement of the mucous membranes and the musculoskeletal, vascular, and digestive systems may lead to a fatal prognosis. Raynaud's phenomenon occurs in about 90 percent of these patients. (24, 106)
- *Sjögren's syndrome*—lymphadenopathy with hypergammaglobulinemia complicated by benign or malignant lymphoma. This chronic autoimmune disease is marked by dryness of the mouth, caused by diminished secretion of saliva, resulting in difficult swallowing, eating, and speaking; dryness of the eyes, with smarting, burning, and itching; and numerous systemic involvements of the pancreas, pleura, pericardium, kidneys, and other organs. (106, 111)

- *systemic lupus erythematosus (SLE)*—collagenous inflammatory multisystem disorder that affects the synovial and serous membranes and vascular system. Clinical manifestations of this disorder include fever, anorexia, malaise, weight loss, joint symptoms, conjunctivitis, and rash over areas exposed to sunlight. Normocytic, normochromic anemia as well as leukopenia and lymphopenia also may be present. SLE is recognized by a typical butterfly lesion on the bridge of the nose and on the cheeks. (106)

Abbreviations

AD—adenovirus
ALG—antilymphocytic globulin
ALS—antilymphocytic serum
ANA—antinuclear antibodies
APC—adenoidal-pharyngeal-conjunctival
Arbo—anthropod-borne
ARC—AIDS-Related Complex
BFP—biologic false positive (reaction)
CF—complement fixation
CID—cytomegalic inclusion disease
CIE—counterimmunoelectrophoresis
CMV—cytomegalovirus
EBV—Epstein-Barr virus
FA—fluorescent antibody
FTA—fluorescent treponemal antibody
FTA-ABS—fluorescent treponemal
     antibody absorption
     (test for syphilis)
FUO—fever of unknown origin
GvH—graft versus host (reactivity)
HAV—hepatitis A virus
HBV—hepatitis B virus
HCV—hepatitis C virus
HI—hemagglutination-inhibition
HIV—human immunodeficiency virus

HSV—herpes simplex virus
LE—lupus erythematosus
MHA—microhemagglutination
    (test for syphilis)
MHA-TP—microhemagglutination for
    Treponema pallidum
    (test for syphilis)
Nt—neutralization test
PPA—Pittsburgh pneumonia agent
RPCF—Reiter protein complement
    fixation
RPR—rapid plasma reagin
RSV—respiratory syncytial virus
SLE—St. Louis encephalitis
SLE—systemic lupus erythematosus
STD—sexually transmitted disease
STS—serologic test for syphilis
TPI—*Treponema pallidum* immobilization
va—variety
VD—venereal disease
VDG—venereal disease gonorrhea
VDRL—Venereal Disease Research
    Laboratories
VZV—varicella-zoster virus

Oral Reading Practice

Herpes Zoster

Herpes zoster, or shingles is an infectious disease caused by the zoster virus. It is characterized by vesicular lesions that follow the course of a **peripheral nerve** in a bandlike fashion. Before the eruption the patient may experience pain for several days without other symptoms. Once the **erythema** and **vesicles** appear in a typical **zoniform** distribution, the diagnosis is readily made. In the beginning the eruption exhibits slightly **edematous,** fairly well-defined **erythematous,** oval, or round areas on which vesicles form in groups. Generally sensory changes along the path of the affected **neutral zones** are associated with the eruption. Pain precedes, accompanies, and follows the appearance of the skin lesion. It varies in duration and intensity from slight, brief **hyperesthesia** to **paroxysmal** attacks or persistent, excruciating **neural-**

gia. Similar to other nerve root involvements, the pain is especially agonizing at night and is intensified by motion. In rare cases it has led to drug addiction and even suicide. **Paresthesia** of the skin may be brought on by touching the affected area or it may develop spontaneously. In addition, the patient may develop tender enlarged lymph nodes, rheumatic pains, and general malaise.

Although the characteristic feature of the disease is the skin eruption, herpes zoster is essentially an inflammation of one or more posterior root ganglia. The rash is confined to the **dermal segment,** supplied by the sensory nerve arising from the involved **posterior (sensory) root ganglion.** The **neurotropic virus** destroys the ganglion cells and fibers. These changes result in a degeneration of the corresponding peripheral nerve.

Evidence now available suggests that herpes zoster virus is identical to the varicella virus that produces chickenpox; the varicella virus enters the body and may be incorporated within the **genome** of many cells, but it does not express itself until later in life as herpes zoster. The factors leading to the activation of herpes are unknown, but are thought to involve immune mechanisms, since the virus becomes active during immunosuppression. Current evidence points to immunologic activity declining during the aging process, which may contribute to the onset of herpes zoster.

One of the most painful forms of herpes is herpes zoster ophthalmicus, caused by a viral infection of the **trigeminal nerve.** This may lead to corneal ulceration, keratitis, iritis, conjunctivitis, and edema of the eyelids.

Herpes zoster oticus results from an inflammation of the **vestibulocochlear** nerve and is associated with deafness, **vertigo, tinnitus,** and severe pain. (28, 66, 114)

References and Bibliography

1. Austen, K. Frank. Diseases of immediate type hypersensitivity. In Braunwald, Eugene, et al., eds., *Harrison's Principles of Internal Medicine*, 11th ed. New York: McGraw-Hill Book Co., 1987, pp. 1407-1447.
2. Beaty, Harry N. Botulism. In Braunwald, Eugene, et al., eds., *Harrison's Principles of Internal Medicine*, 11th ed. New York: McGraw-Hill Book Co., 1987, pp. 561-563.
3. Beaty, Harry N., and Pasculle, A. William. Legionella infections. In Braunwald, Eugene, et al., eds., *Harrison's Principles of Internal Medicine*, 11th ed. New York: McGraw-Hill Book Co., 1987, pp. 620-623.
4. Bennett, John E. Fungal infections. In Braunwald, Eugene, et al., eds., *Harrison's Principles of Internal Medicine*, 11th ed. New York: McGraw-Hill Book Co., 1987, pp. 736-745.
5. ————. Actinomycosis and nocardiosis. Ibid., pp. 745-747.

6. Bisno, Alan B. Streptococcal infections. In Braunwald, Eugene, et al., eds., *Harrison's Principles of Internal Medicine*, 11th ed. New York: McGraw-Hill Book Co., 1987, pp. 543-550.
7. Bradley, Walter G. Dermatomyositis and polymyositis. In Braunwald, Eugene, et al., eds., *Harrison's Principles of Internal Medicine*, 11th ed. New York: McGraw-Hill Book Co., 1987, pp. 2069-2072.
8. Carpenter, Charles C.J. Acute infectious diarrheal diseases and bacterial food poisoning. In Braunwald, Eugene, et al., eds., *Harrison's Principles of Internal Medicine*, 11th ed. New York: McGraw-Hill Book Co., 1987, pp. 502-506.
9. Clyde, Wallace A., Jr. Mycoplasma infections. In Braunwald, Eugene, et al., eds., *Harrison's Principles of Internal Medicine*, 11th ed. New York: McGraw-Hill Book Co., 1987, pp. 757-759.
10. Cooper, Max D., and Lawton, Alexander R., III. Immune deficiency diseases. In Braunwald, Eugene, et al., eds., *Harrison's*

Principles of Internal Medicine, 11th ed. New York: McGraw-Hill Book Co., 1987, pp. 1385-1392.

11. Corey, Lawrence. Herpes simplex viruses. In Braunwald, Eugene, et al., eds., *Harrison's Principles of Internal Medicine*, 11th ed. New York: McGraw-Hill Book Co., 1987, pp. 692-697.

12. ———. Rabies and other rhabdoviruses. Ibid., pp. 712-717.

13. Corey, Lawrence, and Petersdorf, Robert G. Prevention of infection: Immunization and antimicrobial prophylaxis. In Braunwald, Eugene, et al., eds., *Harrison's Principles of Internal Medicine*, 11th ed. New York: McGraw-Hill Book Co., 1987, pp. 524-533.

14. Crystal, Ronald G. Sarcoidosis. In Braunwald, Eugene, et al., eds., *Harrison's Principles of Internal Medicine*, 11th ed. New York: McGraw-Hill Book Co., 1987, pp. 1445-1450.

15. Dale, David C., and Petersdorf, Robert G. Septic shock. In Braunwald, Eugene, et al., eds., *Harrison's Principles of Internal Medicine*, 11th ed. New York: McGraw-Hill Book Co., 1987, pp. 474-478.

16. Daniel, Thomas M. Tuberculosis. In Braunwald, Eugene, et al., eds., *Harrison's Principles of Internal Medicine*, 11th ed. New York: McGraw-Hill Book Co., 1987, pp. 625-633.

17. Dienstag, Jules L., Wands, Jack R., and Koff, Raymond S. Acute hepatitis. In Braunwald, Eugene, et al., eds., *Harrison's Principles of Internal Medicine*, 11th ed. New York: McGraw-Hill Book Co., 1987, pp. 1325-1338.

18. Dolin, Raphael. Influenza. In Braunwald, Eugene, et al., eds., *Harrison's Principles of Internal Medicine*, 11th ed. New York: McGraw-Hill Book Co., 1987, pp. 672-677.

19. Drutz, David J. The mycoses. In Wyngaarden, James B., and Smith, Lloyd H., Jr., eds., *Cecil's Textbook of Medicine*, 18th ed. Philadelphia: W.B. Saunders Co., 1988, pp. 1837-1855.

20. Fauci, Anthony S. The vasculitis syndromes. In Braunwald, Eugene, et al., eds., *Harrison's Principles of Internal Medicine*, 11th ed. New York: McGraw-Hill Book Co., 1987, pp. 1438-1447.

21. Fauci, Anthony S., and Lane, H. Clifford. The acquired immunodeficiency syndrome (AIDS). In Braunwald, Eugene, et al., eds., *Harrison's Principles of Internal Medicine*, 11th ed. New York: McGraw-Hill Book Co., 1987, pp. 1392-1396.

22. Gardner, Morey, MD Personal communication.

23. Gardner, Pierce, and Arnow, Paul M. Hospital-acquired infections. In Braunwald, Eugene, et al., eds., *Harrison's Principles of Internal Medicine*, 11th ed. New York: McGraw-Hill Book Co., 1987, pp. 470-474.

24. Gilliland, Bruce C. Progressive systemic sclerosis (diffuse scleroderma). In Braunwald, Eugene, et al., eds., *Harrison's Principles of Internal Medicine*, 11th ed. New York: McGraw-Hill Book Co., 1987, pp. 1428-1432.

25. Goldsmith, Robert S. Infectious diseases: protozoal. In Schroeder, Steven A., Krupp, Marcus A., and Tierney, Lawrence M., Jr., eds., *Current Medical Diagnosis & Treatment—1988*. Norwalk, CT: Appleton & Lange, 1988, pp. 896-923.

26. ———. Infectious diseases: Helminthic. Ibid., pp. 924-954.

27. Groopman, Jerome E. The acquired immunodeficiency syndrome. In Wyngaarden, James B., and Smith, Lloyd H., Jr., eds., *Cecil's Textbook of Medicine*, 18th ed. Philadelphia: W.B. Saunders Co., 1988, pp. 1799-1808.

28. Grossman, Moses, and Jawetz, Ernest. Infectious diseases: viral and rickettsial. In Schroeder, Steven A., Krupp, Marcus A., and Tierney, Lawrence M., Jr., eds., *Current Medical Diagnosis & Treatment—1988*. Norwalk, CT: Appleton & Lange, 1988, pp. 834-857.

29. ———. Infectious diseases: Bacterial. Ibid., pp. 848-884.

30. ———. Infectious diseases: Spirochetal. Ibid., pp. 885-895.

31. Guerrant, Richard L. Salmonella infections. In Braunwald, Eugene, et al., eds., *Harrison's Principles of Internal Medicine*, 11th ed. New York: McGraw-Hill Book Co., 1987, pp. 592-599.

32. Haynes, Barton, F. Enlargement of lymph nodes and spleen. In Braunwald, Eugene, et al., eds., *Harrison's Principles of Internal Medicine*, 11th ed. New York: McGraw-Hill Book Co., 1987, pp. 272-278.

33. Haynes, Barton F., and Fauci, Anthony S. Introduction to clinical immunology. In Braunwald, Eugene, et al., eds., *Harrison's Principles of Internal Medicine*, 11th ed. New York: McGraw-Hill Book Co., 1987, pp. 328-337.

34. Hirsch, Martin S. Cytomegalovirus infection. In Braunwald, Eugene, et al., eds., *Harrison's Principles of Internal Medicine*, 11th ed. New York: McGraw-Hill Book Co., 1987, pp. 697-699.

35. Hirschmann, Jan V. Rat-bite fever (*Streptobacillus moniliformis* and *spirillum minus* infections). In Braunwald, Eugene, et al.,

eds., *Harrison's Principles of Internal Medicine*, 11th ed. New York: McGraw-Hill Book Co., 1987, pp. 655-656.

36. Hirschmann, Jan V., and Murray, John F. Pneumonia and lung abscess. In Braunwald, Eugene, et al., eds., *Harrison's Principles of Internal Medicine*, 11th ed. New York: McGraw-Hill Book Co., 1987, pp. 1075-1082.

37. Holmes, King K., and Handsfield, H. Hunter. Sexually transmitted diseases. In Braunwald, Eugene, et al., eds., *Harrison's Principles of Internal Medicine*, 11th ed. New York: McGraw-Hill Book Co., 1987, pp. 506-519.

38. Holmes, King K., and Lukenhart, Sheila A. Syphilis. In Braunwald, Eugene, et al., eds., *Harrison's Principles of Internal Medicine*, 11th ed. New York: McGraw-Hill Book Co., 1987, pp. 639-649.

39. Ingram, Roland H., Jr. Adult respiratory distress syndrome. In Braunwald, Eugene, et al., eds., *Harrison's Principles of Internal Medicine*, 11th ed. New York: McGraw-Hill Book Co., 1987, pp. 1134-1137.

40. Isselbacher, Kurt J., and Podolsky, Daniel K. Infiltrative and metabolic diseases affecting the liver. In Braunwald, Eugene, et al., eds., *Harrison's Principles of Internal Medicine*, 11th ed. New York: McGraw-Hill Book Co., 1987, pp. 1353-1356.

41. Jawetz, Ernest, and Grossman, Moses. Introduction to infectious diseases. In Schroeder, Steven A., Krupp, Marcus A., and Tierney, Lawrence M., Jr., eds., *Current Medical Diagnosis & Treatment—1988*. Norwalk, CT: Appleton & Lange, 1988, pp. 817-833.

42. Jawetz, Ernest, Melnick, Joseph L., and Adelberg, Edward A. Immunology: I. Antigens & antibodies. *Review of Medical Microbiology*, 17th ed. Norwalk, CT: Appleton & Lange, 1987, pp. 170-190.

43. ———. Immunology: II. Antibody-mediated & cell mediated (hypersensitivity & immunity) reactions. Ibid., pp. 191-205.

44. ———. Gram-positive bacilli. Ibid., pp. 206-212.

45. ———. Corynebacteria. Ibid., pp. 213-216.

46. ———. The staphylocci. Ibid., pp. 217-222.

47. ———. The streptococci. Ibid., pp. 223-232.

48. ———. Enteric gram-negative rods (enterobacteriaceae). Ibid., pp. 233-246.

49. ———. The neisseriae. Ibid., pp. 268-273.

50. ———. Miscellaneous pathogenic bacteria. Ibid., pp. 274-279.

51. ———. Mycoplasmas (Mollicutes) & cell wall—Defective bacteria. Ibid., pp. 281-284.

52. ———. Mycobacteria. Ibid., pp. 285-292.

53. ———. Spirochetes and other spiral microorganisms. Ibid., pp. 293-300.

54. ———. Rickettsial diseases. Ibid., pp. 301-305.

55. ———. Chlamydiae. Ibid., pp. 306-313.

56. ———. Medical mycology. Ibid., pp. 318-337.

57. ———. Principles of diagnostic medical microbiology. Ibid., pp. 338-361.

58. ———. Detection of viruses & antigens in clinical specimens. Ibid., pp. 401-407.

59. ———. Serologic diagnosis & immunologic detection of virus infections. Ibid., pp. 408-417.

60. ———. Arthropod-borne & rodent-borne viral diseases. Ibid., pp. 418-431.

61. ———. Picornavirus family (enterovirus & rhinovirus groups). Ibid., pp. 432-442.

62. ———. Hepatitis viruses. Ibid., pp. 443-456.

63. ———. Orthomyxovirus (Influenza) and coronavirus families. Ibid., pp. 467-475.

64. ———. Paramyxovirus family & rubella virus. Ibid., pp. 476-486.

65. ———. Adenovirus family. Ibid., pp. 495-501.

66. ———. Herpesvirus family. Ibid., pp. 502-512.

67. ———. Acquired immune deficiency syndrome (AIDS). Ibid., pp. 533-538.

68. Kasper, Dennis L. Infections due to mixed anaerobic organisms. In Braunwald, Eugene, et al., eds., *Harrison's Principles of Internal Medicine*, 11th ed. New York: McGraw-Hill Book Co., 1987, pp. 567-573.

69. Kaye, Donald. Tularemia. In Braunwald, Eugene, et al., eds., *Harrison's Principles of Internal Medicine*, 11th ed. New York: McGraw-Hill Book Co., 1987, pp. 613-615.

70. Kaye, Donald, and Petersdorf, Robert G. Brucellosis. In Braunwald, Eugene, et al., eds., *Harrison's Principles of Internal Medicine*, 11th ed. New York: McGraw-Hill Book Co., 1987, pp. 610-613.

71. Kosek, Margaret S., Medical genetics. In Schroeder, Steven A., Krupp, Marcus A., and Tierney, Lawrence M., Jr., eds., *Current Medical Diagnosis & Treatment—1988*, Norwalk, CT: Appleton & Lange, 1988, pp. 1035-1059.

72. Kuo, G., et al. An assay for circulating antibodies to a major etiologic virus of human non-A, non-B hepatitis. *Science* 244:362-364.

73. Locksley, Richard M. Staphylococcal infections. In Braunwald, Eugene, et al., eds., *Harrison's Principles of Internal Medicine*,

74. Locksley, Richard M., and Plorde, James J. Leishmaniasis. In Braunwald, Eugene, et al., eds., *Harrison's Principles of Internal Medicine*, 11th ed. New York: McGraw-Hill Book Co., 1987, pp. 785-787.

75. Longo, Dan L., and Broder, Samuel. Plasma cell disorders. In Braunwald, Eugene, et al., eds., *Harrison's Principles of Internal Medicine*, 11th ed. New York: McGraw-Hill Book Co., 1987, pp. 1396-1403.

76. McLeod, Rima, and Remington, Jack S. Toxoplasmosis. In Braunwald, Eugene, et al., eds., *Harrison's Principles of Internal Medicine*, 11th ed. New York: McGraw-Hill Book Co., 1987, pp. 791-797.

77. Miller, Richard A. Leprosy (Hansen's disease) In Braunwald, Eugene, et al., eds., *Harrison's Principles of Internal Medicine*, 11th ed. New York: McGraw-Hill Book Co., 1987, pp. 633-637.

78. Nash, Theodore E. Schistosomiasis. In Braunwald, Eugene, et al., eds., *Harrison's Principles of Internal Medicine*, 11th ed. New York: McGraw-Hill Book Co., 1987, pp. 810-814.

79. Pearson, Richard D., and Guerrant, Richard L. Shigellosis. In Braunwald, Eugene, et al., eds., *Harrison's Principles of Internal Medicine*, 11th ed. New York: McGraw-Hill Book Co., 1987, pp. 599-601.

80. Perine, Peter L. Relapsing fever. In Braunwald, Eugene, et al., eds., *Harrison's Principles of Internal Medicine*, 11th ed. New York: McGraw-Hill Book Co., 1987, pp. 656-657.

81. Petersdorf, Robert G., and Root, Richard K. Chills and fever. In Braunwald, Eugene, et al., eds., *Harrison's Principles of Internal Medicine*, 11th ed. New York: McGraw-Hill Book Co., 1987, pp. 50-57.

82. Plorde, James J. The diagnosis of infectious diseases. In Braunwald, Eugene, et al., eds., *Harrison's Principles of Internal Medicine*, 11th ed. New York: McGraw-Hill Book Co., 1987, pp. 459-466.

83. ———. The diagnosis and therapy of parasitic infections. Ibid., pp. 769-771.

84. ———. Amebiasis. Ibid., pp. 773-778.

85. ———. Trypanosomiasis. Ibid., pp. 787-791.

86. ———. Babesiosis. Ibid., pp. 799.

87. ———. Giardiasis. Ibid., pp. 800-801.

88. ———. Cryptosporidiosis and other protozoan infections. Ibid., pp. 801-805.

89. ———. Trichinosis. Ibid., pp. 805-806.

90. ———. Filariasis. Ibid., pp. 807-810.

91. ———. Tissue nematodes. Ibid., pp. 814-816.

92. ———. Intestinal nematodes. Ibid., pp. 816-822.

93. ———. Other trematodes or flukes. Ibid., pp. 822-824.

94. Plorde, James J., and White, Nicholas J. Malaria. In Braunwald, Eugene, et al., eds., *Harrison's Principles of Internal Medicine*, 11th ed. New York: McGraw-Hill Book Co., 1987, pp. 778-785.

95. Prockop, Darwin J. Heritable disorders of connective tissue. In Braunwald, Eugene, et al., eds., *Harrison's Principles of Internal Medicine*, 11th ed. New York: McGraw-Hill Book Co., 1987, pp. 1680-1688.

96. Ramsey, Paul G., and Plorde, James J. Cestode (tapeworm) infections. In Braunwald, Eugene, et al., eds., *Harrison's Principles of Internal Medicine*, 11th ed. New York: McGraw-Hill Book Co., 1987, pp. 825-829.

97. Ray, C. George. Measles (rubeola). In Braunwald, Eugene, et al., eds., *Harrison's Principles of Internal Medicine*, 11th ed. New York: McGraw-Hill Book Co., 1987, pp. 682-683.

98. ———. Rubella ("German measles") and other viral exanthems. Ibid., pp. 684-686.

99. ———. Smallpox, vaccinia, and other poxviruses. Ibid., pp. 686-689.

100. ———. Enteroviruses and reoviruses. Ibid., pp. 703-707.

101. ———. Mumps. Ibid., pp. 709-712.

102. Sanford, Jay P. Leptospirosis. In Braunwald, Eugene, et al., eds., *Harrison's Principles of Internal Medicine*, 11th ed. New York: McGraw-Hill Book Co., 1987, pp. 652-655.

103. ———. Arbovirus infections. Ibid., pp. 717-731.

104. Schaberg, Dennis R., and Turck, Marvin. Diseases caused by gram-negative enteric bacilli. In Braunwald, Eugene, et al., eds. *Harrison's Principles of Internal Medicine*, 11th ed. New York: McGraw-Hill Book Co., 1987, pp. 583-589.

105. Schooley, Robert T. Epstein-Barr virus infections, including infectious mononucleosis. In Braunwald, Eugene, et al., eds., *Harrison's Principles of Internal Medicine*, 11th ed. New York: McGraw-Hill Book Co., 1987, pp. 699-703.

106. Shearn, Martin A. Arthritis and musculoskeletal disorders. In Schroeder, Steven A., Krupp, Marcus A., and Tierney, Lawrence M., Jr., eds., *Current Medical Diagnosis & Treatment—1988*, Norwalk, CT: Appleton & Lange, 1988, pp. 496-532.

107. Sparling, P. Frederick. Sexually transmitted diseases. In Wyngaarden, James B., and Smith, Lloyd H., Jr., eds., *Cecil's Textbook of Medicine*, 18th ed. Philadelphia: W.B.

Saunders Co., 1988, pp. 1701-1722.

108. Stites, Daniel P., et al. Immunologic disorders. In Schroeder, Steven A., Krupp, Marcus A., and Tierney, Lawrence M., Jr., eds., *Current Medical Diagnosis & Treatment—1988*, Norwalk, CT: Appleton & Lange, 1988, pp. 1076-1090.

109. Stamm, Walter E., and Holmes, King K. Chlamydial infections. In Braunwald, Eugene, et al., eds., *Harrison's Principles of Internal Medicine*, 11th ed. New York: McGraw-Hill Book Co., 1987, pp. 759-768.

110. Swierkosz, Ella., PhD. Personal communication.

111. Talal, Norman. Sjögren's syndrome. In Wyngaarden, James B., and Smith, Lloyd H., Jr., eds., *Cecil's Textbook of Medicine*, 18th ed. Philadelphia: W.B. Saunders Co., 1988, pp. 2024-2025.

112. Walzer, Peter D. *Pneumocystis carinii* pneumonia. In Braunwald, Eugene, et al., eds., *Harrison's Principles of Internal Medicine*, 11th ed. New York: McGraw-Hill Book Co., 1987, pp. 797-799.

113. Wands, Jack R., et al. Chronic hepatitis. In Braunwald, Eugene, et al., eds., *Harrison's Principles of Internal Medicine*, 11th ed. New York: McGraw-Hill Book Co., 1987, pp. 1338-1341.

114. Weekly Science News Update. Path to hepatitis C yields tests, clues. *Science News*. 135:246-247, Apr. 22, 1989.

115. Weinstein, Louis. Diseases of the upper respiratory tract. In Braunwald, Eugene, et al., eds., *Harrison's Principles of Internal Medicine*, 11th ed. New York: McGraw-Hill Book Co., 1987, pp. 1111-1115.

116. Whitley, Richard J. Varicella-zoster virus infections. In Braunwald, Eugene, et al., eds., *Harrison's Principles of Internal Medicine*, 11th ed. New York: McGraw-Hill Book Co., 1987, pp. 689-692.

117. Woodward, Theodore E. Rickettsial diseases. In Braunwald, Eugene, et al., eds., *Harrison's Principles of Internal Medicine*, 11th ed. New York: McGraw-Hill Book Co., 1987, pp. 747-757.

P
A
R
T

2

16 | Selected Terms Pertaining to Anesthesiology

17 | Selected Terms Pertaining to Gerontology

18 | Selected Terms Pertaining to Oncology

19 | Selected Terms Pertaining to the Clinical Laboratory

20 | Selected Terms Pertaining to Radiology, Diagnostic Ultrasound, and Magnetic Resonance Imaging

21 | Selected Terms Pertaining to Nuclear Medicine

22 | Selected Terms Pertaining to Physical Therapy

Selected Terms Pertaining to Anesthesiology

CHAPTER 16

Orientation

Origin of Terms

-algia- (G)—pain

anesthesia (G)—loss of sensation or feeling

nacro- (G)—stupor

-spasm (G)—involuntary contractions

General Terms

- *analeptics*—stimulants of the central nervous system, for example, coramine and caffeine.
- *analgesia*—loss of normal sense of pain. (7, 27, 40)
- *analgesics*—drugs that relieve pain. (7, 27)
- *anesthesia*—inability to feel.
    - *general anesthesia*—state of unconsciousness accompanied by varying degrees of muscular relaxation and freedom from physical pain. (61, 35)
    - *local anesthesia*—absence of sensation and consequently of pain in a part of the body; consciousness retained. (10, 42)
- *anesthesiologist*—physician who specializes in anesthesiology. (10)
- *anesthesiology*—the science and study of anesthesia. (10)
- *anesthetic*—an agent producing insensibility to pain.
- *anesthetist*—professional person, not necessarily a physician, who is qualified to administer anesthesia. (10)
- *antiemetic drugs*—drugs that are therapeutically useful for control of nausea or vomiting, such as parasympatholytic agents (belladonna alkaloids), phenothiazines, and butyrophenones. (9, 27)
- *arterial hypotension during anesthesia*—lower arterial blood pressure during anesthesia may result from several causes. These include excessive premedication; potent therapeutic drugs administered prior to anesthesia; overdose of general anesthetics; circulatory effects of spinal and epidural anesthesia; raised airway pressure; compression of the vena cava; hypovolemia; hemorrhage; surgical manipulation; and change in position of the patient. (See Table 21) (29)

Table 21
Causes of Arterial Hypotension Encountered During Anesthesia*

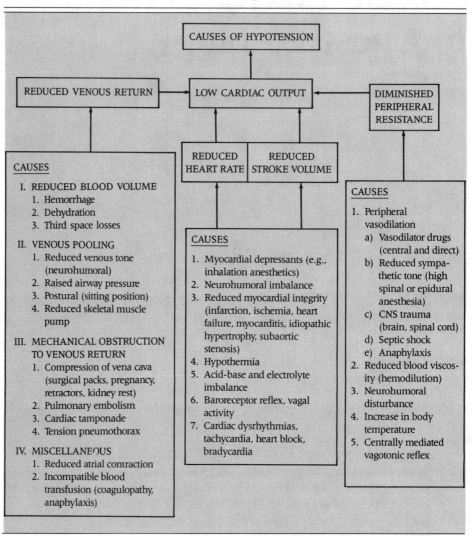

*(Reprinted by permission, from Robert D. Dripps, James E. Eckenhoff, and Leroy D. Vandam. Arterial hypotension during anesthesia. In *Introduction to Anesthesia: The Principles of Safe Practice*, 7th ed. Philadelphia: W.B. Saunders Co., 1988, p. 390.)

- *artificial ventilation*—mechanism (respirator, ventilator, etc.) used to control rate and depth of breathing. The most common indications for artificial ventilation are respiratory failure and deterioration of blood gas levels with progressive signs of tiring. (3, 13, 31, 32)
- *hypercarbia, hypercapnia*—excess of carbon dioxide in the blood.
- *hyperventilation*—excessive respiration, causing an abnormal loss of carbon dioxide from the blood. (31, 32)
- *hypotensive anesthesia*—technique employed to diminish blood loss and oozing to create a dry surgical field and prevent risks of hypertension. It combines elements of pharmacologic blockage, monitoring of blood pressure and patient posture throughout the procedure, and use of the intermittent positive-pressure ventilator, when indicated. (28)
- *hypoxia*—reduction of oxygen supply to the body tissues. (43)

- *inhalation therapy*—administration of inhalant gases such as oxygen or carbon dioxide to relieve oxygen insufficiency or to stimulate respiration. (32)
- *malignant hyperthermia syndrome*—potentially fatal hypermetabolic syndrome that may be induced by any of the inhalation anesthetics such as halothane, methoxyflurane, cyclopropane, and ethyl ether or muscle relaxants, most notably succinylcholine. (See Oral Reading Practice, p. 375 for further information.) (30, 34, 39)
- *neuroleptanalgesics*—potent analgesics and tranquilizers producing detached quiescence and somnolence, used for premedication and general anesthesia or as adjuncts to other anesthetic agents. (8)
- *neuromuscular blocking agents, skeletal muscle relaxants*—drugs that serve as adjuncts to general anesthesia by producing muscular relaxation and thus reducing the need for deep levels of anesthesia.
  - *depolarizing agents*—relaxants that block motor nerve impulses at the myoneural junction, such as succinylcholine chloride (Anectine Chloride) and decamethonium bromide (Syncurine). Depolarizing agents mimic the action of acetylcholine at the nerve-muscle junction, causing a discharge of the end-plate potential.
  - *nondepolarizing agents*—relaxants that inhibit transmission of motor nerve impulses at the myoneural junction, such as gallamine triethiodide (Flaxedil Triethiodide). Pancuronium bromide (Pavulon) is a competitive blocking neuromuscular agent that is longer acting and does not possess histamine or ganglionic blocking properties. (11, 17, 38)
- *preanesthetic medication, premedication*—a combination of drugs, including opium derivatives and barbiturates, tranquilizers, ataraxics, neuroleptanalgesics, and the belladonna group, used in the preanesthetic preparation. The main function of these drugs is to reduce fear and anxiety by better preparing the patient to face the operation with calmness and confidence and to diminish the side effects of the anesthetic agents. Premedication also maintains cardiac stability and prevents convulsive reactions, thus ensuring a smooth recovery from the anesthesia. (12)
- *response evaluation to anesthetics*—a stimulus-response assessment used by most anesthetists and anesthesiologists to classify the adequacy of anesthetic depth in a patient.
  - *presurgical level*—requires more anesthesia. Three signs used to identify surgical anesthesia level are the loss of the eyelid reflex, muscle relaxation, and rhythmic respiration. When these signs are not present, the patient is classified at the presurgical level and additional anesthetization is required.
  - *anesthetic depression*—level identified according to stimulus-response assessment: presurgical anesthesia, surgical anesthesia, and overdose.
  - *surgical anesthesia planes*—planes of surgical anesthesia are classified as too light, adequate, and too deep.
  - *patient's status evaluated*—assessment of afferent input to the nervous system; estimation of observable physiologic responses; and interaction evaluation of patient, stimulus, type of anesthetic administered, and surgical anesthesia plane.
  - *stimulus evaluation*—classification of stimulus ranges between the areas of strong or weak. Local inflammation may heighten the intensity of the stimulus while careful surgical manipulation may lessen the intensity of the stimulus. The stimulus may be lessened by advancing age and/or poor physical state.
  - *Woodbridge Component*—refers to four components of the anesthetic state developed by P.D. Woodbridge. Those four components are sensory, motor, mental, and reflex. (See Table 22, which classifies the intensity of responses that may be observed in these four areas.) (2, 19)

- *stage of analgesia*—period from first inhalations of the anesthetic to beginning of loss of consciousness. The patient is awake, the sensorium is clear, reflexes continue to be active, but the patient is insensitive to surface pain.
- *stage of delirium*—period from loss of consciousness to beginning of surgical anesthesia. There is depression of the cerebral cortex and loss of control of higher centers. Reflexes tend to be exaggerated; struggling, excitement, incoordination, and disorientation may occur. This stage is often absent in children.
- *stage of surgical anesthesia*—period from second stage to cessation of spontaneous respiration. This stage is subdivided into four planes:
  - —*first plane*—muscle tone is unchanged and eyeball movements continue when the lids are raised. The pupil reacts to light.
  - —*second plane*—smaller muscles throughout the body lose their tone and ocular movements cease. The pupils are centrally fixed.
  - —*third plane*—muscular relaxation throughout the body includes large muscles. The corneal reflexes are abolished. Respiration becomes diaphragmatic.
  - —*fourth plane*—the relaxation of large muscles and loss of reflexes are complete. The pupils are widely dilated. Diaphragmatic activity is decreased.
- *stage of toxicity*—period from onset of apnea to circulatory failure. Respiratory movement ceases, the depression of the cardiovascular system increases, and the blood pressure drops rapidly. If artificial respiration is instituted, the condition may be reversible.

The above stages and planes of anesthesia were defined by A.E. Guedel during World War I. He described the respiratory changes, pupillary alterations, eye movements, and swallowing and vomiting responses that provided for the estimation of depth of ether anesthesia in patients. In 1943, N.A. Gillespie added reflex responses: laryngeal and pharyngeal reactivity, lacrimation, and the respiratory response to surgical incision. The above stages and planes of anesthesia represent terminology used in past anesthesia practice but which is used less in current practice because of the development and growth of monitoring devices. Today, most anesthesiologists and anesthetists employ a stimulus-response evaluation. See the above definition for response evaluation to anesthetics. (2, 19)

- *transient global amnesia*—syndrome characterized by an abrupt loss of memory that is self-limited and not recurrent or associated with severe damage of the central nervous system. It occurs in the postanesthetic period and lasts less than 24 hours.
- *vasoconstrictors*—drugs causing a constriction of the blood vessels. They are used in combination with local anesthetics to produce a vasoconstriction locally, thus preventing the anesthetic from being carried away from the site of injection.

Terms Related to Methods of General Anesthesia

- *endotracheal anesthesia*—introduction of a catheter into the trachea for the purpose of conducting the anesthetic mixture directly from the apparatus to the lungs. This may be achieved by oral or nasal intubation. The catheter is then attached to a closed or semiclosed inhaler. In present practice this form of inhalation anesthesia is the method of choice for most major operations, since it permits a patient airway, aspiration of secretions, use of positive pressure, controlled breathing, adequate ventilation, and isolation of the respiratory tract from the gastrointestinal tract. (18, 35)
- *hypercarbic anesthesia*—excess carbon dioxide content of the blood and controlled hypertension causing improved oxygenation and decreased oxygen consumption during general anesthesia. The increased cerebral flow results from vasodilatation of hypercarbia and increased cerebral perfusion of induced hypertension.

Table 22
Evaluation of Response Intensity*

Woodbridge Component	Sensory	Motor	Mental	Reflexes		
				Circulatory	Respiratory	Gastrointestinal
High intensity response	Breath holding Deep breathing Stiff chest Phonation Laryngospasm Tachycardia Rise or fall in BP Movement with stimulus Pupillary dilation Sweating Coughing	Fine or gross movement Abdominal tightness Muscle potentials on ECG	Movement upon stimulation Delirium Uninhibited speech or actions	Bradycardia hypotension Tachycardia hypertension Arrhythmias	Spasm: laryngeal bronchiolar chest wall Salivation	Nausea Retching Vomiting Swallowing
Acceptable response	Minimal response to painful stimuli followed by accommodation Stability of cardiovascular and respiratory systems	Quiet surgical field Relaxation of muscle	Amnesia Ataraxia Sleep	Absence of troublesome cardiovascular, respiratory, and gastrointestinal reflexes		
Low intensity response	No response	Muscle flaccidity Inability to reestablish normal ventilatory function at end of anesthesia	Prolonged obtundation in preanesthetic or post-anesthetic period	Bradycardia Tachycardia Hypotension Arrhythmias Intolerance to position change	Respiratory arrest**	Intestinal atony Postoperative ileus

*(Reprinted by permission, from Robert D. Dripps, James E. Eckenhoff, and Leroy D. Vandam, Evaluation of the response to anesthetics: The signs and stages. In *Introduction to Anesthesia: The Principles of Safe Practice*, 7th ed. Philadelphia: W.B. Saunders Co., 1988, p. 208.)

**In the absence of neuromuscular blockers or hypocarbia.

- *hypocarbic anesthesia*—low carbon dioxide content and deliberate hypertension as an adjunct to general anesthesia.
- *inhalation anesthesia*—general anesthesia produced by the inhalation of vaporized liquids or gases. It is slower than intravenous anesthesia but is more readily controlled and may be safer. Inhalation induction is usually used electively for those patients who have no superficial veins or who are afraid of venipuncture. Several methods are used:
  - *closed method*—technique in which the patient rebreathes the anesthetic mixture, which is contained in a special apparatus composed of a tightly fitting mouth or nose mask or tube, a rebreathing bag, and a device permitting the absorption of carbon dioxide.
  - *open method*—liquid anesthetic drug is dropped on a gauze mask that covers the patient's nose and mouth and permits the inhalation of the vaporized drug.
  - *semiclosed method*—technique that differs from the closed method by use of an exhalation valve, which allows partial rebreathing and carbon dioxide removal with soda lime. (14, 15)
- *intravenous anesthesia*—the intravenous administration of drugs to produce basal anesthesia. A stage of unconsciousness is produced, but analgesia and muscular relaxation may prove unsatisfactory. (16, 23)
- *rectal anesthesia*—the rectal administration of drugs to produce basal anesthesia. The reflexes are partially abolished, and a hypnotic state ensues. Pentothal, Avertin, and ether have been used for this purpose. (25)

Selected Terms Related to Dissociative Anesthesia

- *dissociative anesthesia*—selective blocking of pain conduction and perception, leaving those parts of the central nervous system that do not participate in pain transmission and perception, free from the depressant effects of drugs. The profound analgesia induced by this type of anesthesia is associated with somnolence, in which the patient appears to be disconnected from the environment. (7, 16)
- *neuroleptanalgesia, neuroleptanesthesia*—balanced, highly effective anesthetic state for control of well-defined pain during surgery resulting from the depression of certain corticothalamic systems. It may be used as the sole anesthesia or as adjunct to local, regional, or general anesthesia. Neuroleptanalgesia is a type of dissociative anesthesia. (8, 16)

Selected Reflexes Related to Anesthesia

- *eyelash reflex*—touching the eyelashes to evoke lid movement. The eyelash reflex is a guide to determine the depth of anesthesia. (21)
- *lid reflex*—tapping of the eyelid to evoke its immediate closure. A guide to determine the depth of anesthesia, the lid reflex is lost in the stage of surgical anesthesia. (21)

Local and Regional Anesthesia

Origin of Terms

acus (L)—needle
cata- (G)—down, lower, under
cauda (L)—tail
dura (L)—hard
hypno- (G)—sleep
vas-, vaso- (L)—vessel

Selected Terms Related to Methods of Local Anesthesia

- *acupuncture analgesia*—entails the insertion of stainless steel acupuncture needles at carefully selected points identified as being effective for producing the desired effect.

This practice was developed in China and is widely accepted there as an anesthetic agent. The U.S. medical community views this practice as acupuncture analgesia rather than acupuncture anesthesia. (27)

- *axillary brachial block*—with the patient's arm abducted at right angles and the elbow flexed, the axillary artery is palpated and outlined as high as possible. The anesthetist then places the forefinger of the left hand on the artery and inserts the needle, usually without the syringe attachment, at a right angle to the patient's skin. (23)
- *caudal or sacral anesthesia*—method of epidural anesthesia in which the anesthetic solution is injected into the sacral canal. (14, 15, 21, 22, 42)
- *epidural block*—spinal nerves blocked as they pass through the epidural space. (1, 22, 42)
- *infiltration anesthesia*—injection of a dilute anesthetic agent under the skin to anesthetize the nerve endings and nerve fibers. (22, 42)
- *intravenous regional anesthesia*—method of producing analgesia in the extremities using lidocaine (or other drug) as a regional anesthetic to act at the main nerve trunks. (16, 23)
- *spinal anesthesia*—anesthesia produced by the injection of a local anesthetic solution into the subarachnoid space of the lumbar region to block the roots of the spinal nerves. (1, 21)
- *supraclavicular brachial plexus block*—point of injection is one centimeter above the midpoint of the clavicle. Insertion of the needle is downward and caudally, but not backward or medially. (21, 23)
- *topical or surface anesthesia*—direct application of an anesthetic drug to a mucous membrane to produce insensibility to the nerve endings. Agents employed for topical anesthesia may include benzocaine, cocaine, dibucaine, cyclonine, lidocaine, and tetracaine. (20)

Abbreviations

General

ACh—acetylcholine
Anes.—anesthesiology
C_{10}—decamethonium
C_3H_6—cyclopropane
C_2H_4—ethylene
$CHCl_3$—chloroform
C_2H_5Cl—ethylchloride
C_2HCl_3—trichloroethylene (Trilene)
CO_2—carbon dioxide
HCl—hydrochloride
He—helium
NLA—neuroleptanalgesia
N_2O—nitrous oxide
NR—nonrebreathing

NT—nasotracheal
O_2—oxygen
OD—open drop
OT—orotracheal
Pent.—pentothal
SC—semiclosed
Vin.—vinyl ether (Vinethene)

Standard Pharmacology Texts

ADI—*American Drug Index*
NF—*The National Formulary*
PDR—*Physicians' Desk Reference*
USD—*The Dispensary of the United States of America*
USP—*United States Pharmacopeia*

Oral Reading Practice

Malignant Hyperthermia Syndrome

Malignant hyperthermia syndrome (MHS) is a potentially fatal hypermetabolic syndrome that may be induced by any of the **inhalation anesthetics** such as

halothane, methoxyflurane, cyclopropane, and **ethyl ether** or **muscle relaxants,** most notably **succinylcholine.** The etiology of **MHS** is believed to be an underlying pathophysiologic disorder of the muscle that may affect generalized body membrane dysfunction. Temperature increases rapidly to between 102.2 and 107.6 degrees F. Susceptibility to this disorder is transmitted by **autosomal-dominant inheritance** with variable frequency. Also the syndrome may occur in **myotonic disorders, Duchenne dystrophy, central core disease,** and in a **congenital myopathy** with **dysmorphic** features.

Continued progression of **MHS** depends on a combination of **myogenic, neurologic,** and **endocrinologic** derangements, including generalized membrane dysfunction. At the initiation and during the progression of **MHS,** hyperactivity of the **sympathetic nervous system** with release of **catecholamines** and **thyroid** hormone has been implicated in their effects on muscle cells. In some instances, following the intravenous injection of succinylcholine, muscle rigidity develops, especially **masseter muscle spasm.**

At the height of the syndrome, the **serum creatine phosphokinase (CPK)** increases markedly along with the appearance of **myoglobinuria.** Muscle biopsy usually reveals depletion of **adenosine triphosphate (ATP),** as well as **CPK.**

The clinical sequelae of **MHS** are usually initiated with a hypermetabolic state of muscle followed by a rapid rise in temperature. Most often, the first signal of **MHS** is **tachycardia.** This is followed by **tachypnea** as a result of **metabolic** and **respiratory acidosis.** The patient's skin is hot and **venous** blood in the operative field is dark because of the high oxygen consumption. Tachypnea is noted in the spontaneously breathing patient because of excess **carbon dioxide** production. It is essential to monitor closely the end-expired carbon dioxide and pulse oximetry in order to detect these symptoms.

Dantrolene is administered as soon as **MHS** is suspected, and this is continued until temperature begins to decline and other signs of hypermetabolism disappear. Malignant hyperthermia is a medical emergency. Anesthesia and the operative procedure should be concluded as quickly as possible and cooling mechanisms instituted. With the cooling mechanisms, it is important to avoid the **hypothermic** range. **Pulmonary hyperventilation** with **oxygen** is instituted simultaneously and **sodium bicarbonate** given intravenously to combat both **respiratory** and **metabolic acidosis.** It is important to monitor closely the **arterial blood gases** and **acid-base levels.** An osmotic diuretic is usually given to avoid **vasoconstrictive nephropathy** and **myoglobinemia-induced oliguria.**

Late complications that may develop include **coma,** which may be irreversible and a manifestation of **cerebral ischemia** and **hypoxia,** as well as **disseminated intravascular coagulation** and **vasoconstrictive nephropathy.**

Due to the tendency of this syndrome to run in families, it is essential that the anesthesiologist consider carefully the history of the patient or family members having anesthesia problems, as well as carefully monitoring the temperature of all patients under anesthesia. (30, 33, 34, 36, 37, 39)

Table 23
Classification of Selected General Anesthetics

Anesthetic Agents	Systemic Effects

• Volatile substances, administered by inhalation:
  Liquids producing vapors
    Chloroform
    Enflurane (Ethrane)
    Ether
    Ethyl chloride
    Halothane (Fluothane)
    Methoxyflurane (Penthrane)
    Trichloroethylene (Trilene)
    Vinyl ether (Vinethene)
  Gases
    Cyclopropane
    Ethylene
    Nitrous oxide
	Chemical substances and depressants of the central nervous system; surgically useful because they are complete anesthetics providing:
	  analgesia
	  suppression of reflex activity
	  muscular relaxation, *and*
	  loss of consciousness

• Nonvolatile substances administered intravenously or rectally
  Ultra-short-acting barbiturates:
    Methohexital (Brevital)
    Thiamylal (Surital)
    Thiopental (Pentothal)
  Derivatives of ethyl alcohol:
    Tribromoethanol (Avertin)
    Solution Avertin in Amylene hydrate
	Basal narcotics, medullary depressants, and incomplete anesthetics; these are surgically useful as adjuncts to other anesthetics. They produce:
	  unconsciousness
	  inadequate control of reflex activity
	  unsatisfactory muscular relaxation
	  hypnosis and amnesia (following use of Avertin)

• Nonvolatile substances administered intravenously or intramuscularly:
  Neuroleptics and nonbarbiturates:
    Ketamine (Ketalar)
    Droperidol (Inapsine)
  Neuroleptic and potent narcotic analgesic:
    Innovar (Droperidol and Fentanyl)
	Short-acting anesthetics, depressants of certain corticothalamic systems; useful as sole anesthetic and as adjunct to conventional anesthesia. They produce:
	  profound analgesia
	  amnesia
	  increased cardiovascular activity
	  unsatisfactory muscular relaxation

References and Bibliography

1. Axelsson, Kjell. Motor blockade during spinal anesthesia. In Lofstrom, J.B., and Sjostrand, Ulf, eds., *Local Anesthesia and Regional Blockade*, New York: Elsevier, 1988, pp. 135-156.
2. Ayata, Sadat, M.D. Personal communications.
3. Barnes, Thomas A. Mechanical ventilation. In Barnes, Thomas A., ed., *Respiratory Care Practice*, Chicago: Year Book Medical Publishers, Inc., 1988, pp. 216-248.
4. Corssen, Guenter, Reves, J.G., and Stanley, Theodore H. Pharmacokinetics of narcotic compounds. In *Intravenous Anesthesia and Analgesia*, Philadelphia: Lea & Febiger, 1988, pp. 31-38.
5. ———. Pharmacology of narcotic analgesics. Ibid., pp. 39-66.
6. ———. Barbiturates. Ibid., pp. 67-98.
7. ———. Dissociative anesthesia. Ibid., pp. 99-173.
8. ———. Neuroleptanalgesia and neurolep-

tanesthesia. Ibid., pp. 99-173.

9. ———. Propanidid. Ibid., pp. 263-266.

10. Dripps, Robert D., Eckenhoff, James E., and Vandam, Leroy D. Perspective in Anesthesiology: History, education and clinical practice. In *Introduction to Anesthesia: The Principles of Safe Practice*, 7th ed. Philadelphia: W.B. Saunders Co., 1988, pp. 3-9.

11. ———. Pharmacologic principles. Ibid., pp. 22-36.

12. ———. Premedication and preparation for anesthesia. Ibid., pp. 37-45.

13. ———. Monitoring physiologic function. Ibid., pp. 70-92.

14. ———. Inhalation anesthetics. Ibid., pp. 117-132.

15. ———. Techniques of inhalation anesthesia. Ibid., pp. 133-139.

16. ———. Intravenous anesthetics. Ibid., pp. 141-155.

17. ———. Neuromuscular blocking agents. Ibid., pp. 166-187.

18. ———. Intubation of the trachea. Ibid., pp. 188-204.

19. ———. Evaluation of the response to anesthetics: The signs and the stages. Ibid., pp. 205-210.

20. ———. Local anesthetics. Ibid., pp. 211-222.

21. ———. Spinal anesthesia. Ibid., pp. 223-235.

22. ———. Epidural and caudal anesthesia. Ibid., pp. 236-243.

23. ———. Regional nerve blocks. Ibid., pp. 244-258.

24. ———. Obstetric anesthesia and perinatology. Ibid., pp. 293-313.

25. ———. Pediatric anesthesia. Ibid., pp. 315-334.

26. ———. Cardiopulmonary anesthesia. Ibid., pp. 335-345.

27. ———. The therapy of pain. Ibid., pp. 368-379.

28. ———. Deliberate hypotension. Ibid., pp. 380-387.

29. ———. Arterial hypotension during anesthesia. Ibid., pp. 389-402.

30. ———. Unusual complications of anesthesia. Ibid., pp. 403-416.

31. ———. Respiration and respiratory care. Ibid., pp. 441-468.

32. ———. Inhalation therapy and pulmonary physiotherapy. Ibid., pp. 469-476.

33. Engel, Andrew G. Diseases of muscles (myopathies) and neuromuscular junction. In Wyngaarden, James B., and Smith, Lloyd H., eds., *Cecil's Textbook of Medicine*, 18th ed., vol. 2. Philadelphia: W.B. Saunders Co., 1988, pp. 2269-2288.

34. Malhotra, Vinod. Malignant hyperthermia. In Yao, Fun Sun F., and Artusio, Joseph F., Jr., eds., *Anesthesiology: Problem Oriented Patient Management*, 2d ed. Philadelphia: J.B. Lippincott Co., 1988, pp. 580-591.

35. Miller, Ronald D. Anesthesia. In Way, Lawrence W., ed., *Current Surgical Diagnosis & Treatment*, 8th ed. Norwalk, CT: Appleton & Lange, 1988, pp. 164-173.

36. Olgin, Jeffrey, et al. Non-invasive evaluation of malignant hyperthermia susceptibility with phosphorus nuclear magnetic resonance spectroscopy. *Anesthesiology* 68:507-513, April 1988.

37. Petersdorf, Robert G., and Root, Richard K. Disturbances of heat regulation. In Brunwald, Eugene, et al. eds., *Harrison's Principles of Internal Medicine*, 11th ed., vol. 1. New York: McGraw-Hill Book Co., 1987, pp. 43-50.

38. Rau, Joseph L., Jr. Major drug families. In Barnes, Thomas A., ed., *Respiratory Care Practice*, Chicago: Year Book Medical Publishers, Inc., 1988, pp. 545-549.

39. Schroeder, Steven A., and Chatton, Milton J. General care—symptoms and disease prevention. In Schroeder, Steven A., Krupp, Marcus A., and Tierney, Lawrence M., Jr., eds., *Current Medical Diagnosis & Treatment—1988*, Norwalk, CT: Appleton & Lange, 1988, pp. 1-16.

40. Sjostrand, Ulf. Psychological aspects of regional analgesia. In Lofstrom, J.B., and Sjostrand, Ulf, eds., *Local Anesthesia and Regional Blockade*, New York: Elsevier, 1988, pp. 273-278.

41. Wagner, Dennis L., and Stoetling, Robert K. Hemodynamic monitoring. In Brown, David L., ed., *Risk and Outcome in Anesthesia*, Philadelphia: J.B. Lippincott Co., 1988, pp. 213-234.

42. Willis, Richard J. Caudal epidural blockade. In Cousins, Michael J., and Birdenbaugh, Phillip O., eds., *Neural Blockade in Clinical Anesthesia and Management of Pain*, 2d ed. Philadelphia: J.B. Lippincott Co., 1988, pp. 361-383.

43. Youtsey, John W. Oxygen and mixed gas therapy. In Barnes, Thomas A., ed., *Respiratory Care Practice*, Chicago: Year Book Medical Publishers, Inc., 1988, pp. 131-163.

Selected Terms Pertaining to Gerontology

Orientation

Origin of Terms

asthenia (G)—weakness
gero-, geronto- (G)—old age, the aged
-logy (G)—science or study of

presby- (G)—old, old age
senilis (L)—old age, senile

General Terms

- *ageism*—prejudice against an elderly person because of his or her age. (Ref. 25)
- *aging process, senescence*—refers to the declining years of life or a normal process of growing old: a progressive increase in the probability of an organism continuing to age as time passes. Some authors have defined the physiology of aging as an inability to maintain homeostasis, referring to the body's maintenance of a constant internal environment despite external changes. Major features of the inability may include:
  - —decreased performance of endocrine glands.
  - —changes in the production of reproductive and thyroid hormones, insulin, glucagon, and adrenal glucocorticoids.
  - —changes in the brain and central nervous system.
  - —increases in blood pressure and a decrease in the heart's stroke volume.
  - —reduced tolerance for stress
  - —increase in airway resistance and reduction in vital capacity of the lung
  - —changes in normal immune functions of the body, with increased susceptibility to infections.
    - —*natural immunity*—refers to the production of specific antibodies stimulated by invasion by bacteria or other infective agents.
    - —*artificial immunity*—refers to inoculation weakened or dead bacteria to stimulate antibody production and give protection.
  - —changes in perception, with a decrease in conduction time at the myoneural junction and neurons, which could lead to loss of balance and other subsequent injuries.
  - —impairment of the cardiovascular, neuromuscular, and respiratory systems with subsequent periods of disuse of whole or part of these systems. Examples of such conditions affecting the elderly person include:

-*orthostatic hypotension*, increased work of the heart, and potential thrombus formation.

-osteoporosis, contractures, muscular atrophy, and decubiti.

-decreased respiratory movement, decreased respiratory secretion, and a disturbance in gas exchange, such as in emphysema or chronic bronchitis. (13, 39, 55, 57, 58, 59, 60, 65, 67, 68, 69)

■ *drug interactions*—usually involves two or more drugs; the elderly may be exposed to any number of drug interactions. The drug that precipitates the interaction is called the precipitant drug; the drug whose effect is altered is known as the object drug. Types of interactions can be classified into three categories:

-*pharmaceutical interactions*—usually occur when two drugs are given together in the same infusion solution or when a drug reacts with the infusion or solution.

-*pharmacokinetic interactions*—the disposition of the object drug is altered by the precipitant drug. This may occur as a result of the body's reaction to the drug, so that the defect of the object drug is either diminished or increased by the action of the precipitant drug.

-*pharmacodynamic interations*—may be direct or indirect.

-*direct reaction*—refers to the precipitant or object drugs acting on the same system.

-*indirect reaction*—refers to two aspects: the precipitant drug causes some alteration in fluid or electrolyte balance, which influences the effect of the drug, and the precipitant drug alters the structure of the organ.

The elderly have diminished organ and body clearance for accomplishing proper drug metabolism and are at higher risk to develop higher than usual plasma and tissue levels of a drug. Important aspects that influence the disposition of drugs in the elderly are impairment of renal function and changes in distribution volume. On the other hand, the elderly patient may need to take several drugs for the continued maintenance of good health. This makes it imperative for the practitioner to understand the role played by drug interactions. Examples of two types of medications that require careful monitoring in the older person are:

-*neuroleptic, antipsychotic drugs*—medications that modify psychotic behavior or symptoms by achieving psychomotor slowing, emotional calming, and affective indifference. Three major classes of neuroleptic drugs are:

-butyrophenones

-phenothiazines

-thioxanthenes

Usually, use of these drugs provides improvement in thought disturbances that accompany paranoid ideation. The elderly person may experience such adverse side effects as excess sedation, hypotension, dry mouth, constipation, urinary retention, tardive dyskinesia, cardiac dysrhythmias, some dysphoria, and possible impairment of intellectual performance.

-*tricyclic antidepressant drugs*—drugs whose action is based on their potentiation of the synaptic transmission in the central nervous system, which is mediated by either 4-hydroxytryptamine or norepinephrine. Many of these drugs have sedative effects similar to those produced by the phenothazines; the sedative effect begins immediately but decreases over time. Some of these drugs are:

-amitriptyline

-desipramine

-doxepin

-imipramine

-nortriptyline

-protriptyline

Adverse side effects include constipation, urinary hesitancy or retention, excessive sedation or delirium, dry mouth, impaired visual accommodation, and orthostatic hypotension. These drugs interact adversely with most antidysrhythmic agents because of their quinidine-like effect on the cardiac conduction system and their myocardial depressant activity. (5, 13, 21, 25, 30, 31, 63, 64)

- *evaluation of activities of daily living*—refers to a variety of systems that have been developed to record the progress of these activities. Usually a numeric score is obtained by which the progress or regression of these activities can be gauged. Some of the commonly used systems are:
    - —*Barthel index*—allows a maximum of 100 points and operates on the decimal system.
    - —*Katz index*—classifies patients into one of seven groups; for example, class A: the patient is independent in feeding, continence, transferring, toilet activities, and bathing; class B: the patient is independent in all these functions except one, etc. The Katz index system avoids using the arbitrary point system. Its reliability is based on the assumption that various functions are restored in a precise chronologic order; that is, patients will be able to feed themselves before they bathe independently.
    - —*Kenny system*—uses six major functional subcategories: bed, transfers, locomotion, dressing, personal hygiene, and feeding activities. The patient is scored separately in each of these categories, which are given equal weight, and a total score is then obtained, with a maximum of 24 points. (6, 17, 82)
- *geriatrics*—branch of medical science concerned with the diseases of old age and their treatment. (13)
- *gerontologist*—scientist who studies the process of aging in its biologic, mental, and socioeconomic implications. (25)
- *gerontology*—the scientific study of all facets of aging, including branches of science that contribute to an understanding of older adults, such as physiology, psychology, sociology, and public health. (25)
- *hospice*—refers to a coordinated system of inpatient and outpatient services directed at fostering the emotional and psychologic care of the dying. The hospice approach looks to the needs of both the patient and the family as the dying event culminates. (25)
- *pain*—a symptom of physical hurt or mental or emotional distress. Pain may serve as a warning sign or indicator of disease.
- *podiatrist*—specialist concerned with the diagnosis and treatment of defects, injuries, and diseases of the feet, which are often seen in the elderly. (25)
- *presbyatrics*—the medical treatment of the aging person. (25)
- *psychogerontology*—science that deals with the mental and emotional life of older adults, including their ideation, memory, and level of consciousness. (13, 25)

Some Disorders Affecting the Older Adult

Diagnostic Terms

- *accidental hypothermia (AH)*—the elderly patient's body temperature drops slowly within hours or days to 95° F (35° C) or below; the extremities and abdomen feel cold to touch. The face may be pink and puffy, the blood pressure is low, and the pulse is slow; atrial and ventricular arrhythmias and mental confusion are frequent manifestations. Cardiac arrest (cessation of effective heart action, usually manifested by asystole or ventricular fibrillation) occurs at a temperature of 75° to 85° F (24° to 30° C). Accidental hypothermia refers to environmentally induced hypothermia in contrast to hypothermia that develops secondary to medical conditions or surgical treatment. (25, 49, 51)

- *acute gastrointestinal hemorrhage*—bleeding from the gastrointestinal tract. About 90 percent of acute gastrointestinal bleeding occurs from sites proximal to the ligament of Treitz and is usually manifested by hematemesis or melena. Bright red blood usually indicates a colonic source. In the older adult the cause of lower intestinal hemorrhage may remain obscure, even after standard evaluation. Nonoperative therapies may not control the situation, and more aggressive measures may be recommended, such as right hemicolectomy.. Deaths of elderly persons from gastrointestinal hemorrhage usually occur as a result of:
  —complications of surgery
  —exsanguinating hemorrhage
  —serious cardiovascular, liver, renal, or malignant disease. In these cases the outcome is determined by the disease, with bleeding as the secondary event.
  In the older adult with hemorrhage who experiences an associated illness, the outcome may be compounded by the inability to withstand the effects of shock, massive hemorrhage, or surgical intervention. (25, 28)

- *Alzheimer's disease*—a degenerative disorder beginning in the fifth or sixth decade of life, pathologically characterized by neurofibrillar degeneration, (with silver-staining plaques containing degenerating neuronal products grouped around an amyloid core being randomly pinpointed in the cortex and subcortex); cortical atrophy; and loss of nerve cells. The onset of dementia is insidious. Memory loss in Alzheimer's disease is constant and unvarying. The patient loses interest in social contacts; becomes anxious, depressed, and disoriented; develops aphasia, agnosia, and apraxia; and displays a hesitant shuffle in gait. Incapacitating flexion contractures mark the terminal decerebrate phase of life. Although research studies have investigated roles of aluminum metabolism, immune and autoimmune processes, viruses, and genetic components in explaining the etiology of Alzheimer's disease and its consequences, the cause of Alzheimer's disease remains unknown. This disease is named after Alois Alzheimer, who discovered it in 1907. (1, 52, 57, 83)

- *angina pectoris, classic type*—syndrome characterized by short attacks of substernal precordial pain that radiates to the left shoulder and arm. It is more commonly associated with S-T segment changes than conduction defects. Electrocardiographic (ECG) findings may show atrioventricular defects of conduction, nonspecific S-T segment changes, previous myocardial scar, or other abnormalities; about 30 percent of the ECG studies are likely to be normal. This condition may be provoked by exertion and relieved by rest. (60, 66)

- *apathetic thyrotoxicosis*—an occult form of hyperthyroidism in which apathy and inactivity are prominent features. It is estimated that about 40 percent of elderly thyrotoxic persons fail to present the cardinal signs of exophthalmic goiter: diffuse enlargement of the thyroid gland, prominent eyeballs, tachycardia, and thyroid bruit. This fact may be attributed to the reduced vitality in old age. (7, 16)

- *arteriosclerosis obliterans*—arterial obstruction of the extremities, particularly affecting the lower limbs and causing ischemia. (72)

- *cancer in the elderly*—refers to more than 100 clinically and biologically distinct diseases. Cancer is second only to cardiovascular disease of death in the elderly. (See Chapter 18 for a listing of common malignant neoplasms.) (47)

- *cataract*—an opacity in the lens, usually the acquired type in the older adult. Lenticular opacity is usually linked with the aging process. Insoluble proteins form in the lens and eventually lead to dehydration, lowered metabolism, and tissue necrosis. In the cataractous lens, sodium and calcium content tend to be increased, with potassium protein and ascorbic acid content decreased. Visual impairment is slowly progressive. A so-called ripe cataract has reached the point of marked liquefaction and swelling. Cataracts are usually removed before they reach this stage. (77)

■ *cerebrovascular accident, stroke, apoplexy*—neurologic disorder caused by pathologic changes in extracranial or intracranial blood vessels, primarily atherosclerosis, thrombosis, embolic episodes, hemorrhage, or arterial hypertension. Cerebral infarction or necrosis of brain tissue may occur in the affected lesion. The completed stroke, usually recognized by a rather sudden loss of consciousness, is preceded by:

—*transient ischemic attacks*—symptoms of minor brain damage evidenced by numbness, unilateral weakness, visual defects, motor disability, and similar symptoms. They may last from minutes to hours. A complete return to the preattack status may occur, or there may be residual damage.

—*progressive stroke*—neurologic manifestations are persistent and become more serious, signaling impending stroke. (1, 22, 32)

■ *chronic obstructive pulmonary disease (COPD)*—this refers to a class of diseases of uncertain etiology characterized by persistent slowing of airflow during forced expiration. This prolonged airway obstruction can cause disabling progressive respiratory disease, frequently with irreversible functional deterioration and a fatal prognosis. Examples of disease entities in this category that may affect the older adult include:

—*emphysema*—refers to pathologic destruction of interalveolar septa, including blood vessels, and the fusing of air spaces to form abnormal cystic areas in the lungs that do not function in gas exchange. Destruction of pulmonary elastic tissue occurs with resultant loss of recoil and increased compliance. The most common symptom is progressive dyspnea on exertion. In advanced cases the patient may exhibit wheezing and/or symptoms of cor pulmonale (pedal edema and ascites). Evidence of clubbing of the digits may occur, as well as signs of pulmonary hypertension (increased second heart sound, pedal edema, hepatomegaly, and ascites).

—*chronic bronchitis*—refers to inflammation of the bronchial mucous membranes, which is often sparked by the inhalation of irritant substances such as cigarette or cigar smoke and various forms of air pollution. A chronic cough and sputum production most often signal cases of chronic bronchitis. As the disease progresses, the patient may experience increased cough, change in sputum (from clear to purulent), fever, dyspnea, and possible episodes of respiratory failure. Specifically, the definition for chronic bronchitis requires that chronic cough and expectoration have continued for at least three months or, when there is no other cause such as a neoplasm or tuberculosis, for at least two years. The most important physiologic abnormalities in established chronic bronchitis are hypoxemia and carbon dioxide retention. (3, 27, 69)

■ *congestive heart failure*—condition in which the heart is unable to pump adequate amounts of blood to tissues and organs, generally caused by heart diseases resulting in low cardiac output. It can also result from other conditions (anemia, hyperthyroidism) in which the demand for blood is greater than normal, and the heart fails despite high cardiac output.

—*left-sided heart failure*—failure of the left ventricle precipitated by serious coronary, hypertensive, or valvular heart disease. Except in mitral stenosis, it produces variable degrees of left ventricular dilatation followed by pulmonary congestion and edema, salt and water retention, scanty urinary output, cerebral hypoxia, and coma.

—*right-sided heart failure*—failure of the right ventricle characterized by venous congestion of the portal system with ascites and enlargement of liver and spleen.

In advanced disease left-and right-sided congestive heart failure coexist. Factors that predispose the older adult to coronary heart disease (CHD) include obesity, a sedentary occupation or lack of physical activity, stress, and competitiveness. The major function implication of cardiopulmonary changes is the reduced tolerance for stress; changes in maximal voluntary ventilation, pulmonary gas exchange, blood pressure, and cardiac output add to a neuromuscular picture of an organism slowing down. This reduced capacity of the older adult to adapt to stress may indicate a careful monitoring of vital signs while exercising. (4, 65)

- *cranial arteritis, giant cell arteritis, arteritis of the aged*—a panarteritis of older adults primarily involving the temporal arteries and ophthalmic and retinal arteries and clinically noted for a piercing headache: scalp tenderness; pain; blanching and occasionally gangrene of the tongue, probably due to lingual arteritis; peripheral neuropathy; and sudden blindness. (1, 12, 32)
- *fracture of hip*—a break in upper end of the femur. The two main types are:
    - *femoral neck fracture*—bone broken through the neck of the femur.
    - *trochanteric fracture*—bone broken below, around, or between the greater or lesser trochanters. (11)
- *hypertension*—pathologic elevation of the blood pressure consistently exceeding 160/95 mm Hg. According to the *Statement on Hypertension in the Elderly* from the National Health Institute, hypertension is a major public health problem for the elderly. It is the major risk factor for 500,000 strokes, 37 percent of which are fatal, and is a contributing factor in 1.5 million heart attacks and in approximately 570,000 heart attack deaths each year. Hypertension is more prevalent in women than in men after the age of 65, however the opposite is true before age 55. (68) Hypertension is a major cause of epistaxis (nosebleed) among the elderly population. It usually occurs at night, and the elderly person may awake gagging on a mouthful of blood. Nutritional restrictions and antihypertensive medications tend to lower the blood pressure, thus reducing the elderly person's risk of cardiovascular disorders, particularly cerebrovascular accidents. (18, 46, 66, 68)
- *intestinal obstruction, ileus*—obstruction of the small intestine associated with variable symptoms: abdominal distension, colicky pain, nausea, vomiting, obstipation, or diarrhea. Interference with blood flow to the obstructed intestine demands emergency surgery.
    - *adynamic (paralytic) ileus*—paralysis of intestinal muscles with absence of bowel sounds. It may be caused by electrolyte imbalance or operative handling of the intestines.
    - *dynamic (mechanical) ileus*—intestinal occlusion from adhesions, strangulated hernia, volvulus, intussusception, emboli, or thrombi. (62)
- *myocardial infarction, acute*—clinical syndrome manifested by persistent, usually intense cardiac pain, unrelated to exertion and often constrictive, followed by diaphoresis, pallor, hypotension, dyspnea, faintness, nausea, and vomiting. The underlying disease is usually coronary atherosclerosis that has progressed to coronary thrombosis and occlusion and resulted in a sudden curtailment of blood supply to the heart muscle and myocardial ischemia.
    - *inferior wall infarction, diaphragmatic infarction*—occlusion of the right coronary artery.
    - *lateral wall infarction*—infarction resulting from occlusion of the diagonal branch of the left anterior descending artery or left circumflex artery.
    - *posterior wall infarction*—infarction precipitated by occlusive lesions of the right coronary artery or circumflex coronary artery branch. (50, 65, 66)

A postinfarction (Dressler's) syndrome may develop within the first week or weeks after the patient has sustained a myocardial infarction. It exhibits clinical features of a benign form of pericarditis with or without effusion. (50, 65, 66)

- *normal pressure hydrocephalus (NPH)*—neurologic syndrome of the elderly that occurs without previous identifiable brain disease and is manifested by a peculiar gait (dyspraxia), incontinence, ventricular dilatation, and a normal cerebrospinal fluid pressure. In the early phase NPH may be relieved by shunting of the cerebrospinal fluid from the dilated ventricles. (1, 48, 57)

- *organic brain syndrome*—permanent damage to brain tissue leading to cerebral insufficiency and deterioration of cognitive faculties. In the elderly person it may be associated with senile dementia and advanced cerebral atherosclerosis. It may be classified as:

  —*amnestic syndrome*—dominant aspect of this syndrome is twofold: impairment of short-term memory (the inability to learn new data) and impairment of long-term memory (inability to retain information known in the past).

  —*delirium and dementia*—cognitive impairment is relatively global.

  —*intoxication and withdrawal*—the disorder is associated with ingestion or reduction in use of a drug and does not meet the criteria for any of the syndromes already mentioned.

  —*organic delusional syndromes and organic affective syndrome*—features resemble schizophrenic or affective disorders.

  —*organic personality syndrome*—persistent personality disturbance, either lifelong or representing a change or accentuation of a previously characteristic trait, that results from a specific organic factor. See Chapter 4 for further information regarding these disorders. (5, 25, 44, 52, 80)

- *osteitis deformans, Paget's disease of bone*—skeletal disorder characterized by decalcification, marked bone destruction and rapid bone repair, architectural abnormality of new bone, increased vascularity, and fibrosis. Striking features are intensification with advancing years, proneness to fracture, and the frequency of coexisting osteogenic sarcoma. (7, 34)

- *osteoporosis of the elderly*—disorder of protein metabolism marked by increased porosity of bone that is especially pronounced in the spine and pelvis and leads to spontaneous fractures, deformities, and collapse of vertebrae with reduction in the elderly person's height. (7, 35, 55)

- *paralysis agitans, Parkinson's disease*—slowly progressive neurologic disorder of middle and late life, primarily affecting the nuclei of the brain stem. Rigidity, slow movements, tremors, masklike facies, and a monotonous voice are clinical findings. Characteristic shuffling with increasing pace is evident once locomotion has started. Gait is propulsive or retropulsive. (1, 57)

- *pneumonia*—inflammation of the lungs with exudation into lung tissue and consolidation. Predominant etiologic agents are pneumococci and mycoplasmas or pleuropneumonia-like organisms and less frequently staphylococci, streptococci, meningococci viruses, tubercle bacilli, and others. Hospital-acquired (nosocomial) infections are usually caused by gram-negative organisms. (69)

- *polymyalgia rheumatica*—special type of muscular rheumatism seen more frequently in older women than men, clinically manifested by pain and stiffness in the back, shoulder, neck, and occasionally the pelvic girdle. (11)

- *Raynaud's disease*—painful vascular disorder characterized by peripheral spasms of the digital arterioles of the fingers and toes that may result in gangrene. Digital blanching refers to the fingers and toes becoming pallid due to the vasospasm of the arterioles. (72, 75)

- *senescent (senile) psychiatric disorders*—usually refers to a variety of states affecting the elderly patient. Examples include: (5, 13, 25, 80)

    —*delirium and confusion*—psychotic reaction to fever, dehydration, surgery, and other somatic states. The elderly person appears disoriented and bewildered, hallucinates, and wanders about aimlessly.

    —*depression and agitation*—psychotic state characterized by egocentric behavior, melancholy, intense agitation, defective memory, and mental decline.

    —*paranoia*—common psychotic reaction of senescence in which delusions of persecution tend to predominate.

    —*presbyophrenia*—mental disorder found in elderly persons who previously had a dynamic personality. The presbyophrenic person is constantly busy in an unproductive or destructive way, is out of touch with reality and very forgetful, and covers up memory lapses with confabulations.

    —*senile dementia*—irreversible deterioration of cognitive faculties.

- *senescent (senile) skin disorders:* (56)

    —*ectasia, vascular nevi, cherry angiomas*—elevated red spots caused by dilated capillaries, found on the trunk and extremities of aged persons.

    —*purpura*—hemorrhagic disorder characterized by easy bruising and purple extravasations, chiefly of aging skin on arms and legs.

    —*sebaceous adenomas*—benign lesions, typically appearing on the face of elderly persons as pearly oval papules with a central depression.

- *senescent (senile) visual disorders:*

    —*benign ocular hypertension*—seen in about 15 percent of persons in the 70 to 75 age-group. The intraocular tension is somewhat increased, and the optic disc and visual fields are normal. (77)

    —*chronic blepharitis*—common geriatric problem and seborrheic condition of the eyelashes with accumulation of secretions around the lashes. (77)

    —*chronic primary open-angle glaucoma*—most common type of glaucoma in the 70 to 74 age-group. The outflow obstruction of aqueous humor from the anterior chamber of the eye results from an abnormality in the trabecular meshwork. (77)

    —*diabetic retinopathy*—changes in the blood vessels around the macula cause the visual loss encountered in the onset of diabetes in advanced years. (77)

    —*ectropion*—eversion of the lid margin, attributed to the elongation and laxity of the lid and associated with an overflow of tears. It occurs more readily in advanced years. (77)

    —*entropion*—the lower lid margin turns inward, and the lashes brush against the cornea, injuring the corneal epithelium and predisposing to infection. (67, 77)

    —*degeneration of Bruch's membrane*—irregular thickening of the membrane and a hardening of the choriocapillaris which is composed of one layer of closely spaced capillaries attached to the membrane. The outer third of the retina receives its blood supply from the choriocapillaris, including the fovea centralis. With aging the damage to Bruch's membrane increases, either by detachment or complete atrophy of the pigment epithelium or by formation of new vessels and bleeding. (67, 77)

    —*macular generation*—occurs in the pigment epithelium of the retina; Bruch's membrane is separated from the choriocapillaris and undergoes thickening and hyalinization and breaks, leading to choroidal neovascularization. New vessels may form in the retinal pigment epithelium and penetrate into the subretinal space, producing leakage and detachment. These changes are the primary cause of visual loss in the elderly. (67, 77)

—*retinoschisis*—a splitting of the retina into two layers, resulting from peripheral cystoid degeneration. A self-limited, relatively harmless detachment of the retina may develop. If the retinal splitting encroaches on the macula, treatment is indicated. (40)

Operative Terms

- *blepharoplasty for blepharochalasis*—plastic repair of redundant eyelids.
- *cataract removal*—various procedures for removal of opaque lens, including these four:
    - —*anterior chamber implantation*—preparation of a 7.5-millimeter trephine opening, removal of the cataract by cryoextraction, and insertion of the anterior chamber lens through the trephine opening. (61)
    - —*cryoextraction of cataract*—application of the tip of the cryoextractor to the anterior surface of the lens until the cataract firmly adheres to the instrument. When freezing process has extended two to three millimeters into the lens substance, the probe, with the lens frozen to it, is lifted out. (61)
    - —*extracapsular cataract extraction*—incision into the anterior capsule to express the opaque nucleus of the lens and some of the cortical material. (70)
    - —*intracapsular cataract extraction*—removal of the entire lens in its capsule; a method of choice especially for senescent (senile) cataracts. (61)
- *colon resection and end-to-end anastomosis*—excision of involved colon with or without adjacent lymph glands; joining segments of the colon. (76)
- *dermabrasion and excision of:*
    - —*furrowed brows*—application of dermabrader to frown furrows and removal of skin over the furrowed area. (71)
    - —*perioral wrinkles*—application of dermabrader to each vertical lip line for elimination of wrinkles around mouth. (71)
- *face-lift operation*—reconstructive plastic surgery of the face; the art of surgical sculpture applied to the human face to restore function, remove the marks of time, or correct defects. (71)
- *gastric resection*—removal of 50 to 75 percent of the stomach combined with the following procedures:
    - —*gastroduodenal anastomosis, Billroth I*—joining the resected stomach to the duodenum.
    - —*gastrojejunal anastomosis, Billroth II*—joining the remaining stomach to the jejunum by either the:
        - —*Poly technique*—anterior anastomosis, large stoma *or*
        - —*Hofmeister technique*—posterior anastomosis, small stoma. (45)
- *rhytidectomy*—surgical removal of subcutaneous fat pads and superfluous skin to eliminate wrinkles. (71)
- *rhytidoplasty*—surgical elimination of wrinkles achieved by removal of excess skin and by tightening remaining skin to restore youthful appearance. A dermal fat graft is inserted in the following forms of repair:
    - —*glabellar rhytidoplasty*—operative procedure for removing the vertical furrows between the eyebrows.
    - —*cerviofacial rhytidoplasty*—surgical correction of wrinkles of the neck and face. (71)

Symptomatic Terms

- *agnosia*—sensory inability to recognize objects. (32)
- *alienation*—estrangement felt by the elderly person in a environment that he or she considers undesirable, unpredictable, and detrimental to his or her way of life. (25)
- *aloneness*—feeling of being forsaken or left alone resulting from the loss of family members and friends. (25)
- *aphasia*—difficulty with the use or understanding of words caused by lesions in association areas.
    - —*motor aphasia*—verbal comprehension intact, but patient unable to use the muscles that coordinate speech.
    - —*sensory aphasia*—inability to comprehend the spoken word, if auditory word center is affected, and the written word, if the visual word center is involved. The patient will not understand the spoken or written word if there is an involvement of both centers. Two types of aphasic disorders are:
        - –*Broca's aphasia* (see Fig. 76)—the cerebral lesion is anterior and nearly always associated with hemiplegia or hemiparesis. Spontaneous speech is nonfluent and indistinct, and the vocabulary is limited. Comprehension and reading ability may be intact.
        - –*Wernicke's aphasia* (see Fig. 76)—the cerebral lesion is posterior; spontaneous speech is fluent, but comprehension is defective. There may be logorrheic outpouring of words associated with bizarre, euphoric, or paranoid behavior. (1, 13, 44)
- *apraxia*—inability to carry out familiar, purposeful movements in the absence of paralysis or other motor or sensory impairment. (24)
- *arcus senilis, gerontoxon*—white or grayish opaque ring just within the sclerocorneal junction of the eye seen in elderly persons. If present early in life, it is called arcus juvenilis.
- *ataxia*—motor incoordination. (19, 24)
- *blepharochalasis*—relaxed, baggy eyelids; redundancy may interfere with vision.
- *bradycardia*—slow heart action. (66)
- *bradykinesia*—slowness of all movements; normal in the elderly. (24)
- *cardiogenic shock*—syndrome related to cardiovascular disease, primarily to myocardial infarction, cardiac tamponade, and massive pulmonary embolism. (66)
- *Cheyne-Strokes respirations*—harsh breathing with a prolonged, high pitched increase in depth and rapidity, then a gradual decrease and cessation. After 10 to 20 seconds of apnea, the cycle is repeated. (44, 81)
- *confabulation*—making up tales to fill in memory gaps. The patient is not construing deliberate falsehoods but believes the fantasies to be true. (80)
- *depression*—morbid sadness, melancholy, or dejection that is out of proportion with loss or injury endured; frequently observed in the elderly person. (5)
- *disengagement*—term refers to an inevitable withdrawal of the elderly person, resulting in decreased social interaction. Multiple factors precipitate disengagement, such as sensory deficits, especially loss of hearing and sight; retirement; reduced income; declining physical and mental capacities; and progressive isolation due to the deaths of friends and relatives. Disengagement is only unhealthy in its extreme form. (25)
- *dyskinesia*—abnormal involuntary movement and body posture caused by a brain lesion.
    - —*athetosis*—slow, wormlike, writhing movement, especially in hands and fingers.
    - —*ballism, ballismus*—violent, flinging, shaking, or jerking of extremities.
    - —*chorea*—quick, explosive, purposeless movements.

Figure 76 Broca's area and Wernicke's area of brain

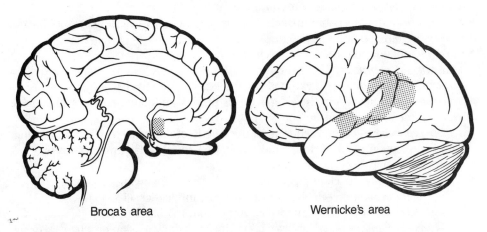

Broca's area   Wernicke's area

—*dystonia*—abnormal posture from twisting movements, usually of limbs and trunk.

—*tardive dyskinesia*—lip smacking, sucking, jaw movements, writhing tongue movements, chorea, athetosis, dystonia, tics, and facial grimacing. This disorder has gradual onset after long-term, high-dose antipsychotic drug use, and research indicates that the elderly are at risk for developing tardive dyskinesia after use of neuroleptic drugs. The abnormal involuntary movements involve the orofacial areas in the older adult, whereas the younger adult exhibits extremity involvement. (5, 30, 57)

- *dyspnea*—difficult breathing. (66, 69)
- *fasciculation*—involuntary twitching of groups of muscle fibers. (23, 24)
- *festination*—quick, shuffling steps and accelerated gait seen in Parkinson's disease. (19)
- *grief reaction*—bereavement caused by the death of or separation from a significant person, which may be first expressed by a feeling of numbness and later profound yearning for the lost one, restlessness, and psychophysiologic responses. Also it may be related to matters of importance, such as enforced retirement or loss of home. (25)
- *hemiplegia*—paralysis affecting one side of the body. (24)
- *Kussmaul breathing*—clinical manifestation in diabetic acidosis marked by unusually deep respirations associated with dyspnea. This type of breathing is caused by an abnormally increased acid content of the blood, resulting in continuous overstimulation of the respiratory center. (81)
- *paraplegia*—paralysis of the lower limbs and, at varying degrees, of the lower trunk. (24)
- *presbylibrium*—loss of balance that occurs with aging, usually manifested in the elderly person as a sensation of unsteadiness or rotary vertigo following head motion. Two movements that may produce these symptoms are getting out of bed and looking upward. (25)
- *presbyopia*—defective vision resulting from changes in accommodation, part of the aging process. (25)
- *presbyacusia, presbycusis*—hearing loss that occurs with aging, usually manifested by impaired perception and discrimination of sounds. (20)

- *progeria of adult*—premature aging, including early graying of hair, baldness, sparse eyebrows, and fine wrinkles around the mouth. (25)
- *regression*—return to infantile patterns of reacting, seen in psychosis, severe illness, and under other circumstances. (5, 25)
- *rigidity*—an abnormal resistance to change. (1)
- *senescent (senile) pruritus*—itching of brittle, dry skin by the elderly person, leading to scratching and followed by excoriations and eczematoid changes. (56)
- *senescent (senile) tremor*—in the elderly, this is usually an intention tremor of variable etiology, rarely a constant tremor. (57)
- *sensory deprivation*—normal sequelae in the elderly of diminished sight and hearing; dulled perception of smell, taste, and touch; and social isolation or restriction.
- *tachycardia*—rapid heart action. (66)
- *urologic symptoms*—the elderly person may exhibit the following:
    - —*urinary incontinence*—inability to hold urine in bladder. (13, 17)
    - —*urinary retention*—inability to pass urine from the bladder. (13)
    - —*stress incontinence*—inability to retain urine under any tension or when sneezing, coughing, or laughing. (13, 17)
    - —*neurogenic incontinence*—may be iatrogenic, produced by administration of drugs that either block the bladder or urethral mechanisms or that interfere with normal urinary function, leading to urinary retention and overflow incontinence. (73)
    - —*neurogenic bladder types:*
        - –*flaccid atonic type*—condition caused by lower motor neuron lesion due to trauma, ruptured intervertebral disk, meningomyelocele, or other disorders and resulting in vesical dysfunction. The bladder has a large capacity, low intravesical pressure, and a mild degree of trabeculation (hypertrophy) of the wall. (73)
        - –*spastic automatic type*—condition caused by upper motor neuron lesion due to injury, multiple sclerosis, or other factors. The bladder capacity is reduced, the intravesical pressure is high, and there is marked hypertrophy of the bladder wall and spasticity of the urinary sphincter. (73)
    - —*dysuria*—difficult or painful urination. (36)
    - —*enuresis*—incontinence or involuntary discharge of urine when asleep at night.
    - —*hesitancy*—dysuria due to nervous inhibition or to obstruction of vesical outlet. (36)
    - —*polyuria*—excessive urinary output. (36)
    - —*tenesmus of vesical sphincter*—painful spasm at end of micturition. (36)
    - —*trabeculation, vesical*—hypertrophy involving all muscle layers of the bladder. It may occur in benign prostatic hypertrophy. (36)

Terms Related to Psychotherapy for the Older Adult

Diagnostic Terms

- *activity therapy*—program of activities prescribed on the basis of psychologic understanding of their specific needs. Types of therapy include:

—educational
—music
—occupational
—play
—recreational
—remotivation (25, 33)

- *attitude therapy*—refers to adapting one of the five basic attitudes to the patient's needs. This type of therapy, designed by James Folsom, calls for a consistency of approach from the staff members toward the client, while allowing them to vary the particular attitude approach, depending on the client's changing needs. The five basic attitudes are:
    —active friendliness for withdrawn and apathetic patients
    —kind firmness for depressed patients
    —matter-of-fact approach to alcoholic and sociopathic patients
    —no demand for destructive patients
    —passive friendliness for suspicious and paranoid patients (25, 33)
- *behavior therapy*—therapeutic approach that attempts to bring about direct change by helping elderly persons unlearn maladaptive and destructive behavior and to enhance their abilities for socially acceptable and productive behavior. (5, 17)
- *group psychotherapy*—method of psychotherapy applied to a group. Group leaders help patients to gain insight into their emotional difficulties and conflicts, to understand the causes, and to translate their defensive reactions into acceptable behavior. (5, 33)
- *individual psychotherapy*—method of psychotherapy applied to the elderly person's mental and emotional problems. By applying various psychologic means, the therapist enables the patient to interact in reliving and restructuring these problems. It is through this type of interaction that the problems of the patient are more effectively resolved. (20)
- *milieu therapy*—the use of a modified and controlled environment in the treatment of mental disease.
- *reality therapy*—provides the patient with an objective evaluation and judgment of the world outside the self. This type of orientation has benefited the older adult following electroshock therapy, during reactions from drugs or alcohol, and during periods of acute confusion. The underlying thrust of this therapy is that even the most severely mentally impaired patient is capable of improvement when exposed to a continuing and consistent program of reality orientation. (4)
- *supportive psychotherapy*—therapeutic efforts directed toward a strengthening of the patient's ego to reduce anxiety. The real problem may remain unsolved and may resurface at a crucial moment. (5, 33)
- *therapy of reminiscence*—refers to a review of past life experiences by the elderly person to establish a renewed sense of identity and self-esteem relative to their present situation and environment. This type of therapy may assist the older adult to face the troubling aspects of life and to facilitate a reshaping of responses to present situations. (25, 38, 41)
- *therapy of remotivation*—refers to using conversation or only a couple of words to stimulate the older adult and bring him or her back to reality. The thrust of this therapy is to remotivate those inner drives and impulses that cause a person to act in a certain way. A structured remotivation program may provide a therapeutic setting in which the older adult can make new assertions of self-respect or independence and gain a renewed dignity of self and others. (25, 29)

Abbreviations

General

AVM—arteriovenous malformation

CHF—congestive heart failure

COPD—chronic obstructive pulmonary disease

ECT—electroconvulsive therapy

GHFT—Gottschaldt hidden figure test

GNP—gerontological nurse practitioner

MOSES—multidimensional observation scale for elderly subjects

NSAID—nonsteroidal anti-inflammatory drug

SAH—subarachnoid hemorrhage

SDAT—senile dementia of Alzheimer's type

SMD—senile macular degeneration

SRRD—sleep-related respiratory disturbances

TIA—transient ischemic attack

TUR—transurethral resection

AMA—American Medical Association

CDC—Centers for Disease Control

DHHS—Department of Health & Human Services

DRG—Diagnostic Related Group

HCFA—Health Care Financing Administration

NCHS—National Center for Health Statistics

NCOA—National Council on Aging

NHI—National Health Insurance

NIA—National Institute on Aging

NIH—National Institute of Health

NSC—National Safety Council

PAHO—Pan American Health Organization

PPS—Prospective Payment System

PRO—Peer Review Organization

QA—Quality Assurance

UR—Utilization Review

USPC—U.S. Peace Corps

USPHS—U.S. Public Health Service

VA—Veterans Administration

VNA—Visiting Nurse Association

WHO—World Health Organization

Other

AARP—American Association of Retired Persons

ACS—American Cancer Society

AHA—American Hospital Association

Oral Reading Practice

Atherosclerotic Occlusive Disease of the Descending Aorta and Its Main Branches

Despite variable pathologic features, **atherosclerotic occlusive** disease exhibits a distinctive pattern, especially as to the extent and location of the occlusion. No matter where the obliterative process occurs, the lesion is generally segmental and well localized. It is significant that a comparatively normal **patent lumen** exists **proximal** and **distal** to the obstructed segment. Confirmatory evidence of these characteristic findings is provided by **arteriography,** which is of primary importance in diagnostic evaluation. (see Fig. 77 to 80)

As in occlusive vascular disease of the heart and brain, the pathologic lesions consist of **intimal atheromatous plaques** with or without **thrombus** formation. Their typical location is the bifurcation of arteries, where they produce arterial obstruction followed by **arterial** insufficiency of the parts distal to the occlusive process. The segmental localization of the **atheromatous** lesions permits a direct surgical attack for restoring the circulation in the major blood vessels.

Figure 77 Normal artery, arterial coats, and lumen.

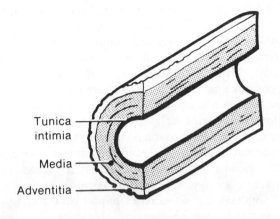

Tunica intimia

Media

Adventitia

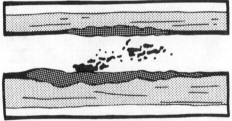

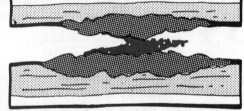

Figure 78 Atheromatous plaques in intima, capillary bleeding, and early mural thrombosis.

Figure 79 Rupture of ulcerated, intimal plaque, mural thrombosis, and occlusion.

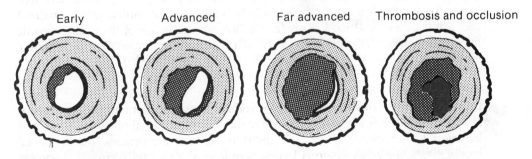

Early   Advanced   Far advanced   Thrombosis and occlusion

Figure 80 Stages of atherosclerosis.

The most common types of **atherosclerotic vascular disease,** apart from **coronary** or **cerebral** involvement, are **aortoiliac** and **femoropopliteal** occlusions and occlusions of the **renal** artery.

Aortoiliac Occlusions

The **aortic bifurcation occlusion syndrome,** or **Leriche's syndrome,** (also known as **thrombotic obliteration** of the **abdominal aorta** and **iliac arteries**) represents a progressive atheromatous occlusive disease of the abdominal aorta, which is seen chiefly in males of middle age or advancing years. Symptoms are those of **ischemia,** including coldness, **intermittent claudication, paresthesias,** and **muscular atrophy** of the lower extremities, and **impotence. Peripheral** pulses of the **femoral, popliteal,** and **pedal** regions tend to be markedly decreased, to the point of being barely palpable, or completely absent. **Arteriosclerotic plaques** in the aorta and iliac arteries may cause **microembolization** of the arteriosclerotic debris to the terminal vessels of the foot, resulting in the presence of blue toe syndrome. **Bruits** heard in the groin can signal presence of proximal occlusive lesions. Utilization of **Doppler** waveform analysis and/or the pulse volume recorder may delineate patterns suggestive of proximal occlusive lesions.

Angiographic studies are imperative, since they provide **visualization** of the entire arterial tree below the area where the **contrast medium** is injected into the aorta, at the level of the twelfth **lumbar vertebra.** This method demonstrates not only an aortoiliac occlusion, but also an associated superficial **femoral** artery occlusion, should it be present.

At the time of angiographic studies, it may be helpful to obtain **pull-back pressures** across the iliac artery lesions of questionable significance since this procedure can demonstrate directly whether or not such lesions are capable of interfering with flow. **Intra-arterial digital subtraction angiography** may be employed for evaluation of the aortoiliac arterial segment. The main advantage of this procedure is that there is good resolution of the vessels studied while very small amounts of contrast medium is utilized. In the presence of minimal **medial** and **adventitial mural lesions** that are well localized, the treatment of choice may be either that of **percutaneous transluminal angioplasty** or a **thromboendarterectomy.** Extensive obstructive lesions are usually treated by excision with graft replacement. These types of interventions prove satisfactory, since normal circulation is restored with subsequent symptomatic relief.

Femoropopliteal Occlusions

The atherosclerotic obstruction in the femoropopliteal region tends to be discrete, locally confined to a segment, and framed on either side by comparatively normal arterial lumen. There may be extensive involvement of the **superficial femoral artery,** with **patency** of the popliteal artery. Sometimes the occlusive lesion is diffuse and spreads to small arteries of the calf, making surgery impossible. Principal manifestations are **intermittent claudication** and **peripheral ischemia.**

Radiographic visualization should not be restricted to the femoropopliteal arteries and should include the iliacs and the abdominal aorta to ensure that no discrete lesions remain undetected. **Saphenous venography** is useful in planning long bypass procedures and is especially indicated in patients who have undergone previous prosthetic bypasses, since these individuals may have sustained injury to their vein while undergoing the first operative procedure.

Femoropopliteal reconstruction may be achieved by removing the **saphenous vein** from the knee to the **saphenofemoral junction.** The obstruction is bypassed by an **autogenous** graft of the saphenous vein. In addition to the **femoropopliteal** bypass, other alternative techniques include **infrapopliteal** bypass and the **axillopopliteal** bypass. Graft materials utilized currently include the **in situ saphenous vein** graft, the reversed **autologous saphenous vein** (ASV) graft, and the tubular expanded **polytetrafluoroethylene** (PTFE) graft, as well as various types of **Dacron** grafts.

Occlusions of the Renal Artery

When atherosclerotic renal artery occlusion is associated with **hypertension,** it requires **antihypertensive** therapy. The occlusive process may occur **unilaterally or bilaterally. Aortography** permits visualization of the renal arteries and their occlusive lesions. The normal circulation to the kidney may be restored by a bypass graft.

Vascular Surgery Considerations

Severe coexisting **cardiac** and **cerebral** disease, as well as far-advanced senescence, are considered contraindications, but elderly persons otherwise in good health are thought to be good candidates for surgical intervention. Low-risk patients with **compensated heart disease, diabetes mellitus,** and **hypertension** also are advised to undergo surgery.

Vascular occlusion presents a major health problem in senescence. Its onset and insidious progression is part of physiologic aging. It assumes pathologic dimensions only after months or years of undetected progress. Modern vascular surgery can offer relief for elderly patients with **atherosclerotic occlusive disease. Percutaneous transluminal angioplasty (PTA)** may be employed as a separate procedure or as an adjunct to **aortofemoral bypass (AFB)** operations in the treatment of **iliac-occlusive disease. PTA** appears to be most effective in those patients with severely limiting claudication due to isolated segmental stenosis or in those afflicted with more extensive lesions, whose poor medical condition increases the risk of major surgical procedures. Despite these benefits, **PTA** may still be considered a temporizing measure because of the progressive natural history of **atherosclerotic peripheral vascular disease** in our population. **AFB** procedures continue to provide the elderly with satisfactory initial and long-term relief of ischemic symptoms due to a wide range of atherosclerotic lesions. (8, 9, 10, 12, 37, 43, 53, 54, 72, 74, 75, 78, 79)

References and Bibliography

1. Aminoff, Michael J. Nervous system. In Schroeder, Steven A., Krupp, Marcus A., and Tierney, Lawrence M., Jr., eds., *Current Medical Diagnosis & Treatment*—1988, Norwalk, CT: Appleton & Lange, 1988, pp. 571-620.

2. Bernier, S. L., and Small, N. R. Disruptive behaviors. *Journal of Gerontological Nursing* 14:8-13, Feb. 1988.

3. Boyars, Michael. COPD in the ambulatory elderly: Management and update. *Geriatrics* 43:29-40, May 1988.

4. Braunwald, Eugene. Heart failure. In Braunwald, Eugene, et al., eds., *Harrison's Principles of Internal Medicine,* 11th ed. New York: McGraw-Hill Book Co., 1987, pp. 905-916.

5. Brophy, James J. Psychiatric disorders. In Schroeder, Steven A., Krupp, Marcus A., and Tierney, Lawrence M., Jr., eds., *Current Medical Diagnosis & Treatment*—1988, Norwalk, CT: Appleton & Lange, 1988, pp. 621-675.

6. Brown, M.D. Functional assessment of the elderly. *Journal of Gerontological Nursing* 14:13-17, May 1988.

7. Camargo, Carlos A., and Kolb, Felix O. Endocrine disorders. In Schroeder, Steven A., Krupp, Marcus A., and Tierney, Lawrence M., Jr., eds., *Current Medical Diagnosis & Treatment*—1988, Norwalk, CT: Appleton & Lange, 1988, pp. 676-748.

8. Cambria, Richard P., et al. Percutaneous an-

gioplasty for peripheral arterial occlusive disease: Correlates of clinical success. *Archives of Surgery* 122:283-287, March 1987.

9. Corson, John D., et al. In-situ saphenous vein bypass. In Bergan, John J., and Yao, James S. T., eds., *Arterial Surgery,* Orlando: Grune & Stratton, Inc., 1988, pp. 507-522.

10. Courbier, Robert, et al. Comparison of PTFE and Dacron bifurcation grafts. In Bergan, John J., and Yao, James S. T., eds., *Arterial Surgery*, Orlando: Grune & Stratton, Inc., 1988, pp. 323-335.

11. Duthie, Robert B., and Hoaglund, Franklin T. Orthopaedics. In Schwartz, Seymour I., ed.-in-chief, *Principle of Surgery*, 5th ed., vol. 2. New York: McGraw-Hill Book Co., 1989, pp. 1879-2020.

12. Fauci, Anthony S. The vasculitis syndromes. In Braunwald, Eugene, et al., eds., *Harrison's Principles of Internal Medicine*, 11th ed. New York: McGraw-Hill Book Co., 1987, pp. 1438-1445.

13. Feigenbaum, Lawrence Z. Geriatric medicine and the elderly patient. In Schroeder, Steven A., Krupp, Marcus A., and Tierney, Lawrence M., Jr., eds., *Current Medical Diagnosis & Treatment—1988*, Norwalk, CT: Appleton & Lange, 1988, pp. 17-26.

14. Frank, Irwin N. Urology. In Schwartz, Seymour I., ed.-in-chief, *Principles of Surgery*, 5th ed., vol. 2. New York: McGraw-Hill Book Co., 1989, pp. 1729-1779.

15. Fry, William J., and Fry, Richard E. Surgically correctable hypertension. In Schwartz, Seymour I., ed.-in-chief, *Principles of Surgery*, 5th ed., vol. 2. New York: McGraw-Hill Book Co., 1989, pp. 1041-1059.

16. Gambert, Steven R., and Escher, Jeffrey E. Atypical presentation of endocrine disorders in the elderly. *Geriatrics* 43:69-71, 76-78, July 1988.

17. Garritson, Susan H. Milieu therapy. In Wilson, H.S., and Kneisl, C.R., eds., *Psychiatric Nursing*. Reading, MA: Addison-Wesley Publishing Co., 1988, pp. 828-849.

18. Gifford, Ray W., Jr. Geriatric hypertension: Chairman's comments on NIH working group report. *Geriatrics* 42: 45-50, May 1987.

19. Gilman, Sid. Ataxia and disorders of equilibrium and gait. In Braunwald, Eugene, et al., eds., *Harrison's Principles of Internal Medicine*, 11th ed. New York: McGraw-Hill Book Co., 1987, pp. 91-96.

20. Goodhill, Victor. Deafness, tinnitus, and dizziness in the aged. In Rossman, Isadore, ed., *Clinical Geriatrics*. Philadelphia: J.B. Lippincott Co., 1986, pp. 410-423.

21. Gordon, Michael, and Periksaitis, H.G. Drugs and the aging brain. *Geriatrics* 43:69-78, May 1988.

22. Gratta, James C. Post-stroke management and outcomes. *Geriatrics* 43:40-46, July 1988.

23. Griggs, R.C. Muscle pains, spasms, cramps and episodic weakness. In Braunwald, Eugene, et al., eds., *Harrison's Principles of Internal Medicine*, 11th ed. New York: McGraw-Hill Book Co., 1987, pp. 96-99.

24. Growdon, John R., and Young, Robert R. Paralysis and other disorders of movement. In Braunwald, Eugene, et al., eds., *Harrison's Principles of Internal Medicine*, 11th ed. New York: McGraw-Hill Book Co., 1987, pp. 79-91.

25. Herold, Sister Duchesne. Personal communication.

26. Imparato, Anthony M., and Riles, Thomas S. Peripheral arterial disease. In Schwartz, Seymour I., ed.-in-chief, *Principles of Surgery*, 5th ed., vol. 2. New York: McGraw-Hill Book Co., 1989, pp. 933-1010.

27. Ingram, Roland H., Jr. Chronic bronchitis, emphysema, and airways obstruction. In Braunwald, Eugene, et al., eds., *Harrison's Principles of Internal Medicine*, 11th ed. New York: McGraw-Hill Book Co., 1987, pp. 1087-1095.

28. Isselbacher, Kurt J., and Richter, James M. Hematemesis, melena, and hematochezia. In Braunwald, Eugene, et al., eds., *Harrison's Principles of Internal Medicine*, 11th ed. New York: McGraw-Hill Book Co., 1987, pp. 180-183.

29. Janssen, J.A., and Giberson, D.L. Remotivation therapy. *Journal of Gerontological Nursing* 14:31-34, June 1988.

30. Jenike, Michael A. Psychoactive drugs in the elderly: Antipsychotics and anxiolytics. *Geriatrics* 43:53-57, 61-62, 67, Sept. 1988.

31. Jenike, Michael A. Psychoactive drugs in the elderly: Antidepressants. *Geriatrics* 43:43-57, Nov. 1988.

32. Kistler, J. Philip, et al. Cerebrovascular diseases. In Braunwald, Eugene, et al., eds., *Harrison's Principles of Internal Medicine*, 11th ed. New York: McGraw-Hill Book Co., 1987, pp. 1930-1960.

33. Kneisl, C.R. Group therapy. In Wilson, H.S., and Kneisl, C.R., eds., *Psychiatric Nursing*, Reading, MA: Addison-Wesley Publishing Co., 1988, pp. 804-827.

34. Krane, Stephen M. Paget's disease of the bone. In Braunwald, Eugene, et al., eds., *Harrison's Principles of Internal Medicine*, 11th ed. New York: McGraw-Hill Book Co., 1987, pp. 1900-1902.

35. Krane, Stephen M., and Holick, Michael F. Metabolic bone disease. In Braunwald, Eugene, et al., eds., *Harrison's Principles of Internal Medicine*, 11th ed. New York: McGraw-Hill Book Co., 1987, pp. 1889-1900.

36. Krupp, Marcus A. Genitourinary tract. In Schroeder, Steven A., Krupp, Marcus A., and Tierney, Lawrence M., eds., *Current Medical Diagnosis & Treatment—1988*, Norwalk, CT: Appleton & Lange, 1988, pp. 533-570.

37. Kwasnik, Edward M., et al. Comparative results of angioplasty and aortofemoral bypass in patients with symptomatic iliac disease. *Archives of Surgery* 1:22:288-291, March 1987.

38. Lappe, Joan M. Reminiscing: The life review therapy. *Journal of Gerontological Nursing* 13:12-16, April 1987.

39. Larson, P. Reed. The thyroid. In Wyngaarden, James B., and Smith, Lloyd H., Jr., eds., *Cecil's Textbook of Medicine*, 18th ed. Philadelphia: W.B. Saunders Co., 1988, pp. 1315-1340.

40. Lincoff, Harvey, et al. Retinoschisis associated with optic nerve pits. *Archives of Ophthalmology* 106:61-67, Jan. 1988.

41. Love, C. Applying the nursing process to the elderly. In Wilson, H.S., and Kneisl, C.R., eds., *Psychiatric Nursing*, Reading, MA: Addison-Wesley Publishing Co., 1988, pp. 996-1033.

42. McCollough, E.G., and English, J.L. Blepharoplasty. *Archives of Otolaryngology—Head & Neck Surgery* 114:645-648, June 1988.

43. Milford, M.A. Femoropopliteal percutaneous transluminal angioplasty for limb salvage. *Journal of Vascular Surgery* 8:292-299, Sept. 1988.

44. Mohr, Jay P., and Adams, Raymond D. Disorders of speech and language. In Braunwald, Eugene, et al., eds., *Harrison's Principles of Internal Medicine*, 11th ed. New York: McGraw-Hill Book Co., 1987, pp. 121-127.

45. Moody, Frank G., et al. Stomach. In Schwartz, Seymour I. ed.-in-chief, *Principles of Surgery*, 5th ed., vol. 1. New York: McGraw-Hill Book Co., 1989, pp. 1157-1188.

46. Moser, Marvin. Diuretics and alternative drugs in geriatric hypertension. *Geriatrics* 42:39-44, Feb. 1987.

47. Morton, Donald L., et al. Oncology. In Schwartz, Seymour I., ed.-in-chief, *Principles of Surgery*, 5th ed., vol. 1. New York: McGraw-Hill Book Co., 1989, pp. 331-386.

48. Mulrow, Cynthia, et al. The value of clinical findings in the detection of normal pressure hydrocephalus. *Journal of Gerontology* 42:277-279, May 1987.

49. Navari, R.M., and Sheehy, T.W. Hypothermia. In Calkins, Evan, et al., eds., *The Practice of Geriatrics*, Philadelphia: W.B. Saunders Co., 1986, pp. 291-301.

50. Pasternak, R.C., Braunwald, E., and Alpert, J.S. Acute myocardial infarction. In Braunwald, Eugene, et al., eds., *Harrison's Principles of Internal Medicine*, 11th ed. New York: McGraw-Hill Book Co., 1987, pp. 982-993.

51. Petersdorf, R.G., and Root, R.K. Disturbances of heat regulation. In Braunwald, Eugene, et al., eds., *Harrison's Principles of Internal Medicine*, 11th ed. New York: McGraw-Hill Book Co., 1987, pp. 43-50.

52. Plum, Fred. The dementias. In Wyngaarden, James B., and Smith, Lloyd H., Jr., eds., *Cecil's Textbook of Medicine*, 18th ed. Philadelphia: W.B. Saunders Co., 1988, pp. 2087-2011.

53. Protrowski, J.J., et al. Aortobifemoral bypass: The operation of choice for unilateral iliac occlusion. *Journal of Vascular Surgery* 8:211-28, Sept. 1988.

54. Quinones-Baldrich, W.J., et al. Is the preferential rise of polytetrafluoroethylene grafts for femoral-popliteal bypass justified? *Journal of Vascular Surgery* 8:219-228, Sept. 1988.

55. Reed, T.A., and Birge, S.J. Screening for osteoporosis. *Journal of Gerontological Nursing* 14:18-20, July 1988.

56. Rees, Rees B., Jr., and Odom, Richard B. Skin and appendages. In Schroeder, Steven A., Krupp, Marcus A., and Tierney, Lawrence M., eds., *Current Medical Diagnosis & Treatment—1988*, Norwalk, CT: Appleton & Lange, 1988, pp. 47-93.

57. Richardson, E.P., Jr., Beal, M.F., and Martin, J.B. Degenerative diseases of the nervous system. In Braunwald, Eugene, et al., eds., *Harrison's Principles of Internal Medicine*, 11th ed. New York: McGraw-Hill Book Co., 1987, pp. 2011-2027.

58. Ross, Russell. The pathogenesis of atherosclerosis. In Braunwald, Eugene, ed., *Heart Disease: A Textbook of Cardiovascular Medicine*, 3rd ed., vol. 2. Philadelphia: W.B. Saunders Co., 1988, pp. 1135-1152.

59. Rossman, Isadore. The anatomy of aging. In Rossman, Isadore, ed., *Clinical Geriatrics*, 3rd ed. Philadelphia: J.B. Lippincott Co., 1986, pp. 3-22.

60. Selwyn, Andrew P., and Braunwald, Eugene. Ischemic heart disease. In Braunwald, Eugene, et al., eds., *Harrison's Principles of Internal Medicine*, 11th ed. New York: McGraw-Hill Book Co., 1987, pp. 975-982.

61. Shock, John P., Lens. In Vaughn, Daniel, and Asbury, Taylor, eds., *General Ophthalmology*, 11th ed. Los Altos, CA: Lange Medical Publications, 1986, pp. 142-140.

62. Silen, William. Acute intestinal obstruction. In Braunwald, Eugene, ed., *Harrison's Principles of Internal Medicine*, 11th ed. New York: McGraw-Hill Book Co., 1987, pp. 1302-1304.

63. Sloan, R.W. Altered drug disposition and drug response. *Practical Geriatric Therapeutics*,

Ordell, NJ: Medical Economics Books, 1986, pp. 12-18.

64. ———. Psychotropic drugs. Ibid,. pp. 264-281.

65. Smith, L. Kent. Cardiac disorders: A guide to assessing risk in the elderly. *Geriatrics* 43:33-38, July 1988.

66. Sokolow, Maurice, and Massie, Barry. Heart and great vessels. In Schroeder, Steven A., Krupp, Marcus A., and Tierney, Lawrence M., Jr., eds., *Current Medical Diagnosis & Treatment—1988*, Norwalk, CT: Appleton & Lange, 1988, pp. 189-265.

67. Soonge, H.K., et al. Clinical significance of common eye changes in older patients. *Geriatrics* 43:49-57, May 1988.

68. Statement on hypertension in the elderly. The working group on hypertension in the elderly. *Journal of the American Medical Association* 256:70-74, July 4, 1986.

69. Stauffer, John L. Pulmonary diseases. In Schroeder, Steven A., Krupp, Marcus A., and Tierney, Lawrence M., Jr., eds., *Current Medical Diagnosis & Treatment—1988*, Norwalk, CT: Appleton & Lange, 1988, pp. 132-188.

70. Steedle, T.O., et al. Cortex removal in extracapsular cataract extraction. In Abrahamson, A.I., ed., *Cataract Surgery*, New York: McGraw-Hill Book Co., 1986, pp. 74-79.

71. Stevenson, Thomas R., and Jurkiewicz, M.J. Plastic and reconstructive surgery. In Schwartz, Seymour I., ed.-in-chief, *Principles of Surgery*, 5th ed., vol. 2. New York: McGraw-Hill Book Co., 1989, pp. 2081-2131.

72. Strandness, D. Eugene, Jr. Vascular diseases of the extremities. In Braunwald, Eugene, et al., eds., *Harrison's Principles of Internal Medicine*, 11th ed. New York: McGraw-Hill Book Co., 1987, pp. 1040-1046.

73. Tanagho, Emil A., et al. Neuropathic bladder disorders. In Tanagho, Emil A., and McAninch, Jack W., eds., *Smith's General Urology*, Norwalk, CT: Appleton & Lange, 1988, pp. 435-451.

74. Taylor, M.L., Jr., and Porter, J.M. Current status of the reversed saphenous vein graft.

In Bergan, J.J., and Yao, James S.T., eds., *Arterial Surgery*, Orlando: Grune & Stratton, Inc., 1988, pp. 438-505.

75. Tierney, Lawrence M., Jr., and Erskine, John M. Blood vessels and lymphatics. In Schroeder, Steven A., Krupp, Marcus A., and Tierney. Lawrence M., Jr., eds., *Current Medical Diagnosis & Treatment—1988*, Norwalk, CT: Appleton & Lange, 1988, pp. 266-293.

76. Townsend, Courtney M., Jr., and Thompson, James C. Small intestine. In Schwartz, Seymour I., ed.-in-chief, *Principles of Surgery*, 5th ed., vol. 1. New York: McGraw-Hill Book Co., 1989, pp. 1189-1223.

77. Vaughan, Daniel. Eye. In Schroeder, Steven A., Krupp, Marcus A., and Tierney, Lawrence M., Jr., eds., *Current Medical Diagnosis & Treatment—1988*, Norwalk, CT: Appleton & Lange, 1988, pp. 94-109.

78. Veith, Frank J., et al. Femoral-popliteal-tibial occlusive disease. In Moore, Wesley, ed., *Vascular Surgery: A Comprehensive Review*, 2nd. ed. Orlando: Grune & Stratton, Inc., 1986, pp. 513-542.

79. Veith, Frank J., et al. Critique of alternatives in utilization of autogenous vein. In Bergan, J.J., and Yao, James S.T., eds., *Arterial Surgery*, Orlando: Grune & Stratton, Inc., 1988, pp. 447-458.

80. Victor, M., and Adams, R.D. Confusion, delirium, amnesia, and dementia. In Braunwald, Eugene, et al., eds., *Harrison's Principles of Internal Medicine*, 11th ed. New York: McGraw-Hill Book Co., 1987, pp. 127-135.

81. West, John B. Disorders of ventilation. In Braunwald, Eugene, et al., eds., *Harrison's Principles of Internal Medicine*, 11th ed. New York: McGraw-Hill Book Co., 1987, pp. 1129-1134.

82. Williams, T.F. Comprehensive assessment of frail elderly in relation to needs for long term care. In Calkins, Evan, et al., eds., *The Practice of Geriatrics*. Philadelphia: W.B. Saunders Co., 1986, pp. 84-92.

83. Young, H.S., et al. Managing nocturnal wandering behavior. *Journal of Gerontological Nursing* 14:6-12, May 1988.

CHAPTER 18

Selected Terms Pertaining to Oncology

Orientation

Origin of Terms

astro- (G)—star
carcino- (G)—cancer
kerato- (G)—horny tissue, cornea

-oma (G)—tumor
onco- (G)—tumor, swelling, mass
sarco- (G)—flesh

General Terms

- *adjuvant*—assisting. Chemotherapy given as an aid to surgery or to radiation in an attempt to reduce or eliminate the cancer cell burden. (23)
- *benign*—mild, not malignant. (17)
- *cancer*—malignant disease characterized by uncontrolled cell growth. (19, 30)
- *carcinogenic agent*—an agent capable of inducing or potentiating carcinoma. (19)
- *carcinolysis*—destruction of cancer cells. (58)
- *carcinoma*—malignant neoplasm that arises from epithelial tissue. (30)
- *carcinoma in situ (CIS)*—true malignant tumor of squamous or glandular epithelium in which no invasion of underlying or adjacent structures has occurred. Lesions may remain in situ (position) for an indefinite period before they become invasive. (19)
- *clone*—population of cells derived from a single cell. This term is commonly used when a number of cells have the same abnormal chromosome complement. Gross colony morphology differs significantly from tumor type to tumor type, similar to differences in bacterial colony formation. (20, 58, 60)
- *deoxyribonucleic acid (DNA)*—genetic substance within the nucleus of a cell responsible for controlling cell division and synthesis. (59)
- *drugs*
    - *antineoplastic drugs*—standard agents serve as the basic regimen in the treatment of neoplastic disease. This type of anticancer treatment involves drug metabolism, method of drug administration, drug stability, drug interactions, and drug incompatibilities and side effects. Common side effects may include pain, nausea, cerebral edema, hypercalcemia, and others. Medical-legal aspects must also be considered in drug investigation and testing, as well as in commercially available anticancer agents. (58, 60)

—*individual drug protocol*—list of commonly used drugs for specific type of tumors (breast, lung, etc.); the resulting tissue culture assay can be ascertained in a short time. Treatment can be initiated or changed according to the individual patient response to drug sensitivity. A direct tissue culture method is now clinically available to measure the sensitivity of human tumor cells to the anticancer drugs. Controversy exists among the medical community as to the actual effectiveness of this procedure at present. If this assay is effective, however, it would eliminate submitting patients to toxic drugs—the only method before this—and speed up the choice of a specific tumor-sensitive drug. This predictive technique to ascertain the selection of effective chemotherapy for individual patients and even similar tumors in different patients is based on one similar to the culture and sensitivity assays used in the management of bacterial infection. (19, 58, 60)

(*See definition of clonogenic assays*, p. 403.)

- *dyskeratosis*—premature keratinization of epidermal cells due to a defect in keratin formation. It may be benign or malignant. (60)
- *encapsulated*—encased in a capsule, usually seen with benign neoplasms.
- *erythroplakia*—well-defined red patches with a velvety appearance and often tiny ulcers that may signal a malignant change in the mucous membrane. (33)
- *fractionation*—radiation is administered to the patient in small repeated doses rather than using large doses. (23, 58)
- *implantation*—the spontaneous passage of tumor cells to a new site with subsequent growth.
- *invasion*—the act of invading or infiltrating and destroying surrounding tissue. (17)
- *lymphocyte*—mononuclear leukocyte whose nucleus contains dense chromatin and a pale-blue-staining cytoplasm. Two major subclassifications of lymphocytes are:
  - —*T-lymphocytes (T-cells)*—acted on by the thymus and concerned with the functional status of cell-mediated immune systems.
  - —*B-lymphocytes (B-cells)*—become antibody-producing cells and are concerned with the functional status of the humoral immune system.

The combined activities of T-cells and B-cells provide immunity against infectious agents and oncogenic agents. For example, the cancer modalities (radiotherapy, surgery, chemotherapy) may affect the immune system, causing either a transitory or prolonged suppression. The severity of such a suppression may be assessed by measuring the levels of T- and B- cells. (42, 49, 58)

- *malignant*—virulent; pertaining to the invasive, metastatic properties of a new growth. (19)
- *medullary*—marrowlike; term used in oncology in reference to soft tumors, such as carcinomas of the breast or thyroid. (19)
- *modality*—refers to type of treatment regimen; for example, chemotherapy, radiation, or surgery or a combination of these approaches. (19)
- *neoplasm*—an actively growing tissue composed of cells that have undergone an abnormal type of irreversible differentiation. The new growth is useless and progressive. Most neoplasms can be divided into three categories: (17, 39)
  - —*benign tumors*—not invasive or metastatic.
  - —*invasive tumors*—not metastatic.
  - —*metastatic tumors*.

Other related terms:

- —*behavior of neoplasm*—biologic interpretation indicating the potentialities of a new growth; for example, ability to spread, histologic appearance, rate of cellular proliferation (rapid cell division), and other aspects. (19)

—*functioning neoplasm*—refers to tumor of endocrine derivation that synthesizes and releases hormones into the bloodstream and may cause some endocrine dysfunction. In a broader sense any well-differentiated neoplasm capable of forming the product of normal parent cell may be considered a functional tumor. (19)

- *oncogene*—viral gene carrying the potential to cause cancer; a transforming gene, since it has the potential to transform the host cell to a neoplastic phenotype. Cellular genes with potential for destabilizing growth regulation are termed proto-oncogenes. When proto-oncogenes become activated, they are termed "oncogenes." Various alterations in these genes such as mutations, amplifications, and chromosomal translocations may serve as mechanisms to activate the proto-oncogenes. The majority of oncogenes can be assigned to gene families based on the relatedness of nucleic acid or amino acid sequences or of enzyme activities of the oncogene product. Examples of some oncogenes implicated in the development of neoplasias are:

    —*ras* oncogene, which has been identified in about 15 percent of the carcinomas affecting the lung, colon, and breast, as well as in several types of leukemias and sarcomas.

    —*myc* oncogene has been implicated in Burkitt's lymphoma, neuroblastomas, retinoblastomas, and small-cell lung carcinomas. Human tumors may contain more than one oncogene. In the case of Burkitt's lymphoma, Lane and associates found a second oncogene which they designated as *B-lym*. Research efforts continue to study the molecular aspects of cellular oncogene involvement with cell proliferation and differentiation and the various alterations affecting these genes, since these represent key elements of the genetic machinery associated with oncogenesis. (5, 8, 15, 35, 49, 52)

- *oncogenesis*—causation of tumors. (5, 8, 35, 49)
- *papillary*—nipplelike or wartlike projection of cells.
- *papilloma*—benign growth that resembles in its histologic structure the parent epithelium from which it is derived. Some skin papillomas are wartlike growths derived from squamous epithelium. Papillomas arising from the larynx, tongue, urinary bladder, or ureter are usually composed of transitional epithelium and tend to undergo malignant changes. Papillomatosis refers to the presence of multiple papillomata. (15)
- *radiocurability*—refers to the tumor-normal tissue relationships; the interaction is such that curative doses of radiation can be regularly applied without excessive damage to the normal tissues. (23, 58)
- *radioresponsiveness*—clinical appearance of a tumor in regression following the initial dose of radiation. (23, 58)
- *radiosensitivity*—refers to innate sensitivity of cells to radiation. (23, 58)
- *remission*—refers to periods when no signs of disease are present. Periods may be described as partial, complete, or stable. Other related terms are:

    —*disease-free interval (DFI)*—refers to period of no active disease.

    —*no evidence of disease (NED)*—refers to periods when no signs of disease are present. (35, 58)

- *sarcoma*—malignant connective tissue tumor. Other related terms are:

    —*leiomyosarcoma*—malignant smooth muscle tumor.

    —*rhabdomyosarcoma*—malignant striated muscle tumor.

    —*Ewing's sarcoma*—highly malignant round cell tumor of the bone that represents the second most common primary bone tumor in children and young adults. (9, 32)

- *scirrhous*—hard; term used in oncology to designate a hard tumor.

- *superior vena caval syndrome (SVCS)*—clinical complication caused by an obstruction of the venous return at the level of the superior vena cava. It is characterized by neck vein and thoracic vein distention, facial edema, tachypnea, and cyanosis. Malignant disease is the main cause of SVCS. This type of oncologic emergency is most often associated with bronchogenic or lung carcinomas and with malignant lymphoma. (58, 60)
- *ulcer*—inflammatory and often suppurating lesion on the skin or an internal mucous surface of the body; may result in necrotic (dead) tissue. (53)
- *verrucous*—wartlike; refers to projection usually occurring in the mouth and cheek areas. (41)

Terms Associated with Neoplastic Growth Patterns

- *anaplasia, dedifferentiation*—loss of differentiation of cells and their orientation to each other, to their axial framework, and to blood vessels. Other related types are: (39, 49)
    - *monophasic anaplasia*—change of cell to embryonic type.
    - *polyphasic anaplasia*—change of cell to more complex cell.
- *differentiation*—specialization of a tissue or organ to perform a particular function. It is accompanied by characteristic morphologic alterations simulating parent tissue. (58, 60)
- *dysplasia*—loss in the regularity and normal arrangement of cells.
- *embryonal, embryonic*—pertaining to an embryo, as well as to marked immaturity. (58, 60)
- *fungating*—cauliflower-shaped pattern of growth. Cells grow rapidly, one on top of another, projecting from a tissue surface. (30)
- *hyperplasia*—abnormal increase in number of cells; cellular proliferation in excess of normal, not progressive (as in neoplasia), but reaching an equilibrium. (58)
- *metaplasia*—refers to a reversible process in which one type of differentiated cell is substituted for another. (17)
- *metastasis formation*—development of secondary centers of neoplastic growth at some distance from the primary tumor. (17, 30)
- *metastasize*—to disseminate or spread via lymphatics, the bloodstream, or body cavities; term used in relation to malignant tumors. (30)
- *sessile polyp*—mass of tissue attached by a broad base. A polyp is a nonspecific term signifying tissue growth of a mucous membrane, which may be an inflammatory lesion or a true tumor. A pedunculated polyp is a mass of tissue attached to an organ by a freely movable, narrow stalk or pedicle. (39)
- *stem cell*—describes a histologically primitive cell with the capacity to give rise to a large number of descendants through a process of self-renewal. (11, 39)

Cancer Grading and Staging Terms

- *grading*—cancer grading refers to the degree of histologic and morphologic differentiation of the tumor, as determined by microscopic sections. (58)
- *staging*—cancer staging refers to the extent of the tumor's geographic spread at the time of the initial diagnosis. The joint efforts of the *International Union Against Cancer* and the *American Joint Committee for Cancer Staging and End Reporting* developed a staging nomenclature entitled the *TNM* system (*T*, tumor; *N*, regional lymph node involvement; *M*, metastatic spread).
    - *TNM System:*
    - *T0*—No evidence of primary tumor.
    - *TIS*—Tumor in situ.
    - *T1, T2, T3, T4*—indicates size progression and involvement of tumor.

-*TX*—tissue cannot be assessed.
-*NO*—regional lymph node abnormality not demonstrated.
-*N1, N2, N3, N4*—indicated degree of node abnormality.
-*NX*—regional lymph node cannot be assessed.
-*MO*—no evidence of lymph node metastasizing.
-*M1, M2, M3, M4*—indicated degree and extent of metastases.

The TNM classification makes it possible to determine in detail the anatomic progression of the disease, but for group staging statistics, this classification tends to divide a series of treated cases into many small groups so that a significant statistical evaluation is not possible. One example of a group staging approach is the classification system for staging malignant tumors in the female pelvis designed by the Cancer Committee of the *International Federation of Gynecology and Obstetrics (FIGO)*. A comparison of the *FIGO* and *TNM* staging systems for carcinoma of the ovary is presented in Table 24, p. 404. Other staging modalities include *computed tomography (CT)* and *magnetic resonance imaging (MRI)*. Both of these radiologic modalities are noninvasive procedures. Another approach to staging of tumors is the *staging laparotomy,* which allows surgical exploration of the abdominal cavity to determine the exact spread of the disease. (1, 12, 13, 38, 58)

Special Studies Related to Cancer

- *bacille Calmette-Guérin (BCG)*—immunotherapeutic agent used to destroy tumors or to prevent new or recurrent tumorigenesis (tumor formation). The immunopotentiating effect of BCG is increased by simultaneous use of antineoplastic agents at regular intervals. (58, 63)
- *clonogenic assays, bilayer or double-agar system*—tissue culture techniques for cloning of tumor cell lines. This technique enhances the growth of malignant tumor cells while inhibiting the growth of normal cells. The in vitro growth of drug-treated tumor cells is compared with untreated "control" cells to determine in vitro sensitivity. Past research studies have indicated that clonogenic assays may be helpful in determining which tumors will fail to respond to chemotherapy. Although routine use of in vitro sensitivity testing cannot be advocated for all tumors (e.g., sarcomas and primary breast cancers display low in vitro growth rates, and/or the scarcity of current antineoplastic drugs limits the clinical value of predictive testing for many common types of neoplasms), these assays do present an important research mechanism that can be used in the continual development of new antitumor drugs, as well as in the ongoing study and development of other research technologies to improve the low in vitro growth rates. (27, 37, 60)
- *exfoliative cytology*—procedure in which cells are scraped from the diseased area, stained, and subsequently viewed under a microscope to detect the presence of cancer. The Papanicolaou (Pap) smear is a sample of this type of cytology: cells are scraped from the cervix or vagina, and the procedure mentioned above is followed. Gastric exfoliative cytology is used to detect gastric malignancy by studying cells shed by the mucosa and obtained by aspiration, lavage, or abrasive brushes following the liquefaction of the mucosal coating. (33, 58)
- *hormonal assays:*
    - *estradiol receptor assay (ERA)*—test predicting the effectiveness of hormone therapy or hormone deprivation (endocrine ablation therapy) in particular breast cancers.
    - *progesterone receptor assay*—test used with estradiol receptor assay to select breast cancer patients who will benefit by hormone therapy.

Table 24
Comparison of FIGO and TNM Staging Systems for Carcinoma of the Ovary*

FIGO		TNM
1A	Neoplasm limited to one ovary	T_{1a}
1B	Neoplasm limited to both ovaries	T_{1b}
1C	Positive peritoneal washings	T_{1c}
IIA	Local extension to the uterus or to the fallopian tubes	T_{2a}
IIB	Local extension to other pelvic tissue	T_{2b}
IIC	Positive peritoneal washings: tumor otherwise would be classified as T_{2a}, T_{2b}	T_{2c}
III	Advanced disease but no distant metastases	T_3
	May involve retroperitoneal nodes, peritoneal seeding outside the true pelvis, omentum/small bowel	
		T_{1-3}, N_+
IV	Widespread metastases	T_{1-3}, M_+

*Reprinted with permission from Dennis M. Balfe, Jay P. Heiken, and Bruce L. McClennan. Oncologic imaging for carcinoma of the cervix, ovary, and endometrium. In David G. Bragg, Philip Rubin, and James E. Youker, eds., *Oncologic Imaging*. New York: Pergamon Press, 1985, pp. 439-475.

Table 25
Classification of Common Neoplasms

Histologic Derivation	Benign Neoplasms	Malignant Neoplasms	Site of Predilection
Epithelial tissue		Carcinomas	
(a) Covering epithelium	Squamous cell papilloma—benign neoplasm composed of squamous epithelial cells, flat and pavementlike in appearance (43)	Epidermoid carcinoma Squamous cell carcinoma—a malignant neoplasm of squamous epithelial cells (43, 40)	Skin, buccal mucosa, tongue, salivary gland, lip, larynx, lung, bladder, anus, and others
		Oat cell carcinoma—very malignant, undifferentiated, small cell tumor (7, 11, 20)	Lung, esophagus, and other sites of low incidence
		Basal cell carcinoma—malignant neoplasm, frequently forming a rodent ulcer and destructive by invasion, rarely by metastasis (40)	Skin; especially face; canthus of eye, tip of nose, chin, lip, and others

Histologic Derivation	Benign Neoplasms	Malignant Neoplasms	Site of Predilection
Epithelial tissue *(Continued)*			
(b) Glandular epithelium	Adenoma—benign neoplasm arising from glands (43, 46)	Adenocarcinoma—malignant neoplasm composed of glandular epithelium and characterized by many variations of anaplasia and metastases. (43, 46)	Breast, bronchi, digestive tract, pancreas, endocrine glands, prostate, and others
	Cystadenoma—cystic neoplasm arising from glandular epithelium	Cystadenocarcinoma—cystic, malignant new growth of glandular epithelium	Ovary, salivary gland, breast, and thyroid
	(a) serous type—uni- or multilocular serous cyst composed of epithelial and connective tissue	(a) serous type—(rare) frequently bilateral loculations characteristic; cyst contains transudate	Ovary
	(b) pseudomucinous type—cystic neoplasm in which lining epithelium produces mucus (46)	(b) pseudomucinous type—malignant changes, cells undergoing stratification; implants on peritoneal surface characteristic of neoplasm; fluid of cyst viscid (46)	Ovary
Embryonal tissue		Choriocarcinoma—a highly malignant tumor of chorionic epithelium; early metastasis common	Uterus, testes, and mediastinum
	Testicular adenoma—glandular tumor derived from germinal epithelium, extremely rare (34)	Embryonal carcinoma of testis—malignant new growth of germinal epithelium (34)	Testes
		Seminoma—testicular neoplasm of distinctive seminoma cells and lymphocytic stroma	Testes, epididymis, pelvic and paraaortic lymph nodes, and others

Histologic Derivation	Benign Neoplasms	Malignant Neoplasms	Site of Predilection
Embryonal tissue *(Continued)*			
	Teratoma, mature—mixed tumor composed of any type of embryonic and adult tissue, as teeth, hair, bone, cartilage, and others (34)	Malignant teratoma, immature—mixed tumor malignant in one or the other tissue elements (34)	Testes, ovaries, and retroperitoneal and sacrococcygeal regions
Connective tissue		*Sarcomas*	
	Chondroma— benign neoplasm composed of cartilaginous elements (58)	Chondrosarcoma— malignant neoplasm of cartilaginous elements usually arising from end of long bones (32)	Bones: femur, humerus, endolarynx, maxillary sinus, nasal fossa, and others
	Lipoma—benign neoplasm composed of adipose tissue (fat) (58)	Liposarcoma—sarcoma composed of adipose tissue (32)	Neck, shoulder, back, gluteal region, thigh, and others
	Fibroma—benign mass or firm nodule of fibroblasts or fibrocytes (58)	Fibrosarcoma—variable degrees of anaplasia and growth rate of tumor in subcutaneous or deeper structures (32)	Extremities, head, neck, breast, and others
	Leiomyoma— benign neoplasm of smooth muscle tissue (58)	Leiomyosarcoma— malignant neoplasm of smooth muscle tissue (4, 64)	Uterus, endometrium, vulva, bladder, small intestine, esophagus, stomach, and others
	Rhabdomyoma— benign tumor arising in skeletal muscle	Rhabdomyosarcoma— malignant, poorly differentiated, bizarre mass in striated muscle (48)	Any skeletal muscles, especially of lower extremities, such as the adductors, biceps, and quadriceps
	Osteoid osteoma—benign tumor derived from osteoblastic tissue	Osteosarcoma Osteogenic sarcoma—malignant tumor of osteoblastic or osseous tissue (9, 32)	Long bones, especially femur, humerus, and fibula; also bones of pelvis and others

Histologic Derivation	Benign Neoplasms	Malignant Neoplasms	Site of Predilection
Reticulo-endothelial tissue		Ewing's sarcoma—malignant tumor of reticuloendothelial tissue; early and wide metastases to other bones (32)	Femur, tibia, fibula, humerus, mandible, pelvic bones, and others
		Multiple myeloma Plasma cell myeloma—malignant tumors derived from plasma cells of bone marrow (50)	Flat bones, ribs, vertebrae, pelvis, skull, and others
Hema-topoietic or hema-tologic tissue		Leukemias—stem cell, undifferentiated or differentiated forms (14, 62)	Blood
Lymph-forming or lymphoid tissue		Lymphomas—stem cell or histiocytic, poorly or well-differentiated forms (21, 24)	Lymph nodes, spleen, liver, and other viscera
		Hodgkin's lymphoma—lymphocytic predominance or depletion, mixed cellularity, or nodular sclerosis (21)	Lymph nodes, spleen, liver, bones, and other viscera
Vascular tissue	Angioma Hemangioma—tumor of blood vessels (48)	Angiosarcoma Hemangiosarcoma—malignant blood vessel tumor (58)	Blood vessels, subcutaneous tissues, muscles, and others
	Lymphangioma—tumor of the lymphatic vessels (48)	Lymphangiosarcoma—sarcoma of the lymphatic vessels (58)	Lymphatic vessels, neck, and others
Nerve tissue or other tissue found in nervous system		Glioma group—primary intracranial tumors composed of glial tissues. Various types of cells are present	Brain
		(a) Astrocytoma—neoplasm of glial tissue containing star-shaped cells or astrocytes	Cerebral hemisphere and brain stem

Histologic Derivation	Benign Neoplasms	Malignant Neoplasms	Site of Predilection
Nerve tissue *(Continued)*		(b) Ependymoma— neoplasm of the lining of the ventricles	Ventricles of the brain
		(c) Glioblastoma multiforme— most malignant form of gliomas, highly invasive and destructive	Cerebrum, cerebellum, brain stem, and spinal cord
		(d) Oligodendro-glioma—relatively rare, slowly growing glioma with areas of calcification (3)	White matter of the frontal lobe
		Medulloblastoma— malignant tumor composed of medullary or neuroepithelial tissue (3)	Cerebellum
	Meningioma— benign tumor arising from the meninges; common tumor (3)		Meninges, cerebral hemisphere, and optic chiasm
Nerve tissue		Neuroblastoma—highly malignant, lethal tumor of neuroblasts occurring in children (3)	Adrenal gland, sympathetic nerve chains, jaw, lip, nose, abdominal viscera, and others
	Ganglioneuroma	Ganglioneuroblastoma —malignant ganglioneuroma composed of ganglionic cells and neuroblasts (3)	Mediastinum and retroperitoneum
	Neurilemoma— benign encapsulated tumor usually arising from peripheral nerve (3)		Peripheral or sympathetic nerves and eighth cranial nerve
	Neurofibroma— tumor of peripheral nerve sheaths (3)	Neurofibrosarcoma— malignant neoplasm of peripheral nerve sheath (58)	Peripheral nerves, hand, mediastinum, ureter, and others

Histologic Derivation	Benign Neoplasms	Malignant Neoplasms	Site of Predilection
Nerve tissue *(Continued)*			
Pigment-forming tissue	Nevus— pigmented mole of developmental origin	Malignant melanoma— malignant pigmented tumor (41)	Skin, eye, and extremities

Reference values:
Estradiol Receptor Assay
—*Positive results*—estradiol greater than 3 fmol/mg (femtomoles per milligram)
—*Negative results*—estradiol equal to or less than 3 fmol/mg
Progesterone Receptor Assay
—*Positive results*—progesterone greater than 5 fmol/mg
—*Negative results*—progesterone equal to or less than 5 fmol/mg (58, 60)

- *monoclonal antibodies*—are homogeneous immunoglobulins directed at a single epitope or antigenic determinant. The most common method for producing monoclonal antibodies involves the use of hybridoma technology initiated in 1975 by Köhler and Milstein. Many tumor-associated antigens have been identified by monoclonal antibodies. Monoclonal antibodies have been developed against breast, colon, prostate, cervical, ovarian, lung, and pancreatic carcinomas. They have become important tools in the study of cell differentiation, tumor progression, and tumor immunology. Monoclonal antibodies can be used as immunodiagnostic agents to discriminate benign from malignant tissues, differentiate histologic subtypes, and perform immunocytologic evaluations. (16, 19, 29, 58, 60)
- *tumor-associated antigen (TAA)*—antigens absent in normal tissues but found in leukemia, lymphoma, myeloma, melanoma, meningioma, neuroblastoma, hepatoma, osteogenic sarcoma, and tumors of urogenital organs. Monoclonal antibodies are ideal reagents for detection of TAA by immunohistochemical staining on biopsy tissue slides and immunocytologic evaluation of cell suspensions. (6, 16, 58, 60)
- *tumor immunity*—the presence of tumor antibodies toward the specific tumor, as detected by immunofluorescence, complement fixation tests, cytotoxicity tests, and immunohistochemistry analysis. (16, 58, 60)
- *tumor marker*—ideally a specific and sensitive index of a microscopic tumor or metastatic lesion. Radioimmunoassay aids in the detection of tumor markers, since they are highly sensitive and measure antigens and hormones in nanograms. Other assays employed may include the enzyme-linked immunoassays (EIA) in which detection is by enzymatic activity rather than by radioactivity. Variations of EIA may include the enzyme-linked immunosorbent assay (ELISA) or the sandwich-type ELISA. Unfortunately, the specificity of tumor markers is very deficient or entirely lacking. Some examples of tumor markers are:
    - *prostate antigen (PA)*—a marker for human prostate epithelial cells used in the diagnosis of prostatic malignancy.
    - *prostatic acid phosphatase (PAP)*—biologic marker used in the diagnosis of metastatic prostatic cancer.

Most metastatic adenocarcinoma of the prostate is positive for both markers; however, occasional metastatic deposits may be positive for one or the other. Current clinical practice encourages staining all cases of metastatic carcinoma of suspected prostatic origins for both markers. (5, 6, 9, 10, 16, 26, 28, 31, 58)

—*ectopic polypeptides*—immunoreactive adrenocorticotropic hormone (ACTH) in tissue extracts of pulmonary cancer; pancreatic polypeptide found in carcinoid tumors and medullary cancer of the thyroid and others. (10, 58)

—*placental proteins*—human chorionic gonadotropin (HCG) and human placental lactogen (HPL); both hormones are normally present in fetal and maternal serum but undetectable 48 hours after delivery. Their continued presence in increasing amounts suggests the growth of a trophoblastic neoplasm in the male or nonpregnant female. (10, 58)

—*oncofetal antigens*—immunologic substances that may serve as tumor markers.

—*alpha$_1$, α_1, fetoprotein, fetal α_1, globulin (AFP)*—alpha$_1$, globulin, synthesized by the embryo in the liver cell, normally present in serum and cord blood of the fetus and absent in the normal infant. If α_1 fetoprotein is found in a child or adult, a hepatoma or embryonal teratoblastoma is suspected.

Reference values: **AFP**

Nonpregnant adult—less than 25 ng/ml (nanograms per milliliter)

Increasing levels suggest tumor growth of primary hepatocellular carcinoma, hepatoblastoma, or embryonal teratoblastoma. This process is thought to be a reversion of the malignant liver cell to the fetal state.

Decreasing levels indicate tumor shrinkage and thus improvement. (10, 16, 58, 60)

—*carcinoembryonic antigen (CEA)*—release of CEA into the underlying tissues of the gastrointestinal tract and its absorption into the blood and lymph channels account for the highly increased CEA concentrations in several entodermal and nonentodermal carcinomas and other disorders.

Reference values: **CEA assay**

In health—plasma level less than 2.5 ng/ml.

Increasing levels of CEA occur in a wide variety of malignant and nonmalignant diseases.

Clinical significance: CEA assay has no diagnostic value. Tests performed before, during, and after surgery, radiotherapy, and chemotherapy point to the benefit or lack of benefit of the treatment and possible need for further therapy. (10, 16, 58, 60)

Terms Related to Cancer Modalities

■ *radiation*—the application of ionizing radiation therapy is aimed at killing malignant cells. By focusing enough radiation damage on the cell, it is hoped that the cell will lose its reproductive integrity. The critical target of this radiation is the DNA (deoxyribonucleic acid), the genetic substance within the nucleus of a cell responsible for controlling cell division and synthesis. Another mechanism, the laser (light amplification by stimulated emission of radiation) beam has had some effect on certain malignant tumors, such as melanomas, achieving some progressive regression. Linear accelerators refer to high-energy and advanced radiotherapy devices that accelerate charged particles in a straight line and provide various x-ray and electron therapy. The radioresponsiveness of tumors may be predictable by histologic grading before therapy. The following tumors have proved to be radiosensitive and in selected cases radiocurable with a dose tolerable by normal tissue: seminomas, lymphosarcomas, Hodgkin's disease, Wilms' tumors, neuroblastomas, medulloblastomas, retinoblastomas, Ewing's sarcomas, and others. (23, 58, 60)

The biologic radiation effect of these mechanisms depends on interfacing several factors: length of radiation time, total dose, and number of treatments used in the delivery of the total dose. These variables are further delineated by consideration of tumor type, size, location, metastases, and the physical condition of the patient. (23, 58, 60)

Other related terms are: (23, 24, 25, 58)

— *boost technique*—giving maximal tolerated dose to the target volume, then using a very localized radiation to raise the dose to the tumor bed.

— *shrinking field technique*—giving the largest potential tumor bed a moderate dose of radiation, then reducing the volume to the tumor and its immediate confines.

— *brachytherapy* (*brachy*, short)—radiation device is placed close or within short range of the target volume. Examples of brachytherapy include interstitial and intracavitary radiation used in the treatment of gynecologic and oral tumors.

— *teletherapy* (*tele*, far)—radiation device is far removed from the target volume. Examples of teletherapy include the majority of orthovoltage or supervoltage machines.

The ranges of radiation utilized in clinical practice are:

— *superficial*—radiation or roentgen rays from 10 to 125 kev (kilo electron volts).

— *orthovoltage*—radiation represents electromagnetic radiation between 125 and 400 kev.

— *supervoltage or megavoltage*—for those energies greater than 400 kev. (58, 60)

The combination of radiation and chemotherapy or radiation and surgery is used to increase the **therapeutic index** (relationship between desired and undesired effects of therapy). This purpose may be achieved by taking advantage of the different mechanisms of action of **systematic chemotherapy** and **regional irradiation.** Another approach toward increasing the therapeutic index is using drugs that specifically affect tumor response to radiation; a third approach is using a combination of drugs and roentgen rays with either independent action or additivity. (23) The combined effect of drugs and radiation or of two drugs may be classified as:

— *independent*—the agent's mechanisms of action are independent, and resulting damage is independent.

— *additivity*—agents focus on the same loci; because of additive sublethal damage, the resulting damage may be greater than the lethal damage of each agent impacting alone.

— *synergism*—two agents achieve a result that is more effective than pure additivity.

— *antagonism*—cell-killing event is less than independent action. (23, 58, 60)

Radiation and surgery modalities may be presented as a combined approach in therapeutic planning. For example, surgery is often limited by the required preservation of vital normal tissues adjacent to the tumor. Radiation can complement this situation, either preoperatively or postoperatively. As with any technique, the value and choice of method, dose of radiation, and the time between radiation and surgery should be viewed in light of goals planned for the patient. (19, 23)

■ *surgery*—is the oldest treatment for cancer and plays a key role in the cancer diagnosis. A variety of techniques are available to obtain tissue for histologic diagnosis. Some of these techniques are:

— *excisional biopsy*—refers to an excision of the entire suspected tumor tissue with little or no margin of surrounding tissue. When it is not necessary to cut directly into the tumor, this procedure is the choice of most surgeons.

— *incisional biopsy*—refers to removal of a small wedge of tissue from a larger tumor mass. This type of procedure is often required for diagnosis of large masses that may require major surgical approaches even for local excision.

— *needle biopsy*—refers to obtaining a core of tissue through a specially designed needle introduced into the suspect tissue. Suction of cells and tissue fragments are obtained through the needle and presented for cytologic analysis. When the tissue obtained is not sufficient for diagnosis, another type of biopsy procedure may be preferred, in which a larger amount of tissue may be obtained. (12, 13, 47, 54)

Surgery can also play a role in the staging of the tumor. For example, **staging laparotomies** allow the surgeon to explore the abdominal cavity to determine the exact spread of the disease. This information is of great assistance to the oncologist in planning treatment. Placement of **radio-opaque** clips during biopsy and staging procedures is important to delineate areas of known tumor mass and to guide later radiation application to these areas. Other surgical procedures may include:

—*cryosurgery*—refers to malignant tissue being destroyed by freezing techniques.

—*electrocauterization*—refers to malignant neoplasm being burned by an electric current. (12, 13, 47, 54, 58)

The exact role of surgery varies with the type and involvement of the tumor. When feasible, the initial type of surgery may be that of biopsy. This may be followed by more radical surgery, such as radical mastectomy and lymph node dissection. Another approach may use other therapeutic modalities in the reduction of the tumor mass, such as chemotherapy, radiation, both of these modalities separately, or both combined. Then a second, less extensive surgery to remove the reduced mass may follow. The interfacing of modalities in cancer treatment may provide the patient with optimal treatment while avoiding extensive radical procedures whenever possible. (13, 51, 54, 58)

■ *chemotherapy*—drugs provide multiple biochemical avenues to destroy tumor cells. They may be used independently, in combination, or as an aid to another modality (adjuvant).

Selective terms pertaining to chemotherapy agents follow: (2, 12, 58)

—*alkylating agents*—highly reactive compounds with the ability to substitute alkyl groups ($R-H_2-Ch_2^+$) for hydrogen atoms of certain organic compounds. The alkylation for DNA is the critical cytotoxic action. Alkylation produces breaks in the DNA molecule and cross-linking of its twin strands, thus interfering with replication and transcription. Even though alkylating agents as a class exert cytotoxic effects on cells throughout the cell cycle, there is a distinct difference in their pharmacokinetic features (chemical reactivity and membrane transport qualities), and these agents do not share cross-resistance in either experimental or clinical chemotherapy. Examples of this group include:

—*nitrogen mustard derivatives*—mechlorethamine, cyclophosphamide, cholorambucil, and melphalan.

—*ethylenimine derivatives*—such as thio-TEPA.

—*alkyl sulfonates*—such as busulfan

—*triazene derivatives*—such as decarbazine.

—*nitrosureas*—such as carmustine (BCNU), lomustine (CCNU), and methyl-CCNU.

—*Streptomyces antibiotics*—produce antibiotic and tumoricidal effects by directly binding to DNA, thus causing a major inhibitory effect on DNA and RNA synthesis.

—*doxorubicin (Adriamycin)*

—*actinomycin-D (Dactinomycin, Cosmegen)*

—*bleomycin (Blenoxane)*

—*mithramycin (Mithracin)*

—*mitomycin-C (Mutamycin).*

—*plants*—may serve as useful antineoplastic agents, such as

—*vincristine (Oncovin)*, and

–vinblastine (Velban).

These alkaloids are extracted from the periwinkle plant.

—*antimetabolites*—structural analogues (analog) of normal metabolites required for cell function and replication. Antimetabolites may interact with enzymes and cause damage to the cells. Examples of this group include:

–methotrexate (MTX, Methotrexate)

–5-fluorouracil (5-FU, Fluorouracil)

–6-mercaptopurine (6 MP, Purinethal)

–6 thioguanine (6-TG, Thioguanine)

—*hormonal therapy*—tends to turn off tumor growth and interrupt hormone synthesis. Biologic antagonism is the primary reason for the application of most hormonal therapies, with the exception of estrogen use in postmenopausal breast cancer. Examples of this group include: (58, 60, 61)

–estrogens (ethingyl estradiol, estradiol, diethylstilbestrol)

–androgens (testosterone, methyltestosterone, oxymethalone)

–progestogens (hydroxyprogesterone, medroxyprogesterone)

–adrenal corticosteroids (prednisone, hydrocortisone)

–antihormonal agents (antiestrogens and antiadrenal agents)

Special uses of chemotherapy may include: (12, 24, 36, 55, 58)

—instillation of drugs into the spinal fluid, directly using a lumbar puncture needle, or into an implanted Ommaya reservoir to treat central nervous system leukemia, lymphoma, and carcinoma.

—instillation of drugs into the pleural or pericardial space to control effusions.

—hepatic artery infusion to treat hepatic metastases.

—carotid artery infusion to treat head and neck cancers.

—use of chemotherapy through the intraperitoneal administration of drugs to treat ovarian cancers.

Special combinations of chemotherapy agents include: (12, 24, 58, 60)

—*AC*—doxorubicin (Adriamycin), cyclophosphamide

—*BACON*—blenomycin, doxorubicin (Adriamycin), lomustine (CCNU), vincristine (Oncovin), mechlorethamine (nitrogen mustard)

—*CAF*—cyclophosphamide, doxorubicin (Adriamycin), 5-fluorouracil (5-FU)

—*CHAD*—cylophosphamide, hexamethylinelamine, doxorubicin, (Adriamycin), cisplatin (DDCP)

—*CMF*—cyclophosphamide, methotrexate, 5-fluorouracil (5-FU)

—*MAP*—melphalan, doxorubicin (Adriamycin), prednisone

—*MCBP*—melphalan, cyclophosphamide, carmustine (BCNU), prednisone

—*MCP*—melphalan, cyclophosphamide, prednisone

—*MOB*—mitomycin, vincristine (Oncovin), bleomycin

—*VBAP*—vincristine, carmustine (BCNU), doxorubicin (Adriamycin), prednisone

—*VCAP*—vincristine, cyclophosphamide, doxorubicin (Adriamycin), prednisone

Oral Reading Practice

Oncology

Oncology is the study or science of tumors. A neoplasm or tumor is a new growth of tissue that may distort the size of an organ. It serves no useful purpose, since it adds nothing to the further development or repair of the organ. Tumors may be divided into **benign** and **malignant neoplasms.** Typical benign tumors are generally **encapsu-**

lated by **connective tissue,** not **invasive,** and slow growing. They never **metastasize.** Benign tumors may cause serious dysfunctions if they encroach on vital organs, obstruct the circulation or air passages, and compress nerves. Microscopically, the pattern of a benign neoplasm is orderly and well organized. In contrast, typical malignant tumors have no capsule, are invasive, grow progressively, metastasize, and endanger physical well-being and even life. Their microscopic pattern exhibits disorder. Benign tumors may persist for years, and then without apparent cause undergo malignant changes. (15, 17, 19, 58)

Another method of classifying tumors is based on their histologic derivation. The majority of tumors arise from **epithelial** and **connective tissues;** others arise from **hemopoietic, vascular** and **nerve tissue;** whereas others are of mixed origin. (9, 44, 48, 58)

The genetic theory that offers evidence that heredity influences susceptibility to neoplastic reactions is linked closely to the viral theory; extensive research has confirmed the possible transmission of the C-type **RNA** virus from parent to offspring. The high incidence of malignancies in patients with **genetic T-cell** defects offers convincing proof of the genetic background. In the elderly, the frequency of malignant growth may be related to the suppression of the immune response T-cells. Genetic analysis has drawn attention to familial predisposition to cancer, as gleaned from the concurrence of **leukemia** in identical twins, or aggregations of **neuroblastoma, Wilms' tumor,** and carcinomas of the liver and adrenal cortex in families. In addition, **Mendelian inheritance** patterns are found in **retinoblastoma, familial polyposis** of the colon, and **Gardner's syndrome,** in which the colon is carpeted with adenomas. In **Turcot's syndrome,** multiple polyps are associated with tumors of the brain and cord. (18, 40, 60, 64, 66)

The virus theory asserts that viruses are an integral part of the malignant transformation of cells. Many of the individuals affected with **acquired immune deficiency syndrome (AIDS),** caused by the **human immunodeficiency virus (HIV)** which attacks **T-lymphocytes** and severely damages the **immune system,** are susceptible to malignancies such as **Kaposi's sarcoma.** (22, 40, 53)

Research has shown that lymphomas induced by **avian leukosis virus (ALV)** display neoplastic transformation resulting from activation of the **cellular gene** *c-myc.* The *myc* gene family has been implicated in various neoplasias, such as Burkitt's lymphoma *(c-myc),* neuroblastomas *(N-myc),* retinoblastomas *(N-myc),* and small cell lung carcinomas *(c-myc, N-myc,* and *L-myc).* (5, 7, 45, 52, 65, 66)

Normal cells contain a chemical lock and key system to govern growth. Small proteins called **growth factors** act as keys while complex structures on the cell's surface called **receptors** are the locks. The proliferation and differentiation of normal cells are regulated by signals derived from the binding of growth factors to receptors on the cell's surface. Waterfield, et al., and Doolittle, et al., showed in 1983 that two peptides that constitute **platelet-derived growth factor (PDGF)** are similar in sequence to the transforming protein encoded by the **sis oncogene** of the **simian sarcoma virus (SSV).** An associated discovery showed that the **epidermal growth factor (EGF)** receptor showed significant homology with the sequence of the **v-erbB oncogene** product. These findings provide the basis for the postulate that alterations involving cellular oncogenes, growth factors, and their receptors may be involved in the **pathogenesis** of cancer by disrupting the mechanism regulating normal cell growth and development. This type of research continues to stimulate investigation in the field of **molecular genetics** and cell regulation. **Seroepidemiologic** studies shed light on **oncogenic herpesviruses** and related antibody production. **Herpesvirus simplex** type II, found in cervical cancer, enters the human body by venereal transmission. The **Epstein-Barr herpesvirus** is an etiologic factor in **nasopharyngeal carcinoma** and **Burkitt's lymphoma.** (5, 7, 11, 15, 45, 53, 56, 57, 58, 65)

Cytogenetics focuses attention on chromosome defects related to malignancies. Primary tumors show more numeric than structural abnormalities, as seen by the **Giemsa's banding method.** (66) Usually less than 60 chromosomes are present. Metastatic tumor cells are likely to reveal nearly **triploid or tetraploid** modes. Marker chromosomes are very restricted in number in primary tumors but abound in metastatic tumors. Chromosome one is most frequently involved in marker formation, and chromosome 2, 3, 5, 7, and 8 are next in frequency. One chromosome, 22, is absent in about 75 percent of the **meningiomas. Leukemia** and **retinoblastoma** occur frequently with trisomy 21 or 13. (49, 60)

Most patients with chronic **myelogenous leukemia (CML)** have chromosomal translocations. In more than 90 percent of cases of **CML,** a **Philadelphia (Ph^1) chromosome** is present in leukemic cells. **Burkitt's lymphomas** are characterized by reciprocal translocations, which in approximately 90 percent of cases involve chromosome 8 and either chromosome 2 or 22. Cytogenetic techniques and their subsequent systemic clinical application have provided evidence that certain chromosomal disorders often precede and therefore predispose to specific types of neoplasms. The findings of recurrent chromosomal defects in numerous human cancers continue to support the theory that chromosomal rearrangements play a crucial role in **carcinogenesis.** (5, 14, 49, 60)

Ionizing radiation and **carcinogenic** chemicals have been incriminated in causing cancer. **Leukemogenic** agents such as **phenylbutazone** are reported to have induced leukemia. (30, 60).

Estrogens are associated with pelvic malignancy, especially **endometrial adenocarcinoma** in the middle and elderly age-groups. In **granulosa cell carcinoma** of the ovary, increased estrogen secretion by this functional tumor is blamed for inducing endometrial adenocarcinoma. The presence of **clear cell carcinoma** of the cervix or vagina may occur in adolescent girls whose mothers had taken **diethylstibestrol.** It is an established fact that malignant neoplasms may be induced by hormones such as **human chorionic gonadotropin,** which is found regularly in large amounts in **gestational choriocarcinoma,** as well as in 50 percent of **testicular tumors.** (58, 60)

The above findings provide ample support for the conclusion that human cancer has a **multifactorial etiology.** Cancer is second only to heart disease as the cause of death in the United States. Epidemiology has added to the knowledge surrounding the origins and causes of human cancer. Although there remains more to be learned about the multifactorial etiology of cancer in the general population, several environmental exposures have been classified as causes of cancer in humans. See Table 26, p. 416. (18, 30, 58, 60)

Table 26
Environmental Causes of Human Cancer

Agent	Type of Exposure	Site of Cancer
Alcoholic beverages	Drinking	Mouth, pharynx, esophagus, larynx, liver, breast
Alkylating agents (melphalan, cyclophosphamide, chlorambucil, semustine)	Medication	Leukemia
Androgen-anabolic steroids	Medication	Liver
Aromatic amines (benzidine, 2-naphthylamine, 4-aminobiphenyl)	Manufacture of chemicals	Bladder
Arsenic (inorganic)	Mining and smelting of certain ores, pesticide manufacturing and application, medication, and contaminated drinking water	Lung, skin, liver (angiosarcoma)
Asbestos	Manufacturing and application	Lung, pleura, peritoneum, gastrointestinal tract
Benzene	Leather, petroleum, and other industries	Leukemia
Bis(chloromethyl)ether	Manufacture of ion exchange resins	Lung
Chlornaphazine	Medication	Bladder
Chromium compounds	Manufacturing	Lung
Estrogens	Medication	
Synthetic (DES)		Vagina, cervix (adenocarcinoma)
Conjugated (Premarin)		Endometrium
Steroid contraceptives		Liver (benign)
Immunosuppressants (azathioprine, cyclosporin)	Medication	Lymphoma (histiocytic), skin (squamous carcinoma), soft tissue sarcoma
Ionizing radiation	Atomic blasts, medical use, radium dial painting, uranium, and metal mining	Nearly all sites
Isopropyl alcohol production	Manufacturing by strong acid process	Nasal sinuses
Mustard gas	Manufacturing in wartime	Lung, larynx, nasal sinuses
Nickel dust	Refining	Lung, nasal sinuses
Phenacetin-containing analgesics	Medication	Renal pelvis
Polycyclic hydrocarbons	Coal carbonization products and some mineral oils	Lung, skin (squamous carcinoma)
Tobacco chews and powder	Snuff dipping and chewing of tobacco, betel, lime	Mouth
Tobacco smoke	Smoking, especially cigarettes	Lung, larynx, mouth, pharynx, esophagus, bladder, pancreas, kidney
Ultraviolet radiation	Sunlight	Skin, including melanoma
Vinyl chloride	Manufacture of polyvinyl chloride	Liver (angiosarcoma)
Wood dusts	Furniture manufacturing	Nasal sinuses

(Reprinted by permission from Joseph F. Fraumeni, Jr. Epidemiology of Cancer. In James B. Wyngaarden, and Lloyd H. Smith, Jr., eds., *Cecil's Textbook of Medicine,* 18th ed. Philadelphia: W.B. Saunders Co, 1988, p. 1093.)

References and Bibliography

1. Abrams, Jeffrey L., et al. Staging, prognostic factors and special considerations in small cell lung cancer. *Seminars in Oncology* 15: 261-277, June 1988.

2. Albers, David S., et al. Phase II trial of mitomycin C plus 5-FU in the treatment of drug-refractory ovarian cancer. *Seminars in Oncology* 15:22-26, June 1988.

3. Aminoff, Michael J. Nervous system. In Schroeder, Steven A., Krupp, Marcus A., and Tierney, Lawrence M., Jr., eds., *Current Medical Diagnosis & Treatment—1988,* Norwalk, CT: Appleton & Lange, 1988, pp. 571-620.

4. Ashley, Stanley W., and Wells, Samuel A., Jr. Tumors of the small intestine. *Seminars in Oncology* 15:116-128, April 1988.

5. Barbacid, Mariano. Human oncogenes. In DeVita, Vincent T., Jr., Hellman, Samuel, and Rosenberg, Steven A., eds., *Important Advances in Oncology—1986,* Philadelphia: J.B. Lippincott Co., 1986, pp. 3-22.

6. Bates, Susan E., and Longo, Dan L. Use of tumor markers in cancer diagnosis and management. *Seminars in Oncology* 14: 102-138, June 1987.

7. Birrer, Michael J., and Minna, John P. Molecular genetics of lung cancer. *Seminars in Oncology* 15:226-235, June 1988.

8. Bishop, J. Michael. Oncogenes. In Wyngaarden, James B., and Smith, Lloyd H., Jr., eds., *Cecil's Textbook of Medicine,* 18th ed. Philadelphia: W.B. Saunders Co., 1988, pp. 1089-1092.

9. Budd, C. Thomas. Soft tissue and bone sarcomas. In Messerli, Franz H., ed., *Current Clinical Practice,* Philadelphia: W.B. Saunders Co. 1987, pp. 361-363.

10. Bunn, Paul A. Tumor markers. In Wyngaarden, James B., and Smith, Lloyd H., Jr., eds., *Cecil's Textbook of Medicine,* 18th ed. Philadelphia: W.B. Saunders Co., 1988, pp. 1099-1100.

11. Carney, Desmond N., and DeLeij, Lou. Lung cancer biology. *Seminars in Oncology* 15:199-214, June 1988.

12. Chabner, Bruce A. Principles of cancer therapy. In Wyngaarden, James B., and Smith, Lloyd H., Jr., eds., *Cecil's Textbook of Medicine,* 18th ed. Philadelphia: W.B. Saunders Co., 1988, pp. 1113-1129.

13. Clark, Susan Ann. New reconstructive techniques in cancer surgery: The use of free and musculocutaneous flaps. In DeVita, Vincent T., Jr., Hellman, Samuel, and Rosenberg, Steven,. eds., *Important Advances in Oncology—1988,* Philadelphia: J.B. Lippincott Co., 1988, pp. 171-216.

14. Clarkson, Bayard. The chronic leukemias. In Wyngaarden, James B., and Smith, Lloyd H., Jr., eds., *Cecil's Textbook of Medicine,* 18th ed.

Philadelphia: W.B. Saunders Co., 1988, pp. 988-1001.

15. Della-Favera, Riccardo, and Cesarman, Ethel. Cellular oncogenes and the pathogenesis of human cancer. In Blasi, F., ed., *Human Genes and Diseases,* New York: John Wiley & Sons, 1986, pp. 503-544.

16. DeLillis, Ronald A., and Yogeshwar, Dayal. The role of immunohistochemistry in the diagnosis of poorly differentiated malignant neoplasms. *Seminars in Oncology* 14:173-192, June 1987.

17. Fidler, Isaiah, and Hart, Ian R. Principles of cancer biology: Cancer metastasis. In DeVita, Vincent T., Jr., Hellman, Samuel, and Rosenberg, Steven A., eds., *Cancer Principles & Practice of Oncology,* 2nd ed., vol. 1. Philadelphia: J.B. Lippincott Co., 1985, pp. 113-124.

18. Fraumeni, Joseph F., Jr. Epidemiology of cancer. In Wyngaarden, James B., and Smith, Lloyd H., Jr., eds., *Cecil's Textbook of Medicine,* 18th ed. Philadelphia: W.B. Saunders Co., 1988, pp. 1092-1096.

19. Gallagher, Neil, MD. Personal communications.

20. Gazdar, A.F., and Linnoila, R.I. The pathology of lung cancer—changing concepts and new diagnostic techniques. *Seminars in Oncology* 15:215-225, June 1988.

21. Glick, John H. Hodgkin's disease. In Wyngaarden, James B., and Smith, Lloyd H., Jr., eds., *Cecil's Textbook of Medicine,* 18th ed. Philadelphia: W.B. Saunders Co., 1988, pp. 1014-1022.

22. Groopman, Jerome E. The acquired immunodeficiency syndrome. In Wyngaarden, James B., and Smith, Lloyd H., Jr., eds., *Cecil's Textbook of Medicine,* 18th ed. Philadelphia: W.B. Saunders Co., 1988, pp. 1799-1808.

23. Hellman, Samuel. Principles of radiation therapy. In DeVita, Vincent T., Jr. Hellman, Samuel, and Rosenberg, Steven A., eds., *Cancer Principles & Practice of Oncology,* 2nd ed., vol. 1. Philadelphia: J.B. Lippincott Co., 1985, pp. 227-255.

24. Hilaris, Basil S., and Nori, Dattatreyudu. Intraoperative radiotherapy in stage I and II lung cancer. *Seminars in Oncology* 3:22-32, 1987.

25. Hilaris, Basil, et al. New approaches to brachy-therapy. In DeVita, Vincent T., Jr., Hellman, Samuel, and Rosenberg, Steven A., eds., *Important Advances in Oncology—1987,* Philadelphia: J.B. Lippincott Co., 1987, pp. 237-261.

26. Israel, Mark A., et al. Patterns of proto-oncogene expression: A novel approach to the development of tumor markers. In DeVita, Vincent T., Jr., Hellman, Samuel, and Rosenberg, Steven A., eds., *Important Ad-*

vances in Oncology—1987, Philadelphia: J.B. Lippincott Co., 1987, pp. 87-104.

27. Kanzawa, F., et al. Human tumor clonogenic assay for carcinoma of the lung. *Oncology* 44:150-155. May-June 1987.

28. Kato, H. Studies on the special tumor marker of cervical cancer of the uterus. *Seminars in Surgical Oncology* 3:55-63, 1987.

29. Larson, Steven M. Cancer imaging with monoclonal antibodies. In DeVita, Vincent T., Jr., Hellman, Samuel, and Rosenberg, Steven A., eds., *Important Advances in Oncology—1986*, Philadelphia: J.B. Lippincott Co., 1986, pp. 223-249.

30. Laszlo, John. Introduction—Oncology. In Wyngaarden, James B., and Smith, Lloyd H., Jr., eds., *Cecil's Textbook of Medicine*, 18th ed. Philadelphia: W.B. Saunders Co., 1988, pp. 1082-1089.

31. Makuch, Robert W., and Muenz, Larry R. Evaluating the adequacy of tumor markers to discriminate among distinct populations. *Seminars in Oncology* 14:89-101, June 1987.

32. Mankin, Henry J. Bone tumors. In Wyngaarden, James B., and Smith, Lloyd H., Jr., eds., *Cecil's Textbook of Medicine*, 18th ed. Philadelphia: W.B. Saunders Co., 1988, pp. 1521-1522.

33. Margolis, Alan J., and Greenwood, Sadja. Gynecology and obstetrics. In Schroeder, Steven A., Krupp, Marcus A., and Tierney, Laurence M., Jr., eds., *Current Medical Diagnosis & Treatment—1988*, Norwalk, CT: Appleton & Lange, 1988, pp. 447-495.

34. Matsumato, Alvin M. The testis. In Wyngaarden, James B., and Smith, Lloyd H., Jr., eds., *Cecil's Textbook of Medicine*, 18th ed. Philadelphia: W.B. Saunders Co., 1988, pp. 1404-1421.

35. Merkel, Douglas E., and McGuire, W.L. Oncogenes and cancer prognosis. In DeVita, Vincent T., Jr., Hellman, Samuel, and Rosenberg, Steven A., eds., *Important Advances in Oncology—1988*, Philadelphia: J.B. Lippincott Co., 1988, pp. 103-117.

36. Monk, Bradley J., et al. Intraperitoneal mitomycin C in treatment of peritoneal carcinomatosis following second-look surgery. *Seminars in Oncology* 15:27-31, June 1988.

37. Morton, Donald L., et al. Oncology. In Schwartz, Seymour I., ed.-in-chief, *Principles of Surgery*, 5th ed., vol. 1. New York: McGraw-Hill Publishing Co., 1989, pp. 331-386.

38. Mountain, Clifton F. Prognostic implications of the International Staging System. *Seminars in Oncology* 15:236-245, June 1988.

39. Pardee, Arthur B. Principles of cancer biology: Biochemistry and cell biology. In DeVita, Vincent T., Jr., Hellman, Samuel, and Rosenberg, Steven A., eds., *Cancer Prin-*

ciples & Practice of Oncology, 2nd ed., vol. 1. Philadelphia: J.B. Lippincott Co., 1985, pp. 3-22.

40. Parker, Frank. Cutaneous manifestations of internal malignancy. In Wyngaarden, James B., and Smith, Lloyd H., Jr., eds., *Cecil's Textbook of Medicine*, 18th ed. Philadelphia: J.B. Lippincott Co., 1988, pp. 1107-1113.

41. Skin diseases. Ibid., pp. 2300-2353.

42. Paul, William E. The immune system: Introduction. In Wyngaarden, James B., and Smith, Lloyd H., Jr., eds., *Cecil's Textbook of Medicine*, 18th ed. Philadelphia: W.B. Saunders Co., 1988, pp. 1932-1937.

43. Pope, Charles E., II. Diseases of the esophagus. In Wyngaarden, James B., and Smith, Lloyd H., Jr., eds., *Cecil's Textbook of Medicine*, 18th ed. Philadelphia: W.B. Saunders Co., 1988, pp. 679-689.

44. Portlock, Carol S. The non-Hodgkin's lymphomas. In Wyngaarden, James B., and Smith, Lloyd H., Jr., eds., *Cecil's Textbook of Medicine*, 18th ed. Philadelphia: W.B. Saunders Co., 1988, pp. 1009-1013.

45. Burkitt's lymphoma. Ibid., pp. 1013-1014.

46. Rebar, Robert W. The ovaries. In Wyngaarden, James B., and Smith, Lloyd H., Jr., eds., *Cecil's Textbook of Medicine*, 18th ed. Philadelphia: W.B. Saunders Co., 1988, pp. 1425-1446.

47. Rosenberg, Steven A. Principles of surgical oncology. In DeVita, Vincent T., Jr., Hellman, Samuel, and Rosenberg, Steven A., eds., *Cancer Principles & Practice of Oncology*, 2nd ed. vol. 1. Philadelphia: J.B. Lippincott Co., 1985, pp. 215-225.

48. Rosenberg, Steven A., et al. Sarcomas of soft tissue. In DeVita, Vincent T., Jr., Hellman, Samuel, and Rosenberg, Steven A., eds., *Cancer Principles & Practice of Oncology*, 2nd ed., vol. 2. Philadelphia: J.B. Lippincott Co., 1985, pp. 1243-1291.

49. Rowley, Janet D. Principles of cancer biology: Chromosomal abnormalities. In DeVita, Vincent T., Jr., Hellman, Samuel, and Rosenberg, Steven A., eds., *Cancer Principles & Practice of Oncology*, 2nd ed., vol. 1. Philadelphia: J.B. Lippincott Co., 1985, pp. 68-78.

50. Salmon, Sydney E. Plasma cell disorders. In Wyngaarden, James B., and Smith, Lloyd H., Jr., eds., *Cecil's Textbook of Medicine*, 18th ed. Philadelphia: W.B. Saunders Co., 1988, pp. 1026-1036.

51. Shipley, William U., et al. The role of radiation therapy and chemotherapy in the treatment of invasive carcinoma of the urinary bladder. *Seminars in Oncology* 15:390-395, Aug. 1988.

52. Sikora, K., et al. c-myc oncogene expression in colorectal cancer. *Cancer* 59:1289-1295, April 1, 1987.

53. Silverman, Sol, Jr. Oral medicine. In Wyngaarden, James B., and Smith, Lloyd H., Jr., eds., *Cecil's Textbook of Medicine*, 18th ed. Philadelphia: W.B. Saunders Co., 1988, pp. 674-679.

54. Snow, James B., Jr. Surgical management of head and neck cancer. *Seminars in Oncology* 15:20-28, Feb. 1988.

55. Spain, Robert C. Neoadjuvant mitomycin C, cisplatin, and infusion vinblastine in locally and regionally advanced non-small cell lung cancer: Problems and progress from the perspective of long-term follow-up. *Seminars in Oncology* 15:6-15, June 1988.

56. Sporn, Michael B., and Roberts, Anita B. Peptide growth factors: Current status and therapeutic opportunities. In DeVita, Vincent T., Jr., Hellman, Samuel, and Rosenberg, Steven A., eds., *Important Advances in Oncology—1987*. Philadelphia: J.B. Lippincott Co., 1987, pp. 75-87.

57. Sporn, Michael B., et al. Principles of cancer biology: Growth factors and differentiation. In DeVita, Vincent T., Jr., Hellman, Samuel, and Rosenberg, Steven A., eds., *Cancer Principles & Practice of Oncology*, 2nd ed., vol. 1. Philadelphia: J.B. Lippincott Co., 1985, pp. 49-65.

58. Tucker, Eugene, M.D. Personal communications.

59. Vande, W., et al. Principles of cancer biology: Molecular biology. In DeVita, Vincent T., Jr., Hellman, Samuel, and Rosenberg, Steven A., eds., *Cancer Principles & Practice of Oncology*, 2nd ed., vol. 1. Philadelphia: J.B. Lippincott Co., 1985, pp. 771-794.

60. Volk, Sr. Leo Rita. Personal communications.

61. Von Roenn, Jamie H. Sequential hormone therapy for advanced breast cancer. *Seminars in Oncology* 15:38-43, April 1988.

62. Weinstein, Howard J. The acute leukemias. In Wyngaarden, James B., and Smith, Lloyd H., Jr., eds., *Cecil's Textbook of Medicine*, 18th ed. Philadelphia: W.B. Saunders Co., 1988, pp. 1001-1007.

63. Williams, Richard D. Tumors of the kidney, ureter and bladder. In Wyngaarden, James B., and Smith, Lloyd H., Jr., eds., *Cecil's Textbook of Medicine*, 18th ed. Philadelphia: W.B. Saunders Co., 1988, pp. 650-655.

64. Winawer, Sidney J. Neoplasms of the large and small intestine. In Wyngaarden, James B., and Smith, Lloyd H., Jr., eds., *Cecil's Textbook of Medicine*, 18th ed. Philadelphia: W.B. Saunders Co., 1988, pp. 766-774.

65. Yamamoto, T., et al. The erbB-related growth factor receptors. In Blasi, F., ed., *Human Genes and Diseases*, New York: John Wiley & Sons, 1986, pp. 571-609.

66. Yunis, Jorge J. Chromosomal rearrangements, genes, and fragile sites in cancer: Clinical and biologic implications. In DeVita, Vincent T., Jr., Hellman, Samuel, and Rosenberg, Steven A., eds., *Important Advances in Oncology—1986*, Philadelphia: J.B. Lippincott Co., 1986, pp. 93-128.

Selected Terms Pertaining to the Clinical Laboratory

Orientation

Origin of Terms

bi-, bio-, (G)—life
hem-, hemo- (G)—blood
hemat-, hemato- (G)—blood
-lysis (G)—dissolution, breaking down
macro- (G)—large
megalo- (G)—big, great size
meli- (G)—sweet, honey

meso- (G)—middle
meta- (G)—change, exchange, transformation
micro- (G)—small
plasmo- (G)—plasma, cell substance
toxico- (G)—poison

General Terms

- *assay*—test or analysis of a substance to determine its biologic, chemical, or physical properties.
- *bioassay*—analysis of a living substance derived from a specific tissue or organ.
- *biochemistry*—chemistry that deals with components and processes of living organisms.
- *conventional values*—traditional way of reporting normal test results.
- *factor*—multiplication number for converting conventional units into International System (SI) units. (17, 67)
- *hematology*—medical science studying the blood and blood-forming organs.
- *immunohematology*—hematologic specialty dealing with antigen-antibody or immune reactions and their effects on the blood. (77)
- *immunopathology*—medical science concerned with diseases caused by antigen-antibody reactions. (77)
- *International System of Units (See Table 28)*—modification of metric system using meter, kilogram, liter, mole, pascal, and second as basic units to ensure worldwide uniformity in presenting laboratory reports or other scientific data. (17, 77)
- *metric system*—a decimal system of measures and weights, using the meter, gram, and liter as basic units. (See Table 27.) (77)
  NOTE: Since measurements of the metric system, especially the International System of Units, are relatively unfamiliar to students, essential data used in reporting laboratory tests are presented here.

- *reference interval*—reference range, formerly normal range. (77)
- *reference values*—set of values of a certain quantity obtained from a person or group of persons and corresponding to a stated description. This description must be spelled out and available if others are to use the reference values. For each type of quantity, a series of reference groups will be necessary, taking into consideration age, sex, race, previous diet, exercise, posture, etc. (17, 67)
- *sensitivity*—the frequency with which a laboratory test yields positive results in patients who have a particular disease. Sensitivity also refers to a state of reacting readily to stimuli or reagents. (77, 81)
- *specificity*—the frequency with which a laboratory test yields negative results in nondiseased persons. Test results apply to a single pathologic state. (77)
- *susceptibility*—decreased resistance to infection or foreign protein caused by impaired immunity. (77)

Table 27
Measurements of the Metric System

Weights in descending order

kg	= kilogram	= 1,000 grams	= 10^3gm	
gm, g	= gram	= 1,000 milligrams	= 10^3mg	
mg	= milligram	= 1,000 micrograms	= 10^{-3}g	
μg	= microgram	= 1,000 nanograms	= 10^{-6}g	
ng	= nanogram	= 1,000 picograms	= 10^{-9}g	
pg	= picogram	= 1,000 femtograms	= 10^{-12}g	
fg	= femtogram	= 1,000 attograms	= 10^{-15}g	

Capacity in descending order

l, L	= liter	= 1,000 milliliters	= 10 deciliters	(dl)
l, L	= liter	= 1,000 cubic centimeters	= 10 deciliters	(dl)
dl	= deciliter	= 100 milliliters	= 0.10 liter	(l)
cl	= centiliter	= 10 milliliters	= 0.10 deciliter	(dl)
ml	= milliliter	= 1,000 microliters	= 0.10 centiliter	(cl)
μl	= microliter	= 1,000 nanoliters	= 0.001 milliliter	(ml)
nl	= nanoliter	= 1,000 picoliters	= 0.001 microliter	(μl)
pl	= picoliter	= 1,000 femtoliters	= 0.001 nanoliter	(nl)
fl	= femtoliter	= 1,000 attoliters	= 0.001 picoliter	(pl)

Length in descending order

m	= meter	= 1,000 millimeters	= 100 centimeters	(cm)
dm	= decimeter	= 100 millimeters	= 10 centimeters	(cm)
cm	= centimeter	= 10 millimeters	= 0.01 meter	(m)
mm	= millimeter	= 1,000 micrometers	= 0.001 meter	(m)
μm	= micrometer	= 1,000 nanometers	= 0.001 millimeter	(mm)
nm	= nanometer	= 1,000 picometers	= 0.001 micrometer	(μm)
pm	= picometer	= 1,000 femtometers	= 0.001 nanometer	(nm)
fm	= femtometer	= 1,000 attometers	= 0.001 picometer	(pm)

Table 28
Traditional Measurements*

Units and subunits

Eq	= equivalent	mEq/l, mEq/L	=	milliequivalent per liter
mEq	= milliequivalent (measure of electrolytes)	μEq/l, μEq/L	=	microequivalent per liter
mμ	= millimicron (same as nanogram)	μU	=	microunit
		IU	=	International Unit
U	= units, units	mIU	=	milliInternational Unit

The International System of Measurements

Basic units

A	= ampere (electric current)	m	=	meter (length)
cd	= candela (luminous intensity)	mol	=	mole (amount of substance)
Hz	= hertz (frequency)	N	=	newton (force)
K	= kelvin (thermodynamic temperature)	s	=	second (time)
kg	= kilogram (mass)	W	=	watt (power, radiant flux)

Some subunits

mmol	= millimole	mmol/l	=	mmol per liter
μmol	= micromole	μmol/l	=	micromole per liter
nmol	= nanomole	nmol/l	=	nanomole per liter
mol/kg	= mole per kilogram	nmol/kg	=	nanomole per kilogram
Pa	= pascal (unit of pressure: newton per square meter)	mOsm	=	milliosmole (measure of osmolarity)
molality	= moles of solute in one kilogram of solvent	molarity	=	moles of solute in one liter of solution

*(17, 67, 71, 81)

Hematology and Immunohematology

Terms Related to Hematology

- *bleeding time*—duration of bleeding from a standardized wound. It measures the platelet function and the integrity of the vessel wall. (39, 77)
- *capillary fragility tourniquet test*—procedure measuring the resistance of the capillaries to pressure and stress. A blood pressure cuff is applied to the upper arm and kept inflated at 80 mm pressure for five minutes. If a number of purpuric spots appear below the cuff area a few minutes after the cuff is released, the test is positive. (40)
- *coagulant*—substance contributing to clot formation. (39)
- *coagulation time, clotting time*—time taken for venous blood to clot. (77)
- *coagulum, blood clot*—lumpy mass formed in static blood in the laboratory and composed of platelets and red and white cells, irregularly scattered in fibrin network. (39)
- *clotlysis*—dissolution of a clot. (39)
- *clot retraction*—formation of a clot and the exuding of serum: a qualitative platelet function test. Normally the retraction of blood begins within 30 to 60 minutes from the time it was drawn. A semiquantitative test method has been devised using platelet rich plasma. Clot retraction depends on an adequate number of functionally

normal platelets. The test is abnormal in thrombocytopenia and in Glanzmann's thrombasthenia. (39)

- *hematocrit (Hct), volume of packed red cells (VPRC)*—measurement of the volume of packed red blood cells in the venous blood. Reference values depend on sex and altitude method used to measure Hct. A similar interdependence is observed in other hematologic findings. (23, 26, 43)

- *hemoglobin concentration (Hb)*—the amount of hemoglobin recorded in grams per deciliter (g/dl) in the conventional system of units and in millimoles per liter (mmol/L) in the International System of Units (SI units). (26, 43)

- *mean corpuscular hemoglobin (MCH)*—weight of hemoglobin in average red blood cells, conventionally expressed in picograms (pg); in the SI System, it is expressed in millimoles per liter (mmol/L). (26, 43)

- *mean corpuscular hemoglobin concentration (MCHC)*—percentage of hemoglobin concentration in the average red blood cell. (32, 43)

- *mean corpuscular volume (MCV)*—mean volume of the average red blood cell, conventionally recorded in cubic microns; in the SI units recorded in femtoliters (fl). (32, 43)

- *osmotic fragility*—measurement of the power of red cells to resist hemolysis in a hypotonic salt solution. (43)

- *platelet aggregation test*—test of the capability of platelets to aggregate in vitro to certain agonists. Aggregation may be measured spectrophotometrically and recorded by a platelet aggregometer. This test may be helpful in patients with prolonged bleeding times in the presence of normal platelet counts and in determining the cause of abnormal platelet function. This test is a useful diagnostic aid in the diagnosis of von Willebrand's disease, Bernard-Soulier's disease and Glanzmann's thrombasthenia. (39)

- *prothrombin*—coagulation factor II present in blood plasma.

- *prothrombin time (PT)*—time in seconds required for thromboplastin to coagulate plasma. PT is a screening test for abnormalities in the extrinsic pathways. It measures factors I, II, V, VII, and X.

> **Reference values:**
> Prothrombin time, two-stage modified, whole blood, (Na citrate)
> PT—18-22 seconds (SIU: 18-22 seconds)
> PT is prolonged in vitamin K deficiency, hypoprothrombinemia, liver disease, and obstructive jaundice. Also, PT is prolonged in heparin administration, in the presence of circulating anticoagulants, in disseminated intravascular coagulation (DIC), and in dysproteinemias. (17, 48, 55, 65)

- *thromboplastin*—coagulation factor III, thought to initiate clotting by converting prothrombin to thrombin in the presence of calcium ions. Tissue thromboplastin is chiefly found in the brain, thymus, placenta, testes, and lungs.
    - *complete thromboplastins*—substances causing clot formation as quickly with hemophilia as with normal blood.
    - *partial thromboplastins*—substances causing clot formation less quickly with hemophilia than with normal blood.
    - *partial thromboplastin time (PTT)*—valuable screening test for abnormalities of blood coagulation, measuring coagulation factors involved in the intrinsic pathways except for platelet factor III, factor VII, and factor XIII. The test is complementary to the prothrombin time and may point out other clotting factors' deficiencies or the presence of a circulating anticoagulant.

—*activated partial thromboplastin time (APTT)*—helpful screening test for the intrinsic coagulation system. Factor XII and cofactors are activated by particulate ingredients of a reagent such as celite. The other proteins are activated by phospholipid in the reagent.

Reference values:
PTT whole blood (Na citrate) 60-85 seconds (SIU: 60-85 seconds)
APTT whole blood (Na citrate) 25-35 seconds (SIU: 25-35 seconds)
Increase in vitamin K deficiency, hepatic disease, von Willebrand's disease, in the presence of circulating anticoagulants, and other disorders. (17, 41)

■ *thrombus*—structure formed in circulating blood; chiefly composed of a head of agglutinated platelets and white cells and a tail of fibrin and entrapped red cells. (41, 90)

Table 29
Selected Hematologic Findings in Disease

Test	Conventional Units (17)	SI Units (17)	Diagnostic Aid in Disease	Pathologic Response
Bleeding time			Thrombocytopenia	Increase
Duke	1-5 min.	1-5 min.	von Willebrand's	Increase
Ivy	2-7 min.	2-7 min.	disease (42)	
Clotting time				
Lee-White	5-8 min.	5-8 min.	Hemophilia (42)	Increase
Clot retraction time	1-24 hr.	1-24 hr.	Thrombasthenia (Glanzmann's disease) (42)	Poor or absent
Hemoglobin				
male	13.5-17.5 g/dL	2.09-2.71 mmol/L	Polycythemia vera (46)	Increase
female	12.0-16.0 g/dL	1.86-2.48 mmol/L	Anemias (5, 38)	Decrease
Mean corpuscular hemoglobin (MCH)	26-34 pg/cell	0.40-0.53 fmol/cell	Hypochromic anemia (38)	Decrease
Mean corpuscular volume (MCV)	80-100 micra^3	80-100 fl	Macrocytic anemia (5) Hypochromic microcytic anemia (38)	Increase Decrease
Mean corpuscular hemoglobin concentration (MCHC)	31-37% Hb/cell	4.81-5.74 mmol/Hb/L RBC	Hypochromic microcytic anemia (38)	Decrease

Test	Conventional Units (17)	SI Units (17)	Diagnostic Aid in Disease	Pathologic Response
(Continued)				
Platelet count	$150\text{-}400 \times 10^3/\mu L$ (mm³)	$150\text{-}400 \times 10^9/L$	Idiopathic thrombocyto-penic purpura (ITP) (42)	Decrease

Terms Related to Blood Groupings

- *ABO system*—the international system of Landsteiner, in which the four main blood groups are designated by the letters A, B, AB, and O. This system is universally used. (84, 86)
- *blood group or blood type*—inherited characteristic of human blood that remains unchanged throughout life. (86)
- *blood grouping systems*—the classification of blood based on hemagglutinogens in red blood corpuscles. There are different types of blood factors (hemagglutinogens) requiring special methods of typing. The blood group systems refer to these serologic factors; for example:

  ABO system to A, B, AB, and O factors

  MN system to M, N, and MN factors

  Rh-Hr system to Rh and Hr factors.*

  The recent discovery of subgroups (A_1, A_2, A_3, A_4, and others for the ABO system) explains why the incompatibility of types of blood may occur within the same blood group.

  —*incompatible blood*—blood not capable of being mixed without causing hemolysis or clumping of red blood cells.

  —*type O*—universal donor—blood has no agglutinogens, hence no clumping. (86, 89)
- *cross-matching*—procedure done to determine the compatibility between the recipient's blood and donor's blood to prevent blood transfusion reaction. (84, 86, 87)

(See Table 30).

- *MN system*—classification based on the presence of MN factors in erythrocytes. This system is used in genetic blood group analysis and in medical-legal paternity studies when parental claims are disputed. (86, 89)
- *Rh-Hr system*—a system of complex antigen structure. The Rh factor is an agglutinogen that occurs in the red blood corpuscles of 87 percent of white people. Originally only Rh-positive and Rh-negative agglutinogens were known; at present subgroups of Rh factors are recognized. The Rh determinations are of clinical importance in blood transfusion and obstetrics. There is a reciprocal relationship between Hr and Rh factors. (86, 89)

Terms Related to Serologic and Immunologic Tests

- *agglutination*—clumping of erythrocytes when mixed with incompatible blood or antisera. (81, 85)

---

*For more information on other blood group systems, such as Duffy, Kell, and Lewis, etc., consult reference 86, pp. 145-200. Rh studies are done routinely on all blood transfusions. In addition, subgroups may be checked to prevent reactions. Universal donor blood is only used for recipients of group A or B or AB in emergency when their respective type is not available.

Table 30
Compatibility of Blood for Transfusion*

Recipient's Blood	Donor's Blood
A	A or O
B	B or O
AB	AB, A, B, or O
O	O only

*(83, 86, 87)

- *agglutination test*—serologic reaction in which the antibody combines with an antigen in agglutination. (81)
- *agglutinin*—specific antibody in blood serum that causes agglutination.
  - *—autoagglutinin*—resembles cold agglutinin, reacts at temperature below 37°C with person's own cells and those of other groups.
  - *—cold agglutinin*—antibody causes clumping of human group O red cells at zero 5°C or below 37°C. (41, 81)
- *agglutinogen*—substance that stimulates the production of agglutinins when introduced into the body.
- *antibody*—molecule belonging to a special group of proteins known as gamma globulins (IgG, IgM, others).
- *antibody labeling with fluorescein*—histochemical technique for identifying antigen and antibody within tissues.
  - *—direct immunofluorescent staining*—sensitive serologic test in which the specific antibody is labeled with fluorescein and the fluorescing antigen-antibody complex is viewed in the tissues.
  - *—indirect immunofluorescent method*—procedure in which fluorescein-labeled anti-human globulin is employed in the detection of unlabeled antibody in human tissues. Since plasma cells show marked fluorescence, they are thought to be antibody-producing cells. Examples: immunofluorescent skin test in systemic lupus erythematosus and rheumatoid factor by indirect immunofluorescence. (9)
- *antibody screen*—combination of tests for detecting anti-red cell antibodies in serum, routinely used for transfusion cross-matching. An indirect Coombs test is included in the antibody screen. (32, 83, 87)
- *antigen*—a substance that causes the formation of antibodies.
  - *—ABO antigens*—genetically determined, specific glycoproteins, primarily located on the surface of red blood cells but also in other body tissues. (86)
  - *—human leukocyte antigens (HLA)*—antigens found on the surface of nucleated cells, including most body tissues and cellular components of the circulating blood, with exception of red cells. Peripheral blood leukocytes are often suitable to assess the HLA antigenic composite of a person. It is imperative that HLA typing is done for the detection of HLA antibodies before platelet or leukocyte transfusions or transplant procedures of bone marrow, kidney, heart, and other organs.
  - *—platelet antigens*—antigens specific for platelets and associated with ABO and HLA antigens. Matching for platelet transfusions is complex and problematic. (9, 88)
- *antinuclear antibodies (ANA), antinuclear factor (ANF)*—serum antibodies to cellular components, including:

—*autoantibodies*—antibodies formed by the patient against his or her own nuclear components, such as red cell antigens of the blood.

—*non-organ-specific antibodies*—antibodies found in connective tissue diseases. The most characteristic finding in almost all patients with active lupus erythematosus is antinuclear antibodies directed against deoxyribonucleoprotein (DNP).

—*organ-specific antibodies*—antinuclear antibodies present in pernicious anemia, ulcerative colitis, and others. (77)

- *antinuclear antibody (ANA) determination*—test performed by indirect fluorescent microscopy as a two-stage antigen-antibody reaction. Negative results show antinuclear antibody titer between 1:20 or less, and positive results indicate antinuclear antibody titer between 1:320 or over, which is strongly suggestive of systemic lupus erythematosus (SLE). (77)
- *blood factor for hemagglutinogen*—serologic factor that occurs on the surface of red blood corpuscles. (77)
- *complement fixation (CF) test*—antigen-antibody reaction requiring a complement for the union of antigen and antibody. (85)
- *counterimmunoelectrophoresis (CIE)*—a combination of the double immunodiffusion method of Ouchterlony and electrophoresis for detecting microbial antigens in body fluids. (73, 75)
- *direct microscopy*—identification of pathogens by microscopic examination of tissues, exudates, and body fluids. (73)
- *electron microscopy*—method for identifying various viral infections such as vesicular fluid and scabs of febrile skin eruptions by using an electron microscope because of its extremely high magnification.
- *enzyme-linked immunosorbent assay (ELISA)*—a purified enzyme bound in a stable way to a specific antibody. To some extent ELISA has replaced electron and light microscopy. The procedure is safe, and there is no fading as with fluorescent tests and light microscopy. (9, 85)
- *hemagglutination-inhibition (HI) test*—the detection of the presence of specific antibodies capable of inhibiting agglutination of red cells by agents such as viruses. (77)
- *immunofluorescence*—the tagging of antibodies with a fluorescent dye to detect or localize antigen-antibody combinations (see *antibody labeling*). (9)
- *immunomicroscopy*—a procedure for localization of immunologic reactions (antigen-antibody) at the cellular level. (77, 87)
- *latex agglutination*—highly sensitive test of special value in detecting cryptococcal antigen in meningoencephalitis. Its many false-positive reactions detract from its usefulness.
- *latex tests*—tests that are rather nonspecific for rheumatoid arthritis but highly sensitive for rheumatoid factors. (68)
- *neutralization test*—detection of the presence of antibodies capable of inactivating an infective agent, thus rendering it noninfective or neutral. (87)

Hematologic and Serologic Tests for Specific Disorders

- *infectious mononucleosis:* (23, 33)

    —*serologic tests:*

    –*Paul-Bunnell test*—serologic test for heterophil agglutinins is positive in infectious mononucleosis after the first week of illness and usually reaches a peak titer at two or three weeks.

    –*sheep cell differential test*—a specific and qualitative test based on the fact that anti-sheep agglutinins in infectious mononucleosis are completely removed with beef cells and are incompletely or not removed with Forssman antigen (guinea pig or horse kidney). Other disorders are associated with production of heterophil antibodies, which also may agglutinate sheep red cells. The Davidsohn's differential test is helpful in increasing the specificity of this test (one aliquot of serum is absorbed with beef erythrocytes and another aliquot is absorbed with guinea pig kidney cells before reacting the serum with sheep red cells).

—*spot test for infectious mononucleosis, Monospot*—a complete one-minute differential slide test for the detection of the specific heterophile antibodies associated with infectious mononucleosis.

- *lupus erythematosus:* (11, 15, 82)

—*anti-DNP, antinucleoprotein*—the most typical antinuclear antibody (ANA) that causes the LE-cell phenomenon and is present in untreated systemic lupus erythematosus (SLE). Antinuclear factors may also be found in rheumatoid arthritis, other connective tissue diseases, and disseminated malignancies.

—*Farr assay*—an ammonium sulfate precipitation assay adapted for detection and study of antibodies specific for DNA. Both anti-ssDNA (anti-single-stranded DNA) antibodies and anti-dsNA (anti-double-stranded DNA) antibodies have been demonstrated with the Farr assay. Anti-ssDNA antibodies have been found in a variety of diseases other than SLE. As well as being specific for SLE, anti-dsNA antibodies in sera correlated with onset and decline of clinically active disease.

—*LE-cell*—large granulocyte containing purplish stainable inclusions (Wright stain) thinly rimmed with cytoplasm. The nucleus is pushed aside.

—*LE-cell factor, LE-serum factor*—one of several autoantibodies reacting against nucleoprotein to transform nuclei into homogenous globular bodies, which are then phagocytized by intact granulocytes to form typical LE-cells.

—*LE-cell phenomenon*—the presence of the LE serum factor (antinucleoprotein factor), causing an agglutination reaction between antigen-treated particles and the serum containing antinuclear globulins.

—*LE-test*—rapid slide test for antinucleoprotein factors associated with systemic lupus erythematosus. The test specimen is compared with control serums.

- *rheumatoid arthritis:* (68)

—*rheumatoid factor*—proteins belonging to a family of IgM antibodies that evolved in response to antigenic stimulation by an altered immunoglobulin. Consequently they are antiglobulins. Currently used tests detect IgM rheumatoid factor. Examples of associated tests are:

—*bentonite flocculation test*—pooled human gammaglobulin is used as antigen for coating particles.

—*latex fixation test*—pooled human gammaglobulin is absorbed to standard latex particles.

—*Rheumanosticon*—a rapid slide test for the detection of the rheumatoid factor, performed on serum or whole blood. The rheumatoid factor reacts with the coating material, causing a visual agglutination of the inert latex particles.

Terms Related to Obstetrical, Fetal, and Neonatal Tests and Procedures

- *ABO incompatibility*—incompatibility in the A, B, AB, and O blood types. Usually the mother is type O and the baby type A or B. This incompatibility occurs in a considerable number of pregnancies, but erythroblastosis develops in a relatively small percentage of them. (34, 83, 86)
- *amniotic fluid analyses*—spectrophotometric tracings or other determinations on amniotic fluid in the antepartum management of Rh incompatibility, diabetes, etc.

Fetal involvement exists if there is an abnormal increase in the pigments that absorb light at wavelengths between 450 and 460 mμ.* Repeated amniotic fluid analyses are valuable guides for timing intrauterine transfusion or induction of labor. (61)

- *antiglobulin reaction, Coombs test*—test for antibodies.

  —*direct Coombs test*—test for the antibody coating of erythrocytes.

  > **Negative reaction:** direct Coombs, no antibody coating on newborn's red cells.
  > **Positive reaction:** direct Coombs, antibody coating on newborn's red cells, indicative of hemolytic disease.

  —*indirect Coombs test*—test determines presence of antibodies in serum. (41, 43, 47, 87)

- *bilirubin*—pigment in the bile derived from degenerated hemoglobin of destroyed blood cells. In newborns and particularly in premature and erythroblastic babies the liver is unable to cope with the large amount of bilirubin liberated by destroyed erythrocytes. This results in an excess of bilirubin in the blood. (41, 61, 67)

- bilirubin determinations using cord blood of neonate. (47)

  Reference values:
  serum bilirubin, total—0.2-1.0 mg/dl (SIU: 3.4-17.1 μmol/L)
  Increase in serum bilirubin is seen in physiologic jaundice, hyperbilirubinemia, and kernicterus. The more immature the neonate, the more marked is suspectibility to kernicterus.

  Phototherapy for the neonate is an effective method of lowering unconjugated bilirubin levels by exposing the newborn to fluorescent or other light, according to need. Infants with physiologic jaundice resulting from mildly elevated serum bilirubin benefit by the fluorescent lighting system of the nursery. Infants with hyperbilirubinemia who may develop encephalopathy are exposed to intense fluorescent light therapy in special incubators to reduce their excessive bilirubin. (12, 17, 59, 65, 77)

- *blood group analysis of prospective parents*—study of the parental blood groups in order to detect maternal and paternal grouping differences, predictive of mother-child incompatibilities. Routine procedures include ABO grouping, Rh typing, and screening for irregular antibodies.

- *blood group analyses for exclusion studies*—tests used in medical-legal practice on the basis that parental blood groups are inherited by the child.

  The American Medical Association accepts only the findings of the ABO, MN, and Rh-Hr analyses for legal purposes, except when experts use other systems. Determinations are made to exclude allegation or denial of paternity. To clarify the issue, an example of the MN system of blood typing should be of interest.

Disputed Father	Mother
Type M	Type N

Child

Type N—Genotype NN

Since the child does not have the gene M, the person in question is not the father. (83, 86)

---

*1mμ = 1 millimicron = 0.001 of a micron = 1 nm = 1 nanometer.

- *blood group genetic marker*—inherited characteristic determined by genes located on a pair of chromosomes. Markers are of value in paternity testing. Exclusion of paternity is based on the following:
  - —the child cannot have a genetic marker which is missing in both parents.
  - —the child inherits one of a pair of genetic markers from the mother and father.
  - —the child cannot possess a pair of identical markers (aa) if both parents do not have the marker (a). (86, 87, 88)
- *glucuronyl transferase*—enzyme absent from the liver of premature infants at birth and incompletely developed in full-term newborns. This enzyme lack seems to account for the liver's inability to handle the load imposed by the increased destruction of red cells in the first days of life.
- *Guthrie test*—simple screening test for the detection of phenylketonuria, requiring several drops of blood from the heel of the newborn before the baby is taken home from the hospital.

  Negative test: phenylketonuria is unlikely to develop.
  Positive test: diagnosis to be confirmed by other tests.

  In states where mandatory testing of the neonate for phenylketonuria is done, the Guthrie test is considered legally acceptable. Thus the detection of this hereditary disorder is becoming a legal as well as a professional obligation in medicine. (71)
- *phenylalanine*—essential amino acid present in protein foods. A blocking of its conversion into tyrosine causes phenylalanine blood levels to rise and phenylketone bodies to be excreted in the urine. As a result, brain development ceases. Mental retardation is preventable by early treatment with a low-phenylalanine diet. A serum phenylalanine test measures phenylalanine levels in blood serum. Plasma phenylalanine concentrations are maintained between 3 and 12 mg/dL. In classic phenylketonuria, plasma phenylalanine values are greater than 20 mg/dL. (71)
- *Rh isoimmunization*—sensitization that occurs when red cells containing Rh antigens, not present in the cells of the recipient, enter the circulation. This develops most commonly in Rh-negative women carrying Rh-positive babies or receiving transfusion with Rh-positive blood. It usually occurs during the second Rh-positive pregnancy or subsequent pregnancies. (86)
- *rubella, German measles, in early pregnancy*—relatively mild disease with fever, rash, and lymph node involvement that causes serious deformities in the growing fetus when it occurs during the first trimester. Preventive measures are presented:
  - —*active immunization against rubella*—live virus vaccine prepared in tissue cell culture derived from various sources and given as a single subcutaneous injection to nonpregnant, nonimmune women.
  - —*hemagglutination inhibition (HI) test for rubella*—routine test to be performed within 10 days of exposure to rubella. An antibody titer of 1:10 or above usually indicates the patient is immune and will not develop rubella. An antibody titer below 1:10 suggests that the patient may develop rubella.
  - —*immune serum globulin (ISG)*—prophylactic agent thought to prevent maternal and congenital rubella and rubella-induced congenital malformations. This passive immunization against rubella should be given to pregnant, nonimmune women within 7 or 8 days after exposure.
  - —*postpartum rubella immunization*—procedure performed on nonimmune women during the puerperium to prevent rubella infection in future pregnancies. (23, 31)
- *sickle cell disease screening tests*—screening procedures for sickle cell hemoglobin (HbS)

during the first months of life, preferably at the infant's first checkup. Tests primarily indicated include the tube solubility or microscopic test for HbS and the sickling test, a blood smear to detect sickled cells. (45)

Terms Related to Some Essential Blood Tests

- *acid hemolysis test, Ham test*—test diagnostic for paroxysmal nocturnal hemoglobinuria (PHN), in which lysis of red cells occurs in acidified fresh serum. (46)
- *blood culture*—method of isolating the causative microorganisms in specific infectious diseases by placing blood withdrawn from a vein in a suitable culture media. (21, 24, 77)
- *blood gas determinations*—sensitive indicators of physiologic changes of lung function and tissue perfusion in acute illness. Measurements are obtained from hydrogen, carbon dioxide, and oxygen tensions (pressures) of arterial or venous blood. The "p" refers to partial pressure. (77)

    —*PCO_2*—pressure of tension of carbon dioxide measured in millimeters of mercury.

    Reference values:
    arterial PCO_2—35-50 mm Hg
    venous PCO_2—40-45 mm Hg
    Increase in PCO_2 (hypercarbia): CO_2 retention in respiratory acidosis and metabolic alkalosis.
    Decrease in PCO_2 (hypocarbia): Excessive loss of carbon dioxide in hyperventilation due to respiratory alkalosis or metabolic acidosis. (3, 77, 79)

    —*pH*—hydrogen ion concentration or acidity value of blood (urine).

    Reference values:
    arterial pH—7.38 to 7.44
    venous pH—7.36 to 7.41
    Increase in acidosis.
    Decrease in alkalosis. (3, 77, 79)

    —*PO_2*—pressure or tension of oxygen expressed in millimeters of mercury.

    Reference values:
    arterial PO_2—95 to 100 mm Hg
    Patients with chronic lung disease normally have an arterial PO_2 of 70 mm Hg or less
    Decreased values in arterial PO_2 in advanced lung or heart disease, venous PO_2 due to inadequate blood volume, exchange of gases, cardiac output, and tissue perfusion. (3, 77, 79)

- *continuous transcutaneous blood gas measurement*—noninvasive determination of oxygen tension (PO_2) at the skin surface using a membrane system that permits diffusion of oxygen from the epidermal surface into an electrode chamber. Continuous monitoring of PO_2 is achieved by electronic recording. No blood samples are needed. Carbon dioxide tension (PCO_2) may be measured in a similar way. (77)
- *C-reactive protein antiserum*—nonspecific test for tissue breakdown and disseminated inflammatory conditions. It is often used to follow the clinical course of the disease. Results are usually positive in rheumatic fever and carditis, rheumatoid arthritis, arteriosclerotic heart disease with myocardial infarction, Hodgkin's disease, widespread invasive malignancies, and infections. (28)

Table 31
Characteristic Reference Values of Arterial Blood Gases*

Component	Conventional units	Increase	Decrease
PCO_2	45-50 mm Hg (arterial)	Hypercarbia CO_2 retention in respiratory acidosis and metabolic alkalosis	Hypocarbia CO_2 loss in hyperventilation due to respiratory alkalosis and metabolic acidosis
pH	7.38-7.44 (arterial)	Acidosis	Alkalosis
PO_2	95-100 mm Hg (arterial)	——————	Advanced lung and heart disease

*(3, 77, 79)

- *erythrocyte sedimentation rate (ESR)*—speed with which red blood cells settle when mixed with antiocoagulant. (26)

    Reference values: (method varies)
    ESR (Wintrobe method)
    Males: 0-9 mm/hr
    Females: 0-20 mm/hr
    (SIU: Males: 0-9 mm/hr
            Females: 0-20 mm/hr)
    Increase (marked) in multiple myeloma, macroglobulinemia, polyclonal hyperglobulinemia due to inflammatory disease, and hyperfibrinogenemia.
    Increase (moderate) in rheumatoid arthritis, chronic infections, collagen disease, and neoplastic disease. (17, 26)

- *fibrin-fibrinogen degradation products (FDP)*—protein fragments resulting from the digestive action of plasmin or related enzymes on fibrin or fibrinogen. (48)
- *fibrinogenolysis*—the proteolytic destruction of fibrinogen and other clotting factors in the circulating blood. (48)
- *fibrinolysis*—the destruction of fibrin in blood clots or the dissolution of fibrin due to enzymatic action. (48)
- *FDP detection*—direct latex test (Thrombo-Wellco test) and rapid slide test based on a latex reagent that is sensitized with anti-FDP antibodies. These are capable of detecting degradation products and fibrin in serum and urine. (48)

    Reference values:
    Fibrin degradation products (FDP)
        (Agglutination, Thrombo-Wellco test)
        Whole blood—less than 10 µg/mL (SIU: less than 10 mg/mL)
        Urine—less than 0.25 µg/mL (SIU: less than 10 mg/mL)
    Increased values of serum FDP in thromboembolic disease, with peak level of 400 µg/ml and a drop to normal in about 24 hours; acute myocardial infarction with serum FDP rising 2 to 4 days after the attack. If, after the peak level subsides, a second rise of serum occurs, this signals extension of myocardial infarction or complications. (17, 48)

- *serum iron level*—iron concentration in serum. Iron is normally bound to transferrin.

  Reference values:
  serum iron:
  　　Males: 50-160 μg/dL
  　　Females: 40-150 μg/dL
  　　(SIU: Males—8.95-28.64 μmol/L
  　　　　　　Females—7.16-26.85 μmol/L) (17, 27, 44)

- *total iron-binding capacity (TIBC)*—valuable diagnostic test in anemia and related disorders to determine iron excess or iron deficit. The calculation of percentage saturation of iron provides additional information for differential diagnosis.

  Reference values:
  TIBC serum—250-400 μg/dL
  Iron saturation—20%-55%
  (SIU: TIBC—44.75-71.60 μmol/L
  Fraction of iron saturation—0.20-0.55) (17, 27, 44)

- *transferrin, siderophilin*—an iron-binding glycoprotein primarily synthesized by functional liver cells and referred to as transport iron due to its iron-transferring activity. Transferrin saturated with iron is known as iron-binding capacity (IBC) or total iron-binding capacity (TIBC). (24, 27, 44)

Special Studies Related to Cancer
(See Chapter 18).

Some Terms Related to Tests for Syphilis
(See Chapter 15.)

Biochemistry: Serum, Plasma, Whole Blood

Terms Related to Electrolytes in General

- *anion*—ion carrying a negative electric charge that travels toward the positive pole or anode. (79)
- *anode*—the positive pole or electrode toward which negatively charged ions (anions) or particles are attracted. (79)
- *cathode*—negative pole or electrode toward which positively charged ions (cations) or particles are attracted. (79)
- *cation*—ion carrying positive electric charge that travels toward the negative pole or cathode. (79)
- *electrolyte*—substance that conducts an electric current. (79)
- *electrolyte balance*—particular electrolyte performs its physiologic task, has the appropriate concentration in serum, body fluids, or tissues, and uses the proper channels of entry and exit, thus regulating its serum concentration. (79)
- *electrolyte imbalance*—particular electrolyte in the blood, body fluids, or tissues in too high or too low a concentration, which may adversely affect the body tissues and fluids. (79)
- *ion*—part of an electrolyte, an atom, or number of atoms carrying a positive or negative electric charge. (79)
- *molality*—concentration of a solution expressed in moles per kilogram of pure solvent. (77)

- *molarity*—concentration of a solution expressed in moles per liter of solution. (77)
- *pascal (Pa)*—derived unit of pressure in SIU system expressed in newtons per square meter. (77)
- *valence*—the number of charges on an electrolyte. The valence of the ion must be considered in the relationship of moles and equivalents. For example:
  —*univalent, monovalent ions (Na^+, K^+, Cl^-, HCO_3^-)*—molarity is equivalent.
  —*divalent, bivanet ions (Ca^{++}, Mg^{++}, SO_4^{--})*—these have two equivalents per mole.
  —*trivalent ions (Fe_3^+, Po_4^{3-})*—the relationship is three equivalents per mole. (77)

Terms Related to Specific Electrolytes

- *bicarbonate (HCO_3^-)*—univalent anion that is part of the carbonate-bicarbonate buffering system for the maintenance of the pH (hydrogen ion concentration) and acid-base balance.

  Reference values:

  serum bicarbonate—18-23 mEq/L (SIU: 18-23 nmol/L)

  Increase in metabolic alkalosis resulting from protracted vomiting, gastric suction, hypokalemia, excessive aldosterone, renal artery stenosis, malignant hypertension, Cushing's syndrome, and other causes.

  Increase in respiratory acidosis caused by deficient elimination of carbon dioxide and subsequent rise of PCO_2 as occurs in severe lung emphysema, heart failure, or any other marked interferences with ventilatory function.

  Decrease in metabolic acidosis resulting from prolonged diarrhea, starvation, diabetic ketosis, renal failure, and other causes.

  Decrease in respiratory alkalosis caused by hyperventilation. (3, 17, 67)

- *calcium (Ca^{++})*—divalent calcium cations play an important role in several major physiologic processes, including:
  —ion transfer, cell division, and growth
  —bone mineralization and turnover
  —maintenance or hemostasis and blood coagulation
  —electric excitation of muscular contraction and cellular secretion
  —electric activity of the heart.

  Reference values:

  serum calcium, total—8.4-10.2 mg/dL (SIU: 2.10-2.55 mmol/L)

  urine calcium, 24 hr: 100-300 mg/d (SIU: 2.5-7.5 mmol/d)

  Increase in serum calcium in metastatic bone cancer, multiple myeloma, Paget's disease of bone, hyperparathyroidism, and other diseases.

  Decrease in serum calcium in rickets, hypoparathyroidism, osteomalacia, malabsorption syndrome, and severe pancreatitis with necrosis. (17, 67)

- *chloride (Cl^-)*—important inorganic anion of extracellular fluid that maintains electrolyte and acid-base balance. Chloride retention or ingestion may initiate acidosis, chloride loss, and alkalosis. Sodium chloride aids in the control of osmolarity of body fluids.

  Reference values:

  serum chloride—98-106 mEq/L (SIU: 98-106 mmol/L)

  Increase in serum chloride, or hyperchloremia, in dehydration, overuse of intravenous saline solution, selected cases of hyperventilation, renal disease, and other disorders.

Decrease in serum chloride, or hypochloremia, in chronic diarrhea, protracted vomiting, excessive sweating, renal failure, diabetic ketosis, and other conditions. (17, 67)

- *magnesium (Mg^{++})*—divalent cation occurring in high intracellular concentration and serving as an activating ion to certain enzymes involved in carbohydrate, lipid, and protein metabolism.

  Reference values:
  serum magnesium—1.3-2.1 mEq/L (SIU: 0.65-1.05 mmol/L)
  Increase in magnesium levels may be present in renal failure and excessive magnesium salt treatment.
  Decrease in magnesium levels may occur in prolonged intravenous feeding, alcohol intoxication, hyperaldosteronism, hyperparathyroidism, malabsorption syndromes, diabetic coma, and other states. (13, 17, 77)

- *potassium (K$^+$)*—a univalent, essentially intracellular cation found in platelets and leukocytes. At present determinations of potassium within human cells have *not* been achieved. Plasma or serum potassium measures the extracellular potassium concentration. When muscle weakness and paralysis develop, early potassium disturbance is suspected. It may progress to serious ventricular fibrillation and cardiac arrest, confirmed by electrocardiographic patterns. The ECG (EKG) is of diagnostic importance in the detection of hyperkalemia and hypokalemia.

  Reference values:
  serum potassium—3.5-5.1 mEq/L (SIU: 3.5-5.1 mmol/L)
  plasma potassium—3.5-4.5 mEq/L (SIU: 3.4-4.5 mmol/L)
  Increase in renal failure, adrenal insufficiency, Addison's disease, and excessive potassium ingestion.
  Decrease in starvation, severe diarrhea, protracted vomiting, malabsorption syndromes, metabolic alkalosis, and factors involved in hypokalemia. (17, 77, 79)

- *sodium (Na$^+$)*—univalent ion and major cation in extracellular fluid (ECF). Serum sodium concentration may serve as index of osmotic pressure of extracellular fluid (water) in healthy persons.

  Reference values:
  plasma sodium—136-146 mEq/L (SIU: 136-146 mmol/L)
  Increase in dehydration, disease or trauma of central nervous system, and excess of aldosterone.
  Decrease in low-salt intake; in sodium shift caused by burns or trauma; and with marked sodium loss via digestive tract or from fistula, obstruction, or other conditions. (17, 77)

Terms Primarily Related to Myocardial Enzymes and Isoenzymes

- *enzyme*—catalytic protein that increases biochemical reactions in living cells, may possess marked specificity, and if present in the blood in large amount, usually indicates tissue damage. (77, 98)
- *isoenzyme*—distinct molecular fraction of a certain enzyme found in various tissues and separated by electrophoresis of serum. Of clinical significance are cardiac isoenzymes released into the serum in myocardial injury:

  —*creatine kinase (CK-2) isoenzyme or (CK-MB) formerly creatine phosphokinase (CPK-2)*

or (CPK-MB) isoenzyme—a more specific test for myocardial infarction than the serum enzyme (CK).

—*lactate dehydrogenase isoenzymes (LD-1), (LD-2)*—both fractions prove to be useful indicators of myocardial infarction. LD-3 level is high in lung disease and LD-4 and LD-5 are moderately increased in liver disease. (77, 90)

- *serum enzymes of the heart muscle*, but also present in other organs.

  —*aspartate aminotransferase (AST), glutamate oxaloacetate transaminase (GOT)*—enzyme widely distributed in body tissues but found in its highest concentration in the liver and heart muscle.

  —*creatine kinase (CK), creatine phosphokinase (CPK)*—enzyme released into the blood following injury to the heart muscle or skeletal muscles.

  —*lactate dehydrogenase (LD, LDH)*—enzyme primarily found in the heart muscle, skeletal muscles, liver, and kidney. (77, 90)

- *serum enzyme tests in myocardial infarction (MI)*—determinations based on the principle that high levels of enzyme activity reflect the evolution and extent of damage to the heart muscle. Since the enzymes are also present in other organs, the tests are nonspecific.

  —*serum aspartate aminotransferase (SAST), formerly serum glutamate oxaloacetate transaminase (SGOT)*—valuable diagnostic aid in myocardial infarction.

Reference values:

Serum aspartate aminotransferase (AST, SGOT):

  10-30 UL (SIU: 10-30 UL)

High increase of AST (GOT) serum levels suggest massive heart damage and poor prognosis.

Moderate increase of AST (GOT) serum levels may occur in congestive heart failure with infarcts, tachyarrhythmias, pericarditis, pulmonary infarction, or embolism and liver disease.

No increase of AST (GOT) serum levels may be present in coronary insufficiency and angina pectoris.

Decrease of AST (GOT) may be found in pregnancy. (17, 79, 90)

—*serum creatine kinase (SCK), serum creatine phosphokinase (SCPK)*—determination of serum CK activity, a very useful test due to the early CK rise after myocardial infarction and the absence of the enzyme from the liver and blood.

Reference values:

serum creatine kinase

  Females: 38-174 U/L

  Males: 96-140 U/L

  (SIU: Females: 38-174 U/L

  Males: 96-140 U/L)

Increase in myocardial infarction and acute lung disease. Since CPK appears in skeletal muscle, muscular dystrophy of Duchenne may have to be ruled out. (17, 77, 90)

—*serum lactate dehydrogenase (SLD, SLDH) test*—determination of LD activity in serum, a valuable test because of its late enzyme rise and its prolonged elevation in myocardial infarction. A disadvantage is its lack of specificity, resulting from the enzyme release into red blood cells, liver, lungs, and skeletal muscles.

Reference values:

(method varies)

Serum lactate dehydrogenase (SLDH): 210-420 U/L (SIU: 210-420 U/L)

Increase in myocardial infarction, progressive muscular dystrophy, megaloplastic anemia, and cancer. (17, 77, 90)

Table 32 compares the occurrence of the characteristic rise, maximal peak elevation, and decline to normal levels of the chief enzymes released into the serum after myocardial injury.

Table 32

Serum Enzyme Activity Postmyocardial Infarction

Serum Enzyme	Activity		
	Rise after Onset	Peak	Return to Normal
CK	4-8 hrs.	24-36 hrs.	3-4 days*
AST (GOT)	6-10 hrs.	24-48 hrs.	4-5 days†
LDH	12-48 hrs.	72-144 hrs.	8-14 days*

* Reprinted with permission from Richard C. Pasternak, et al. Acute myocardial infarction. In Eugene Braunwald, et al. eds., *Heart Disease,* 3rd ed., vol. 2. Philadelphia: W.B. Saunders Co., 1988, pp. 1222-1313.
†Reprinted with permission from Regina Daley Ford, ed., *Diagnostic Tests Handbook.* Springhouse, Pennsylvania: Springhouse Corporation, 1987, pp. 134-136.

Terms Related to Other Serum Enzyme Abnormalities

- *serum enzymes primarily concerned with digestion*
    - *amylase (AMS), diastase*—digestive enzyme acting on starches. It is found in the salivary glands, pancreatic juice, liver, and adipose tissue.
    - *amylase isoenzymes*—electrophoretic fractionation of salivary gland and pancreatic amylase, which fall into two general classes: 1) those arising from the pancreas (P isoamylases), and 2) those arising from nonpancreatic sources (S isoamylases).
    - *amylase (AMS) determination*—test of diagnostic value in pancreatic disorders.

Reference values: (varies with method)

Method of Somogyi: serum amylase—60-160 units/dl (SIU: 111-296 U/L)

Increase usually in acute pancreatitis, chronic recurrent pancreatitis, carcinoma of the head of the pancreas, and renal failure.

Decrease in chronic hepatic disease and in starvation. (22, 63, 77, 79)

- *serum gamma glutamyl transferase (GGT)*—digestive enzyme probably involved in protein synthesis. It is found in kidney, lung, and prostate and in high concentration in the liver. GGT is an exquisitely sensitive indicator of hepatic disease and valuable in the detection of alcoholic liver disease and in monitoring alcoholics who are involved in an abstention program.

Reference values: (varies with method)

Serum gamma glutamyl transferase (GGT)

Males: 9-50 U/L

Females: 8-40 U/L

(SIU: Males: 9-50 U/L

Females: 8-40 U/L)

Increase in chronic hepatitis, obstructive hepatic disease, alcoholic cirrhosis of the liver, and hepatobiliary and pancreatic malignancies. (17, 77, 79)

—*serum leucine aminopeptidase (SLAP) determination*—measurement of LAP, a protein-splitting enzyme in the blood.

Reference values:

SLAP at 30°C—14-40 mIU/ml (SIU: 14-40 units L)

Increase in most types of liver disease but values are highest in biliary obstruction. Serum leucine aminopeptidase is sensitive in detecting obstructive infiltrative space-occupying lesions of the liver. (29, 77)

—*serum lipase (SLPS)*—measurement of a lipase, a lipolytic (fat-splitting) enzyme in the blood.

Reference values:

Method of Cherry-Crondall: serum lipase—0-1.5 units (SIU: 0-1.5 units)

Increase in serum lipase activity in mumps, indicative of marked salivary gland and pancreatic involvement. (17, 22)

■ *serum glycolytic enzymes*—chiefly enzymes that catalyze the breakdown of glycogen to glucose in serum. Glycolytic enzymes are present in many tissues, and some are of diagnostic importance.

   —*serum aldolase (SALS)*—highly sensitive glycolytic enzyme.

Reference values:

serum aldolase—1.5-12.0 U/L (SIU: 1.5-12.0 U/L)

Increase in muscle disease, hepatic necrosis, megaloblastic anemia, neoplastic disease, myocardial infarction, and pulmonary infarction. (17)

   —*serum phosphohexoisomerase (SPHI)*—increasing serum levels of this glycolytic enzyme reflect metastases, especially in patients with cancer of the prostate and breast.

   —*serum pyruvate kinase (SPK)*—abnormally low glycolytic enzyme activity in red cells causes PK deficiency, a chronic hemolytic anemia. (77)

■ *serum hemic enzymes*—enzymes of the formed elements of the blood; the abnormality is acquired or genetic.

   —*serum alanine aminotransferase (SALT)*—an acquired red cell defect of ALT is present in pyridoxine deficiency.

   —*serum alkaline phosphatase (SALP)*—acquired white cell defect of ALP occurs in granulocytic leukemia.

   —*serum catalase*—genetic red cell deficiency of catalase is found in acatalasia, in which the oral tissues become ulcerated and gangrenous. (77)

   —*serum phosphorylase, hepatophosphorylase*—genetic white cell defect of this enzyme is present in glycogenosis type 4, one of the glycogen storage diseases. Measurement of the activity of phosphorylase of leukocytes confirms hepatophosphorylase deficiency.

■ *serum glucose-6-phosphate dehydrogenase (G-6-PD)*—deficiency of G-6-PD results in a mild or severe form of hemolytic anemia, which may be drug induced. If enzyme levels depress both erythrocytes and leukocytes, the disease is more serious. (41)

■ *serum phosphatases*—these enzymes are widely distributed throughout the body. The action of their isoenzymes has not been defined.

*—serum acid phosphatase (SACP) measurement—*concentration of ACP in the prostate, red cells, platelets, spleen, liver, and kidney, as reflected in the serum.

Reference values:

Method of King-Armstrong: SACP—1-5 units (SIU: 1-5 units)

Increase in metastatic cancer of the prostate, particularly if the lesion has extended beyond the capsule of the prostate gland. SACP may also be elevated in Gaucher's disease, bone malignancy, and liver and kidney disease. (41, 77, 79)

*—serum alkaline phosphatase (SALP) measurement—*enzyme first noted for its high concentration in osteoblastic bone disease, since osteoblasts are rich in phosphatase. The present emphasis is on SALP levels in hepatobiliary disease.

Reference values:

Method of King-Armstrong: SALP—5-13 units (SIU: 5-13 units)

Increase is usually present in hepatic jaundice, posthepatic obstruction caused by gallstones or tumor, congenital atresia of intrahepatic bile ducts, biliary cirrhosis, metastases of prostatic carcinoma to bone, bone growth and repair, bone injury, Paget's disease of the bone, and other disorders. (22, 77, 79)

Biochemistry: Hormones and Metabolism

Terms Primarily Related to Endocrine Function Studies

- *adrenal hormones:*
  - *—adrenal cortex—*outer portion of adrenal gland. The cortex produces hormones, including three major groups:
    - –steroids controlling the salt and water metabolism, such as aldosterone.
    - –steroids regulating the glucose metabolism and promoting gluconeogenesis, such as hydrocortisone.
    - –steroids affecting androgenic activity, such as androsterone.
  - *—adrenal medulla—*inner portion of adrenal gland; which secretes adrenalin (epinephrine) and noradrenalin (norepinephrine).
  - *—aldosterone—*potent salt-retaining hormone of adrenal cortex that affects electrolyte balance.
  - *—aldosterone in urine—*quantitative measurement of aldosterone excreted in urine.

Reference values:

urinary aldosterone level—3-20 µg/24 hr (SIU: 8.3-55 nmol/24 hr)

Increase in primary and secondary aldosteronism, nephrosis with edema, congestive heart failure with edema, hepatic cirrhosis with ascites, and in the second and third trimesters of normal pregnancy. (77, 78, 79)

*—catecholamines in urine—*determination of excretion of epinephrine, norepinephrine, total free catecholamines, and metanephrines.

Reference values:

epinephrine—10 µg/24 hr (SIU less than 55 nmol/24 hr)

norepinephrine—less than 100 µg/24 hr (SIU: less than 590 nmol/24 hr)

total free catecholamines—4 to 126 µg/24 hr (SIU: 24-745 nmol/24 hr)

total metanephrines—0.1 to 1.6 mg/24 hr (SIU: 0.5-8.1 µmol/24 hr)

Increase in pheochromocytoma, neuroblastoma (30%) (77, 78, 79)

—*corticosteroids*—steroid hormones secreted by the adrenal cortex.

—*corticotropin, adrenocorticotropic hormone (ACTH)*—hormone of the hypothalamus under the negative feedback control of cortisol. ACTH and cortisol plasma levels are increased in the morning and low at night.

Reference values:

plasma ACTH—0800 hr: 25-100 pg/mL (SIU: 25-100 ng/L)

          —1800 hr: less than 50 pg/mL (SIU: less than 50 ng/L)

plasma cortisol—0800 hr: 5-23 µg/dl (SIU: 138-635 nmol/L)

          —1600 hr: 3-15 µg/dl (SIU: 82-413 nmol/L) (17, 77, 78, 79)

—*17-hydrocorticosteroids*—hormones regulating gluconeogenesis, the production of sugar from protein.

Reference values: 17-OH corticosteroids, 17-OH-CS, glucocorticoids

men—3.9 mg/24 hr (SIU: 8.3-25 µmol/24 hr)

women—2-8 mg/24 hr (SIU: 5.5-22 µmol/24 hr)

Increase usually in Cushing's syndrome, marked stress, acute pancreatitis, and eclampsia.

Decrease in hypopituitarism and Addison's disease. (77, 78, 79)

■ *anterior pituitary hormones:*

—*follitropin, follicle-stimulating hormone (FSH)*—a glycopeptide hormone of the anterior pituitary that, together with the luteinizing hormone (LH), promotes the development and function of the sex organs. In the female, FSH stimulates the ripening of the ovarian follicle and thus prepares for ovulation; in the male, FSH stimulates the maturation of the sperm.

Reference values:

serum FSH (radioimmunoassay [RIA])

men—4-24 mIU/ml

women—4-30 mIU/ml

    midcycle—two times baseline

    postmenopause—40-250 mIU/ml

Increase of FSH in primary gonadal failure, ovarian or testicular agenesis, castration, seminiferous tubule failure, Klinefelter's syndrome, and other disorders.

Decrease of FSH in children before puberty; panhypopituitarism; anorexia nervosa; estrogen or androgen-secreting neoplasms of the adrenals, ovaries, or testes; and other conditions. (20, 77, 79)

—*lutropin, luteinizing hormone (LH)*—potent hormone of the anterior pituitary. It exerts multiple effects on its target organ, the ovary; brings about follicular maturation, rupture of the follicle, and release of the mature ovum; develops the corpus luteum and progesterone; and stimulates estrogenic secretions. In the male it is primarily concerned with testosterone production and in conjunction with FSH promotes the maturation of sperms in the seminiferous tubules.

Reference values:

serum LH (RIA)

men—7-24 mIU/ml

women—6-30 mIU/ml

    midcycle peak—greater than three times baseline

    postmenopause—greater than 30

Increase in primary gonadal dysfunction in men and in women with amenorrhea, if caused by ovarian failure. (77, 78, 79)

—*prolactin (HPRL)*—pituitary hormone that initiates and maintains lactation. (20, 77)

- *placental hormones and related tests:*
  —*human choriogonadotropin (HCG), human chorionic gonadotropin*—glycopeptide secreted by the placenta during gestation. In one or two weeks after the implantation of the fertilized ovum, HCG is found in both blood and urine. Its rapidly rising levels reach a peak at 8 to 12 weeks of pregnancy, which is followed by a decline. After delivery, HCG becomes undetectable within two or three days.

  Reference values: (RIA)
  serum chorionic gonadotropin—less than 3 mIU/ml
  urine chorionic gonadotropin—less than 30 mIU/ml. (20, 77, 79)

  —*immunologic pregnancy tests, immunoassays for pregnancy*—sensitive tests for human chorionic gonadotropin (HCG) in serum and urine. Excess HCG is present in pregnancy. Techniques are simple, and results are read in two hours or less. The tests are designed for office use. Immunologic tests, however, also yield positive results in choriocarcinoma and hydatidiform moles. In menopause elevated pituitary gonadotropin may product a false-positive test.

  The following commercial immunologic pregnancy tests are in current use:
  —*Gravindex 90*—slide test for pregnancy
  —*Neocept*—hemagglutination inhibition test
  —*Pregnosis*—slide test for pregnancy
  —*Sensi-Tex*—latex agglutination inhibition tube test for pregnancy (13, 77, 79)
  —*human placental lactogen (HPL)*—this hormone has been isolated in considerable amounts from human placentas at term. It maintains the pregnancy and initiates lactation. The HPL concentration of maternal serum is a sensitive indicator of placental function and invaluable in monitoring high-risk pregnancies. The higher the blood pressure of hypertensive toxemia patients, the lower their placental lactogen.

  Reference values: serum HPL (RIA)
  men—less than 0.5 μg/ml*
  nonpregnant women—less than 0.5 μg/ml
  pregnant women (weeks of pregnancy on left)
     5-27—less than 4.6 μg/ml
     28-31—2.4-6.1 μg/ml
     32-35—3.7-7.7 μg/ml
     36-term—5.0-8.6 μg/ml
  Increase or normal urinary HPL and decrease of serum HPL after eight weeks of menstrual cessation suggest the growth of a hydatidiform mole. (20, 77, 79)

- *steroid hormone*—chemically interrelated organic compounds possessing a four-ring carbon structure.

---

*μg same as mcg (microgram)

—*androgenic hormones*—biologic substances that stimulate secondary sex characteristics in the male.

—*17-ketosteroids (17-KS) in urine*—in men measurement of the adrenocortical steroids and adrenal and gonadal androgens; in women and children primarily measurement of adrenal gland secretion. The level of the 17-KS in urine aids in the detection of endocrine disorders.

Reference values:
17-KS excretion (significant daily variation in urine secretion)
   men—6-18 mg/24 hr (SIU: 21-62 μmol/24 hr)
   women—4-13 mg/24 hr (SIU: 14-45 μmol/24 hr)
Increase in adrenocortical tumor, especially if malignant, interstitial neoplasm of testes, adrenogenital syndrome, and occasionally Cushing's disease.
Decrease in Addison's disease and myxedema. (14, 77, 78, 79)

—*testosterone*—steroid hormone and very potent androgen.

Reference values:
plasma testosterone
men—275-875 ng/dl (SIU: 9.5-30 nmol/l)
women—23-75 ng/dl (SIU: 0.8-2.6 nmol/l)
Increase in adrenal hyperplasia or tumor, polycystic ovaries, and ovarian tumors.
Decrease in estrogen therapy, hypogonadism, hypopituitarism, Klinefelter's syndrome, and orchidectomy. (77, 79)

—*estrogenic hormones*—internal secretions of the gonads, adrenal glands, and placenta that prepare the uterus and tubes for progesterone stimulation.

—*clomiphene*—antiestrogen used in diagnosis and therapy to detect anovulation and initiate a normal menstrual cycle, thus making pregnancy possible.

—*estriol (E$_3$)*—estrogenic hormone, synthesized in the placenta and highly elevated in pregnancy. Determinations of estriol are of clinical significance, since they reflect the status of the fetoplacental complex and may serve as treatment guides in a high-risk pregnancy. A marked decline in pregnancy estriol during the second or third trimester signals placental insufficiency and impending fetal death.

—*total estrogens*—these include (E$_1$), estradiol (E$_2$), and estriol (E$_3$). They are measured to evaluate ovarian function. Estrogen excretion in urine is variable, with low levels at the menstrual period and peak levels at the midperiod of the cycle.

Reference values:
total estrogens:
—serum—men—40-115 pg/mL (SIU: 40-115 ng/L)
      —female cycle:
1-10 days 61-394 pg/mL (SIU: 61-394 ng/L)
11-20 days 122-437 pg/mL (SIU: 122-437 ng/L)
21-30 days 156-350 pg/mL (SIU: 156-350 ng/L)
prepubertal and postmenopausal 40 pg/mL (SIU: 40 ng/L)
—urine—men—5-25 μg/24 hr (SIU: 15-90 nmol/24 hr)
      —women—5-100 μg/24 hr (SIU: 18-360 nmol/24 hr)
Increase in pregnancy, ovarian tumors, testicular atrophy, and testicular tumors.
Decrease due to absence of ovulation, ovarian hormones, and corpus luteum function; amenorrhea, sterility; and other conditions. (17, 77)

■ *progestational hormones:*

—*progesterone*—steroid hormone formed by the corpus luteum and rapidly metabolized to pregnanediol; consequently there is little progesterone in the blood. Plasma progesterone determinations aid in the detection of ovulatory and luteal deficiencies and hormonal imbalance in pregnancy.

—*pregnanediol*—hormone produced in the liver by progesterone metabolism and excreted in urine.

Reference values:
(method varies)
—men—0.6-1.5 mg/d (SIU: 1.9-4.7 μmol/d)
—female cycle:
   follicular less than 1.0 mg/d (SIU: less than 3.1 μmol/d)
   luteal 2-7 mg/d (SIU: 6.2-22 μmol/d)
   postmenopausal 0.2-1.0 mg/d (SIU: 0.6-3.1 μmol/d)

After delivery, pregnanediol excretion returns gradually to nonpregnant levels. (17)

Terms Primarily Related to Metabolic Studies

■ *basal metabolic rate (BMR)*—measurement of the number of calories needed for the support of basic metabolic functions, such as respiration, circulation, and body temperature, in a resting person. The normal range is from −10 to +10 percent. (79)

■ *blood sugar level*—concentration of glucose in the blood. (57)

■ *calcitonin*—calcium-reducing hormone derived from thyroid, parathyroids, and sometimes the thymus. It affects calcium metabolism and regulates plasma calcium levels and bone remodeling. Calcitonin secretion is excessive in medullary carcinoma of the thyroid.

■ *carbohydrate tolerance tests:* (77)

—*glucose tolerance tests*—the intravenous or oral administration of a measured glucose load to discover disorders of the carbohydrate metabolism.

Reference values:
glucose tolerance test, oral

Serum	conventional units	
	Normal	Diabetic
Fasting:	70-105 mg/dL	>140 mg/dL
60 min:	120-170 mg/dL	≥200 mg/dL
90 min:	100-140 mg/dL	≥200 mg/dL
120 min:	70-120 mg/dL	≥140 mg/dL

Serum	international units (SIU)	
	Normal	Diabetic
Fasting:	3.9-5.8 mmol/L	> 7.8 mmol/L
60 min:	6.7-9.4 mmol/L	≥11 mmol/L
90 min:	5.6-7.8 mmol/L	≥11 mmol/L
120 min:	3.9-6.7 mmol/L	≥ 7.8 mmol/L

(17)

—*postprandial blood sugar determination*—screening procedure for the detection of diabetes mellitus. Blood to determine sugar content is drawn two hours after the patient started to eat a meal containing 50 to 100 grams of carbohydrates.

Reference values:

2 hr. postprandial glucose serum—less than 120 mg/dL (SIU: less than 6.7 mmol/L) (17, 57)

■ *carbon dioxide combining power*—test for determining the acid-base balance in the blood. In health and with normal activity, the acid waste products of metabolism exceed the basic levels.

Reference values:

Carbon dioxide, total (TCO$_2$)
   serum or plasma—23-29 mEq/L (SIU: 23-29 mmol/L) (3, 17)
Carbon dioxide content in serum:
   Adults: *Increase* in alkalosis, hypercorticoadrenalism, and excessive alkali therapy.
         Decrease in acidosis, diabetes, nephritis, and eclampsia.
   Infants: *Increase* in respiratory conditions.
         Decrease in severe diarrhea. (77, 79, 81)

■ *glucagon*—polypeptide hormone secreted by the alpha-cells of the pancreatic islets.
■ *glucose tolerance*—the more sugar a healthy person takes, the more is utilized. The reverse is true in the diabetic person.
■ *insulin antibody, anti-insulin Ab*—immunoglobin that may be present in diabetic persons receiving insulin and may account for allergic reactions and insulin resistance. (77, 81)
■ *insulin resistance*—tolerance to high daily dosage (200 units) due to obesity or to the development of antibodies that bind insulin. (77, 81)
■ *insulin secretion radioimmunoassay*—test determines insulin secretion response to glucose. Reference values are increased in insulinoma, acromegaly, and Cushing's syndrome. (77, 81)
■ *ketone bodies*—acetone bodies, products of faulty metabolism in diabetic acidosis. Since sugar is not utilized normally in diabetes mellitus, excessive fat is mobilized and employed in energy production. Other clinical states characterized by faulty fat metabolism that result in ketoacidosis are starvation, prolonged diarrhea and vomiting, and von Gierke's disease. In ketoacidosis ketone bodies accumulate in the blood (ketonemia) and are excreted in the urine (ketonuria).

Reference values: no ketone bodies in blood and urine
Ketoacidosis
      serum ketone test (serum acetone test)—greater than 2.0 mg/dl.
      urine ketone test (Acetest or Ketostix)—purple color reaction with diabetic acid 5-10 mg/dl. (3, 57, 77, 79)

■ *lactic acidosis*—excess lactic acid in the blood due to its inadequate removal in circulatory, respiratory, renal, and hepatic failure; septic shock; and terminal cancer. Its clinical manifestations are hyperventilation and mental confusion followed by coma and collapse. (3)
■ *lipids*—group of organic substances, mostly composed of carbon, hydrogen, and some oxygen; they may also contain nitrogen and phosphorus. Lipids are soluble in hydrocarbon and ether and insoluble in water.

Reference values: serum lipids
total lipids—450-1000 mg/dL
   (SIU: 4.5-10 g/l)
cholesterol—150-265 mg/dL
   (SIU: 3.9-6.85 mmol/L)
triglycerides—10-190 mg/dL
   (SIU: 1.09-20.71 mmol/L)
phospholipids—150-380 mg/dL
   (SIU: 1.50-3.80 g/L)
fatty acids (free) 9.0-15.0 mM/l
   (SIU: 9.0-15.0 mmol/L)
phospholipid phosphorus—8.0-11.0 mg/dL
   (SIU: 2.85-3.55 mmol/L) (17, 21, 30)

- *lipoproteins*—lipids and proteins combined. Lipids alone cannot enter the circulation, but lipoproteins can be transported by the bloodstream.
    - —*alpha lipoproteins*—tiny particles containing large amount of protein; do not predispose to atherosclerosis.
    - —*beta lipoproteins*—tiny particles with high cholesterol content, predisposing to atherosclerosis.
    - —*pre-beta lipoproteins*—particles are relatively large and appear to be active in the transport of triglycerides.
    - —*chylomicrons*—large particles present in serum during digestion of fat-containing foods. Chylomicrons undergo rapid metabolic transformations and are cleared from circulation within a few minutes and therefore are not detected in fasting plasma. (1, 30)
- *metabolite*—any product of metabolism; for example, the mineral metabolites: sodium, potassium, and chloride, which are profoundly influenced by the activity of the adrenal cortex.
    - —*chloride salts*—chiefly bound to sodium. In the gastric juice chlorides are present in the form of hydrochloride.

Reference values:
plasma chloride—98-106 mEq/L (SIU: 98-106 mmol/L)
Increase in many conditions resulting from decreased excretion or increased intake. (3, 17)

    —*potassium salts: as potassium chloride, phosphates, and bicarbonates*—found within tissue cells, especially in muscle cells and blood plasma.

Reference values:
plasma potassium—3.5-4.5 mEq/L (SIU: 3.5-4.5 mmol/L)
Increase in Addison's disease.
Decrease in Cushing's syndrome. (3, 17)

    —*sodium salts, as sodium chloride and sodium bicarbonate*—present in the blood plasma and extracellular fluids.

Reference values:
plasma sodium—136-146 mEq/L (SIU: 136-146 mmol/L)
Increase in Cushing's syndrome.
Decrease in Addison's disease. (3, 17)

- *osmolality*—solute concentration per unit of water, usually expressed in milliosomols per liter of a solution (mOsm/L).

    Reference values:
    serum osmolality—275-295 mOsmol/kg (SIU: 275-295 mOsmol/kg) (3, 17)

- *phenotype*—the external expression of the genetic constitution of an organism. (77)
- *transferrin*—glycoprotein that transports iron in plasma. (77)
- *triglycerides*—simple or neutral fats composed of three molecules of fatty acid that are esterified to glycerin. (1, 67)

Urine Findings and Renal Function

Terms Related to Urine Findings

- *urinalysis*—examination of physical and chemical properties of urine. Physical properties comprise quantity, color, specific gravity, odor, and other qualities. Chemical properties are concerned with quantitative or qualitative tests dealing with protein, glucose, bile pigments, ketone bodies, blood, calculi, and similar substances. In conditions of the urinary sysem albumin and casts are frequently present, and the pH concentration is altered.

    —*albumin, protein*—abnormal constituent of urine in renal and febrile diseases and toxemias of pregnancy. It is caused by increased permeability of the glomerular filter.

    —*Bence-Jones protein*—peculiar type of protein molecule that is excreted in the urine in the majority of cases of multiple myeloma (plasma cell myeloma), amyloidosis and in certain bone tumors.

    —*calcium in urine (and feces)*—these tests are concerned with the calcium balance in the body. In health the calcium intake exceeds the calcium excretion in urine and feces.

    —*casts*—cells abnormally formed in the renal tubules and shed in the urine as hyaline, granular, epithelial, blood, and pus casts.

    —*hydrogen ion concentration* (chemical symbol: pH)—the reaction of the urine.

    –*pH concentration of 7*—normal neutrality

    –*pH concentration less than 7*—acid in reaction

    –*pH concentration greater than 7*—alkaline in reaction.

    In acidosis the urine is strongly acid; in chronic cystitis and in urinary retention the urine is usually alkaline in reaction. (2, 13, 16, 35, 77)

    —*porphyrins (corproporphyrin, uroporphyrin, porphobilinogen)*—pigments resembling bilirubin and apparently derived from the hemoglobin of the blood. Minute amounts of porphyrins are normally present in the urine. An increase is abnormal.

    —*corproporphyrin urinary excretion*—a valuable test in the detection of lead poisoning, acute porphyria, pellagra, and liver damage.

    —*uroporphyrin urinary excretion*—diagnostic aid in acute porphyria and acute intermittent porphyria. (8, 44)

- *Sulkowitch test*—approximate estimate of amount of calcium in urine. Calcium excretion is increased in hypercalciuria, hyperthyroidism, and urinary calcium calculi. Calcium excretion is decreased in hypocalciuria and hypoparathyroidism. (18, 77)

- *urinary calculi*—stones found in the pelvis of the kidney, ureter, and bladder in the forms of:

—*crystine stones*—white or pale yellow granules.
—*oxalate stones (calcium oxalate)*—crystalline structure.
—*phosphate and carbonate stones*—compact balls.
—*uric acid stones*—smooth, round pebbles. (58)

Terms Related to Proprietary Urine Tests

- *Clinistix, Clinitest*—reagent strip or tablet for testing glucose in urine. (30)
- *Combistix*—three separate reagent areas: pH, protein, and glucose in urine, providing information on acid-base balance, renal function, and carbohydrate metabolism. (16)
- *Keto-Diastix*—reagent strip for detecting glucose and ketones in urine. (30)
- *Ketostix*—reagent strip for checking ketones in urine, serum, and plasma. (30)

Terms Related to Renal Function Studies

- *blood urea nitrogen (BUN)*—renal function test that measures the concentration of urea in the blood. In health the blood levels are low, since urea, an end product of protein metabolism, is freely excreted in the urine. In renal impairment and failure, urea nitrogen accumulates in the blood, and the patient may lapse into coma.

  References values:
  BUN—8 to 18 mg of urea nitrogen per 100 ml of blood.
  Increase in nephritis, urinary obstruction, and uremia.
  Decrease in amyloidosis, nephrosis, and pregnancy. (16, 65, 77)

- *concentration and dilution test*—measures the functional capacity of the kidney to concentrate and dilute urine. Failure to concentrate urine indicates kidney damage. It may be partially caused by a faulty mechanism of the antidiuretic hormone (ADH) released from the pituitary gland.

  Reference values:
  creatinine, urine, 24 hr—men—14-26 mg/kg/d
               —women—11-20 mg/kg/d
     (SIU: men—124-230 μmol/kg/d
           women—97-177 μmol/kg/d (16, 17, 77, 79)

- *endogenous creatinine clearance*—renal function test that measures the removal of creatinine from plasma, as reflected by the glomerular filtration rate (GFR). (35, 54)
- *Howard test; excretion of water, salt, and creatinine*—renal function study to detect ischemia of the kidney caused by stenosis of the renal artery or its branch or by chronic pyelonephritis with arteriolar involvement. A low-urine volume and a low-sodium and high-creatinine concentration are positive findings and indicate that the patient may benefit by renovascular surgery.
- *phenolsulfonphthalein (PSP)*—dye test for detection of kidney impairment. About 90 percent of the PSP is eliminated through the renal tubules and only 10 percent through glomerular infiltration.

  Reference values: PSP
  first hour—40%-50%
  second hour—20%-25%
  A low urinary excretion of the dye of 40 percent or less in two hours is usually associated with nitrogen retention in the blood. Elimination of the dye is delayed in hypertrophy of the prostate gland complicated by hydronephrosis, malignant hypertension, and cystitis with urinary retention. (12, 77, 79)

- *plasma renin activity (PRA)*—bioassay method of Gunnels measuring the enzyme activity of renin to screen patients for renovascular hypertension or malignant hypertension. (78)
- *renin*—enzyme originating in the glomerulus. Renin levels rise with lowered perfusion pressure and lowered delivery of water and sodium to the glomerulus. High levels of renin formed by the diseased kidney may lead to renal hypertension and primary aldosteronism. (78)
- *Stamey test, sodium chloride—urea—ADH—PAH—(para-aminohypuric acid) test*—demonstrates the abnormally increased water reabsorption by the renal tubules in kidney ischemia, resulting in decreased urinary output and increased PAH concentration. (77)
- *urea clearance*—test measures the glomerular function of the kidney to remove urea from the blood. It is calculated as plasma cleared of urea in one minute. (35)

Gastrointestinal and Hepatobiliary Tracts and Pancreas

Terms Related to Tests of the Digestive System

- *gastric analysis and related tests:*
    - —*augmented histalog test*—procedure in which the histalog dose has been calculated according to body weight to induce maximal gastric acid secretion. If no acid is released, anacidity is present.
    - —*augmented histamine test*—an optional histamine dose is used to evoke a maximal gastric acid response, thus providing quantitative measurement of the secretory capacity of the stomach.
      NOTE: To avoid the undesirable side effects of histamine, the augmented histamine test may be replaced by the pentagastrin test, which results in a similar magnitude of acid output with considerably fewer side effects. Pentagastrin is a synthetic pentapeptide derivative that contains four C-terminal amino acids of gastrin linked to substituted alanine. Pentagastrin retains a good portion of the biologic activity of gastrin and serves as a potent stimulus to the secretion of acid pepsin and the intrinsic factor of the stomach. Pentagastrin stimulates secretion of both bicarbonate and enzymes by the pancreas, as well as stimulating relaxation of the sphincter of Oddi and gallbladder contraction. (66, 77)
    - —*basal acid output (BAO)*—quantitative measurement of gastric acid secretion under basal conditions that is without histamine or Histalog stimulation. (64, 66)
    - —*maximal acid output (MAO)*—quantitative measurement of gastric acid secretion after stimulation with an augmented dose of histamine or Histalog. (64, 66)
    - —*gastric analysis (tube)*—aspiration of gastric contents for the purpose of determining the secretory ability and motility of the stomach.
- *gastric exfoliative cytology*—valuable method for detecting gastric malignancy by studying cells shed by the mucosa and obtained by aspiration, lavage, or abrasive brushes following the liquefaction of the mucosal coating. (77)
- *gastric juice*—composite of water, hydrochloric acid, electrolytes, enzymes, blood group components, and the intrinsic factor of Castle. (64)

- *gastrin*—hormone formed by cells of the antral mucosa of the stomach and carried by the blood to the gastric fundus, stimulating the release of hydrochloric acid and evoking the secretion of pepsin, pancreatic enzymes, and the intrinsic factor of Castle. (64)
- *gastrin secretory test*—use of a purified gastrin preparation in gastric secretory studies analogous to those of histamine and Histalog. (60)
- *guaiac test*—test for occult blood in feces (also in urine).

  > Reference values:
  > guaiac test:
  > *negative reaction*—no blood, no greenish to blue color.
  > *positive reaction*—blood present, greenish to blue color.

- *Hemoccult test*—test for occult blood in feces that can be done at home. Test depends on the presence of peroxidase activity of the heme in the sample. Usually two small fecal specimens are applied to prepared slides from three consecutive bowel movements. Bleeding from the upper gastrointestinal tract and oral doses of vitamin C diminish the sensitivity of the test.

  > Reference values:
  > *Hemoccult test:*
  > *negative reaction*—no blood, no bluish color present.
  > *positive reaction*—blood present, bluish color present.

  Ulcerated carcinomas of the colon or stomach usually yield a positive reaction with use of the guaiac or Hemoccult tests. (32, 77)

- *histamine*—powerful stimulant to gastric secretion used clinically in gastric function tests. (64)
- *Hollander insulin hypoglycemia test*—use of insulin-induced hypoglycemia to evaluate the outcome of vagotomy. Positive results, a few months after surgery, may indicate that vagal nerve fibers are regenerating or that the vagotomy was incomplete. The Hollander test is no longer recommended because of the reported hypoglycemic seizures, strokes, and myocardial infarctions that are associated with it. The sham feeding test is employed for establishing the diagnosis of incomplete vagotomy. The contents of a meal are chewed but not swallowed. Acid output is determined during the test by aspirating gastric secretions through a nasogastric tube. If the acid output caused by the sham feeding is greater than 10 percent of the pentagastrin-stimulated peak acid output, this implies that the vagal innervation of the stomach is intact. (75, 77, 81)
- *intestinal absorption test, urinary D-xylose test*—test that distinguishes between malabsorption due to small intestinal disease and that due to pancreatic exocrine insufficiency. Decreased urinary D-xylose values are seen in ascites. The urinary D-xylose test helps to differentiate whether steatorrhea is secondary to pancreatic disease or to small bowel disease. (76, 77, 79)
- *pepsin, protease*—digestive enzyme present in gastric juice and capable of converting proteins into peptones and proteoses. (64)
- *proteolytic*—protein-splitting.
- *secretin*—hormone produced by the duodenal mucosa and acting as a potent stimulus to the release of pancreatic secretions. (64)
- *secretin test (Dreiling and Hollander)*—the intravenous injection of secretin following the removal of the duodenal contents. The secretin stimulates pancreatic secretions,

which enter the duodenum and are removed. The study of the duodenal aspirate, which includes volume of output, amylase activity, and content of bicarbonate, bile, and proteolytic enzymes, aids in the diagnostic evaluation of pancreatic and biliary disorders. (76)

■ *serum alpha-fetoprotein (SAFP)*—useful test for the detection of hepatic cancer, despite its nonspecificity.

■ *stool examination*—macroscopic and microscopic studies, chemical analysis, and examinations for parasites and protozoa; used as diagnostic aids, especially for detecting diseases of the digestive tract. (35, 37)

■ *sweat test, Gibson-Cooke technique*—sweat electrolytes by pilocarpine iontophoresis into the skin to stimulate an increased secretion of the sweat glands. The laboratory diagnosis is based on the abnormally high content of sodium chloride (NaCl) in sweat. (46, 51)

> Reference values:
> *sodium chloride concentration*—greater than 60 mEq per liter. Increased sodium and chloride concentration in sweat, exceeding 60 mEq per liter in children and 70 mEq per liter in adults is indicative of cystic fibrosis. (17, 51)

Terms Related to Liver Function

■ *aminotransferases (formerly called transferases)*—enzymes that catalyze the transfer of biochemical substances. They are sensitive indicators of liver cell injury and other hepatocellular diseases such as hepatitis. They include:

  —*serum alanine aminotransferase* (SALT) or serum glutamate pyruvic transaminase (SGPT)

> Reference values:
> SALT or SGPT (at 30°C)—8-50 U/ml (SIU: 4-24 U/L)
> *Increase* in hepatitis, hepatic cirrhosis, metastatic cancer, obstructive jaundice, and other disorders. (29, 77, 79)

  —*serum aspartate aminotransferase* (SAST) or serum glutamate oxaloacetate transaminase (SGOT).

> Reference values:
> SAST or SGOT (at 30°C)—16-60 U/ml (SIU: 8-33 U/L)
> *Increase* in hepatitis, cirrhosis of liver, obstructive jaundice, myocardial infarction, and other disorders. (29, 55, 77, 79)

  —*serum gamma glutamyl transferase* (SGGT) or *serum gamma glutamyl transpeptidase* (SGGTP).

> Reference values:
> SGGT or SGGTP (at 37°C)—5-40 IU/1 (SIU: 5-40 U/I)
> *Increase* in hepatitis, obstructive jaundice, hepatic cirrhosis, alcoholic hepatitis, certain malignancies of liver and pancreas. (29, 55, 77, 79)

■ *liver function tests*—are of great importance not only in discovering the severity of hepatic disease, but also in determining the amount of liver damage caused by pathologic conditions of the gall bladder and pancreas. (29, 55)

(See Table 33.)

Table 33
Liver Function Tests

Hepatic Function	Tests	Comments
Excretory function, chiefly related to bile pigments	Bromsulphalein (BSP) (29) Retention of dye indicative of liver damage, metastatic carcinoma of liver, and others	Most sensitive test of liver function, but use discontinued because of reactions
Detoxification and excretion	Serum bilirubin (7, 29) Increase in hepatogenous jaundice, obstructive jaundice, portal cirrhosis, and hepatic carcinoma	Highly valued hepatic test
	Bilirubin in urine Present in hepatitis and hepatogenous and obstructive jaundice	Test of considerable use
	Urobilinogen in urine Present in hepatogenous jaundice and obstructive jaundice	Very helpful test
	Urobilinogen in feces Increase in hemolytic jaundice Decrease in obstructive jaundice	Helpful test
Regulation of composition of blood	Prothrombin determination Increased in seconds Decreased in percent in obstructive jaundice, liver cell damage, and vitamin K deficiency	Usefulness of test established
Protein metabolism	Total serum proteins (49) Serum albumin Serum globulin Serum gamma globulin Increase of globulin in infectious hepatitis Decrease of total proteins and albumin in liver disease Serum immunoglobulins IgA increased in alcoholic hepatitis IgG increased in chronic hepatitis IgM increased in biliary cirrhosis	Of value in detection of hepatic and nonhepatic disorders
	Blood ammonia levels Increased in hepatic coma	Of diagnostic importance

Hepatic Function	Tests	Comments

(Continued)	Alpha-fetoprotein
	  Increased in the presence
	    of hepatocellular cancer
	    in adults
		Helpful clue—not liver func-
		tion test

	Alpha-1-antitripsin	Of value in detection of meta- bolic error

Carbohydrate metabolism	Oral galactose test (4, 49)
	  Excretion in a 5-hour
	    period
	  Increased in toxic hepatitis
	    and galactosemia
		Decreasing use

	Oral glucose tolerance test
	  Excretion of glucose within
	    30 to 60 minutes
	  Increased in obstructive
	    jaundice
		Rarely of value in hepatic dis-
		ease

	Glucagon tolerance (111)	Diagnostic aid in glycogenoses

	Epinephrine tolerance
	  Decreased in cirrhosis,
	    hepatitis, and glycogen
	    storage disease
		Useful in clinical research

Lipid metabolism	Determination of serum cholesterol (4, 36)	Use restricted in liver function study

	Determination of serum cho-
	  lesterol esters
	  Both increased in obstruc-
	    tive jaundice
	  Both decreased in liver fail-
	    ure and hepatic necrosis
		Limited clinical application

Enzyme activity	Serum alkaline phosphatase
	  (13, 27, 50)
	  Increased in obstructive
	    jaundice, congenital in-
	    trahepatic biliary atresia,
	    and cancer of liver
		Wide application in study of
		hepatic disease

	Serum alanine amino trans-
	  ferase (SALT or SGPT)
	  Highly elevated in acute
	    hepatitis, toxic hepatitis,
	    and hepatocellular
	    damage
		Of greater value than SAST in
		liver disease—very sensi-
		tive test

	Serum aspartate aminotrans-
	  ferase (SAST or SGOT)
		Clinical usefulness
		  comfirmed

	Serum gamma glutamyl transferase (SGGT)	Highly sensitive measure of hepatic pathology

Hepatic Function	Tests	Comments
Metals and electrolytes	Serum iron and iron-binding capacity (10) Increased in acute hepatitis and hemochromatosis Decreased in cirrhosis	Diagnostic aid Clinical usefulness confirmed
	Serum copper and ceruloplasmin (84) Decreased in Wilson's disease (hepatolenticular degeneration) Urine copper Increased in Wilson's disease	Helpful in diagnostic investigation

Special Laboratory Studies

Terms Related to Amniotic Fluid Analysis

- *alpha-fetoprotein (AFP)*—major protein (glycoprotein) in fetal serum. It is synthesized by the embryonic liver. An elevated AFP in amniotic fluid is present in neural tube anomalies such as fetal anencephaly, myelocele, and spinal bifida. AFP also is increased in Turner's syndrome, tetralogy of Fallot, and other non-neural tube defects. (60, 77, 81)
- *amniotic fluid*—fluid contained in the amniotic sac. (61)
- *amniotic fluid analysis*—study of the components of amniotic fluid to assess fetal health and maturity. It may be done at early gestation (20 weeks) or as the need arises in high-risk pregnancy or at term. A complete analysis involves spectrophotometric, biochemical, cytologic, genetic, and cytogenetic evaluation of the fetus. (61)
- *bilirubin in amniotic fluid*—spectrophotometric tracings detect bilirubin elevation in the Rh isoimmunization syndrome and predict the progress of fetal hemolysis and the risk of intrauterine death. When repeated amniocentesis signal a severely affected fetus, labor should be induced in 33 to 34 weeks to prevent perinatal death. (61)
- *bilirubin scan of amniotic fluid*—this scan shows correlation with severity of hemolytic disease. (61)
- *creatinine levels of amniotic fluid*—increasing levels provide information concerning fetal muscle development and renal concentration ability. They aid in the assessment of the fetal age.
- *evaluation of the pulmonary maturity of the fetus*—the development of the lungs is lined to the functional adequacy of the surfactant, a phospholipoprotein matrix that lines each alveolus and reduces the pulmonary surface tension during expiration. Since the fetal air passages communicate with the amniotic fluid, the surfactant is found in the amniotic fluid. Its presence in sufficient amount signals lung maturity of the fetus; its absence or an insufficient amount signals lung immaturity. The following tests are done to detect the fetal pulmonary status:
  - —*amniotic fluid lung profile*—test to evaluate lung maturity. The lung profile detects lecithin, as well as two other phospholipids, namely phosphatidylglycerol (PG), and phosphatidylinositol (PI). PG appears after the thirty-fifth week of gestation and continues to increase until term. PI increases in the amniotic fluid after the

twenty-sixth to thirtieth week of gestation and then slowly decreases. PI and PG act as surfactant—stabilizing substances, assisting to prevent alveolar collapse. The presence of PG in an amniotic fluid specimen, when the L/S ratio exceeds 2, is a strong indicator that respiratory distress syndrome (RDS) will not occur. PG is important in high-risk pregnancies such as those complicated by diabetes, isoimmunization, or by hydrops fetalis to document stable pulmonary stability. Recently, a slide agglutination test to determine the presence of PG has been established. (56, 60)

—*foam stability index (FSI)*—test based on the surfactant being a foaming agent and ethanol inhibiting foam production. Ethanol (95% or 100%) is placed in a tube, 500 μl of amniotic fluid are added, and the tube is shaken for 30 seconds.

Positive reaction: presence of a complete ring of bubbles predictive of lung maturity of neonate; no respiratory distress syndrome will develop.

Negative reaction: no bubbles or an incomplete ring of bubbles predictive of lung immaturity of neonate with or without respiratory distress syndrome. (56, 60)

—*lecithin-to-sphingomyelin (L/S) ratio*—the ratio of these phospholipids reflects the extrusion of the surfactant into the amniotic fluid. L/S ratio greater than 2.0 suggests adequate lung development in the third trimester. L/S ratio less than 2.0 indicates lung immaturity, which is normal in early pregnancy but not before term. (56)

■ *fetal chromosome analysis*—after 15 to 18 weeks of gestation fetal cells can be grown in a satisfactory cell culture. Chromosomal abnormalities such as balanced translocation in either parent may be transmitted to the offspring. The incidence of Down's syndrome, trisomy 21, and spontaneous abortions increases with maternal age. The fetal chromosome analysis establishes an exact antenatal diagnosis of chromosome aberrations. (60)

■ *fetal sex*—determination of the sex of the fetus is possible at 15 to 18 weeks of gestation. Amniotic fluid studies commonly performed are:

—the Barr test of nuclear sex

—Y chromosome staining in uncultured cells

—tissue culture of human cells and karyotyping (60)

■ *inherited disorders*—numerous inborn errors of metabolism are identifiable by amniotic fluid analysis; for example, Gaucher's disease, galactosemia, and cystinosis, representing metabolic errors of lipid, carbohydrate, and amino acid metabolism. (60)

Terms Related to Seminal Fluid

■ *semen*—secretion containing spermatozoa, the male cells of reproduction. (69, 77)

■ *semen culture*—study of the seminal flora, useful in confirming a diagnosis of bacterial prostatitis.

■ *seminal fluid*—fluid chiefly secreted by the prostate and in minute amount by the testes.

■ *sperm count*—60 to 150 million/ml (SIU: 60 to 150 $\times$ 10^9/L) spermatozoa present in the seminal fluid of a healthy male. (69)

■ *sperm morphology*—shape of cells indicating that more than 70 percent are normal mature spermatozoa. (69)

■ *sperm motility*—sperm movement is greater than 60 percent.

■ *volume of seminal fluid*—1.50 to 5.0 ml is the amount of seminal fluid produced by a healthy male. (69)

Terms Related to Cerebrospinal Fluid

- *cerebrospinal fluid (CSF)*—produced in the capillaries of the choroid plexus, CSF circulates through the ventricles of the brain and enters the subarachnoid space. Its functions are:
    - —to protect the brain and cord from sudden pressure changes
    - —to maintain a stable environment for both structures
    - —to remove waste products of brain metabolism (73, 74, 75)
- *collection of CSF:*
    - *cisternal puncture*—removal of CSF from the cisterna magna; for example, in the case of blocking of the central canal of the spinal cord.
    - *lumbar puncture*—needle puncture of subarachnoid space of the lumbar cord used in determining CSF pressure and removing CSF for diagnostic evaluation or other purposes. (56, 62)
    - *ventricular puncture*—removal of ventricular fluids, rarely done on adults except for ventriculography, but a more common procedure for infants with open fontanels.
- *cytology of CSF*—cell count and differential count of CSF may aid in the detection of neurologic disease. Neutrophils in CSF signal an acute inflammatory process such as bacterial meningitis, and malignant cells shed in CSF may be derived from primary or metastatic brain tumors, lymphomas, or leukemias. (73)
- *examination of CSF by chemical analysis:*
    - *CSF glucose*—elevated CSF glucose is of no diagnostic importance. Values less than 40 mg/dl may be present in tuberculous, bacterial, or fungal meningitis or malignant infiltration of meninges.
    - *CSF glutamine*—determination indirectly suggests the ammonia level in the central nervous system. Elevated ammonia concentrations have a toxic effect on nerve tissue. As a protective response, ammonia is converted to glutamine. Glutamine levels higher than 35 mg/dl indicate hepatic encephalopathy (hepatic coma).
    - *CSF lactate dehydrogenase (LD)*—test useful in distinguishing between aseptic and bacterial meningitis.
    - *CSF lactic acid concentrations*—if greater than 35 mg/dl, results suggest tuberculous or bacterial infection.
    - *CSF total protein*—reliable but nonspecific index of neurologic disease and a common abnormality in chemical analysis. Elevated immunoglobulin (IgG) levels are found in multiple sclerosis, neurosyphilis, and other central nervous system pathology. (70, 72, 73)
- *microbiology of CSF*—bacterial, fungal, tuberculous, protozoal or viral infections may result from:
    - —infiltration of CSF with microorganisms
    - —hematogenous dissemination of microorganisms *or*
    - —direct inoculation due to trauma or surgery (70, 73)
- *Queckenstedt test*—diagnostic maneuver consisting of compression of one or both jugular veins, which normally results in a quick, brief rise in CSF pressure. With blockage of the vertebral canal the rise in CSF is minimal or absent. (77)
- *turbidity of CSF*—cloudy appearance caused by the presence of microorganisms, granules, or flaky material in spinal fluid. (70, 73)
- *Venereal Disease Research Laboratories (VDRL) test of CSF*—flocculation test for syphilis. A positive reaction confirms the diagnosis of neurosyphilis. (25)
- *xanthochromic*—canary yellow. Xanthochromic CSF may occur in cerebral hematoma, subarachnoid hemorrhage, toxoplasmosis, abscesses, and tumors. (77)

Terms Related to Toxicology Testing

- *alcohol abuse, ethanol abuse*—excessive consumption of alcoholic beverages.

  Reference values: alcohol abuse
  marked intoxication—0.3%-0.4% (SIU: 65-87 mmol/L)
  alcoholic stupor—4.0%-0.5% (SIU: 87-109 mmol/L)
  coma—greater than 0.5% (SIU: greater than 109 mmol/L) (71, 79)

- *carbon monoxide poisoning (CO)*—occurs in suicide attempts or accidental inhalation.

  Reference values: CO poisoning
  up to 5% saturation
  (SIU: up to 0.5 saturation)
  symptoms occur with 20% saturation
  (SIU: symptoms occur with 0.20 saturation) (77, 79)

- *lead poisoning*—chronic toxic state, usually seen in children of teething age and caused by biting of crib or bedstead with paint containing lead.

  Reference values:
  lead, blood—0-40 µg/dl (SIU: 0-2 µmol/L)
  lead, urine—less than 100 µg/24 hr (SIU: less than 0.48 µg/24 hr) (77, 79)

Terms Related to Therapeutic Drug Monitoring (43, 47, 52, 53, 54)

- *drug monitoring*—using the therapeutic range as a guideline, a serum drug level is obtained and interpreted in the context of clinical and pharmacokinetic criteria.
- *drug toxicity*—toxic effects of medication caused by incorrect dosage and related to age, impaired metabolism, faulty absorption or detoxification, renal dysfunction, and subsequent retention and cumulative effects of the drug.
- *overdose*—may result from overtreatment with medication by physician or intentional overuse of medicine by a suicidal patient or one with psychiatric problems.
- *pharmacokinetics*—discipline dealing with the action of drugs on the body, including their absorption, distribution, metabolism, elimination, and pharmacologic response.
- *pharmacology*—discipline that studies the action of drugs on the body.
- *therapeutic drug monitoring (TDM)*—measurement of serum drug levels to:
  - —ascertain if the drug regimen achieves the therapeutic serum concentrations with a narrow therapeutic ratio; for example, in administration of lithium and digoxin.
  - —observe high-risk patients for:
    - —drug interactions; for example, with tricyclic antidepressants, lithium, and digoxin.
    - —impaired renal clearance; for example, with theophylline and digoxin.
    - —potential toxic reactions; for example, with theophylline and lithium.

Terms Related to Testing Methods

- *drug assay*—procedure used to detect the therapeutic value of a particular drug based on criteria of specificity, sensitivity, precision, time to run the test, cost, and instrumentation. (77)
- *immunoassay*—assay requiring antibody production, which is achieved by injecting an animal with a chemical or drug bound to a macromolecule. The complex of the drug molecule stimulates antibody formation. Several animal injections with the drug create a high antibody titer. The animal is bled, and the antibodies are removed

and exposed to the particular drug in vitro, thus stimulating drug antibody-interaction. This drug antibody interaction is the underlying principle of enzyme immunoassays, fluorescent immunoassays, and radioimmunoassays. (77)

—*enzyme immunoassay (EIA)*—an enzyme binds the drug. Antibodies interacting with the drug-enzyme complex modify the activity of the enzyme. This change in enzyme activity is considered a measure of drug concentration.

—*fluorescent immunoassay, fluoroimmunoassay (FIA)*—in this procedure the drug is bound to a fluorogenic enzyme. A standard curve relates the intensity of fluorescence to the drug level. Commercial kits for FIA contain an antibody-enzyme reagent, fluorogenic drug reagents, a buffer, and drug standards. FIAs have a greater sensitivity (2 μg/ml) than enzyme immunoassays.

—*radioimmunoassay (RIA)*—specified amount of a radioactive drug is added to the antibody solution, and the serum sample for testing is added to the mixed solution. If the drug under study is found in the serum, the following reaction takes place:

Drug + Radioactive drug = (Drug − Antibody) + (Radioactive drug − Antibody)

The radioactive drug bound to the antibody is removed from the free drug to be measured. (4)

Abbreviations

Related to Tests

ABO—A, B, AB, and O blood types
ACP—acid phosphatase
ACTH—adrenocorticotropic hormone
ADH—antidiuretic hormone
AFP—alpha-fetoprotein
AI—atherogenic index
ALP—alkaline phosphatase
ALS—aldolase
ALT—alanine aminotransferase
AMS—amylase
AST—aspartate aminotransferase
BAO—basal acid output
B-cell—B-lymphocyte
C^{++}—calcium (electrolyte)
CK—creatine kinase
CK-MB—creatine kinase isoenzyme
CK-2—creatine kinase isoenzyme
E_1—estrone
E_2—estradiol
E_3—estriol
EIA—enzyme immunoassay
ELISA—enzyme-linked immuno-sorbent assay
FDP—fibrin-fibrinogen degradation products
FIA—fluoroimmunoassay

5-HIAA—5-hydroxyindole acetic acid
FSH—follicle-stimulating hormone
FSI—foam stability index
GGT—gamma glutamyl transferase
GGTP—gamma glutamyl transpeptidase
GOT—glutamate oxaloacetate transaminase
GTT—glucose tolerance test
Hb—hemoglobin concentration
HCG—human chorionic gonadotropin
Hct—hematocrit
HDL—high-density lipoprotein
HI—hemagglutination inhibition
HLA—human leukocyte antigen
HPL—human placental lactogen
IBC—iron-binding capacity
IgA—immunoglobulin A
IgD—immunoglobulin D
IgG—immunoglobulin G
IgM—immunoglobulin M
ISG—immune serum globulin
K^+—potassium (electrolyte)
LAP—leucine aminopeptidase
LD, LDH—lactate dehydrogenase
LDL—low-density lipoprotein
LD-1—lactate hydrogenase isoenzyme

LH—luteinizing hormone
LPS—lipase
L/S ratio—lecithin-to-sphingomyelin ratio
MAO—maximal acid output
MCH—mean corpuscular hemoglobin
MCHC—mean corpuscular hemoglobin
    concentration
MCV—mean corpuscular volume
Mg^{++}—magnesium (electrolyte)
mm Hg—millimeters of mercury
Na^{+}—sodium (electrolyte)
NAPA—N-acetyl procainamide
OCT—oxytocin challenge test
Pco_2—pressure (tension) of carbon
    dioxide
pH—hydrogen ion

PHI—phosphohexoisomerase
PK—pyruvate kinase
PO_2—pressure (tension) of oxygen
PRA—plasma renin activity
PSP—phenolsulfonphthalein
PT—prothrombin time
PPT—partial prothrombin time
T-cell—T-lymphocyte
TDM—therapeutic drug monitoring
TIBC—total iron-binding capacity
VLDL—very-low-density lipoprotein

Organizations

AABB—American Association of Blood
    Banks
ACS—Association of Clinical Scientists

References and Bibliography

1. Alpers, David H., and Sabesin, Seymour M. Fatty liver: Biochemical and clinical aspects. In Schiff, Leon, and Schiff, Eugene R., eds., *Diseases of the Liver,* 6th ed. Philadelphia: J.B. Lippincott Co., 1987, pp. 949-978.
2. Andreoli, Thomas E. Approach to the patient with renal disease. In Wyngaarden, James B., and Smith, Lloyd H., Jr., eds., *Cecil's Textbook of Medicine,* 18th ed. Philadelphia: W.B. Saunders Co., 1988, pp. 502-508.
3. ———. Disorders of fluid volume, electrolyte, and acid-base balance. Ibid., pp. 528-558.
4. Balisteri, William F., and Schubert, William K. Liver disease in infancy and childhood. In Schiff, Leon, and Schiff, Eugene R., eds., *Diseases of the Liver,* 6th ed. Philadelphia: J.B. Lippincott Co., 1987, pp. 1337-1426.
5. Beck, William S. Megaloblastic anemias. In Wyngaarden, James B., and Smith, Lloyd H., Jr., eds., *Cecil's Textbook of Medicine,* 18th ed. Philadelphia: W.B. Saunders Co., 1988, pp. 900-907.
6. Berk, Paul D. Erythrocytosis and polycythemia. In Wyngaarden, James B., and Smith, Lloyd H., Jr., eds., *Cecil's Textbook of Medicine,* 18th ed. Philadelphia: W.B. Saunders Co., 1988, pp. 975-984.
7. Billings, Barbara H. Bilirubin metabolism. In Schiff, Leon, and Schiff, Eugene R., eds., *Diseases of the Liver,* 6th ed. Philadelphia: J.B. Lippincott Co., 1987, pp. 103-127.
8. Bissell, D. Montgomery. Porphyria. In Wyngaarden, James B., and Smith, Lloyd H., Jr., eds., *Cecil's Textbook of Medicine,* 18th ed.

Philadelphia: W.B. Saunders Co., 1988, pp. 1182-1187.
9. Blanchette, Victor S. Neonatal alloimmune thrombocytopenia. In Stockman, James A., III, and Pochedly, Carol. eds., *Developmental and Neonatal Hematology,* New York: Raven Press, 1988, pp. 145-168.
10. Bothwell, Thomas H., Charlton, Robert W. Hemochromatosis. In Schiff, Leon, and Schiff, Eugene R., eds., *Diseases of the Liver,* 6th ed. Philadelphia: J.B. Lippincott Co., 1987, pp. 1001-1035.
11. Bourdage, James S., and Voss, Edward, Jr. Comparative immunological analysis of anti-deoxynucleotide and anti-single-stranded DNA antibodies. In Voss, Edward W., Jr., ed., *Anti-DNA Antibodies in SLE,* Boca Raton, FL: CRC Press, Inc., 1988, pp. 17-67.
12. Bowman, John M. Alloimmune hemolytic disease of the neonate. In Stockman, James A., III, and Pochedly, Carl. eds., *Developmental and Neonatal Hematology,* New York: Raven Press, 1988, pp. 223-248.
13. Brody, Jerome S. Diseases of the pleura, mediastinum, diaphragm, and chest wall. In Wyngaarden, James B., and Smith, Lloyd H., Jr., eds., *Cecil's Textbook of Medicine,* 18th ed. Philadelphia: W.B. Saunders Co., 1988, pp. 466-473.
14. Camargo, Carlos A., and Kolb, Felix O. Endocrine disorders. In Schroeder, Steven A., Krupp, Marcus A., and Tierney, Lawrence M., Jr., eds., *Current Medical Diagnosis & Treatment—1988,* Norwalk, CT: Appleton & Lange, 1988, pp. 676-748.
15. Casperson, Gerald F., and Voss, Edward W.,

Jr. Specificity of anti-DNA antibodies in systemic lupus erythematosus. In Voss, Edward W., Jr., ed., *Anti-DNA Antibodies in SLE,* Boca Raton, FL: CRC Press, Inc., 1988, pp. 69-111.

16. Dennis, Vincent W. Investigations of renal function. In Wyngaarden, James B., and Smith, Lloyd H., Jr., eds., *Cecil's Textbook of Medicine,* 18th ed. Philadelphia: W.B. Saunders Co., 1988, pp. 520-528.

17. Elin, Ronald J. Reference intervals and laboratory values of clinical importance. In Wyngaarden, James B., and Smith, Lloyd H., Jr., eds., *Cecil's Textbook of Medicine,* 18th ed. Philadelphia: W.B. Saunders Co., 1988, pp. 2394-2404.

18. Fishback, Frances Talaska. Urine studies. In *A Manual of Laboratory Diagnostic Tests,* 3rd ed. Philadelphia: J.B. Lippincott Co., 1988, pp. 116-197.

19. Ford, Regina Daley, ed. Blood chemistry testing. In *Diagnostic Tests Handbook,* Springhouse, PA: Springhouse Corporation, 1987, pp. 43-158.

20. Frohman, Lawrence A. The anterior pituitary. In Wyngaarden, James B., and Smith, Lloyd H., Jr., eds., *Cecil's Textbook of Medicine,* 18th ed. Philadelphia: W.B. Saunders Co., 1988, pp. 1290-1305.

21. Gotto, Antonio M., Jr. Cholesterol: New approaches to screening management. *Diagnosis* 10:40-41, 45, 49-53, Jan. 1988.

22. Greenberger, Norton J., and Toskes, Phillip P., and Isselbacher, Kurt J. Diseases of the pancreas. In Braunwald, Eugene, et al. eds., *Harrison's Principles of Internal Medicine,* 11th ed. New York: McGraw-Hill Book Co., 1987, pp. 1372-1384.

23. Grossman, Moses, and Jawetz, Ernest. Infectious diseases: viral and rickettsial. In Schroeder, Steven A., Krupp, Marcus A., and Tierney, Lawrence M., Jr., eds., *Current Medical Diagnosis & Treatment—1988,* Norwalk, CT: Appleton & Lange, 1988, pp. 834-857.

24. ———. Infectious diseases: Bacterial. Ibid., pp. 858-884.

25. ———. Infectious diseases: Spirochetal. Ibid., pp. 885-895.

26. Jandl, James H. Blood and bloodforming tissues. In *Blood Textbook of Hematology,* Boston: Little, Brown & Co., 1987, pp. 1-48.

27. ———. The hypochromic anemias and other disorders of iron metabolism. Ibid., pp. 181-235.

28. ———. Granulocytes. Ibid., pp. 441-471.

29. Kaplan, Marshall M. Laboratory tests. In Schiff, Leon, and Schiff, Eugene R., eds., *Diseases of the Liver,* 6th ed. Philadelphia: J.B. Lippincott Co., 1987, pp. 219-260.

30. Karam, John H. Diabetes mellitus, hypoglycemia, and lipoprotein disorders. In Schroeder, Steven A., Krupp, Marcus A., and Tierney, Lawrence M., Jr., eds., *Current Medical Diagnosis & Treatment—1988,* Norwalk, CT: Appleton & Lange, 1988, pp. 749-783.

31. Katz, Samuel L. Rubella (German measles). In Wyngaarden, James B., and Smith, Lloyd H., Jr., eds., *Cecil's Textbook of Medicine,* 18th ed. Philadelphia: W.B. Saunders Co., 1988, pp. 2394-2404.

32. Keitt, Alan S. Introduction to anemias. In Wyngaarden, James B., and Smith, Lloyd H., Jr., eds., *Cecil's Textbook of Medicine,* 18th ed. Philadelphia: W.B. Saunders Co., 1988, pp. 878-884.

33. Kieff, Eliott. Infectious mononucleosis (Epstein-Barr virus infection). In Wyngaarden, James B., and Smith, Lloyd H., Jr., eds., *Cecil's Textbook of Medicine,* 18th ed. Philadelphia: W.B. Saunders Co., 1988, pp. 1786-1788.

34. Kim, Haewon C. Blood-component therapy in the neonate. In Stockman, James A., III, and Pochedly, Carol. eds., *Developmental and Neonatal Hematology,* New York: Raven Press, 1988, pp. 169-198.

35. Klahr, Saulo. Structure and function of the kidneys. In Wyngaarden, James B., and Smith, Lloyd H., Jr., eds., *Cecil's Textbook of Medicine,* 18th ed. Philadelphia: W.B. Saunders Co., 1988, pp. 508-520.

36. Koff, Raymond S., and Galambos, John T. Viral hepatitis. In Schiff, Leon, and Schiff, Eugene R., eds., *Diseases of the Liver,* 6th ed. Philadelphia: J.B. Lippincott Co., 1987, pp. 457-581.

37. Krejs, Guenter J. Diarrhea. In Wyngaarden, James B., and Smith, Lloyd H., Jr., eds., *Cecil's Textbook of Medicine,* 18th ed. Philadelphia: W.B. Saunders Co., 1988, pp. 725-732.

38. Kushner, James B. Hypochromic anemias. In Wyngaarden, James B., and Smith, Lloyd H., Jr., eds., *Cecil's Textbook of Medicine,* 18th ed. Philadelphia: W.B. Saunders Co., 1988, pp. 892-900.

39. Larson, Linda. Primary hemostasis. In McKenzie, Shirlyn B. *Textbook of Hematology,* Philadelphia: Lea & Febiger, 1988, pp. 363-379.

40. ———. Disorders of hemostasis. Ibid., pp. 417-475.

41. Linker, Charles. Blood. In Schroeder, Steven A., Krupp, Marcus A., and Tierney, Lawrence M., Jr., eds., *Current Medical Diagnosis & Treatment—1988,* Norwalk, CT: Appleton & Lange, 1988, pp. 294-338.

42. Marcus, Aaron J. Hemorrhagic disorders: Abnormalities of platelet and vascular function. In Wyngaarden, James B., and Smith,

Lloyd H., Jr., eds., *Cecil's Textbook of Medicine,* 18th ed. Philadelphia: W.B. Saunders Co., 1988, pp. 1042-1060.

43. McKenzie, Shirlyn B. General aspects and classification of anemia. In McKenzie, Shirlyn B., *Textbook of Hematology,* Philadelphia: Lea & Febiger, 1988, pp. 81-108.

44. ———. Anemia of defective heme and porphyrin synthesis. Ibid., pp. 109-130.

45. ———. Anemias by abnormalities in globin biosynthesis. Ibid., pp. 131-165.

46. ———. Hemolytic anemias caused by intrinsic red cell defects. Ibid., pp. 201-219.

47. ———. Hemolytic anemias caused by extrinsic factors. Ibid., pp. 221-249.

48. ———. Secondary hemostasis. Ibid., pp. 381-416.

49. Mendenhall, Charles L. Alcoholic hepatitis. In Schiff, Leon, and Schiff, Eugene R., eds., *Diseases of the Liver,* 6th ed. Philadelphia: J.B. Lippincott Co., 1987, pp. 669-685.

50. Mosher, Deane F. Disorders of blood coagulation. In Wyngaarden, James B., and Smith, Lloyd H., Jr., eds., *Cecil's Textbook of Medicine,* 18th ed. Philadelphia: W.B. Saunders Co., 1988, pp. 1060-1081.

51. Newth, Christopher J.L. Cystic fibrosis. In Wyngaarden, James B., and Smith, Lloyd H., Jr., eds., *Cecil's Textbook of Medicine,* 18th ed. Philadelphia: W.B. Saunders Co., 1988, pp. 440-442.

52. Niles, Alan S. Principles of drug therapy. In Wyngaarden, James B., and Smith, Lloyd H., Jr., eds., *Cecil's Textbook of Medicine,* 18th ed. Philadelphia: W.B. Saunders Co., 1988, pp. 97-98.

53. ———. Interaction between drugs. Ibid., pp. 98-101.

54. ———. Adverse reactions to drugs. Ibid., pp. 102-104.

55. Ockner, Robert K. Laboratory tests in liver disease. In Wyngaarden, James B., and Smith, Lloyd H., Jr., eds., *Cecil's Textbook of Medicine,* 18th ed. Philadelphia: W.B. Saunders Co., 1988, pp. 814-817.

56. O'Grady, John P., and Veille, Jean Claude. Obstetric management of prematurity. In Fanaroff, Avroy A., and Martin, Richard J., eds., *Neonatal-Perinatal Medicine—Diseases of Fetus and Infants,* St. Louis: The C.V. Mosby Co., 1987, pp. 123-141.

57. Olefsky, Jerrold M. Diabetes mellitus. In Wyngaarden, James B., and Smith, Lloyd H., Jr., eds., *Cecil's Textbook of Medicine,* 18th ed. Philadelphia: W.B. Saunders Co., 1988, pp. 1360-1381.

58. Pak, Charles Y.C. Renal calculi. In Wyngaarden, James B., and Smith, Lloyd H., Jr., eds., *Cecil's Textbook of Medicine,* 18th ed. Philadelphia: W.B. Saunders Co., 1988, pp. 638-644.

59. Pasternak, Richard C., et al. Acute myocardial infarction. In Braunwald, Eugene, et al., *Heart Disease,* 3rd ed., vol. 2. Philadelphia: W.B. Saunders Co., 1988, pp. 1222-1313.

60. Polin, Richard A., and Mennuti, Michael T. Genetic disease and chromosomal abnormalities. In Fanaroff, Avroy A., and Martin, Richard J., eds., *Neonatal-Perinatal Medicine—Diseases of Fetus and Infants,* St. Louis: The C.V. Mosby Co., 1987.

61. Queenan, John T. Erythroblastosis fetalis. In Fanaroff, Avroy A., and Martin, Richard J., eds., *Neonatal-Perinatal Medicine—Diseases of Fetus and Infants,* St. Louis: The C.V. Mosby Co., 1987, pp. 153-162.

62. Rapoport, Samuel. Neurologic diagnostic procedures. In Wyngaarden, James B., and Smith, Lloyd H., Jr., eds., *Cecil's Textbook of Medicine,* 18th ed. Philadelphia: W.B. Saunders Co., 1988, pp. 2056-2058.

63. Ray, C. George. Mumps. In Braunwald, Eugene, et al. eds., *Harrison's Principles of Internal Medicine,* 11th ed. New York: McGraw-Hill Book Co., 1987, pp. 709-712.

64. Richardson, Charles T. Pathogenesis. In Wyngaarden, James B., and Smith, Lloyd H., Jr., eds., *Cecil's Textbook of Medicine,* 18th ed. Philadelphia: W.B. Saunders Co., 1988, pp. 692-696.

65. Schiff, Leon. Jaundice: A clinical approach. In Schiff, Leon, and Schiff, Eugene R., eds., *Diseases of the Liver,* 6th ed. Philadelphia: J.B. Lippincott Co., 1987, pp. 209-217.

66. Schiller, Lawrence R. Epidemiology, clinical manifestations, and diagnosis. In Wyngaarden, James B., and Smith, Lloyd H., Jr., eds., *Cecil's Textbook of Medicine,* 18th ed. Philadelphia: W.B. Saunders Co., 1988, pp. 696-703.

67. Schroeder, Steven A., Krupp, Marcus A., and Tierney, Lawrence M., Jr., eds., Appendix. In *Current Medical Diagnosis & Treatment—1988,* Norwalk, CT: Appleton & Lange, 1988, pp. 1091-1123.

68. Shearn, Martin A. Arthritis and musculoskeletal disorders. In Schroeder, Steven A., Krupp, Marcus A., and Tierney, Lawrence M., Jr., eds., *Current Medical Diagnosis & Treatment—1988,* Norwalk, CT: Appleton & Lange, 1988, pp. 496-532.

69. Sherins, Richard J., and Howards, Stuart S. Male infertility. In Walsh, Patrick C., et al. eds., *Campbell's Urology,* 5th ed., vol. 1. Philadelphia: W.B. Saunders, 1986, pp. 640-697.

70. Silberberg, Donald H. The demyelinating diseases. In Wyngaarden, James B., and Smith, Lloyd H., Jr., eds., *Cecil's Textbook of Medicine,* 18th ed. Philadelphia: W.B. Saunders Co., 1988, pp. 2211-2217.

71. Smith, Lloyd H., Jr. The hyperphenylalani-

emias. In Wyngaarden, James B., and Smith, Lloyd H., Jr., eds., *Cecil's Textbook of Medicine,* 18th ed. Philadelphia: W.B. Saunders Co., 1988, pp. 1155-1157.

72. Swartz, Morton N. Bacterial meningitis. In Wyngaarden, James B., and Smith, Lloyd H., Jr., eds., *Cecil's Textbook of Medicine,* 18th ed. Philadelphia: W.B. Saunders Co., 1988, pp. 1604-1611.

73. ———. Meningococcal disease. Ibid., pp. 1611-1617.

74. ———. Infections caused by hemophilus species. Ibid., pp. 1617-1621.

75. Thirlby, Richard C. Surgical therapy. In Wyngaarden, James B., and Smith, Lloyd H., Jr., eds., *Cecil's Textbook of Medicine,* 18th ed. Philadelphia: W.B. Saunders Co., 1988, pp. 703-706.

76. Toskes, Philip. Malabsorption. In Wyngaarden, James B., and Smith, Lloyd H., Jr., eds., *Cecil's Textbook of Medicine,* 18th ed. Philadelphia: W.B. Saunders Co., 1988, pp. 732-745.

77. Tucker, Eugene, MD. Personal communications.

78. Tyrell, J. Blake, and Baxter, John D. Disorders of the adrenal cortex. In Wyngaarden, James B., and Smith, Lloyd H., Jr., eds., *Cecil's Textbook of Medicine,* 18th ed. Philadelphia: W.B. Saunders Co., 1988, pp. 1340-1360.

79. VanKley, Harold, MD. Personal communications.

80. Van Thiel, David H., et al. The liver and its effect on endocrine function in health and disease. In Schiff, Leon, and Schiff, Eugene R., eds., *Diseases of the Liver,* 6th ed. Philadel-phia: J.B. Lippincott Co., 1987, pp. 129-162.

81. Volk, Sr. Leo Rita. Personal communications.

82. Voss, Edward W., and Casperson, Gerald F. Anti-DNA antibodies in SLE: Historical perspective. In Voss, Edward W., Jr., ed., *Anti—DNA Antibodies in SLE,* Boca Raton, FL: CRC Press, Inc., 1988, pp. 1-15.

83. Wallerstein, Ralph O. Blood transfusions. In Schroeder, Steven A., Krupp, Marcus A., and Tierney, Lawrence M., Jr., eds., *Current Medical Diagnosis & Treatment—1988,* Norwalk, CT: Appleton & Lange, 1988, pp. 338-341.

84. Walshe, J.M. The liver in Wilson's disease. Hepatolenticular degeneration. In Schiff, Leon, and Schiff, Eugene R., eds., *Diseases of the Liver,* 6th ed. Philadelphia: J.B. Lippincott Co., 1987, pp. 1037-1049.

85. Weisz-Carrington, Paul. Immunology. In *Principles of Clinical Immunohematology,* Chicago: Year Book Medical Publishers, Inc., 1986, pp. 102-144.

86. ———. Blood group antigens. Ibid., pp. 145-200.

87. ———. Laboratory aspects of blood banking. Ibid., pp. 201-217.

88. ———. The HLA system. Ibid., pp. 218-235.

89. ———. Paternity testing and forensic immunohematology. Ibid., pp. 409-417.

90. Willerson, James T. Acute myocardial infarction. In Wyngaarden, James B., and Smith, Lloyd H., Jr., eds., *Cecil's Textbook of Medicine,* 18th ed. Philadelphia: W.B. Saunders Co., 1988, pp. 329-337.

Selected Terms Pertaining to Radiology, Diagnostic Ultrasound, and Magnetic Resonance Imaging

CHAPTER 20

Orientation

Origin of Terms

echo- (G)—return of sound
-genic (G)—origin
-gram (G)—a writing, a mark
-graphy (G)—to write or record
lamina (pl. laminae) (L)—layer
radio- (L)—ray
scolio- (G)—twisted or crooked

-scopy (G)—to examine, inspection
stereo- (G)—solid
sonus (L)—sound
tomo- (G)—section, cutting
ultra- (L)—beyond
xero- (G)—dry, dryness

Radiology

General Terms

- *absorption of x-rays*—one of the two main processes by which x-rays passing through an object are reduced in their intensity. The other main process is called scattering. (98)
- *algorithm*—procedure for solving a mathematical problem by a series of operations that may be repetitive. (67, 98)
- *archival storage*—long-term storage of information on digital magnetic tape or floppy disk or as images on x-ray film.
- *artifact*—an error in the reconstructed image that has no counterpart in reality. (98)
- *attenuation of x-rays*—the term covering both absorption and scattering of x-rays as they pass through an object. (98)
- *axial*—referring to the axis of a part or structure.
- *back projection*—refers to both a process and a method of reconstructing an image. (98)
- *bit*—the smallest unit of digital information expressed in binary system of notation (either a 0 or a 1)
- *calcification*—deposit of lime salts in the tissue seen on a radiograph.
- *collimator*—device that shapes the x-ray beam. (98)

- *computed, computerized*—calculated.
- *computed tomography (CT)*—the reconstruction by computer of a tomographic plane (slice) of a part of the human body. It is developed from multiple x-ray absorption measurements collected by detectors after the passage of the x-ray beam through the patient's body. The planes that can be visualized include axial, coronal, sagittal, and oblique sections. The computer is used to make the necessary calculations and synthesize the images. (57, 64)
- *conventional tomography*—body section radiography that delineates a thin layer of tissue of an organ; thus the structures lying anteriorly and posteriorly are more or less blurred out. (98)
- *data acquisition system (DAS)*—the components of a computed tomography (CT) machine used to produce and collect the x-ray attenuation information: x-ray tube, detectors, and detector preamplifiers. These are mounted on the gantry. (98)
- *density*—the compactness of structure or a substance. (98)
- *digital*—pertaining to a function or process of discrete quantities or bits in computers. (19)
- *digital computer*—computer that uses numbers representing digits in a decimal or other system. (98)
- *digital radiography*—radiographic imaging in digital form, including various procedures applicable to angiography and radiography in general. Electronic digital recordings are used instead of film techniques. (19, 60, 67)
- *discrete*—well defined and clear-cut in appearance.
- *display monitor*—the television screen used to display the CT image. A monitor is distinct from a TV set in that it normally does not include the tuner that allows the selection of a particular channel. Monitors therefore are used in closed-circuit applications. (54)
- *emission computed tomography (emission CT)*—technique for obtaining cross-sectional images of the head or the body based on the detection of the geometric distribution of the emissions or activity of radionuclides. The emissions may be single photons or coincidental photons arising from position decay. (64, 73)
- *fibrosis*—replacement of normal tissue with fibrous tissue. Fibrotic lesions are seen on the x-ray film.
- *filter*—technique for shaping the x-ray beam's intensity. An example of this technique is placing an aluminum plate between the x-ray tube and the patient. Usually different filters are used for head and body scanning. (98)
- *filter function*—mathematical function incorporated into the CT algorithm. Filter functions modify the spatial frequency content of the signal information by limiting or enhancing information of different spatial frequencies. (98)
- *fluorescence*—the property of becoming luminous through the influence of x-rays or other agents.
- *fluoroscopy*—direct x-ray examination using a fluoroscopic screen. (37)
- *floppy disk*—flexible vinyl disk, approximately eight inches in diameter, on which digital information can be recorded magnetically. It can be used as the archival storage for the electronic CT images. (98)
- *gantry*—the movable frame on a CT machine that holds the x-ray tube, collimators, and detectors.
- *gated computed tomography*—process for synchronizing scanning or data collection with some physiologic process; technique employed for imaging the heart in different phases of the cardiac cycle by accumulating data for discrete portions of the cardiac cycle. The cardiac cycle is gated on the basis of the electrocardiogram.

- *image intensifier*—an electronic vacuum-tube device for increasing the intensity of a two-dimensional light image from a fluoroscopic screen. (64, 98)
- *inspissated*—thickened by absorption of fluid content.
- *invasive technique*—injection of contrast medium for enhancement of radiographic images. Types of contrast medium may include barium, diatrizoate meglumine, and diatrizoate sodium injection, USP (Renografin-76), diatrizoate sodium, USP (Hypaque), and metrizamide, USP (Amipaque). (67)
- *laminograph, planograph, tomograph*—body section radiographs imaging a thin layer of body tissue of varying depths without interference with the intervening structures. (67, 98)
- *law of tangents*—the radiographic image is determined primarily by the portions of the x-ray beam that pass tangentially or nearly tangentially along the borders between objects of different densities and thickness. (64)
- *linear accelerators*—high-energy and advanced radiotherapy devices that accelerate charged particles in a straight line and provide various x-ray and electron therapies. Their primary usefulness is in the field of radiation oncology. The radioresponsiveness of tumors may be predictable by histologic grading before therapy. The following tumors have proved to be radiosensitive and in selected cases radiocurable with a dose tolerable by normal tissue: seminomas, lymphosarcomas, Hodgkin's disease, Wilms' tumors, neuroblastomas, medulloblastomas, retinoblastomas, Ewing's sarcomas, and other disorders.
- *linear amplifier*—electric device producing an output signal proportioned to the input signal. The amplifier may be a transistor or electric tube. (72)
- *linear tomography*—form of conventional tomography in which the x-ray tube and film move at the same time, so that the central ray of the x-ray beam moves in a single plane. To accomplish rectilinear motion, the x-ray tube and film each move in a straight line; while in curvilinear motion, the x-ray tube and film both move in an arc within a given plane. (37, 72)
- *noninvasive technique*—no injection of contrast material needed for radiographic procedures. (72)
- *pixel*—short term for picture element cell. The pixel is a representation of the volume element on the display. (98)
- *positions of the body*—refers to the manner in which the patient is placed in reference to the surrounding space. Terms to describe body positions may include:
    - *dorsal recumbent*—supine.
    - *lateral recumbent*—lying on side.
    - *ventral recumbent*—prone.

    Terms used to describe part location or position may include:
    - *anterior, ventral*—designates forward part of body or organ.
    - *distal*—designates away from the source.
    - *lateral*—designates parts away from the median plane of the body or away from the middle of a part to the right or left.
    - *proximal*—designates nearness to the source. (4)
- *profile*—the plot of detector readings versus position made during a linear transverse of the scanning gantry (or its equivalent in a continuous rotation multi-element detector system). Another word for profile is projection. The term projection can also be used in a different sense; see definition of back projection. (98)
- *radiograph, radiogram, roentgenograph, roentgenogram*—picture of an internal structure made on photographic film by means of x-rays. (67, 98)
- *radiography, roentgenography*—the making of x-ray photographs of internal structures.

- *radiologist*—physician who uses roentgen rays, radium, and other forms of radiant energy for diagnostic, therapeutic, and research purposes. (98)
- *radiology*—the study or science concerned with the use of various forms of radiant energy. It includes:
    —diagnostic radiology.
    —interventional or therapeutic radiology.
    —investigational, experimental, or research radiology. (64)
- *radium*—radioactive substance used in treating certain diseases, usually malignancies. (64)
- *radon*—heavy radioactive gas given off in the disintegration of radium. (64)
- *rarefaction*—process of decreasing density.
- *rarefied area*—area of lessened density.
- *raw data, scan data, x-ray data*—refers to data or information representing the intensity of x-rays entering the detectors after digitization. (98)
- *reconstruction*—an estimate of the density distribution or variation in x-ray attenuation; finite dimensional approximation of the x-ray attenuation distribution in a transverse section of the patient. (98)
- *resolution*—in diagnostic radiology the perception of two adjacent objects or points as being separate. (57, 98)
- *roentgen rays, x-rays*—form of radiant energy capable of penetrating solid and opaque objects and named after Wilhelm Conrad Roentgen (1845-1923), a German physicist who discovered x-rays in 1895. (67)
- *scan*—the mechanical motion required to produce a CT image.
- *scan enhancement*—increasing the clarity of a radiologic image by injecting a contrast medium. (54)
- *scattering of x-rays*—one of the two ways in which the x-ray beam intensity is diminished in passing through an object. The x-rays are scattered in a direction different from the original beam direction and do not add to the production of the radiologic image. (98)
- *slice*—the cross-sectional portion of the body that is scanned for the production of the CT image. (98)
- *slit-beam radiography*—refers to any imaging technique that uses a slitlike detector, in contrast to the large area used in conventional radiography.
- *subtraction angiography*—procedure that images arteries without their overlying or surrounding structures. (50)
- *thermography*—refers to an imaging technique based on the detection of the naturally occurring body emission of infrared radiation. (71)
- *tomography (from the Greek, "to write; a slice or section")*—the process of imaging a particular body section or slice. (64)
- *xeroradiography*—radiographic imaging by using a selenium-coated plate and developing it without liquid chemicals. (64)

Selected Radiologic Studies

Terms Related to Arthrography

- *air arthrogram, pneumoarthrogram*—air injection used as the contrast medium in a joint for radiologic evaluation. (74)
- *arthrography*—contrast study of joints as an aid in establishing the diagnosis and selection of treatment modality for joint diseases and injuries. The most common joints evaluated by this technique include the knee, hip, and shoulder. (74)

—*hip arthrography*—this includes:

—evaluation of congenital hip dysplasias of infants and children to determine the type of corrective surgery needed while the bones are still partially cartilginous.

—examination of complications of Legg-Calvé-Perthes disease, such as avascular necrosis and a detached hip fragment that may be covered by intact cartilage. (74)

—detection of cartilaginous and synovial abnormalities of certain joint diseases in children and adults. Arthrograms are especially useful in prepuberty due to partial ossification of the skeleton. (74)

—visualization of total hip arthroplasty immediately after surgery to determine the success or failure of the operation or year later when pain indicates infection or a loosening of the prosthesis. (74)

—*knee arthrography*—may include:

—*meniscal injuries*—common knee injuries that may disrupt the meniscal cartilage and split the meniscus into fragments. Evaluation of meniscal abnormalities may be achieved by single- or double-contrast arthrography.

—*extrameniscal injuries*—abnormalities that include tears of ligaments, defects of articular cartilage such as loose bodies, synovial disorders, and popliteal cysts (Baker's cyst). Double-contrast arthrography of the knee aids in the diagnosis of these injuries. (74)

—*shoulder arthrography*—of the several bursal cavities and articulations present in the shoulder, arthrograms of the glenohumeral joint provide valuable information on various disorders, such as adhesive capsultitis, tears of the rotator cuff, recurrent dislocations and subluxations of the joint, bicipital tendon abnormalities, and articular diseases. (74)

Other types of arthrography may include:

—*ankle arthrography*—to assess injury or disease of the ankle joint area, such as severe sprains with rupture of the ankle ligament. (74)

—*temporomandibular joint (TMJ) arthrography*—the anatomic and physiologic complexity of TMJ requires careful arthrographic techniques to detect the possible cause of clicking, grinding, and locking of jaw; detachments; and perforations. (74)

Terms Related to Musculoskeletal Imaging

- *computed tomography in musculoskeletal diagnosis*—CT scanning performed by a recently developed machine that possesses capabilities for high-contrast resolution and three-dimensional imaging and usually allows a low-rad dose, thus reducing radiation exposure to the patient. Major applications are the assessment of solid or cystic tumors; benign, malignant, recurrent, or metastatic musculoskeletal masses; trauma; back pain; and metabolic bone disease. (34)
- *plain radiographs of skeleton*—conventional radiographs of bones that image fractures, orthopedic deformities, metabolic or neoplastic bone disease, and backache. (74)
- *scanography*—method of x-ray examination for accurate measurement of the length of structures of the body, usually of the long bones; for example, to determine a discrepancy in a leg length. (64)
- *stereoradiography, stereoroentgenography*—obtaining an x-ray picture from two similar positions to give the object an appearance of relief, depth, and solidity. (64)
- *tomography of skeleton*—sectional radiography for the diagnosis of bone disorders. Extraneous structures overlying the region under study are blurred, enabling the tomograms to clearly demonstrate osteolytic and inflammatory lesions, joint derange-

ments, erosions, and ischemic necrosis, which cannot be seen on the conventional radiograph. (34)

Terms Related to Neuroradiography, Including Endocrine Glands

- *cerebral angiography*—conventional procedure or method of demonstrating the cervical and cerebral blood vessels by taking a series of radiograms during the injection of a contrast medium. Extracranial atheromatous occlusions of the carotid, vertebral, and subclavian arteries producing cerebrovascular insufficiency can be readily detected and are surgically correctable. A radiographic visualization of the intracranial vasculature may be of diagnostic value in locating space-occupying lesions, brain tumors, cerebral aneurysms, embolisms, and thrombosis. Various techniques have been devised. (10, 11, 12, 13)

    —*aortic arch catheterization, thoracic aortography*—this procedure includes a percutaneous puncture with insertion of a catheter, with retrograde advancement into the aortic arch (usually by the transfemoral route) and an arterial injection of a contrast medium for each of the serial angiograms. In occlusive disease or tortuosity of the iliacs, a brachial, axillary, or subclavian artery may be used. The procedure demonstrates the site and extent of vascular occlusions and of collateral blood vessels and permits the determination of the regional circulation time.

    —*vertebrobasilar angiography*—visualization of the vertebral arteries is achieved in various ways. For example, a right vertebral artery can be identified by introducing a contrast medium into the brachiocephalic trunk via a percutaneous puncture of the right subclavian artery, followed by a series of angiograms. The procedure is used primarily in detecting subarachnoid hemorrhage and subtentorial abnormalities. (10, 50)

- *computed intracranial tomography*—radiologic method using an automatic computerized tomographic scanner for establishing a diagnosis. The patient's head is placed in the center of the scanning ring, and the x-ray beam is directed to scan the brain from a number of different angles. Contiguous slices show differential tissue absorption, which is calculated by a computer and presented in a series of images of the cerebral structures. Computed tomography of the brain tends to detect:

    —primary or metastatic brain lesions, brain abscesses, and subdural hematomas.

    —strokes resulting from cerebral hemorrhage, as well as distinguishing strokes resulting from cerebral infarction. In computed tomograpy (CT) evaluation of a stroke condition, additional data may be obtained when CT scans are performed both before and after the intravenous administration of contrast material. The delayed contrast enhancement in CT is more informative than the immediate scan. Although cerebral angiography may be the only technique other than direct pathologic examination to determine specifically the nature of a vascular disease process, it does appear that the CT alterations may be strongly suggestive in aiding the physician to determine the etiology of the vascular disease process, e.g., in the case of a stroke patient. Computed tomography scanning, when concerned with endocrine disorders, tends to identify:

    –pinealomas, including solid and cystic teratomas, pineal blastomas, cystomas, and gliomas.

    –cystic changes within the pituitary gland; or a craniopharyngioma, an avascular mass in the suprasellar area with calcification and cystic components. (4, 7, 11, 42)

- *computed tomography of cord*—procedure demonstrating the spinal cord, nerve roots and sheaths, nerves, ganglia, and intervertebral disks. (19, 74)

- *discography*—diagnostic aid in the detection of a herniated lumbar or cervical disk followed by radiographs of the spine. Discography may be performed prior to lower lumbar spinal fusions as a mechanism to evaluate the integrity of the disk immediately above the level of planned fusion. Also, discography may be performed in conjunction with chemonucleolysis and disk aspiration. (19, 74)
- *dynamic computed tomography*—rapid scanning technique that delineates vascular perfusion and enhancement patterns of normal vessels, as well as abnormal lesions indicative of neoplasia, vascular occlusions, or other disorders. (54, 96)
- *epidural venography*—indirect technique for investigating intervertebral disks, vertebrae, spinal cord, and other neural components by visualizing the anterior epidural veins and their relationship to these structures. The epidural venous plexus can be opacified by catheterization and injection of contrast material into an ascending lumbar, presacral, radicular, intervertebral, or internal iliac veins. The anterior internal vertebral veins lie between the nerve roots and the intervertebral disks and may display compression by a herniating disk before there is impingement upon the dural sac. The main indication for lumbar epidural venography is to confirm the presence and location of a suspected disk herniation. (35)
- *myelography*—the injection of a radiopaque substance into the subarachnoid space by lumbar or cisternal puncture. The procedure permits the fluoroscopic observation of the contrast medium in the spinal canal as it rises and falls when the patient's position is changed. (62, 63)
- *ventriculography*—the introduction of air into the ventricular system following the removal of cerebrospinal fluid. This procedure allows the radiographic examination of the brain.
- *xeroradiography of the thyroid*—radiographic imaging of the thyroid gland by using a selenium-coated plate and developing it without liquid chemicals. This technique is considered superior to plain soft tissue radiographs in the detection of calcifications of the thyroid in papillary adenocarcinoma. (7)

Terms Related to Cardiovascular Imaging

- *angiocardiography:*
  - *peripheral angiocardiography*—injection of contrast medium into the basilic or cephalic veins of the arm for examining the chambers of the heart and pulmonary circulation. (50, 84)
  - *selective angiocardiography*—injection of contrast material through a catheter placed into the chamber or vessel of interest. (84)
  - *selective retrograde aortography and left ventriculography*—retrograde aortic catheterization for passing a radiopaque catheter across the aortic valve into the left ventricle. The correct position of the catheter is ascertained either by fluoroscopic or television guidance or a radiogram. This method discloses ventricular septal defects, aneurysms, mitral and aortic regurgitation, and other pathology. (53, 84)
  - *selective right ventricular angiography*—visualization of the anatomic structures involved in tetralogy of Fallot, transposition of the great vessels, patent ductus arteriosus, and similar conditions. (84)
  - *sequential angiocardiography*—serial films taken at accurately recorded intervals. They reveal the time and sequence of filling of the great vessels and chambers of the heart, as well as their position, size, and configuration. (84)
- *angiocardiographic film techniques:*
  - *angiocardiography with large films*—technique using regular x-ray films with rapid

film changers of 2 to 12 films per second. Rapid filming of heart and vessels may be either single plane or biplane.

—*cineangiocardiography*—technique of recording the radiographic image of the heart and great blood vessels on motion picture film. This complex procedure combines cardiac catheterization and selective angiocardiography. Under fluoroscopic guidance the cardiac catheter is maneuvered through the heart chambers and pulmonary artery. An image amplifier visualizes the cardiovascular structures. The frame speed of the motion picture camera ranges from a few frames up to 200 frames. Both cineangiographic and large film techniques require a power injector with or without timing devices. (64)

- *angiocardiographic injection technique*—injection of contrast media via a catheter or needle, using a suitable pressure injector.

  —*standard injection of opaque substance*—injection with automatic high-pressure injector regardless of the time in the cardiac cycle.

  —*time injection of contrast material*—technique in which beginning of the injection may be triggered by electronic timing devices at any point in the cardiac cycle, using the electrocardiogram as a reference. It can be limited to the duration of either systole or diastole, depending on the lesion of the opacified chamber of interest, such as a systolic injection into the atrium and a diastolic injection into the ventricle.

- *aortography*—injection of opaque solution for x-ray examination of the aorta.

  —*abdominal aortogram*—injection of opaque solution into the abdominal aorta through a catheter that is introduced through the femoral artery or a needle puncture of the aorta in the lumbar region.

  —*thoracic aortogram*—injection of opaque solution into the ascending aorta via retrograde introduction of catheter, either through femoral or axillary arteries or by a cutdown of the brachial artery. (50, 78)

- *arteriography*—radiographic examination of arteries following the injection of a contrast medium. (50)

- *cardiac computed tomography*—sectional imaging of the heart using a computerized machine to demonstrate the size and shape of cardiac chambers, intracavitary masses, septal defect, aneurysm, and graft patency or occlusion after coronary bypass.

- *cardiac fluoroscopy*—x-ray examination of the heart using a fluoroscope, preferably an image intensifier coupled with closed-circuit television monitor that permits visualization of fine details because of contrast and increased brightness; useful in delineating cardiac motion and intracardiac calcifications. (64)

- *cardiac series with barium swallow*—the patient drinks a barium solution while fluoroscopic and radiographic examinations are performed to reveal abnormalities of the cardiac outline and esophageal displacement. (78)

- *cardiac tomography*—sectional radiography of the heart.

- *digital angiography, digital subtraction cardiography (DSA)*—vascular imaging with a digital subtraction apparatus following the intravenous or, infrequently, intraarterial injection of a contrast medium. DSA has been successfully used to demonstrate vascular abnormalities of the aorta and carotid and renal arteries. (50)

- *digital computer*—calculator using numbers that represent a decimal or other system. (60)

- *digital fluorography*—digital capabilities added to the conventional fluoroscopic procedure to provide clear, sharp images with the injection of a low-dose contrast medium.

- *digital video radiography device*—apparatus composed of an x-ray generator and tube, TV system, image intensifier, display device, and computer disk recorder, which serves real-time functions. (50)

- *digital video subtraction angiography*—the video imaging system applied to digital subtraction angiography. It may be used to detect renovascular abnormalities. (50)

Terms Related to Radiography of the Chest

- *bronchography*—radiographic examination of the bronchial tree following the intratracheal injection of an opaque solution. (37)
- *chest radiographs*—series of x-ray projections designed to evaluate chest, heart, lungs, and thoracic cage. These projections may demonstrate pulmonary diseases, blunt trauma to the chest, some congenital cardiac defects, and acquired heart disease. (37)
- *computed tomography of the bronchial tree*—by computerized device to visualize diseases and tumors of the bronchi. (37)
- *computed tomography of the lungs*—radiographic imaging of thin slices of lung tissue for diagnostic evaluation using a machine with an automatic electronic calculator. (37)
- *conventional tomography of the lungs*—body section radiographs that delineate a thin layer of lung tissue; thus the structures lying anteriorly and posteriorly are more or less blurred out. Tomographs demonstrate the presence of lung lesions. (38)
- *dynamic computed tomography of the lungs*—rapid sequence (dynamic) CT following the injection of an opaque medium into a peripheral vein for contrast enhancement to differentiate vascular and nonvascular lung lesions. (38)

Terms Related to Abdominal Imaging

- *air-contrast enema, double-contrast enema*—examination of the colon using a small amount of barium to coat the walls of the mucosa and air to distend the colon. This procedure may demonstrate intestinal polyps and rectal carcinoma. (64)
- *barium enema examination*—fluoroscopic and radiographic examination of the colon after administering a barium sulfate mixture rectally. Barium enemas are used in the treatment of intussusception, which is often reduced by the rectal instillation of barium under fluoroscopic guidance. (64)
- *barium upper gastrointestinal examination*—radiologic study of the integrity of esophagus, duodenum, and upper small intestine. Study also may indicate some changes in the pancreatic or biliary system, alerting the radiologist to possible obstructive or disease processes in those areas. (8)
- *cholangiography*—introduction of radiopaque material into the bile ducts for x-ray examination of the biliary system.
    - *endoscopic retrograde cholangiography (ERC)*—provides direct injection of the common bile duct with contrast material. This study is of value in detecting common duct stones, inflammatory abnormalities, and neoplastic ductal abnormalities.
    - *percutaneous transhepatic cholangiography*—allows the injection of contrast material under fluoroscopic vision through a narrow gauge needle positioned in the parenchyma of the liver. Like the ERC procedure, this procedure is of value in detecting common duct stones, inflammatory problems, and neoplastic ductal abnormalities. However, this procedure does provide the opportunity to institute biliary drainage if needed. Usually, this procedure is reserved for patients with biliary obstruction who require permanent or temporary biliary drainage. (2, 61)
- *cholecystokinin cholecystography (CCK-CCG)*—procedure valuable in the diagnosis of chronic acalculous cholecystitis or biliary dyskinesia. The gallbladder is opacified, and serial radiographs are obtained after intravenous administration of cholecystokinin. (2)

■ *computed tomography of the pancreas*—CT procedure of value if correlated with pancreatic ductography. Procedure demonstrates presence of pancreatitis and pancreatic cyst.

Terms Related to Urogenital Imaging

■ *plain radiograph of abdomen (KUB)**—radiograph made without injection of air or radiopaque solution to serve as contrast medium. The procedure is a preliminary step when urologic diagnosis is anticipated. (2, 61)

■ *urograph*—any radiograph, either of the entire tract or of a particular organ. A radiopaque solution is used for the visualization of the organs. (61)

■ *urography*—radiography concerned with detection of urologic disorders. Some special procedures are:

—*cineradiography of urinary tract*—urographic motion picture record of successive images appearing on a fluoroscopic screen to demonstrate transient or persistent vesicoureteral reflux after having gradually filled the bladder with radiopaque medium. (64)

—*computed renal tomography*—use of an automated electronic scanner with a calculator to differentiate between normal renal tissue, and renal tumors and cysts and to provide cancer staging. (92)

—*cystourethrography*—cystography combined with urethrography to visualize abnormalities of the bladder and urethra following blunt pelvic trauma. (92)

—*excretory urograph*—urograms demonstrating renal excretory function. They are obtained by intravenous injection of a contrast medium or, less frequently, by retrograde filling of a renal calices and pelves with radiopaque solution. Excretory urograms visualize tumors, cysts, hydronephrosis, pyelonephritis, calculi, and other obstructive lesions of the urinary tract; vesicoureteral reflux; and renal ischemia. (4, 92)

—*lymphangiography; pedal*—delineation of the lymphatic system after the injection of radiopaque material into both feet to visualize the lymphatic structures of the lower extremities: the groin, pelvis, periaortic region, and thoracic duct. (25)

—*nephrotomography*—body section radiography of the kidney, primarily for differentiating renal cysts and tumors. (92)

—*retrograde cystography*—vesical filling with opaque solution to detect bladder perforation due to injury and to study the neurogenic bladder. (92)

—*retrograde pyelography*—roentgenograms are obtained following direct instillation of contrast material into the pelvis via the catheters. The first roentgenograms are obtained after 3 to 5 ml of the contrast medium have been introduced through the ureteral catheter into the renal pelvis, and the second roentgenograms are obtained after the catheters are withdrawn. The main advantage of this procedure is that a dense contrast substance can be injected directly under controlled pressure resulting in good visualization. This procedure usually is employed when excretory urography has been inconclusive. (92)

Terms Related to Obstetric Imaging

■ *amniography*—radiography of the pregnant uterus after injecting a radiopaque substance into the amniotic fluid. The procedure permits an evaluation of the fetus, placenta, and amniotic sac. (64)

---

*KUB—kidney, ureter, and bladder

- *fetography*—radiographic study of the fetus in utero using a contrast medium with lipid affinity that coats the vernix and thus outlines the fetus. (64)
- *neonatal radiography*—radiologic investigation of the newborn to diagnose a major health problem such as congenital heart disease, increased size of the head and cerebral ventricles, esophageal atresia, tracheobronchial fistula, and urinary tract or large bowel disorder.* (64)
- *pelvimetry*—radiographic measurement of various obstetric diameters of the bony pelvis. (100)
- *pelvimetry and cephalometry*—radiographic measurement of the size of the fetal head in relation to the size of the pelvic diameters.* (100)
- *simple roentgenogram of abdomen and pelvis*—plain abdominal x-ray film may identify the fetal skeleton after 16 weeks of gestation.

Terms Related to Breast Imaging

- *ductography*—radiography procedure performed after injecting the mammary ducts with radiopaque contrast material. This technique is used to identify the discharging ductal system in three dimensions. It may provide a diagnosis, e.g., mass or suspicion of carcinoma, and it is helpful in localizing the origin of discharge prior to biopsy. (93)
- *mammography*—soft tissue mammary radiography based on varying degrees of absorption of the x-ray beam by fatty, fibroglandular, and cancerous tissue in the breast, in decreasing order of translucency. (40, 41, 72)
- *mammograms*—three radiographic views of the breast that outline:
  —benign lesions, nodules, or cysts, well circumscribed and usually surrounded by a thin halo of radiolucent fat.
  —malignant lesions, spicular, ragged and irregular in shape and poorly circumscribed, frequently associated with thickening and retracting of skin, nipple deformity, axillary lymph node involvement, microcalcifications, and venous congestion. Since the presence of fat serves to identify lesions, no radiopaque substance is injected into the lactiferous ducts. As a result, the breast is not distorted, and pathologic conditions are clearly delineated. Mammography may also be used in screening studies of asymptomatic women and in postmastectomy follow-up examinations. (40, 41)
- *thermography*—the recording of infrared radiations of the skin as a cancer detection tool. Black or dark areas of the thermogram register abnormally increased skin temperature, which may be indicative of the presence of a malignant lesion. (71)
- *xeroradiography of breast*—an x-ray method of obtaining images of breast structures on selenium-coated metal plates. (31)

Terms Related to Imaging of the Sense Organ of Vision

- *angiography of ophthalmic artery*—radiographic visualization of the ophthalmic artery for the detection of primary and metastatic tumors of the orbit, extraorbital neoplasms, vascular malformations, and occlusions and aneurysms of the ophthalmic artery. (10)
- *computed tomography in ophthalmology*—use of an automatic electronic machine that provides scans of tissue planes at a given thickness. In ophthalmology, scans are made of the orbit, including the lateral and third ventricles, to detect orbital disease or tumors as well as intracranial lesions: optic glioma, metastasis, or brain injury.

---

*These radiographic procedures are rarely done today, since they expose the unborn child to the danger of ionizing radiation. They are replaced by obstetric ultrasonic imaging, which has no known health hazards.

Computed tomography used in ocular motility disorders can demonstrate the anatomy and (to some degree) the physiology of extraocular muscles, as well as any intracranial neurologic cause. Extraocular muscle enlargement in Graves' disease and associated compressive neuropathy also may be visualized by computed tomography scanning. (10, 65)

- *distention dacryocystography*—forceful injection of contrast medium into a canaliculus during x-ray exposure to outline that nasolacrimal duct system in its distended state. Direct x-ray magnification aids in the detection of the obstructive lesion. (6)
- *orbital arteriography*—serial angiograms of the orbital arteries, primarily via the ophthalmic branch of the internal carotid artery and secondarily via branches of the external carotid artery. The technique is used to detect arterial malformation or arteriovenous fistula of orbital vessels. (10)
- *orbital tomography*—tomographic sections of the orbit delineating its extent, size and relation to adjoining structures. (10, 97)
- *orbital venography*—procedure used to localize space-occupying lesions within the orbit. The rise of computed tomography usage to demonstrate these lesions has decreased markedly the use of orbital venography. Currently, orbital venography is used to demonstrate orbital venous malformations and cavernous sinus thrombosis. (43)
- *orbitography*—useful diagnostic procedure for localization of retrobulbar tumors before visual damage has become irreparable. Two types of the procedure are:
    - *negative contrast orbitography, orbital pneumotomography*—radiographic visualization of the orbit using air or oxygen as the contrast medium. It is indicated primarily when tumors of the optic nerve are suspected. (10, 97)
    - *positive contrast orbitography*—radiographic visualization of the orbit using water-soluble preparations as contrast media. Retrobulbar lesions may be found in the muscle cone of the superior rectus. (10, 97)

Terms Related to Imaging of the Sense Organ of Hearing

- *polytomography, tomography, otic*—multiple serial section views of the ear that are of diagnostic value in middle and inner ear disorders, such as pure cochlear otosclerosis, Meniére's disease, and others. It is also helpful in detecting the site of facial nerve injury by cholesteatoma or glomus jugulare, intracranial extension of glomus tumor, translucent areas of temporal bone, malformations of the middle and inner ear, and ossicular chain injury. (94)
- *posterior fossa myelography*—radiologic procedure that aids in the detection of space-occupying lesions, particularly acoustic neuroma, meningioma, and primary cholesteatoma. (96)
- *retrograde jugular venography*—venogram that demonstrates either a normal jugular vein or a venous narrowing caused by external pressure of a partial or total occlusion of the jugular vein within the jugular fossa. The procedure is indicated when a glomus jugular tumor is suspected. (82)

Terms Related to Radiation Injury

- *overirradiation*—excessive radiation therapy. It may cause a syndrome characterized by nausea, vomiting, diarrhea, anorexia, and malaise within hours after overexposure, followed by blood dyscrasia within weeks or months. (64)
- *radiation anemia*—usually aplastic anemia; no red blood cells are formed due to suppression of bone marrow activity. It occurs following excessive whole body radiation. (64)
- *radiodermatitis*—inflammation of skin resulting from exposure to radiation. (64)

- *radioepithelitis*—disintegration of epithelial tissue due to radiation, notably to that of the mucous membrane. (64)
- *radionecrosis*—disintegration or death of tissue caused by radiation. (64)
- *radionephritis*—acute condition caused by overexposure of the kidney to radiation. It is manifested by hypertension, edema, casts, and protein in the urine. (64)
- *radioneuritis*—nerve involvement resulting from overexposure to radioactivity. (64)
- *radiation sickness*—untoward effects of radiotherapy, usually manifested by nausea, vomiting, and diarrhea, resulting from the breakdown of body tissue. (64)

Diagnostic Ultrasound

General Terms

- *diagnostic ultrasonography*—the recording of ultrasonic waves as they pass through deep structures of different density to locate pathologic lesions. (45, 102)
    - *—gray-scale ultrasound*—an ultrasound image containing various shades of gray rather than only black and white. A gray-scale image contains more complete information, since echoes of the intermediate strength are recorded. (24, 45)
    - *—real-time imaging*—method of representation that displays images almost as fast as they are produced, permitting them to be viewed without delay. (45, 102)
    - *—real-time ultrasound computer*—instrument that provides diagnostic data for application in abdominal ultrasound, echocardiography, and peripheral vascular studies. (102)
- *echography*—reflected ultrasound imaging. Related terms are:
    - *—anechoic, sonolucent*—echo-free, nonproductive of echoes.
    - *—echogenic*—echo-producing, productive of echoes.
    - *—echogenicity*—ability to produce echoes.
    - *—echogram*—graphic record of reflected ultrasound imaging. (102)
    - *—echographic elements:*
        - *—attenuation sign*—decrease in reflective sound or echoes in solid tissue to differentiate solid from cystic fluid-filled lesions. (102)
        - *—posterior echo accumulation sign*—an indication of the fluid-filled cystic nature of an anechoic pattern. (102)
        - *—reflection*—the return of an echo from a surface, the strength of return being related to impedance. (24, 102)
        - *—strength of echo*—sensitivity of sound beam, capable of delineating differences in tissue density with minute precision. (67, 102)
        - *—ultrasonic tissue differentiation*—echogenicity of tissue is variable, since stiffness or bulk influence the sonographic beam; for example, thick barium prevents ultrasound transmission, and thin barium allows some ultrasound transmission. (102)
        - *—collagen*—supporting tissue of various organs is thought to be a source of echogenicity. When a tumor replaces normal collagen, the echogenicity is decreased in the organ.
        - *—fat*—this tissue is of considerable echogenicity.
        - *—fluid*—cell-free fluid is sonolucent. Tumors are echogenic; cysts are echo-free. (102)
- *general measurements:*
    - *—density*—mass per unit of volume.
    - *—frequency*—number of cycles per second. (45, 51)
        - *—Hertz (Hz)*—a unit of frequency equivalent to one cycle per second.

—*megaHertz*—1,000,000 Hertz or one million cycles per second (Hz = 1 cycle per second).

—*impedance*—product of the density and velocity of a material. (102)

—*sonic*—pertaining to the audible range; sound is heard by the human ear.

  –*infrasonic, subsonic*—below the audible range; sound is too weak to be heard.

  –*ultrasonic, ultrasound*—"above the audible range" refers to sound beams of frequencies over 20,000 per second, which are inaudible to human hearing. (22, 102)

—*sound wave*—mechanical disturbance propagating through a liquid, solid, or gas medium. Sound waves are produced by vibrating sources that are in contact with the medium.

  –*longitudinal wave*—occurs as a sound wave travels through air, water, or soft tissue; the particles in the medium vibrate parallel to the direction of propagation of the sound wave.

  –*sound wave frequency*—determined by the number of oscillations per second made by the vibrating source. (45, 102)

—*velocity*—product of frequency times the wave length.

—*wave*—distance traveled per unit of time.

—*wave length*—distance between one given point and the next similar point of a wave measured in the direction of propagation. (45)

■ *ultrasonic scan*—any procedure that moves the sonic beam and is simultaneously followed by the trace. (102)

■ *ultrasonic transducer*—electronic instrument that converts electric energy into mechanical energy. Some related terms are:

  —*coupling agent*—agent needed to keep the ultrasound transducer in contact with the skin, such as a soluble aqueous gel.

  —*crystal*—component of transducer that sends out vibrations, producing sound. (102)

■ *ultrasound imaging methods:*

  —*modes*—methods of display or imaging. (See Fig. 81.)

  –*A-mode*—amplitude modulation that portrays echoes as vertical spikes and reflects the height of the spike in proportion to the strength of the echoes. The transducer remains stationary. In the A-mode a single beam of sound waves and its reflection creates a simple linear display on an oscilloscope. (45, 102)

  –*B-mode*—brightness modulation that depicts echoes on a linear trace as dots differing in size and intensity relative to the strength of the echoes and producing a two-dimensional cross-sectional display. Two methods are used:

    B-mode in time motion (TM)—the transducer remains in a fixed position while used to reflect echoes of a moving structure. Difference in strength of echoes may be portrayed by various shades of gray. The gray-scale scan is static.

    B-mode, B scan, ultrasonography—the transducer is guided across the body region under study producing a transsectional, two-dimensional image of the structures. This method, known as real-time scanning, is dynamic. (45, 102)

  –*M-mode*—motion modulation that displays the changing pattern in echoes, with the transducer in a fixed position and the trace moving sideways. (76, 102)

  —*Doppler ultrasound*—continuous ultrasonography, concerned with the change in the frequency of sound waves, which are reflected from a pulsating target or circulating blood in a vessel and are transmitted as audible sounds. (45, 57, 102)

Figure 81 Three methods of ultrasound imaging. (The B and M modes are schematic.)

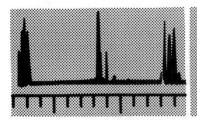 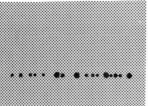 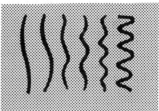

A-mode: amplitude, spikes   B-mode: brightness, dots   M-mode or T-mode: time motion

Selected Ultrasonic Studies

Terms Related to Diagnostic Ultrasound of the Brain and Thyroid

- *echoencephalography*—rapid determination of intracranial midline displacements using ultrasonic pulse echo techniques. As soon as the density of the brain tissue is altered, a pulse beam of high-frequency sound, emitted by the transmitter, will echo back and be recorded on an oscillographic screen. The procedure aids in the detection of pressure-producing and space-occupying brain lesions, cerebrovascular disease, seizure disorder, hydrocephalus, mental retardation, and brain death. (64)
- *transcranial Doppler (TCD) sonography*—ultrasonographic technique for recording blood flow velocities in the basal cerebral arteries. Also, this technique is utilized to assess the time course and severity of vasospasm following subarachnoid hemorrhage, as well as to detect stenosis and occlusions of intracranial arteries and to study the intracranial hemodynamics in carotid artery disease. (44, 68)
- *ultrasonography (Doppler) in supraorbital region*—blood flow measurements by the transmission of a sound wave of ultrasonic frequency.
    - *—normal blood flow*—the direction of the blood flow is from the ophthalmic artery into the supraorbital artery and over some ramifications into the external carotid artery.
    - *—retrograde blood flow*—reversal of the blood flow occurs in occlusion of the internal carotid artery and is detectable by ultrasonography. (6, 43, 45, 97)
- *ultrasonography of the thyroid gland*—diagnostic ultrasound, a simple noninvasive method for ascertaining the size of the thyroid gland and nodule and differentiating solid from cystic lesions. B-mode ultrasonography offers information about hypofunctioning thyroid nodules and aids in establishing patterns for cystadenoma, multinodular goiter, and thyroiditis. It is a safe procedure in the assessment of pediatric and pregnant patients with thyroid lesions. (7)

Terms Related to Diagnostic Ultrasound of Cardiovascular Disorders

- *continuous-wave Doppler technique*—method involving continuous transmission of ultrasound waves coupled with continuous ultrasound reception. The principal advantage of continuous-wave Doppler is its ability to measure high blood cell velocities. The main disadvantage of this method is its lack of depth discrimination. Usually, this method is not incorporated into color flow systems. (59, 90)
- *pulsed Doppler technique*—noninvasive, nontraumatic method of comprehensive and quantitative assessment of blood flow to a structure or organ. A primary concern is the detection of blood flow disturbances in mitral stenosis, aortic, mitral, and pulmonic regurgitation, and in congenital defects such as patent ductus arteriosus and ventricular septal defect. (59, 90)

- *Doppler ultrasonic flowmetry*—ultrasound techniques for obtaining phasic, continuous, and instantaneous measurement of velocity (speed) of blood flow in various cardiovascular disorders, especially in aortic valvar disease and venous thrombosis. (59, 90)
- *Doppler color flow mapping*—method whereby the characteristics of blood flow (direction, velocity, and size) are displayed on the two-dimensional echocardiographic image by means of color encoding of the Doppler-generated flow signal. The usual method to visualize Doppler color flow data is in real-time at the time of the examination. However, images may also be recorded on video tape for review and analysis after examination. In color flow imaging, the colors red and blue represent the direction of a given jet, while the various hues from dull to bright represent the velocities. The brighter the hue, the faster the velocity; the duller the hue, the slower the velocity. Doppler color flow mapping is noninvasive, relatively inexpensive, with little patient risk in comparison to other imaging methods, and makes flow information readily available for patient care. (59)
- *echoaortography*—ultrasonic study of the aorta. (45)
  - *—B-mode imaging*—ultrasound technique for detecting atheromatous lesions, calcifications, or aneurysms of the aorta. A thrombus may produce fine echoes; a dissecting aneurysm, thin linear echoes; and advanced calcifications, strong echoes.
  - *—gray-scale imaging*—echographic method for detecting abdominal aortic aneurysm and measuring the vascular lumen distinct from the thrombus, which transmits denser internal echoes than the lumen.
  - *—echography of aortic root*—screening technique for assessing bicuspid aortic valve, a congenital defect that predisposes to serious aortic disorders. The normal aortic valve has three cusps. (45, 69)
- *echocardiography*—graphic recording of ultrasound waves reflected from the heart for the purpose of determining the development and severity of mitral stenosis, delineating such conditions as pericardial effusion, congenital, and acquired heart disease. Intraoperative echocardiography includes assessment of left ventricular size and function: monitoring of left ventricular performance; imaging of coronary arteries; and assessment of coronary flow velocity, myocardial perfusion, and adequacy of mitral valve operations. (32, 90)
  - *—Doppler echocardiography*—utilizes ultrasound to record blood flow within the cardiovascular system. This technique focuses primarily on cardiac function in contrast to emphasis primarily on structure. Doppler echocardiography provides excellent noninvasive hemodynamic information. It may be used as a screening mechanism for suspected valvular disease. Doppler echocardiography is the technique of choice for assessing the pressure gradient in valvular stenosis. Doppler echocardiography is a very effective instrument in detecting valvular regurgitation and intracardiac shunt lesions. (1, 32, 48, 90, 91)
  - *—two-dimensional echocardiography*—reliable study of the heart in cross-section for detecting asynergy of the left ventricle in ischemic heart disease. It is useful in establishing the diagnosis of congenital, valvular, and coronary heart disease, as well as acute myocardial infarction and its complications. (1, 32, 76, 90)
  - *—two dimensional real-time echocardiography*—valuable noninvasive technique that uses a multiple transducer for imaging positions and permits appreciation of spatial relationships of cardiac anatomy.   (32, 76)
- *ultrasound in pulmonary disease*—lung echograms aiding in the diagnosis of pulmonary embolism and thromboembolism, pleural effusion, pleural thickening, and calcification.
- *preoperative saphenous ultrasonic venography*—use of a high resolution B-mode imager

to map the saphenous vein. This is a safe and accurate method of providing the surgical team with valuable anatomic and physiologic data about the saphenous vein and is an effective tool to be employed in preoperative planning and decision making. This data may assist the surgeon to decrease the length of skin incision required in performing an *in situ* bypass, identify the location of major tributaries that may produce arteriovenous fistulae, identify valves that are not competent and need to be excised. In addition, the data may enable the surgeon to evaluate the adequacy of the vein, either for reversed vein bypass or coronary bypass as well as to determine the presence of old disease and to permit the maximal amount of vein to be preserved for later use. (14)

Terms Related to Diagnostic Ultrasound of the Urinary Tract

- *renal sonogram, nephrosonogram*—record of ultrasonic waves passing through the renal tissue for the purpose of determining the size and location of the kidney. Sonograms may detect congenital anomalies, such as horseshoe kidney, agenesis, and renal ectopy; aid in differentiating between hydronephrosis, unilateral multicystic kidney, and polycystic kidney; and demonstrate cyst-tumor deformity and leukemic infiltration of the kidney. (5, 80)
- *ultrasonic scanning of renal transplant*—serial volume measurements of kidney transplant by ultrasound to detect changes in size, such as:
    - —an increase in renal size with or without scattered echoes from collecting tubules in acute rejection of transplant. (83)
    - —a decrease in size, usually present in chronic rejection of transplant.
- *ultrasonic vesical scanning*—echographic imaging of intravesical calculi, clots, diverticula, papillomas, primary or metastatic bladder tumors, prostatic hypertrophy, chronic granulomatous cystitis, and other disorders. (5, 83)
- *urologic ultrasonography*—the diagnostic use of sound beam echoes in the detection of renal tumors or cysts, perirenal abscess, retroperitoneal mass or hemorrhage, polycystic kidneys, testicular torsion, and prostatic disorder. Infantile polycystic kidney disease may be diagnosed by in utero sonography. (21, 46, 80)

Terms Related to Diagnostic Ultrasound of the Abdomen

- *abdominal echography*—the use of noninvasive diagnostic ultrasound for studying the liver, gallbladder, and pancreas, spleen, kidney, aorta, and retroperitoneal space. It aids in the detection of intraabdominal abscesses, cysts, or tumors. (61)
- *biliary echography*—ultrasound imaging of the gallbladder and biliary ducts, which may be anechoic or display variable echoes: small, thin or coarse, strong, reflected, or few or multiple, depending on the biliary pathology, such as dilated bile ducts and gallbladder obstructed by cancer of the ampulla; hydrops of the gallbladder due to obstruction of the cystic duct; fluid-filled gallbladder portrayed by acoustic lucency, or gallstones seen by acoustic shadows. (8)
- *hepatic echography*—ultrasonic investigation revealing either a normal liver or specific echogenicity, as present in hepatic cirrhosis, ascites, liver abscess, fluid-filled cysts, hepatoma, cancer, and metastasis.
- *pancreatic echography*—noninvasive ultrasound technique producing characteristic echoes that aid in the differential diagnosis of pancreatic cysts and pseudocysts, tumors, cancer, and pancreatitis. (61)
- *sonographic bowel examination*—ultrasound imaging employed in finding and differentiating neoplastic masses, cysts, and abscesses. (61)
- *ultrasound guidance of abdominal biopsy*—ultrasound is one of the imaging modalities used for guiding percutaneous biopsy of the abdomen. The other methods are computed tomography and fluoroscopy. (64)

Table 34
Ultrasonic Findings Related to Ovarian Lesions

Ovarian Cysts and Tumors	Ultrasonic Identification*
Follicular cysts, luteal cysts	Complete cystic adnexal mass; demonstrates no internal echoes; appearance is anechoic.
Endometriomas	Completely cystic adnexal mass. Echogenic material's internal consistency ranges from completely anechoic to homogenously echoic depending on the presence and amount of the internal clot. Sometimes, endometriomas can be differentiated from other benign cystic adnexal masses by their irregular borders, which are the result of fibrosis occurring around the mass.
Mucinous cystadenomas	Predominately cystic mass but with some thin internal septations. The mucinous secretions within the cyst may appear as echogenic layering material within the mass.
Dermoid cysts	Cystic and solid components with echogenic material that does not demonstrate a change in configuration.
Hemorrhagic corpus luteum cysts	Complex mass with cystic and solid components. Echogenic material within these masses represents organized hemorrhage that may be attached to the wall of the mass by several thin synechiae.
Fibroma	Completely solid mass. These masses are echogenic because of the dense collagen contained within them. Areas of internal hemorrhage can be encountered in this type of solid mass.
Granulosa cell tumor	Complex mass, predominately solid with some hypoechoic areas caused by internal hemorrhage or necrosis. This type of mass may also exhibit irregular septations and may be multiloculated.

*Adapted from Arthur C. Fleischer and Stephen S. Entman. Sonographic evaluation of the ovary and related disorders. Rudy E. Sabbagha, ed., *Diagnostic Ultrasound Applied to Obstetrics and Gynecology,* 2nd ed. Philadelphia: J.B. Lippincott Co., 1987, pp. 497-520.

Terms Related to Diagnostic Ultrasound in Gynecology and Obstetrics

- *fetal echocardiography*—ultrasound examination of human fetal cardiac development and function in utero. By the early second trimester, the fetal heart is seen as a distinct, contracting fluid-filled structure. By the midsecond trimester, the cardiac chambers and valves can be depicted and studied. Cardiac structures are usually imaged by cross-sectional echocardiography and augmented by a combination of range-gated pulsed Doppler ultrasonography and M-mode echocardiography. The joining of Doppler ultrasonographic techniques with the two-dimensional echocardiogram, and the representation in color of abnormalities in flow, volume, and direction serve to aid the physician in establishing a definitive diagnosis. Pulsed Doppler ultrasound examination combined with findings from fetal echocardiographic examination often detect such defects as hypoplastic left heart syndromes or Ebstein's malformation of the tricuspid valve. (33, 90, 91)
- *gynecologic ultrasonography*—the diagnostic use of ultrasound in detecting ovarian masses, pelvic inflammations, abnormalities of uterus, and tubo-ovarian abscesses. (See Table 34.) (86, 100)

- *obstetric echocardiography*—cardiac evaluation of maternity patient with pericardial effusion, mitral valve disease, or cardiomyopathy by using ultrasound to assess the cardiac status and estimate the volume overload to the heart. (32)
- *obstetric ultrasonography*—ultrasound technique for detecting fetal abnormalities, such as fetal hydrops, anencephaly and maternal disorders: hydramnios, ectopic pregnancy, hydatidiform mole, fibroids, or cysts associated with pregnancy. Ultrasound is used in normal placental localization and the detection of placenta previa, and twin placentas, as well as pinpointing the best placental puncture site before amniocentesis. (56, 86, 100)
- *pulse echosonography in early pregnancy*—detection of intrauterine gestation.
    - —after five to six weeks of amenorrhea, a white ring delineating the gestational sac is visible on sonograph.
    - —at eight weeks of pregnancy distinct echoes from the embryo are present within the sac and it is possible to estimate the gestational age from the length of the embryo. A poorly defined or small gestational sac or absent echoes suggest a blighted ovum, dead embryo, and threatened abortion.
    - —after 11 weeks gestation fetal heart action is detected by real-time sonography or Doppler instrument. (89)
- *ultrasonic cephalometry*—A-mode and B-mode ultrasonic techniques combined for determining the biparietal diameter (BPD) as a means of estimating the size, weight, and probable gestational age of the fetus. (100)
- *ultrasonography in abortion*—ultrasonic detection is a useful diagnostic test in making a differential diagnosis, which usually consists of missed or incomplete abortion, threatened abortion, spontaneous abortion, ectopic pregnancy, or gestational trophoblastic disease. In some cases, solid echogenic material is detected within the endometrial cavity, possibly indicating an incomplete abortion with the echogenic material representing clotted blood and retained products of conception. This could also represent the presence of early gestational trophoblastic disease. A quantitative serum B-hCG level is helpful in distinguishing between these two disorders; the level is elevated in gestational trophoblastic disease and low in an incomplete abortion. (100)
- *ultrasound monitoring of fetus*—real-time ultrasound provides assessment of fetal well-being by documenting fetal activity. This type of sonographic biophysical data assesses variations of fetal heart rate, fetal breathing activities, coarse and fine motor activity, fetal tone, and amniotic fluid volume. (100)
- *ultrasound scan of the fetal spine*—direct visualization of neural tube defects using a high-resolution real-time scanner for obtaining longitudinal and transverse sections of the fetal spine. (86)
- *ultrasound scan of the neonatal brain*—safe, noninvasive imaging modality providing detailed visualization of the ventricles and intracranial structures of the neonate and promoting the assessment of hydrocephalus, cystic lesions, and cerebral hemorrhage. The skull defect in encephalocele is also delineated by ultrasound. (86)

Magnetic Resonance Imaging

General Terms (3)*

- *artifacts*—false features in the image produced by the imaging process. The random fluctuation of intensity due to noise can be considered separately from artifacts.

---

*Reprinted by permission, from the American College of Radiology. *Glossary of MR Terms*, 2nd ed. Reston, VA: American College of Radiology, 1986.

- *Carr-Purcell (CP) sequence*—sequence of a 90° radio frequency (RF) pulses to produce a train of spin echoes; if useful for measuring T2.
- *Carr-Purcell-Meiboom-Gill (CPMG)*—modification of Carr-Purcell RF pulse sequence with 90° phase shift in the rotating frame of reference between the 90° pulse and subsequent 180° pulses. Suppression of effects of pulse error accumulation can alternatively be achieved by switching phases of the 180° pulses by 180°.
- *chemical shift reference*—a compound with respect to whose frequency the chemical shifts of other compounds can be compared. The standard can either be internal or external to the sample. Because of the need for possible corrections due to differential magnetic susceptibility between an external standard and the sample being measured, the use of an internal standard is generally preferred.
- *chemical shift imaging*—a magnetic resonance imaging technique that provides mapping of the regional distribution of intensity (images) of a restricted range of chemical shifts, corresponding to individual spectral lines or groups of lines.
- *continuous wave NMR (CW)*—a technique for studying nuclear magnetic resonance (NMR) by continuously applying RF radiation to the sample and slowly sweeping either the RF frequency or the magnetic field through the resonance values; now largely superceded by pulse MR techniques.
- *dipole interaction*—interaction between a spin and its neighbors due to their magnetic dipole moments. This is an important mechanism contributing to relaxation times. In solids and viscous liquids this can result in broadening of the spectral lines.
- *eddy currents*—electric currents induced in a conductor by a changing magnetic field or by motion of the conductor through a magnetic field; these represent one source of concern (among others) about potential hazard to subjects in very high magnetic fields or rapidly varying gradient or main magnetic fields.
- *electron spin resonance (ESR)*—magnetic resonance phenomenon involving unpaired electrons, e.g., in free radicals. The frequencies are much higher than corresponding NMR frequencies in the same static magnetic field.
- *Faraday shield*—electrical conductor interposed between transmitter and/or receiver coil and patient to block out electric fields.
- *Fast Fourier transform (FFT)*—an efficient computational method of performing a Fourier transform.
- *Fourier transform (FT)*—a mathematical procedure to separate out the frequency components of a signal from its amplitudes as a function of time, or visa versa. The Fourier transform is used to generate the spectrum from the FID or spin echo in pulse MR techniques and is essential to most MR imaging techniques.
- *free induction decay (FID)*—if transverse magnetization of the spins is produced, e.g., by a 90° pulse, a transient MR signal will result that will decay toward zero with a characteristic time constant T2 (or T-two-star); this decaying signal is the FID. In practice, the first part of the FID is not observable because of residual effects of the powerful exciting RF pulse on the electronics of the receiver, the receiver dead time.
- *gradient*—the amount and direction of the rate of change in space of some quantity, such as magnetic field strength. Also commonly used to refer to magnetic field gradient.
- *gradient coils*—current carrying coils designed to produce a desired magnetic field gradient (so that the magnetic field will be stronger in some locations than others). Proper design of the size and configuration of the coils is necessary to produce a controlled and uniform gradient.
- *gradient echo*—spin echo produced by reversing the direction of a magnetic field gradient or by applying balanced pulses so as to cancel out the position-dependent

phase shifts that have accumulated because of the gradient. In the latter case, the gradient echo is generally adjusted to be coincident with the RF spin echo.

- *gyromagnetic ratio (γ)* — the ratio of the magnetic movement to the angular momentum of a particle. This is a constant for a given nucleus.
- *Hertz (Hz)* — the standard (SI) unit of frequency; equal to the old unit, cycles per second.
- *interpulse time* — time between successive RF pulse used in pulse sequences. Particularly important are the inversion time (TI) in inversion recovery, and the time between 90° pulse and the subsequent 180° pulse to produce a spin echo, which will be approximately one half the spin echo time (TE). The time between repetitions of pulse sequences is the repetition time (TR).
- *Kilohertz (kHz)* — unit of frequency; equal to one thousand hertz.
- *Larmor equation* — states that the frequency of precession of the nuclear magnetic moment is proportional to the magnetic field

$$\omega_o = -\gamma B_o \qquad \text{(radians per second)}$$

or

$$f_o = -\gamma B_o/2\pi \qquad \text{(hertz)}$$

Where ω_o or f_o is the frequency, γ is the gyromagnetic ratio, and B_o is the magnetic induction field. The negative sign indicates the direction of the rotation.

- *magnetic dipole* — north and south magnetic poles separated by a finite distance. An electric current loop, including the effective current of a spinning nucleon or nucleus, can create an equivalent magnetic dipole.
- *magnetic field gradient* — a magnetic field that changes in strength in a certain given direction. Such fields are used in NMR imaging with selective excitation to select a region for imaging and also to encode the location of NMR signals received from the object being imaged. Measured in teslas per meter.
- *magnetic moment* — a measure of the net magnetic properties of an object or particle. A nucleus with an intrinsic spin will have an associated magnetic dipole moment, so that it will interact with the magnetic field (as if it were a tiny bar magnet).
- *magnetic resonance (MR)* — resonance phenomenon resulting in the absorption and/or emission of electromagnetic energy by nuclei or electrons in a static magnetic field, after excitation by a suitable RF magnetic field. The peak resonance frequency is proportional to the magnetic field and is given by the Larmor equation. Only unpaired electron nuclei with a non-zero spin exhibit magnetic resonance.
- *magnetic resonance imaging (MRI)* — use of magnetic resonance to create images of objects such as the body. Currently, this primarily involves imaging the distribution of mobile hydrogen nuclei (protons) in the body. The image brightness depends jointly on the spin density (N(H)) and the relaxation times (T1 and T2), with their relative importance depending on the particular imaging technique and choice of interpulse times. Image brightness is also affected by any motion such as blood flow, respiration, etc.
- *megahertz (MHz)* — unit of frequency, equal to one million hertz.
- *pulse sequences* — set of RF (and/or gradient) magnetic field pulses and time spacings between these pulses; used in conjunction with magnetic field gradients and NMR signal reception to produce NMR images. See also interpulse times definition. A recommended shorthand designation of interpulse times used to generate a particular image is to list the repetition time (TR), the echo time (TE), and, if using inversion-recovery, the inversion time (TI), with all times given in milliseconds. For

example, 2500/30/1000 would indicate an inversion-recovery pulse sequence with TR of 2500 msec, TE of 30 msec, and TI of 1000 msec. If using multiple spin echoes, as in CPMG (Carr-Purcell-Meiboom-Gill), the number of spin echoes used should be stated.

- *radiofrequency (RF)*—wave frequency intermediate between auditory and infrared. The RF use in NMR studies is commonly in the megahertz (MHz) range. The RF used in ESR studies is commonly in the gigahertz (GHz) range. The principle effect of RF magnetic fields on the body is power deposition in the form of heating, mainly at the surface; this is a principal area of concern for safety limits.

- *RF pulse*—burst of RF magnetic field delivered to object by RF transmitter. For RF frequency near the Larmor frequency, it will result in rotation of the macroscopic magnetization vector in the rotating frame of reference (or a more complicated nutational motion in the stationary frame of reference). The amount of rotation will depend on the strength and duration of the RF pulse; commonly used examples are $90°$ ($\pi/2$) and 180 (π) pulses.

- *shim coils*—coils carrying a relatively small current that are used to provide auxiliary magnetic fields in order to compensate for inhomogeneities in the main magnetic field of NMR system.

- *SIU (International System of Units)*—the preferred international standard system of physical units and measures.

- *solenoid coil*—a coil of wire wound in the form of a long cylinder. When a current is passed through the coil, the magnetic field within the coil is relatively uniform. Solenoid RF coils are commonly used when the static magnetic field is perpendicular to the long axis of the body.

- *spin density (N)*—the density of resonating spins in a given region; one of the principal determinants of the strength of the NMR signal from the region. The SI units would be moles/m^3. For water, there are about 1.1×10^5 moles of hydrogen per m^3, or .11 moles of hydrogen/cm^3. True spin density is not imaged directly, but must be calculated from signals received with different interpulse times.

- *spin echo*—reappearance of an NMR signal after the FID has apparently died away, as a result of the effective reversal of the dephasing of the spins (refocusing) by techniques such as specific RF pulse sequences, e.g, Carr-Purcell sequence (RF spin echo), or pairs of magnetic field gradient pulses (gradient echo), applied in times shorter than or on the order of T2. Unlike RF spin echos, gradient echos will not refocus phase differences because of chemical shifts or in homogeneities of the magnetic field.

- *spin echo imaging*—any of many MR imaging techniques in which the spin echo is used rather than the FID. Can be used to create images that depend strongly on T2 if TE has value approximately greater than T2 of the relevant image details. Note that spin echo imaging does not directly produce an image of T2 distribution. The spin echoes can be produced as a train of multiple echoes, e.g., using the CPMG pulse sequence.

- *T1 ("T-one" or T_1)*—spin-lattice or longitudinal relaxation time; the characteristic time constant for spins to tend to align themselves with the external magnetic field. Starting from zero magnetization in the z direction, the z magnetization will grow to 63% of its final maximal value in a time TI.

- *T2 ("T-two" or T_2)*—spin-spin or transverse relaxation time; the characteristic time constant for loss of phase coherence among spins oriented at an angle to the static magnetic field, due to interactions between spins, with resulting loss of transverse magnetization and NMR signal. Starting from a nonzero value of the magnetization in the xy plane, the xy magnetization will decay so that it loses 63% of its initial value in a time T2.

- *T2* ("T-two-star")*—the observed time constant of the FID due to loss of phase coherence among spins oriented at an angle to the static magnetic field, commonly due to a combination of magnetic filed inhomogeneities. ΔB, and spin-spin transverse relaxation with resultant more rapid loss in transverse magnetization and NMR signal. NMR signals can usually still be recovered as spin echo in times less than or on the order of T2. $1/T2^* \cong 1/T2 + \Delta\ \omega/2; \Delta\omega = \gamma\ \Delta\ B.$
- *Tesla (T)*—the preferred International System of Units measurement of magnetic flux density. One tesla is equal to 10,000 gauss, the older unit of measurement.
- *TI*—inversion time. In inversion recovery, the time between the middle of the inverting (180°) RF pulse and the middle of the subsequent exciting (90°) pulse to detect amount of longitudinal magnetization.
- *TR*—repetition time. The period of time between the beginning of a pulse sequence and the beginning of the succeeding (essentially identical) pulse sequence.
- *transmitter coil*—coil of the RF transmitter, used in excitation of spins.
- *zeugmatography*—term for MR imaging, coined from Greek roots, suggesting the role of the magnetic field gradient in joining the RF magnetic field to a desired local spatial region through magnetic resonance.

Oral Reading Practice

Selected Magnetic Resonance Imaging Studies
Brain, Skull Base, and Spinal Cord MR Imaging

Magnetic resonance imaging (MR or MRI) is capable of differentiating between **gray** and **white matter** within the brain substance and to provide excellent contrast between blood vessels and surrounding structures. The diagnosis of tumors in the **posterior fossa** region is greatly enhanced with MR imaging. **Primary hemangioblastomas** of the posterior fossa are easily depicted by MRI. The separate cystic and solid components may be easily differentiated. Hemangioblastomas are a primary characteristic of **von Hippel-Lindau disease.** Individuals with this familial neurocutaneous disorder may exhibit multiple site tumors. Any type of change or insult to the structure of the brain associated with alteration in water content or myelin can be depicted in abnormal signal intensity on MR imaging. MRI is a sensitive instrument to be utilized in the detection of a wide variety of **non-neoplastic processes** that affect the brain. Within a short period (usually a few hours) following vascular occlusion, MRI is capable of detecting and localizing the **cerebral infarction.** Due to MRI sensitivity to flowing blood, it has proven to be quite effective in detecting and localizing **arteriovenous malformations.** Also, MRI has detected **intracranial hemorrhage,** including hemorrhagic contusions and shearing injuries. (9, 15, 26, 49, 87)

MR imaging of the **skull base** offers several benefits such as lack of artifact from bone, multiple plane imaging, and minimal artifacts from dental fillings. Anatomic landmarks identified in the orbit by MR imaging are the **globe, rectus muscles, optic nerve,** and **blood vessels.** MR imaging detects **optic nerve** and **chiasmal gliomas;** however, it may be difficult to distinguish **optic nerve sheath tumors** from **optic nerve gliomas.** The MR imaging of anatomic landmarks in the **cerebellopontile angle cistern** and **temporal bone** include the **cranial nerves** VII **(facial nerve),** VIII **(vestibulocochlear nerve),** and the **vestibulocochlear apparatus.** MR imaging is effective in detecting **acoustic neuromas,** other cerebellopontine angles masses, and facial nerve tumors. (15, 26)

MR imaging is gradually becoming the procedure of choice used in the evaluation of abnormalities of the spinal axis. MRI has been helpful in the assessment of **intramedullary disease** (congenital, neoplastic, or demyelinating in origin). The ability to image the spinal cord in its entirety with MRI facilitates the diagnosis of intramedullary neoplasms. This is also important in patients with **vertebral metastatic disease,** since multiple lesions are usually present in these patients. MR imaging is site specific in defining the **demyelinating plaques** associated with **multiple sclerosis.** MR imaging is effective in detecting syringomyelia. Spinal cord abnormalities associated with **congenital spinal dysraphism** are well depicted by MR imaging. (23, 66, 75)

Musculoskeletal, Thoracic and Mediastinal Imaging

MR imaging depicts **aneurysmal bone cyst** as a well-defined expansile mass, occasionally with multiple internal septations. MR imaging demonstrates the severe marrow disorder of **Gaucher's disease** more effectively than other conventional methods. MRI can provide information on the extent of vascular invasion of **osteosarcoma** that is often difficult to assess on computed tomography. The skeletal and muscular components of the **pelvis** are well detected on T1-weighted images where the high-signal fat depicts the various muscle groups. MR imaging of the **iliopsoas** and other muscle groups appears to be superior to other modalities. The knee cartilage, ligaments, menisci, and regional bone marrow can be imaged quite effectively with MRI. Sagittal view provide visibility of the anterior and posterior **cruciate ligaments, menisci, popliteal vessels,** and surrounding tissues. Coronal views display collateral ligaments and lateral aspects of the menisci, while transaxial views display **tendons, patellae, collateral ligaments,** and **diaphyseal** bone marrow spaces. The MRI's capability of using multiple planes of view provides for precise definition of the anatomic structures of the wrist and hand. The nerves, blood vessels, and tendons can be depicted through the **carpal tunnel** better than other imaging techniques. MRI's transaxial and coronal planes are used most in the evaluation of the hips. The coronal view is well suited for determining pathologic involvement along the vertically oriented muscle planes and the femoral heads, while the transaxial plane is more suited for the evaluation of long bone marrow involvement. In the shoulder area, MRI's coronal and transaxial views are usually utilized for viewing the muscles and tendons of the **rotator cuff.** (17, 29, 30, 47, 81, 101)

MR imaging provides a method of evaluating the **acetabular** and **epiphyseal cartilage** of the hip affected by **Legg-Calvé-Perthes disease,** permitting assessment of femoral head containment, congruity of the acetabular and femoral articular surfaces, and intracapsular soft-tissue irregularities. (85)

MR imaging is an excellent modality for depicting the normal anatomy of the thorax, and MRI is being employed more and more in the evaluation of **intrathoracic** abnormalities. **Cardiac** and **respiratory gating techniques** may be utilized to help reduce motion artifacts. Fast imaging techniques are also used to decrease motion artifacts. The views reflected by the sagittal plane most often are applied to the mediastinal portion of the thorax, unless **apical** or **diaphragmatic** disease is suspected, although the sagittal plane also may be used to demonstrate pathologic processes in the anterior, middle, and posterior compartments of the mediastinum. Substernal and pretracheal lesions may best be delineated with this view. The oblique projections are particularly effective for cardiac imaging. The **thoracic wall** is easily visualized, however, there may be some loss of detail surrounding the lower thorax due to greater respiratory motion and cardiac activity. MR imaging reflects the ribs as a bright marrow signal surrounded by black cortical bone. MR imaging data for determining the anatomic association between mediastinal masses and great vessels is not always present with other types of modalities. Although computed tomography is the modality used for the detection of **pulmonary nodules,** MRI's ability to visualize flowing blood is preferred to determine whether **hilar** or **parenchymal** masses are solid or vascular. (16, 18, 23, 39)

Great Vessel and Cardiovascular Imaging

MR imaging utilizing electrocardiographic gating techniques in conjunction with obtaining multisection single-echo images in the transverse plane best depicts the entire **aorta** from the **aortic root** to the **aortic bifurcation;** it is also very effective in demonstrating **aortic dissection.** Aortic dissections are identified as definite when the characteristic **intimal flap** is visualized on the MR image. Additional views in the sagittal or coronal planes provide helpful assistance in determining branch vessel involvement, especially in the aortic arch. MRI can identify the most hazardous complication of dissection, namely, leakage of blood from the aorta resulting in **pleural effusion, pericardial effusion,** and **periaortic fluid collection.** MR imaging of congenital abnormalities of the aorta provides structural image detail that is useful in the evaluation of congenital abnormalities of the aorta including **double aortic arch, vascular rings, supravalvular aortic stenosis,** and **coarctation.** (51, 52, 58, 79)

MR imaging has the capability to readily visualize the great vessels. The **brachiocephalic vessels** appear to angle in a slightly oblique direction through the various coronal planes. MR imaging of the vena cava is an excellent technique to evaluate the presence of a **superior vena cava syndrome,** particularly in terms of differentiating extrinsic compression from the presence of a superior vena cava clot or tumor. Segments of the superior and inferior vena cava can be well defined, as well as their entry into the right atrium. The **descending aorta** and the **azygos vein** can be visualized easily. The main, left, and right **pulmonary arteries** may be followed throughout their mediastinal course. The **pulmonary veins** intermittently can be visualized inserting into the left atrium.

MR imagings detect **thoracic aortic aneurysms,** displaying concentric enlargement of the ascending or descending aortic aneurysms. Transverse MR images visualize the size of the residual lumen as well as the outer diameter of the aneurysm. Because of this, MR imaging can provide an accurate measure of the diameter of the aneurysm even in the presence of wall thickening or **mural thrombus.** MR imaging is capable of defining cardiac structures and anatomic details clearly. The development of **cine MRI** permits rapid dynamic imaging that allows evaluation of **ventricular performance,** as well as estimating the severity of **valvular regurgitation.** The cine MRI technique may be utilized to detect **myocardial infarction.** Cine MRI can be used to define the regional contractile abnormality caused by **ischemic heart disease.** Cine MRI may be used to determine **patency** of **coronary artery bypass grafts.** Flow through the patent graft produces high signal intensity in the grafts so that they may be easily identified. Cine MR is able to demonstrate the abnormal flow pattern associated with **stenotic** and **regurgitant lesions.** The greater temporal and spatial resolution of cine MRI is one of its distinct advantages over radionuclide imaging in the evaluation of **cardioventricular** anatomy and function. Radionuclide imaging does not have the capability of demonstrating intracardiac flow patterns caused by shunt and regurgitant flow. (16, 23, 50, 51, 52, 55, 79, 88, 95)

Adrenal Glands and Kidney Imaging

MR imaging is utilized to assess patients with **adrenal cortical hyperfunction.** **Adrenal adenomas** larger than two centimeters in diameter can be detected by MRI. **Adrenal cortical carcinomas** that are usually larger than ten centimeters in diameter and produce **Cushing's syndrome** can be depicted easily by MRI. Computed tomography (CT) appears at present to be better than MRI in assessing **primary hyperaldosteronism,** because **aldosteronomas** and lesions of **nodular hyperplasia** tend to be very small and are poorly resolved on MR images. Both CT and MRI show high sensitivity for detection of **adrenal pheochromocytoma.** MRI possesses good sensitivity for detecting extra-adrenal and recurrent malignant pheochromocytomas. Views in the coronal plane offer an effective technique for scanning the **sympathetic chain,** thus increasing further the modality's ability to detect extra-adrenal lesions. The high soft tissue contrast of MR imaging provides easy discrimination between adrenal gland and adjacent organs. One disadvantage of MRI is that it is unable to detect adrenal calcification. (23, 27, 36, 70)

The kidneys are well delineated with MRI. MR imaging demonstrates morphological changes. Coronal views clearly define the renal veins, inferior vena cava and enable extrarenal metastases to the **retroperitoneum, mediastinum,** and **liver** to be more effectively demonstrated. A major disadvantage of renal MRI is the poor demonstration of calcification and calculi. MR imaging of known **renal cell carcinoma** has advantages over computed tomography because of its better detection of tumor **thrombus** in major vessels and distinction of collateral vessels in the **renal hilus** from **renal hilar lymph nodes.** However, the staging process with MR imaging also has several limitations, such as its inability to allow reliable determination of tumor in lymph nodes, and MRI cannot currently be used to identify tumor spread through the **renal capsule.** (23, 28, 36, 55, 70)

Abbreviations

Related to Diagnostic Radiology

ACG—angiocardiography, apex cardiogram
AP—anterior-posterior (projection of x-rays)
BMT—barium meal test
CAT—computed axial tomography
CCK-CCG—cholecystokinin cholecystography
CUG—cystourethrogram
DGE—delayed gastric emptying
DSA—digital subtraction angiography
DVI—digital vascular imaging
DVSA—digital video subtraction angiography
EDD—end-diastolic dimension
EDV—end-diastolic volume
ESD—end-systolic dimension
ESV—end-systolic volume
IRS—integrated radiography system

LSB—left sternal border
OCG—oral cholecystography
SNR—signal-to-noise ratio
SPR—scanned projection radiography
TID—time interval difference (imaging)

Related to Therapeutic Radiology

EF—extended field (radiotherapy)
IF—involved field (radiotherapy)
MDF—multiple daily fractionation (therapy)
RTP—radiation treatment planning
SSI—segmental sequential irradiation (same as TNI)
TANI—total axial lymph node irradiation
TBI—total body irradiation
TNI—total nodal irradiation
TNM—classification;

T—primary tumor
N—lymph node involvement
M—distal metastasis
TR—therapeutic ratio

Related to Ultrasonography

A-mode—amplitude modulation
B-mode—brightness modulation
M-mode—motion modulation
TM—time motion
TP—time position

Related to Doppler Techniques

AoR—aortic root
FFT—fast Fourier transform
LAD—left anterior descending (artery)
LAO—left anterior oblique (artery)
LCA—left circumflex artery
LMC—left main coronary (artery)
RAO—right anterior oblique (artery)
RCA—right coronary artery
TIH—time interval histogram

Related to Symbols and Measurements

A—area of blood vessel lumen
    expressed in square centimeters

Bev—one billion electron volts
Δf—difference in frequency spectrum
DFS—digital field store
E—energy in ergs
erg—one unit of work
ev—one electron volt
f—frequency
Hz—Hertz
Kev, keV—1,000 electron volts
Mev, MeV—one million electron volts,
    megavolt, megavoltage
mHz—megaHertz, one million Hertz
mw per cm^2—milliwatts per square
    centimeter
Q—volumetric flow rate
r—roentgen
Rad, rad—radiation absorbed dose
    (100 ergs/g tissue)
Rem, rem—roentgen equivalent, physical
SV—sample volume
V—velocity

Related to Scientific Organizations

ABR—American Board of Radiology
ACR—American College of Radiology

References and Bibliography

1. Albdoliras, Ernerio T., et al. Impact of two-dimensional and Doppler echocardiography on care of children aged two years and younger. *American Journal of Cardiology* 61:166-169, Jan. 1988.
2. Amberg, John R., and Juhl, John H. The gallbladder and biliary ducts. In Juhl, John H., and Crummy, Andrew B., eds., *Paul and Juhl's Essentials of Radiologic Imaging*, 5th ed. Philadelphia: J.B. Lippincott Co., 1987, pp. 492-504.
3. American College of Radiology. *Glossary of MR Terms*, Reston, VA: American College of Radiology, 1986.
4. Ballinger, Philip W. General anatomy and radiographic positioning terminology. In *Merill's Atlas of Radiographic Positions and Radiologic Procedures*, 6th ed., vol. 1. St. Louis: The C.V. Mosby Co., 1986, pp. 31-44.
5. Baltarowich, Oksana H., and Kurtz, Alfred B. Sonographic evaluation of renal masses. *Urologic Radiology* 9:79-87, 1987.
6. Becker, Melvin H. The lacrimal drainage system. In Gonzalez, Carlos F., et al. eds., *Diagnostic Imaging in Ophthalmology*, New York: Springer-Verlag, 1986, pp. 81-91.
7. Blum, Manfred. Ultrasonography and computed tomography of the thyroid gland. In Ingbar, Sidney H., and Braverman, Lewis E., eds., *Werner's The Thyroid*, 5th ed. Philadelphia: J.B. Lippincott Co., 1987, pp. 276-591.
8. Bowley, N.B., and Malmud, L.S., The biliary tract. In Grainger, Ronald G., and Allison, David J., eds., *Diagnostic Radiology*, vol. 2. New York: Churchill Livingstone, Inc., 1986, pp. 955-987.
9. Brandt-Zawadzki, Michael. MR imaging of the brain. *Radiology* 166:1-10, Jan. 1988.
10. Brismar, J., et al. The skull and brain: Methods of examination: Diagnostic approach. In Grainger, Ronald G., and Allison, David J., eds., *Diagnostic Radiology*, vol. 3. New York: Churchill Livingstone, Inc., 1986, pp. 1671-1704.
11. ———. Cranial pathology (1). Ibid., pp. 1705-1737.
12. ———. Cranial pathology (2). Ibid.,

pp. 1739-1767.

13. ———. Cranial pathology (3). Ibid., pp. 1769-1796.

14. Buchbinder, Dale, et al. B-mode ultrasonic imaging in the preoperative evaluation of saphenous vein. *The American Surgeon* 53:368-372, July 1987.

15. Bushong, Stewart C. MRI anatomy: Central nervous system. In *Magnetic Resonance Imaging Physical and Biological Principles*, St. Louis: The C.V. Mosby Co., 1988, pp. 225-257.

16. ———. MRI anatomy: Thorax and abdomen. Ibid., pp. 248-283.

17. ———. MRI anatomy: Pelvis and extremities. Ibid., pp. 284-307.

18. ———. MRI artifacts. Ibid., pp. 308-325.

19. Capp, M.P., Roehrig, H., and Ovitt, T.W. Digital radiography. In Grainger, Ronald G., and Allison, David J., eds., *Diagnostic Radiology*, vol. 1. New York: Churchill Livingstone, Inc., 1986, pp. 93-98.

20. Cogswell, Terrence L., Sagar, Kiran B., and Wann, L. Samuel. Echocardiographic evaluation of cardiac function during exercise. In Pohost, Gerald M., ed.-in-chief, *New Concepts in Cardiac Imaging—1987*. Chicago: Year Book Medical Publishers, Inc., 1987, pp. 13-33.

21. Cohen, Harris L., and Haller, Jack O. Diagnostic sonography of the fetal genitourinary tract. *Urologic Radiology* 9:88-98, 1987.

22. Cole-Beuglet, Catherine. Ultrasound. In Bassett, Lawrence W., and Gold, Richard H., eds., *Breast Cancer Detection: Mammography and Other Methods in Breast Imaging*, 2nd ed. Orlando: Grune & Stratton, Inc., 1987, pp. 153-167.

23. Consensus Conference Report. Magnetic Resonance Imaging. *Journal of American Medical Association* 259:2132-2138, April 8, 1988.

24. Cosgrove, David O. Ultrasound: General principles. In Grainger, Ronald G., and Allison, David J., eds., *Diagnostic Radiology*, vol. 1. New York: Churchill Livingstone, Inc., 1986, pp. 25-37.

25. Crummy, Andrew B., and Peters, Mary Ellen. The superficial soft tissues. In Juhl, John H., and Crummy, Andrew B., eds., *Paul and Juhl's Essentials of Radiologic Imaging*, 5th ed. Philadelphia: J.B. Lippincott Co., 1987, pp. 347-384.

26. Daniels, David L., et al. Skull base. In Stark, David D., and Bradley, William G., Jr., eds., *Magnetic Resonance Imaging*. St. Louis: The C.V. Mosby Co., 1988, pp. 524-569.

27. Demas, Barbara E., and Hricak, Hedvig. Adrenal glands. In Stark, David D., and Bradley, William G., Jr., eds., *Magnetic Reso-*

nance Imaging. St. Louis: The C.V. Mosby Co., 1988, pp. 1164-1186.

28. Demas, Barbara E., Stafford, Susan A., and Hricak, Hedvig. Kidneys. In Stark, David D., and Bradley, William G., Jr., eds., *Magnetic Resonance Imaging*. St. Louis: The C.V. Mosby Co., 1988, pp. 1187-1232.

29. Dooms, George C., and Hricak, Hedvig. Magnetic resonance imaging of the pelvis: Prostate and urinary bladder. *Urologic Radiology* 8:156-165, 1986.

30. Ehman, Richard, et al. MR Imaging of the musculoskeletal system: A 5-year appraisal. *Radiology* 166:313-320, Feb. 1988.

31. Feig, Stephen A. Xeromammography. In Bassett, Lawrence W., and Gold, Richard H., eds., *Breast Cancer Detection: Mammography and Other Methods in Breast Imaging*, 2nd. ed. Orlando: Grune & Stratton, Inc., 1987, pp. 89-109.

32. Feigenbaum, Harvey. Echocardiography. In Braunwald, Eugene, ed., *Heart Disease: A Textbook of Cardiovascular Medicine*, 3rd ed., vol. 1. Philadelphia: W.B. Saunders Co., 1988, pp. 83-139.

33. Friedman, William F. Congenital heart disease in infancy and childhood. In Braunwald, Eugene, ed., *Heart Disease: A Textbook of Cardiovascular Medicine*, 3rd ed., vol. 2. Philadelphia: W.B. Saunders Co., 1988, pp. 83-139.

34. Gentant, Harry K. CT scanning. In Grainger, Ronald G., and Allison, David J., eds., *Diagnostic Radiology*, vol. 2. New York: Churchill Livingstone, Inc., 1986, pp. 1523-1534.

35. Gershater, Raziel, and St. Louis, Eugene L. Lumbar epidural venography. In Kricun, Morrie E., ed., *Imaging Modalities in Spinal Disorders*. Philadelphia: W.B. Saunders Co., 1988, pp. 538-556.

36. Glazer, Gary M. MR Imaging of the liver, kidneys, and adrenal glands. *Radiology* 166:303-312, Feb. 1988.

37. Goddard, Paul R. Investigations of value with regard to the chest. In *Diagnostic Imaging of the Chest*. New York: Churchill Livingstone, Inc., 1987, pp. 1-5.

38. ———. Pleural and chest wall lesions. Ibid., pp. 112-124.

39. ———. The mediastinal mass. Ibid., pp. 132-167.

40. Gold, Richard H. Bassett, Lawrence W., and Coulson, Walter F. Mammographic features of malignant and benign disease. In Bassett, Lawrence W., and Gold, Richard H., eds., *Breast Cancer Detection: Mammography and Other Methods in Breast Imaging*, 2nd ed. Orlando: Grune & Stratton, Inc., 1987, pp. 15-65.

41. Gold, Richard H., Bassett, Lawrence W.,

and Kimme-Smith, Carolyn. Introduction to breast imaging: State of the art and future directions. In Bassett, Lawrence W., and Gold, Richard H., eds., *Breast Cancer Detection: Mammography and Other Methods in Breast Imaging*, 2nd ed. Orlando: Grune & Stratton, Inc., 1987, pp. 3-13.

42. Goldberg, Herbert I., and Lee, Seungho Howard. Stroke. In *Cranial Computed Tomography and MRI*, 2nd ed. New York: McGraw-Hill Book Co., 1987, pp. 643-716.

43. Gonzalez, Carlos F. Investigation of the orbit by contrast techniques. In Gonzalez, Carlos F., et al., eds., *Diagnostic Imaging in Ophthalmology*. New York: Springer-Verlag, 1986, pp. 71-79.

44. Grolimund, P., et al. Evaluation of cerebrovascular disease by combined extracranial and transcranial Doppler sonography. *Stroke* 18:1018-1024, Nov.-Dec. 1987.

45. Hagen-Ansert, Sandra L. Diagnostic ultrasound. In Ballinger, Philip W. *Merrill's Atlas of Radiographic Positions and Radiologic Procedures*, 6th ed., vol. 3. St. Louis: The C.V. Mosby Co., 1986. pp. 245-274.

46. Haller, Jack O., and Cohne, Harris L. Pediatric urosonography: An update: *Urologic Radiology* 9:99-107, 1987.

47. Harms, Steven E., and Greenway, Guerdon. Musculoskeletal system. In Stark, David D., and Bradley, William G., Jr., eds., *Magnetic Resonance Imaging*. St. Louis: The C.V. Mosby Co., 1988, pp. 1323-1433.

48. Harrison, Michael R., et al. A practical application of Doppler echocardiography for the assessment of severity of aortic stenosis. *American Heart Journal* 115:622-628, March 1988.

49. Hasso, Anton N., et al. Tumors of the posterior fossa. In Stark, David D., and Bradley, William G., Jr., eds., *Magnetic Resonance Imaging*. St. Louis: The C.V. Mosby Co., 1988, pp. 425-450.

50. Higgins, Charles B. Newer cardiac imaging techniques: Digital subtraction angiography; computed tomography; magnetic resonance imaging. In Braunwald, Eugene, ed., *Heart Disease: A Textbook of Cardiovascular Medicine*, 3rd ed., vol. 1. Philadelphia: W.B. Saunders Co., 1988, pp. 356-382.

51. Higgins, Charles B. The vascular system. In Higgins, Charles B., and Hricak, Hedvig, eds., *Magnetic Resonance Imaging of the Body*. New York: Raven Press, 1987, pp. 309-345.

52. Higgins, Charles B., et al. Cine magnetic resonance. In Higgins, Charles B., and Hricak, Hedvig, eds., *Magnetic Resonance of the Body*. New York: Raven Press, 1987, pp. 295-307.

53. Hillis, L. David, and Grossman, William. Cardiac ventriculography. In Grossman, William, ed., *Cardiac Catheterization and Angiography*, 3rd ed. Philadelphia: Lea & Febiger, 1986, pp. 200-212.

54. Husband, Janet E. Whole body computed tomography. In Grainger, Ronald G., and Allison, David J., eds., *Diagnostic Radiology*, vol. 1. New York: Churchill Livingstone, Inc., 1986, pp. 39-59.

55. Isherwood, Ian, and Jenkins, Jeremy P.R. MRI—The body. In *Textbook of Radiology and Imaging*. New York: Churchill Livingstone, Inc., 1988, pp. 1810-1845.

56. Kazzi, George M., et al. Placenta maturation. In Sabbagha, Rudy E., ed., *Diagnostic Ultrasound Applied to Obstetrics and Gynecology*, 2nd ed. Philadelphia: J.B. Lippincott Co., 1987, pp. 209-218.

57. Kelsey, Charles A. Introduction. In Juhl, John H., and Crummy, Andrew B., eds., *Paul and Juhl's Essentials of Radiologic Imaging*, 5th ed. Philadelphia: J.B. Lippincott Co., 1987, pp. 1-18.

58. Kersting-Sommerhoff, Barbara A., et al. Aortic dissection: Sensitivity and specificity of MR imaging. *Radiology* 166:651-655. March 1988.

59. Kisslo, Joseph, Adams, David B., and Belkin, Robert N. *Doppler Color Flow Imaging*. New York: Churchill Livingstone, Inc., 1988, pp. 1-10.

60. Kruger, Robert A. Digital radiography. In Ballinger, Philip W. *Merrill's Atlas of Radiographic Positions and Radiologic Procedures*, 6th ed., vol. 3. St. Louis: The C.V. Mosby Co., 1986, pp. 225-232.

61. Lunderquist, Anders, and Cotton, P.B. The pancreas. In Grainger, Ronald G., and Allison, David J., eds., *Diagnostic Radiology*, vol. 2. New York: Churchill Livingstone, Inc., 1986, pp. 999-1008.

62. McAllister, V.L., et al. The spine: methods of examination: diagnostic approach. In Grainger, Ronald G., and Allison, David J., eds., *Diagnostic Radiology*, vol. 3. New York: Churchill Livingstone, Inc., 1986, pp. 1798-1819.

63. ———. Spinal pathology. Ibid., pp. 1821-1855.

64. McNamara, John J., MD. Personal communications.

65. Mafee, Mahmood F., and Miller, Marilyn T. Computed tomography scanning in the evaluation of ocular motility disorders. In Gonzales, Carlos F., et al., eds., *Diagnostic Imaging in Ophthalmology*. New York: Springer-Verlag, 1986, pp. 40-54.

66. Maravilla, Kenneth R. Multiple sclerosis. In Stark, David D., and Bradley, William G., Jr., eds., *Magnetic Resonance Imaging*. St.

Louis: The C.V. Mosby Co., 1988, pp. 344-358.

67. Margulis, Alexander R. Introduction: Developments in imaging. In Grainger, Ronald G., and Allison, David J., eds., *Diagnostic Radiology*, vol. 1. New York: Churchill Livingstone, Inc., 1986, pp. 3-11.

68. Mattle, Heinrich, et al. Transcranial Doppler sonographic findings in middle artery disease. *Archives of Neurology* 42:289-295, March 1988.

69. Meire, Hylton B. Vascular ultrasound. In Grainger, Ronald G., and Allison, David J., eds., *Diagnostic Radiology*, vol. 3. New York: Churchill Livingstone, Inc., 1986, pp. 2113-2120.

70. Mezrich, Ruben, Banner, Marc P., and Pollack, Howard M. Magnetic resonance of the adrenal glands. *Urologic Radiology* 8:127-138, 1986.

71. Milbrath, John R. Thermography. In Bassett, Lawrence W., and Gold, Richard H., eds., *Breast Cancer Detection: Mammography and Other Methods in Breast Imaging*, 2nd ed. Orlando: Grune & Stratton, Inc., 1987, pp. 145-152.

72. Mosley, Ivan. Methods of examination: 1-Noninvasive methods using X-rays. In *Diagnostic Imaging in Neurological Disease*. New York: Churchill Livingstone, Inc., 1986, pp. 14-41.

73. ———. Noninvasive methods of investigation. II Methods which do not use X-rays. Ibid., pp. 42-54.

74. Murphy, William A. Joint disease. In Grainger, Ronald G., and Allison, David J., eds., *Diagnostic Radiology*, vol. 2. New York: Churchill Livingstone, Inc., 1986, pp. 1473-1508.

75. New, Paul F. J., and Shoukimas, Gregory. Thoracic spine and spinal cord. In Stark, David D., and Bradley, William G., Jr., *Magnetic Resonance Imaging*. St. Louis: The C.V. Mosby Co., 1988, pp. 632-665.

76. Pandis, Ionnis P., and Morganroth, Joel. The role of M-Mode and two dimensional echocardiography in detection of cardiac masses. In Pohost, Gerald M., ed.-in-chief, *New Concepts in Cardiac Imaging—1987*. Chicago: Year Book Medical Publishers, Inc., 1987, pp. 61-102.

77. Papanicolaou, Nicholas, et al. Magnetic resonance imaging of the kidney. *Urologic Radiology* 8:139-150, 1986.

78. Paulin, Sven. Aortography. In Grossman, William, ed., *Cardiac Catheterization and Angiography*, 3rd ed. Philadelphia: Lea & Febiger, 1986, pp. 227-247.

79. Peshock, Ronald M. Heart and great vessels. In Stark, David D., and Bradley, William G., Jr., eds., *Magnetic Resonance Imaging*. St.

Louis: The C.V. Mosby Co., 1988, pp. 902-910.

80. Piccirillo, Mark, et al. Sonography of renal inflammatory disease. *Urologic Radiology* 9:66-73, 1987.

81. Picus, Daniel, and Lee, Joseph K. T. Magnetic resonance imaging of the female pelvis. *Urologic Radiology* 8:166-174, 1986.

82. Powell, Thomas. The ear, nose and throat. In Grainger, Ronald G., and Allison, David J., eds., *Diagnostic Radiology*, vol. 3. New York: Churchill Livingstone, Inc., 1986, pp. 1937-1983.

83. Rabinovici, Reuven, et al. Ultrasonographic diagnosis of vesical leakage in a renal transplant recipient. *Urologic Radiology* 8:112-113, 1986.

84. Raphael, M. J. Cardiac radiology: Techniques—normal appearances. In Grainger, Ronald G., and Allison, David J., eds., *Diagnostic Radiology*, vol. 1. New York: Churchill Livingstone, Inc., 1986, pp. 379-392.

85. Rush, Barbara Hall, et al. Legg-Calvé-Perthes disease: Detection of cartilaginous and synoval change with MR imaging. *Radiology* 167:473-476, May 1988.

86. Sabbagha, Rudy E., et al. Correlative anatomy. In Sabbagha, Rudy E., ed., *Diagnostic Ultrasound Applied to Obstetrics and Gynecology*, 2nd ed. Philadelphia: J.B. Lippincott Co., 1987, pp. 264-289.

87. Sato, Yutaka, et al. Hippel-Lindau disease: MR imaging. *Radiology* 166:241-246, Jan. 1988.

88. Sechtem, Udo, et al. Mitral or aortic regurgitation: Quantification of regurgitant volumes with Cine MR imaging. *Radiology* 167:425-430, May 1988.

89. Sholl, John S. Placental position. In Sabbagha, Rudy E., ed., *Diagnostic Ultrasound Applied to Obstetrics and Gynecology*, 2nd ed. Philadelphia: J.B. Lippincott Co., 1987, pp. 195-208.

90. Stewart, William J., and Schiavone, William A. Doppler echocardiographic evaluation of valvular stenosis. In Pohost, Gerald M., ed.-in-chief. *New Concepts in Cardiac Imaging—1986*. Chicago: Year Book Medical Publishers, Inc., 1986, pp. 41-64.

91. Switzer, Donald F., Maulik, Debarata, and Nanda, Navin C. Advances in the use of echocardiography in congenital heart disease. In Pohost, Gerald M., ed.-in-chief, *New Concepts in Cardiac Imaging—1986*. Chicago: Year Book Medical Publishers, Inc., 1986, pp. 41-64.

92. Thornbury, John R., and Weiss, Stan L. The urinary tract. In Juhl, John H., and Crummy, Andrew B., eds., *Paul and Juhl's Essentials of Radiologic Imaging*, 5th ed.

Philadelphia: J.B. Lippincott Co., 1987, pp. 565-657.

93. Threatt, Barbara. Ductography. In Bassett, Lawrence W., and Gold, Richard H., eds., *Breast Cancer Detection: Mammography and Other Methods in Breast Imaging*, 2nd ed. Orlando: Grune & Stratton, Inc., 1987, pp. 119-129.

94. Unger, June M. The temporal bone. In Juhl, John H., and Crummy, Andrew B., eds., *Paul and Juhl's Essentials of Radiologic Imaging*, 5th ed. Philadelphia: J.B. Lippincott Co., 1987, pp. 1079-1094.

95. Utz, Joseph A., and Herfkens, Robert J. Dynamic and physiologic cardiac MR. In Stark, David D., and Bradley, William G., Jr., eds., *Magnetic Resonance Imaging*. St. Louis: The C.V. Mosby Co., 1988, pp. 921-933.

96. Valavanis, A., Schubiger, O., and Naidich, T. P. CT examination: Techniques for evaluation of the Cerebello-Pointine Angle. In *Clinical Imaging of the Cerebello-Pontine Angle*. Berlin: Springer-Verlag, 1987, pp. 4-9.

97. Vignaud, J., et al. The orbit. In Grainger, Ronald G., and Allison, David J., eds., *Diagnostic Radiology*, vol. 3. New York: Churchill Livingstone, Inc., 1986, pp. 1875-1897.

98. Villafana, Theodore. Physics and instrumentation: CT and MRI. In Lee, Seungho, Howard, and Rao, Krishna C.V.G., eds., *Cranial Computed Tomography*, 2nd ed. New York: McGraw-Hill Book Co., 1987, pp. 1-69.

99. Weissman, Barbara N.W., and Sledge, Clement B. General principles. In *Orthopedic Radiology*. Philadelphia: W.B. Saunders Co., 1986, pp. 1-69.

100. Wicks, Jeffrey D. Obstetric and gynecologic imaging. In Juhl, John H., and Crummy, Andrew B., eds., *Paul and Juhl's Essentials of Radiologic Imaging*, 5th ed. Philadelphia: J.B. Lippincott Co., 1987, pp. 658-692.

101. Young, Stuart W. Clinical applications of MRI. In *Magnetic Resonance Imaging: Basic Principles*, 2nd ed. New York: Raven Press, 1988, pp. 101-189.

102. Zagazebski, James A. Basic physics. In Sabbagha, Rudy E., ed., *Diagnostic Ultrasound Applied to Obstetrics and Gynecology*, 2nd ed. Philadelphia: J.B. Lippincott Co., 1987, pp. 2-32.

Selected Terms Pertaining to Nuclear Medicine

CHAPTER 21

Orientation

Origin of Terms

atom (G)—indivisible
fission (L)—cleft, split
iso- (G)—equal

kine-, kinesio- (G)—movement
prot-, proto- (G)—first
tele- (G)—distant, far away

General Terms

- *activated water*—water containing radioactive elements. (42)
- *activation analysis*—method for identifying and measuring the chemical elements in a sample to be analyzed. The sample is first made radioactive by bombardment with neutrons, charged particles, or other nuclear radiation. The newly radioactive atoms in the sample give off characteristic nuclear radiations that can identify the atoms and indicate their quantity. Activation analysis is frequently more sensitive than chemical analysis. It is being used more and more in research. (42)
- *acute exposure*—a brief, intense radiation exposure, in contrast to prolonged or chronic exposure.
- *alpha particle*—positively charged helium nucleus characterized by poorly penetrating but strongly ionizing radiation. (47)
- *annihilation reaction*—the interaction of a positron and electron, resulting in conversion of the masses of the two particles into gamma radiation.
- *atom*—smallest unit of any element that consists of a central nucleus and outer orbital electrons. The nucleus is composed of protons and neutrons, except that all of the hydrogen atom, which has no neutrons.
   —*electrons*—negatively charged particles revolving around the nucleus.
   —*neutrons*—electrically neutral particles present in the nucleus of an atom.
   —*protons*—positively charged particles present in the nucleus of an atom. (42)
- *atomic weight*—relative weight of an atom compared to that of one carbon atom, which is 12. (42, 47)
- *background radiation*—the radiation of the natural environment, consisting of radiation from cosmic rays and from the naturally radioactive elements of the earth, including that from within the human body. The term may also mean radiation extraneous to an experiment. (44, 47)

- *becquerel (Bq)*—adopted by the International System of Units as the official unit of radioactivity. One Bq is defined as one nuclear transformation per second. One disintegration or decay per second (dps) equals one Bq. (34)
- *beta particle*—nuclear particle either positively or negatively charged. When positively charged, the positron is useful for the gamma radiation produced when it interacts with a negatively charged beta particle. When negatively charged, the beta particle is essentially an electron, more penetrating and less ionizing than an alpha particle. The effect of beta particles is moderately destructive and usually limited to the first few millimeters of tissue. (47, 48)
- *body burden*—the amount of radioactive material present in the body of human beings or animals.
- *bone seeker*—a radionuclide that tends to lodge in the bones when it is introduced into the body; for example, strontium-90, which behaves chemically like calcium. (24)
- *by-product material*—any radioactive material (except source or fissionable material) obtained in the process of producing or using source or fissionable material. Includes fission products and many other radioisotopes produced in nuclear reactors. (47)
- *contamination, radioactive*—the spread of radioactivity to places where it can have adverse effects on persons, experiments, and equipment.
- *counter*—device for making radiation measurements or counting ionizing events. The term is used loosely as a synonym of detector. (23)
- *curie*—the unit for measuring the activity of all radioactive substances, or the quantity of radioactive material that undergoes 3.7×10^{10} disintegrations per second (dps). Recently, the International System of Units has adopted the becquerel (Bq) as the official unit of radioactivity. See above for becquerel definition. (34)
- *cyclotron*—a particle accelerator in which charged particles receive repeated synchronized accelerations of "kicks" by electric fields as the particles spiral outward from their source. The particles are kept in the spiral by a powerful magnet. Cyclotrons are a valuable source of radionuclides for medical diagnosis and research. (22, 23, 34)
- *decontamination*—the removal of harmful radioactive material from persons, equipment, instruments, rooms, and so on. Some articles may be decontaminated by thorough washing with detergents or other chemicals. (34)
- *dose (clinical radionuclides)*—the amount of radionuclides for diagnostic evaluation, known as tracer dose, or for treatment, referred to as therapeutic dose. (23, 34)
- *dosimeter*—an instrument for measuring the dose of radiation. (23)
- *emission computed tomography*—consists of numerous techniques that produce a three-dimensional representation of the distribution of radionuclide within the patient. This technique eliminates the superimposed artifacts found in conventional two-dimensional gamma camera imaging, thus facilitating the monitoring of body physiologic changes and detecting abnormal pathologic lesions. In radionuclide emission computed tomography, photons are emitted from the patient. Two technologies associated with this concept are:
  - *positron emission tomography (PET)*—a form of transaxial computed tomography utilized in the study of physiologic processes. With this process, it is possible to "label" compounds that have positron-emitting isotopes with proton emitters and subsequently "image" their distribution in the living body over time.
  - *single photon emission computed tomography (SPECT)*—a form of transaxial computed tomography in which a set of planar views (projections) is obtained. These projections are stored in the computer memory and subsequently reconstructed into transaxial slices by algorithms. The projections are obtained by one or two conventional gamma camera detectors with parallel-hole collimation. (12, 23, 33, 39, 43)

- *external hazards*—exposure to ionizing radiation from radioactive sources outside the body. (34)
- *film badge*—photographic, dental size x-ray film worn on the person for detecting radiation exposure. (10, 34, 48)
- *gamma ray*—short wavelength eletromagnetic radiation of nuclear origin. Gamma rays are more penetrating than alpha and beta particles, are similar to x-rays, and are very useful in diagnostic nuclear medicine. (34)
- *Geiger-Müller counter*—a sensitive radiation detector composed of a tube filled with gas and a scaler. It is used to detect nuclear radiation. (23, 34)
- *half-life, biologic*—the time required for a biologic system, such as a human being or an animal, to eliminate, by natural processes, half the amount of a substance that has entered it.
- *half-life, radioactive*—time required for a radioactive substance to lose 50 percent of its activity by decay. (34) For example:

  —*Radiophosphorus* (^{32}P)—has a half-life of 14 days. This means that a quantity of ^{32}P having a radioactivity of:
  250.0 mCi (millicuries) on a certain day will have an activity of:
  125.0 mCi (millicuries) 14 days later and
  62.5 mCi (millicuries) 28 days later. (33)

- *internal hazards*—those caused by exposure to ionizing radiation from radioactive substances deposited inside the body. (34)
- *ion*—an atomic particle, charged atom, or chemically bound group of atoms. (23)
- *ionization*—the process of producing ions. (23)
- *isotopes*—atoms having the same number of protons (atomic number) but differing by their atomic weight.
- *labeled compound*—a compound composed in part of a radionuclide. For example:

  sodium radioiodide ....Na^{131}I
  radiocobalt B^{12} ....^{60}CoB$_{12}$
  chromic radiophosphate ....Cr^{32}PO$_4$. (47)

- *mass number*—the sum of the neutrons and protons in a nucleus. The mass number of uranium-235 is 235. It is the nearest whole number to the atom's actual atomic weight. (42)
- *maximum permissible concentration*—that amount of radioactive material in air, water, and foodstuffs that competent authorities have established as the maximum that would not create undue risk to human health. (47)
- *maximum permissible dose*—that dose of ionizing radiation that competent authorities have established as the maximum that can be absorbed without undue risk to human health. (34)
- *median lethal dose* (MLD, LD$_{50}$)—radiation that kills, in a given period, 50 percent of a large group of animals or other organisms. (47)
- *microcurie (nuclear medicine)*—unit for measuring the energy of a radionuclide in a tracer dose. One microcurie is one millionth of a curie. (34, 47)
- *millicurie (nuclear medicine)*—unit for measuring the energy of a radionuclide in a therapeutic dose. One millicurie equals a thousand microcuries. (34, 47)
- *monitoring*—area monitoring, a procedure for determining the amount of radioactive contamination present in a certain locality and at a given time. In personnel monitoring, individuals are monitored; namely, their breath, excreta, clothing, and so on to detect health hazards and provide environmental safety. (34)
- *nuclear fission*—the splitting of a heavy nucleus into two or more nuclei, resulting in nuclear conversion and the release of powerful energy. (47)

- *nuclear numbers:*

  Symbol
  - *atomic number* Z—number of protons in the nucleus of an atom.
  - *neutron number* N—number of neutrons in the nucleus of an atom.
  - *mass number* A—sum of neutrons and protons in the nucleus of an atom.
  $A = Z + N$ (34, 42)

- *nuclear transformation, radioactive decay*—diminished nuclear properties (activity) of a radioactive substance in the course of time. (34)
- *nucleon*—an essential part of a nucleus, synonym for protons or neutrons. (47)
- *nucleus of an atom*—central part of atom containing protons, or positively charged particles, and neutrons, or neutral particles. (42)
- *nuclide (see Fig. 82)*—term denoting all nuclear species of chemical elements, both stable and unstable. It is used synonymously with isotope. (34)
- *overexposure to radiation*—excessive contamination by ionizing radiation that has deleterious effects on a person's health. In massive overexposure, symptoms of radiation injury develop in hours, days, or weeks; in chronic overexposure to small amounts of radiation, symptoms appear within months or years. (47)
- *photon*—a discrete quantity of electromagnetic energy. Photons have momentum but no mass or electric charge. (34)
- *positron*—a positively charged nuclear electron. (22)
- *proton*—an elementary particle with a single positive electric charge and a mass approximately 1,847 times that of the electron. The atomic number of an atom is equal to the number of protons in its nucleus. (23, 34)
- *radiation*—the propagation of energy through matter or space in the form of waves. In atomic physics the term has been extended to include fast-moving particles (alpha and beta rays, free neutrons, etc.). Gamma rays and x-rays, of particular interest in atomic physics, are electromagnetic radiation in which energy is propagated in packets called photons. (34)
- *radiation protection guide*—the total amounts of ionizing radiation dose over certain periods that may safely be permitted to exposed industrial groups. These standards, established by the National Council on Radiation Protection and Measurements, are equivalent to what was formerly called the "maximum permissible exposure." (10, 47, 48)
- *radiation protection procedures*—techniques used to safeguard patients and personnel from external and internal exposure. Principles of safety are concerned with:
  - *time*—the shorter the period of exposure, the lower the radiation dose.
  - *distance*—the further away from the radioactive substance, the less radiation received. Distance is a more important factor than time, and it varies inversely as the square of the distance.
  - *shielding*—the denser the material between the person and the radioactive material, the lower the radiation hazard. Protection from the internal exposure is achieved by avoiding ingestion, inhalation, and direct contact with radioactive materials. Monitoring records must be kept on all persons exposed to nuclear radiation in their employment. (10, 35, 47, 48)
- *radioactive tracer*—radionuclide used in minute amounts for diagnostic testing. (34)
- *radioactivity*—the spontaneous decay or disintegration of an unstable atomic nucleus, accompanied by the emission of radiation. (34, 35)
- *radioassay*—quantitative analysis of substances using radionuclide tracer techniques to detect minute quantities not easily measured by other means. (23)
- *radioautograph, autoradiograph*—record of radiation from radioactive material in an

Figure 82   Stable nuclides and radioactive nuclides. (Courtesy of the U.S. Atomic Energy Commission)

What are nuclides?

Nuclides are atoms of an element distinguishable by their weight.

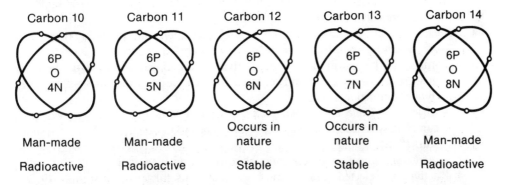

Carbon 10	Carbon 11	Carbon 12	Carbon 13	Carbon 14
6P O 4N	6P O 5N	6P O 6N	6P O 7N	6P O 8N
		Occurs in nature	Occurs in nature	
Man-made	Man-made	nature	nature	Man-made
Radioactive	Radioactive	Stable	Stable	Radioactive

object, made by placing its surface in close proximity to a photographic emulsion. By this technique differences in cell function are discernible. (33)

- *radiobiology*—branch of biology dealing with the effects of radiation on biologic systems.
- *radioimmunoassay (RIA)*—technique of measuring minute amounts of substances by employing antigens and/or antibodies labeled with radioactive tracers. This technique has been applied to other biologically active substances, including nonimmune systems. Commonly used radioassay procedures measure serum levels of:
    - —cardiac glycosides such as digoxin
    - —cortisol
    - —folic acid
    - —triiodothyronine (T_3)
    - —thyrotoxine (T_4)
    - —vitamin B_{12}

Radioimmunoassays offer reliable data and excel in specificity and sensitivity. (23, 33, 56)

- *radioisotopes*—chemical elements that have been made radioactive by bombardment with neutrons in an atomic pile or cyclotron. Some occur in nature. By giving off radiation, they provide a valuable means for diagnosis and treatment. Radioisotopes differ from their nonradioactive partners by their atomic weight. (1, 47)

For example: Potassium, the stable isotope, has an atomic weight of 39.

Radiopotassium, the unstable isotope, has an atomic weight of 42.

- *radionuclides, radioactive nuclides*—comprehensive terms including isobars, isomers, isotones, and isotopes, which exist for a measurable length of time and differ by atomic weight, atomic number, and energy state. The term *radioisotope* has become obsolete and radionuclide is the accepted term.
    - —*isobars*—atoms have the same mass number (A) but have different atomic numbers (Z) and neutron numbers (N).
    - —*isomers*—atoms have the same atomic numbers (Z) and the same mass numbers (A) but differ in nuclear energy states.
    - —*isotones*—atoms have the same number of neutrons in the nucleus (N) but differ in atomic numbers (Z) and number of mass particles (A).

— *isotopes*—atoms have the same atomic numbers (Z), and therefore, the same number of nuclear protons; but different numbers of mass particles (A), and therefore have a different number of nuclear neutrons (N).

A daughter radionuclide is a decay product produced by a radionuclide. The element from which the daughter was produced is called the "parent". Radionuclidic purity refers to the amount of total radioactive species in a sample that represents the desired radionuclide. (7, 34, 35, 42, 49)

- *radionuclidic imaging devices*—currently several instruments are in common use:
  — *Anger camera, scintillation camera, gamma camera*—an instrument for presenting images of the distribution of radioactivity in any organ or part of the body. Its greatest assets are speed and sensitivity, which are of particular significance in dynamic function studies.
  — *Anger multiplane tomographic scanner*—nuclear instrument that provides six complete synchronized images or readouts of variable depth or plane on a single scan (film).
  — *rectilinear scanner*—the conventional scanner and a moving detector of radio-activity in selected areas of the body that is useful for static studies. (9, 22, 23, 34, 42)

- *reactor*—a device in which a fission chain reaction can be initiated, maintained, and controlled. Its essential component is a core with fissionable fuel. It usually has a moderator, a reflector, shielding, and control mechanisms. (47)

- *relative biologic effectiveness* (RBE)—the relative effectiveness of a given kind of ionizing radiation in producing a biologic response as compared with x-rays. (47)

- *scaler*—an electronic instrument for counting radiation-induced pulses from Geiger counters and other radiation detectors. (23, 34)

- *scan*—image of the deposit of a radionuclide.
  — *photoscan*—the pattern of radioactivity presented on x-ray film by a photo-recorder.
  — *scintillation scan*—image made by a scintillation counter to determine the size of a tumor, goiter, or other involvement and to locate aberrant, metastatic lesions. (23, 34)

- *scanning (nuclear medicine)*—method of mapping out the deposition of a radionuclide in an organ using a rectilinear or other scanning device. (23, 51)

- *scintillation counter*—a highly sensitive detector for measuring ionizing radiation capable of counting scintillations (light flashes) induced by radiation in certain materials. (23)

- *scintiphotography, gammaphotography*—the use of the Anger scintillation camera for obtaining photographs of the distribution of gamma-emitting radionuclides in living subjects.

Scintiphotography may be employed for:
  — dynamic studies portraying rapidly changing images, as in the visualization of blood flow, vascular filling, or of ventilation.
  — static studies requiring highly technical performance of individual images (views) and comparability of tracer concentration in related organs; for example, the intensity of radioactivity concentration in the spleen and marrow compared with that in the liver to demonstrate portal-systemic shunting of venous blood flow after surgery. (9, 34, 50)

- *teletherapy with* ^{60}CO—treatment of tumors within the body using an external source of cobalt 60 that is heavily shielded. The therapy beams may be rotated and shaped to permit a high dose to the tumor while sparing adjacent normal structures. (9, 47)

- *tracer*—an element or compound that has been made radioactive so that it can be easily followed (traced) in biologic and industrial processes. Radiation emitted by the radioisotope pinpoints its location. (25)
- *waste, radioactive*—equipment and materials (from nuclear operations) that are radioactive and have no further use. Wastes are generally referred to as high level (having radioactivity concentrations of hundreds to thousands of curies per gallon or cubic foot), low level (in range of one microcurie per gallon of cubic foot), and intermediate (between these extremes). (34, 47, 48)
- *whole body counter*—device used to identify and measure the radiation in the body (body burden) of human beings and animals; uses heavy shielding to keep out background radiation and ultrasensitive scintillation detectors and electronic equipment. (9, 23)
- *zipper effect*—overlapping of two or more images. (1, 23)

Special Studies

Terms Related to Radionuclide Imaging

- *blood flow imaging, perfusion studies*—noninvasive, dynamic, nuclear uptake measurements to detect occlusive or stenotic vascular lesions or malformations of the brain, heart, lungs, kidneys, skeletal muscles, and other organs. (7)
- *bone marrow imaging*—delineation of areas of active bone marrow to detect abnormal expansion of bone marrow and areas of bone marrow destruction. (29, 30, 50)
- *bone imaging*—scintillation imaging following the intravenous injection of a bone-seeking radionuclide, such as one of the technetium-99m phosphate complexes, to detect metastases to osseous tissue and help to determine the extent of pathologic bone lesions or healing processes. Bone scintillation imaging has been used in the early detection of stress fractures and other fractures not demonstrated by usual radiographs. This particular type of imaging has detected minimal osseous trauma areas where radiographs of the same areas reflected normal findings in some child abuse cases. This technique serves as a diagnostic tool in the early detection of osteomyelitis, Legg-Calvé-Perthes disease, and other hip abnormalities. (13, 24, 51)
- *brain imaging*—radionuclide uptake studies, dynamic or static, to detect intracerebral space-occupying lesions, malformations, trauma, or cerebrovascular disease. Diagnostic tracers frequently used are technetium 99m bound to diethylenetriamine pentaacetic acid and referred to as ^{99m}Tc DTPA, as well as ^{99m}Te-pertechnetate, ^{99m}-Tc glucoheptonate, and others. (5, 21). *Iofetamine HCL I-123* (SPECTamine) is the first lipid soluble radiopharmaceutical for functional brain imaging approved by the FDA. Unlike earlier brain-imaging agents, SPECTamine easily crosses the intact blood-brain barrier because of its unique lipid solubility. Extraction efficiency is high, washout is slow, and blood-brain ratios are high. The initial distribution of SPECTamine is maintained for at least one hour despite slow washout. Transverse, coronal, and sagittal views may be obtained during brain imaging. Regional changes in brain physiology indicating impaired brain function are revealed, and this procedure is useful in documenting the site and extent of cerebrovascular accident (CVA). (1)
    - —*cerebral circulation imaging*—dynamic brain imaging to visualize cerebral blood flow to compare values in different regions and to analyze cerebrovascular disease or other vascular abnormalities. Images are taken in a sequential manner at one- to three-second intervals. (32)

—*radionuclide cisternography*—intrathecal injection of a tracer for diagnostic evaluation. Scans of cisterns are useful in delineating obstructive, nonobstructive, or *ex vacuo* types of hydrocephalus. This is the only diagnostic test used for establishing the diagnosis of normal pressure hydrocephalus. This test is also used to determine patency and drainage of neurosurgical shunts and to visualize the point of leakage associated with this type of shunt. (32)

- *heart and circulation imaging:*

—*arterviovenous shunts*—^{99m}Tc human albumin microspheres (^{99m}Tc-HAM) particle perfusion studies demonstrate collateral circulation when the surgically created shunts occlude. (25)

—*infarct-avid myocardial imaging*—increased uptake of a radiopharmaceutical within an area of myocardial injury that permits its visualization as a "hot spot." Technetium 99m stannous pyrophosphate, ^{99m}Tc-labeled PYP, is commonly used as an imaging agent. The hot spot may be indicative of a subendocardial infarction, if increased uptake is two plus, and acute transmural infarction, if it is three or four plus. (11, 25)

—*myocardial perfusion studies*—evaluation of blood flow through the heart muscle. The determination of regional blood flow depends on the tracers being uniformly mixed in the blood, extracted, and retained in the perfusion bed of the myocardium long enough to obtain static images. Blood flow and extraction are greatly reduced in ischemic and injured myocardium areas. This area is reflected as a "cold spot" or defect. Thallium 201 (^{201}Tl) scintigraphy is a sensitive technique for the detection of perfusion defects of the heart muscle in myocardial infarction. The larger the perfusion abnormality, the poorer the prognosis. Those patients with large perfusion defects may benefit from intracoronary streptokinase infusion or insertion of an intraaortic balloon pump to avert further hemodynamic deterioration. (14, 25, 53)

—*blood pool studies of the heart:*

—*multigated (MUGA) blood pool studies*—these studies deal with ventricular wall motion and the ejection fraction and require that a tracer remain within the blood vessels during imaging. Technetium 99m-labeled red blood cells, ^{99m}Tc RBC, *in vitro* or *in vivo*, fulfill this condition. This study determines systolic, diastolic, and stroke volumes, cardiac output, ejection fraction, and regional and global wall motion abnormalities. (25, 51, 54)

—*other radionuclide cardiovascular studies:*

—*exercise thallium 201, ^{201}Tl scintigraphy*—thallium 201 imaging in patients with exercise electrocardiograms for:

—localizing and estimating the extent of significant coronary artery disease.

—evaluating the patient before and after myocardial revascularization. Serial studies are done to evaluate the patency or occlusion of postoperative grafts. This type of study is usually repeated one year after the graft procedure. (16, 25)

—*venous thrombosis radionuclide studies*—nuclear medicine procedures available for the detection of deep-vein thrombosis include the following: (3, 7, 25, 39, 55)

—*radionuclide venography*—bilateral injection of either ^{99m}Tc-human albumin microspheres (HAM) or ^{99m}Tc microaggregated albumin (MAA) into the dorsal veins of the foot. Application of tourniquets at the ankles assist to facilitate filling of the deep venous system.

—*iodinated ^{125}I-fibrinogen-uptake test*—presence of fibrinogen labeled with iodine-125 in the bloodstream will be attracted to the forming clot so that the thrombus will show a higher concentration of radioactivity than the adjacent areas.

—*radiolabeled platelets technique*—employs indium-111 labeled autologous platelets to detect forming blood clots. This rather new technique looks promising
as a method for diagnosing focal atherosclerotic and thrombotic lesions, and
for imaging vascular grafts.

■ *kidney imaging, renal imaging*—radionuclide visualization of the kidney to study its
structural and functional status and detect congenital abnormalities, perfusion
defects, renovascular disease, obstructive lesions, kidney trauma, or other renal
disorders. Radiopharmaceuticals for urologic diagnosis are various technetium-99m
compounds, which label the renal cortex, define renal blood flow, or determine the
rate of glomerular filtration. Abscesses and occult neoplasms may be detected by
nuclear scans using gallium-67 citrate (^{67}Ga citrate). (31, 38)

■ *kidney scintiphotography*—use of a scintillation camera to visualize renal position and
structure and evaluate renal function and blood flow distribution. Iodohippurate
sodium ^{131}I (radioactive iodine) and technetium-99m cortical agent are diagnostic
aids in evaluating renal blood flow in transplants, acute tubular necrosis, and
uremia. (31, 38)

■ *kidney-related urologic techniques:*
   —*nuclear cystograms*—accurate method of imaging bladder reflux.
   —*testicular scanning*—procedure for detecting testicular and scrotal disorders.
   —*whole-body bone imaging*—use of technetium—99m phosphate for skeletal
   scanning to demonstrate the extent of metastatic bone involvement of urologic
   malignancies. (34)

■ *liver imaging and hepatobiliary imaging*—nuclear method of evaluating the liver or both
liver and gallbladder. (28, 37)
   —*xenon-133 (^{133}Xe)*—retention in hepatic fatty infiltration due to alcohol abuse
   confirmed by scintigrams.
   —*technetium-99m (^{99m}Tc) sulfur colloid*—scintigram showing abnormal hepatic
   uptake in chronic alcoholics. Radionuclide demonstrates functioning of reticuloendothelial cells in liver, bone marrow, and spleen.
   —*technetium-99m (^{99m}Tc) diethyl-IDA imaging*—useful in noninvasive evaluation of
   hepatobiliary disorders. Nuclear cholescintigraphy provides accurate information
   about the biliary and hepatocellular function and the patency of the cystic duct
   and common bile duct. This is a reliable and often used test to demonstrate
   acute cholecystitis before surgery. This test may be used to evaluate postoperative status following cholecystectomy.

■ *lung imaging*—pulmonary imaging by:
   —*technetium-99m aggregated human serum albumin*—injected intravenously and
   carried into the pulmonary circulation for perfusion studies. The particles lodge
   in the capillaries of the lung, except in areas of embolic obstruction or other
   blockage (about 70 percent of emboli are multiple). (30)
   —*xenon-133 (^{133}Xe)*—for ventilatory studies inhaled to differentiate between
   emphysematous involvement or pulmonary emboli. Perfusion defects on lung
   scintigrams without any ventilation abnormality in the region are highly
   suggestive of pulmonary emboli. The diagnosis of pulmonary emboli is based
   on evaluation of blood flow to the lungs. Clearance of the perfusion defects after
   four to five days of anticoagulation therapy is presumptive evidence of recovery
   from embolic disease. No change in serial lung scans suggests presence of
   obstructive lung disease, such as emphysema, carcinoma, or other disorders.
   (30)
   —*gallium-67 (^{67}Ga)*—used for staging of lung neoplasms (tumors less than 1.5 cm
   in diameter are not detectable), infections, and inflammatory conditions.
   Abnormal uptake of ^{67}Ga in the mediastinum increases the prospect that

mediastinal disease is present. ^{67}Ga scans have been effectively used in patients with acquired immunodeficiency syndrome (AIDS) and the AIDS-related complex to identify *Pneumocystis carinii* pneumonia. (2, 30, 40)

Terms Related to Radionuclides in Diagnostic Tests

- *blood studies:*
  - —*blood volume*—sum total of red cell volume and plasma volume using chromium (^{51}Cr) labeled red cells or technetium-99m (^{99m}Tc) labeled red cells for measuring the blood volume. These findings are helpful in the diagnosis of polycythemia vera and in the management of fluid balance after surgery and severe burns. (6, 19)
  - —*iron studies*—ferrokinetic tests include:
  - –*incorporation of iron (^{59}Fe) into red blood cells*—in normal subjects this is 60 to 80 percent of the dose administered in seven to ten days. (52)
  - —*plasma iron clearance*—iron (^{59}Fe) disappearance in half the time in plasma, which is normally 60 to 120 minutes. (52)
  - —*plasma iron pool (in milligrams)*—determination by multiplying serum iron in milligrams by plasma volume per milliliter. Results may indicate iron deficiency anemias, polycythemias, and other disorders. (56)
  - —*red blood cell sequestration, RBC sequestration*—measurement of rate of accumulation of chromium-51 (^{51}Cr) tagged red cells in spleen, liver, and pericordium by scintillation counting. The test aids in the diagnosis of hypersplenism due to any cause. (19, 33)
  - —*red blood cells survival*—determination of rate of disappearance of labeled erythrocytes from the circulating blood. Chromium-51 (^{51}Cr) is usually the tagging agent. The normal rate of RBC disappearance from circulation is 28 to 32 days. A decreased rate of cell survival is present in hemolytic anemias. (6, 10, 19, 33, 52)
- *clot formation studies:*
  - —*fibrinogen uptake test ^{125}I*—detection of thrombi in their formative stage by locating the vascular lesion where the fibrinogen is being used.
  - —*fibrinogen uptake test ^{131}I*—same as above except for the tracer, ^{131}I.

These tests are valuable diagnostic tools for defining deep venous thrombosis developing in the calf or popliteal and femoral veins, which can be followed by daily testing. Compared to the use of ^{131}I, ^{125}I presents a lower radiation dose to the patient and an increased shelf life. A distinctive disadvantage of ^{125}I is its soft photon emissions, which hinder or make almost impossible the diagnosis of thrombosis in the veins of the upper thighs and pelvis. Although ^{131}I could provide imaging capability, the accompanying high-radiation dose to the patient precludes using an adequate scanning dose. ^{125}I represents the most commonly used agent in clinical practice. (25, 56)

- *gastrointestinal studies:*
  - —*fat absorption test, lipid absorption test*—measurement of fat digestion and absorption with radioiodine-labeled triolein and oleic acid, useful in distinguishing malabsorption syndromes. (15)
  - —*gastrointestinal (GI) blood loss*—localization of gastrointestinal bleeding by using technetium-99m-labeled red blood cells (^{99m}Tc-labeled RBCs) or sulfur colloid for evaluation of GI bleeding. Serial images of the abdomen are done; if normal, the abdomen is clear; if bleeding is present, the activity can be localized. (15, 27)

—*GI protein loss determination*—measurement of albumin leakage into the gastrointestinal tract using intravenous injection of chromium-51 (^{51}CR) labeled albumin.

—*vitamin B$_{12}$ absorption test, method of Schilling*—determination of vitamin B$_{12}$ absorption as an aid in diagnosis of pernicious anemia and malabsorption of B$_{12}$ due to other causes. Using cobalt 57, 58, or 60 as a tracer, the amount of B$_{12}$ absorbed is indirectly measured by determining the percentage of the test dose that is excreted in the urine in 24 hours. Since the pathophysiology of pernicious anemia is the inability to absorb vitamin B$_{12}$ the urinary excretion in these patients is low (less than 10 percent). If a potent intrinsic factor is administered with the test dose B$_{12}$, it will permit absorption of B$_{12}$ from the intestine in pernicious anemia but will not increase the absorption of B$_{12}$ in the presence of malabsorption caused by diseases other than pernicious anemia. (15, 33)

■ *renal clearance study*—functional renal imaging based on the fact that different radionuclear tracers measure the physiologic ability of specific areas of the kidney, such as:
  —effective renal plasma flow (ERPF) through glomeruli and proximal tubules.
  —glomerular filtration rate (GRF). (4, 46)

■ *renography*—a graphic demonstration of both kidneys following the intravenous injection of a radioactive tracer and the placement of a sensitive detector over the kidneys. In the presence of unilateral disease the curve of the moving nuclear bolus reflects reduced or increased tracer uptake by the affected kidney. (38)

■ *thyroid studies* (major tests):
  —*FTI, free thryoxine index, free T$_4$, index, FTE, free thyroxine estimate*—an indirect measure of thyroxine-binding protein. FTI is increased in hyperthyroidism and decreased in hypothyroidism. (26, 60)
  —*RAIU, radioactive iodine uptake determination (see Fig. 83)*—this test measures the ability of the thyroid gland to trap and organify the nuclide following the oral ingestion of a radioiodine tracer dose. A scintillation detector is used to determine the percentage of the thyroidal uptake of the radioiodine, usually 6 and 24 hours after administration of the tracer dose. There tends to be an increase of radioactive iodine uptake in pregnancy and hyperthyroid and euthyroid states and a decrease in hypothyroidism. (8, 20)
  —*TBG, thyroxine-binding globulin serum level*—measurement of circulating levels of TBG. It is not to be confused with thyroxine-binding index (TBI). An increase of TBG may occur in hypothyroidism, estrogen therapy, oral contraceptives, pregnancy; a decrease of TBG may occur in nephrotic syndromes, genetic hepatic disease, and other disorders. (57, 60)
  —*TBI, thyroxine-binding index*—a test of thyroxine-binding globulin levels in the patient's serum. A major problem is that the use of the contraceptive pill has become so prevalent that it interferes with the clinical interpretation of the test by elevating the level of the thyroxine-binding globulin (TBG) similar to pregnancy. (45)
  —*TRH, thyotropin-releasing hormone*—hormone produced by the hypothalamus, extrahypothalamic cerebral regions, and extracentral nervous system regions. TRH testing is an invaluable diagnostic procedure that is gradually replacing thyroidal stimulation and suppression studies. (20, 26, 58)
  —*TSH-RIA*—this radioimmunoassay of the thyroid-stimulating hormone (TSH) is a highly sensitive test for detecting primary hypothyroidism. TSH may be increased in a goiter deficient in iodine, such as in myxedema. (20, 57, 58)

Figure 83 Radioiodine and the thyroid gland.

Radioactive iodine—for diagnosing and treating gland disorders.

Medical action: 1. Diagnosis and treatment of hyperthyroidism.
2. Location of thyroid cancer and metastases.

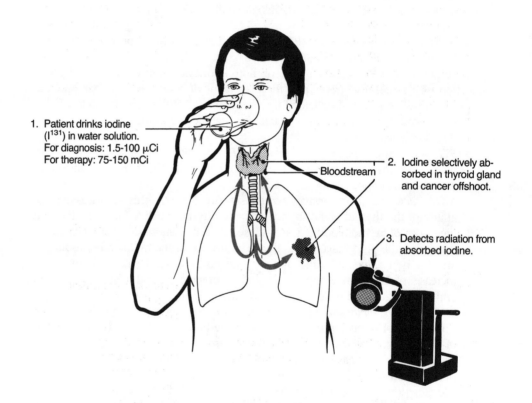

1. Patient drinks iodine (I^{131}) in water solution.
For diagnosis: 1.5-100 μCi
For therapy: 75-150 mCi

Bloodstream

2. Iodine selectively absorbed in thyroid gland and cancer offshoot.

3. Detects radiation from absorbed iodine.

—*TSH, thyroid stimulation hormone test*—measurement of the thyroid response to the administration of the thyroid-stimulating hormone (TSH). The test aids in the differential diagnosis of thyroidal hypothyroidism, in which a diseased thyroid fails to respond to TSH. In pituitary hypothyroidism the thyroid gland may begin to function after a TSH injection, since the gland may be simply dormant rather than diseased. (58)

—*T_3 or T_3 RIA serum level*—measurement of tridothyronine (T_3) in human serum by radioimmunoassay. An elevated T_3 serum level in the presence of normal T_4 (thyroxine) concentration may indicate T_3 toxicosis or toxic nodular goiter. (20, 26, 41)

—*T_3 or T_4 suppression test*—measurement of the thyroidal uptake of radioiodine and a scan following the oral administration of triiodothyronine (T_3) or thyroxine (T_4). In euthyroid patients there is usually a 50 percent suppression of the thyroidal uptake. In thyrotoxicosis, it does not drop below the normal range. The test is useful in distinguishing neurotic persons with borderline uptake from true hyperthyroidism. T_3 or T_4 suppression tests and TSH stimulation tests are gradually being replaced by TRH testing, since the procedure is safer for the patient. (20, 41, 58, 60)

—*Tg, thyroglobulin RIA*—measurement of the protein thyroglobulin (Tg) in human serum by means of a radioimmunoassay. Serum Tg levels are elevated in Graves' disease, toxic adenomas, toxic multinodular goiter, and in nontoxic diffuse or multinodular goiter. (59)

Table 35 presents a summary of radionuclides used in diagnostic evaluation.

Table 35
Some Radionuclides in Diagnosis*

Radionuclide	Labeled Tracer	Diagnostic Procedures	Clinical Use
Indium-111 ^{111}Ind	Leukocytes (WBC)	Abscess localization	Chronic abscess and other infections
Iodine-123 ^{123}I	Iofetamine	Brain imaging	Brain function Cerebrovascular accident Dementia Epilepsy
Iodine-131 or 123 ^{131}I ^{123}I	Sodium Iodide	Thyroid scan and uptake RAIU	Thyroid carcinoma Thyroid adenoma Thyroid nodule Others
^{131}I	Hippuran	Measurement of effective renal plasma flow-ERPF	Renal clearance
Iodine-125 ^{125}I		TBI (Thyroxine-binding index) FTI (Free thyroxine index) T_3 (Triiodothyronine uptake test)	T_3 toxicosis

*(1, 8, 9, 20, 26, 34, 42, 45, 52, 55, 58)

Radionuclide	Labeled Tracer	Diagnostic Procedures	Clinical Use
Iodine-125 ^{125}I *(Continued)*			
	Others	TSH (Thyroid - stimulating hormone)	Others
	Fibrinogen	Clot formation study ^{125}I fibrinogen uptake	Detection of thrombi in formative stage
	Human serum albumin	Blood volume determination, cardiac output, and circulation time	Vascular and cardiac disease
		Others	Others
Technetium-99m ^{99m}Tc	Diethylenetriamine pentaacetic acid DTPA or DTPA chelate	Brain scan Perfusion studies Nuclear cisternography	Brain lesion Vascular disorder Hydrocephalus Others
	Pertechnetate	Renography or imaging	Renal disorder unilateral or bilateral obstructive renovascular hypertensive
		Perfusion studies	Transplanted kidney
	Pertechnetate	Cerebral circulation studies	Cerebrovascular disorders
	Human serum albumin	Nuclear cisternography	Hydrocephalus Others
	Red blood cells	Nuclear cardiology Angiocardiographic studies—blood pool imaging	Congenital cardiac defects Myocardial infarction Ventricular aneurysm Ischemic heart disease
	Aggregated human serum albumin	Lung perfusion studies	Pulmonary embolism Pulmonary venous hypertension Arteriovenous shunt Response to anticoagulation therapy
	Erythrocytes	Erythrocyte venography	Deep vein thrombosis Thrombophlebitis
Technetium-99m ^{99m}Tc	Sulfur colloid	Imaging for functioning of reticuloendothelial cells in spleen, liver, and bone marrow	Evaluation of functional status of reticuloen-dothelial cells—chronic alcoholism
	Stannous pyrophosphate	Bone imaging to detect osteogenic alterations Cardiac imaging Infarct-avid imaging Blood pool imaging	Metastatic bone lesions Osteomyelitis Acute myocardial infarction
Thallium-201 ^{201}TI and Technetium-99m ^{99m}TC		Parathyroid scan	Parathyroid adenoma

Radionuclide	Labeled Tracer	Diagnostic Procedures	Clinical Use
Thallium-201 ^{201}TI	Thallous chloride	^{201}TI scintigraphy	Perfusion defects Myocardial ischemia or infarction
		Exercise ^{201}TI myocardial scintigraphy	Evaluation of coronary artery disease Results of myocardial revascularization Postoperative graft occlusion
Chromium-51 ^{51}Cr	Human red cells	Blood volume determination Red cell survival	Hemolytic disease
	Human serum albumin	Fecal analysis for blood loss protein loss	Intestinal protein loss in hypoproteinemia
Iron-52 or 59 ^{52}Fe ^{59}Fe	Ferrous citrate	Determination of plasma iron clearance plasma iron turnover rate plasma iron pool	Aplastic anemia Hemolytic anemia Iron deficiency anemia Others
Cobalt-57 or 60 ^{57}Co ^{60}Co	Cyanocobalamine (vitamin B_{12})	Determination of intestinal absorption of vitamin B_{12}	Pernicious anemia Sprue

Radionuclides in Therapy

In nuclear medicine radionuclides are primarily used for tracer studies, and their significance in diagnostic evaluation has been firmly established. The application of radionuclides in therapy is more restricted. In the treatment of carcinomas, radionuclides serve as palliative agents with potential for prolonging life, and they have a low capacity for inhibiting or destroying malignancies other than certain thyroid or ovarian cancers. Radionuclides also are employed in the treatment of polycythemia vera and in selected cases of leukemia and lymphoma (see current therapeutic uses of some radionuclides listed in Table 36).

Table 36
Some Radionuclides in Therapy*

Radionuclide	Method	Clinical Use
Cesium-137 ^{137}Cs	Brachytherapy Intracavity insertion of cesium sources	Cancer of uterine cervix
Cobalt-60 ^{60}Co	Teletherapy External high-energy irradiation by telecobalt unit	Cancer of breast and other malignancies

*(1, 16, 36, 42, 47, 56)

Radionuclide	Method	Clinical Use
Phosphorus-32 ^{32}P	Intravenous administration of disodium phosphate	Polycythemia vera and selected cases of leukemia or lymphoma Palliation of pain in some bone metastases
	Intracavitary infusion of colloidal chromic phosphate	Therapeutic or palliative treatment of pleural and peritoneal malignancy or resulting effusion
Iodine-131 ^{131}I	Oral administration of sodium radioiodine	Hyperthyroidism adenocarcinoma of thyroid Selected cases of angina pectoris and heart failure

Abbreviations

Symbols of Radionuclides in Nuclear Medicine

^{111}Ag—radiosilver
^{72}As, ^{74}As—radioarsenic
^{198}Au—radiogold
^{57}Co, ^{60}Co—radiocobalt
^{51}Cr—radiochromium
^{137}Cs—radiocesium
^{61}Cu, ^{64}Cu—radiocopper
^{18}F—radiofluorine
^{52}Fe, ^{59}Fe—radioiron
^{67}Ga—radiogallium
^{197}Hg, ^{203}Hg—radiomercury
^{113m}In—radioindium
^{125}I, ^{131}I—radioiodine
^{192}Ir—radioiridium
^{42}K—radiopotassium
^{81}Kr—radiokrypton
^{52}Mn—radiomagnesium
^{24}Na—radiosodium
^{32}P—radiophosphorus
^{86}Rb—radiorubidium
^{35}S—radiosulfur
^{85}Sr, ^{87}Sr—radiostrontium
^{99m}Tc—radiotechnetium
^{201}Tl—radiothallium
^{169}Yb—radioytterbium
^{90}Y—radioyttrium

Tests and Miscellaneous Symbols

A—mass number
FTI—free thyroxine index
FUT—fibrinogen uptake test
GM—Geiger-Müller (counter)
MAA—macroaggregated albumin
MHP—mercuryhydroxypropane
MPC—maximum permissible concentration
MPL—maximum permissible level or limit
N—neutron
RAIU—radioactive iodine uptake
RBE—relative biologic effectiveness
RIA—radioimmunoassay
TBG—thyroxine-binding globulin
TBI—thyroxine-binding index
TRH—thyrotropin-releasing hormone
TSH—thyrotropin, thyroid-stimulating hormone
Z—atomic number

Multiples of Curie Units

1 Ci	curie	1 curie
1mCi	millicurie	10^3 curie
1μCi	microcurie	10^4 curie
1nCi	nanocurie	10^9 curie
1pCi	picocurie	10^{13} curie

Other Units of Measurement

Bev—1 billion electron volts
E—energy in ergs
erg—1 unit of work
ev—1 electron volt
Kev, keV—1,000 electron volts
Mev, MeV—1 million electron volts
r—roentgen
RAD, rad—radiation absorbed dose,
        100 ergs/gm tissue
REM, rem—roentgen equivalent, man

REP, rep—roentgen equivalent, physical

Scientific Organizations

ABNM—American Board of
        Nuclear Medicine
ACNM—American College of
        Nuclear Medicine
ACNP—American College of
        Nuclear Physicians
NRC—Nuclear Regulatory Commission
SNM—Society of Nuclear Medicine

Oral Reading Practice

The Thyroid Gland and Radioiodine

The **thyroid gland** lies in the anterior part of the neck, immediately in front of the trachea and below the thyroid cartilage. The two lobes of the thyroid are united by an **isthmus** in the form of a shield. The avidity of the thyroid for **iodine** is an interesting and unique characteristic of this **endocrine gland.** It is the basis of many thyroid function studies and the medical treatment of many thyroid diseases. (9, 16, 36, 56)

Associated with the development of **nuclear reactors** as part of the atomic weapons program, **radionuclides** became abundantly available as by-products. Investigations proved that many of these were useful in clinical medicine. **Nuclides** are varieties of a chemical element that differ in their atomic weights but possess the same chemical properties. Some elements are available as both stable and **radioactive nuclides.** For example:

> Iodine-127, the stable element with an atomic weight of 127.
> Iodine-131, one of the radionuclides, with an atomic weight of 131.

The latter is a widely used radionuclide of iodine and is generally the one implied by the term "radioiodine." (36, 42)

The value of radioiodine (^{131}I) in the diagnosis and treatment of **hyperthyroidism** and in **thyroid carcinoma** is well established. ^{131}I does not differ chemically from iodine, but differs physically in that it emits **beta particles** and **gamma rays.** Since the beta particles penetrate only two millimeters of tissue, they are almost all absorbed within the gland. On the other hand, about 90 percent of the gamma rays escape and can be accurately measured outside the body with a radiation detector such as a **scintillation counter.**

^{131}I has a **half-life** of eight days. This means that every eight days its radioactivity is reduced to half the intensity present eight days previously. The half-life is of clinical importance, since the nuclide must not exert its effect too long, to avoid excessive radiation damage, and not too short, to ensure adequate results. (34, 42)

When a radioiodine uptake study is ordered, the patient receives a calibrated dose of ^{131}I, either in a capsule or in a solution. The tracer dose ranges from 5 to 25 microcuries (μCi), whereas therapeutic doses are measured in **millicuries** (1 mCi = 1,000 μCi). After oral administration radioiodine is rapidly absorbed from the **gastrointestinal (GI) tract** and selectively picked up by thyroid tissue. Within four to six hours the gland has become the depot for about one fourth of the nuclide ingested. In 24 hours thyroid function can be estimated by the amount of radioiodine retained. The thyroidal uptake of ^{131}I by the normal gland in 24 hours is 15 to 40 percent of the tracer dose. In **hyperthyroidism** it is 50 to 100 percent. (8, 9, 36, 42, 56)

Pregnancy is an absolute contraindication to the administration of ^{131}I because of the danger of radiation to the fetus. Usually women of childbearing age are advised to avoid pregnancy for at least one year following ^{131}I therapy, should there be need to have ^{131}I retreatment. (36, 42, 56)

The major indications for radioiodine therapy include the treatment of hyperthyroidism and the elimination of metastases from thyroid carcinoma. Forms of hyperthyroidism that may be treated with radioiodine therapy are **Graves' disease (diffuse toxic goiter), Plummer's disease (toxic multinodular goiter),** and **toxic adenoma.** (1, 16, 36)

References and Bibliography

1. Ahmad, Munir, MD. Personal communications.
2. Bitran, Jacob, et al. Patterns of gallium-67 scintigraphy in patients with acquired immunodeficiency syndrome and the AIDS related complex. *Journal of Nuclear Medicine* 28:1103-1106, July 1987.
3. Bonow, Robert O., and Bacharach, Stephen L. Left ventricular diastolic function: Evaluation by radionuclide ventriculography. In Pohost, Gerald M., ed.-in-chief, *New Concepts in Cardiac Imaging—1987.* Chicago: Year Book Medical Publishers, Inc., 1987, pp. 103-137.
4. Brenner, Barry M., Hostetter, Thomas H., and Hebert, Steven C. Disturbances of renal function. In Braunwald, Eugene, et al. eds., *Harrison's Principles of Internal Medicine,* 11th ed. New York: McGraw-Hill Book Co., 1987, pp. 1143-1149.
5. Brillman, J., et al. The diagnosis of skull brain metastases by radionuclide bone scan. *Cancer* 59:1887-1891, June 1987.
6. Bunn, H. Franklin. Anemia. In Braunwald, Eugene, et al. eds., *Harrison's Principles of Internal Medicine.* 11th ed. New York: McGraw-Hill Book Co., 1987, pp. 262-266.
7. Carretta, Robert F., and Matin, Philip. Thrombus detection with radionuclides. In Matin, Philip, ed., *Clinical Nuclear Medicine Imaging.* New York: Elsevier Science Publishing Co., Inc., 1986, pp. 262-275.
8. Cavalieri, Ralph R. Quantitative in vivo tests. In Ingbar, Sidney H., and Braverman, Lewis E., eds., *Werner's The Thyroid,* 5th ed. Philadelphia: J.B. Lippincott Co., 1986, pp. 445-458.
9. Charkes, N. David. Thyroid and whole-body imaging. In Ingbar, Sidney H., and Braverman, Lewis E., eds., *Werner's The Thyroid,* 5th ed. Philadelphia: J.B. Lippincott Co., 1986, pp. 458-478.
10. Code of Federal Regulations, Title 10, Part 20. *Standards for Protection against Radiation.* Section 20, 303, 1983.
11. Cooper, Richard A., and Bunn, H. Franklin. Hemolytic anemias. In Braunwald, Eugene, et al. eds., *Harrison's Principles of Internal Medicine,* 11th ed. New York: McGraw-Hill Book Co., 1987, pp. 1506-1518.
12. Corbus, Howard F., and Touya, Jean J. Emission computed tomography. In Matin, Philip, ed., *Clinical Nuclear Medicine Imaging.* New York: Elsevier Science Publishing Co., Inc., 1986, pp. 305-354.
13. Durzinsky, Dennis, et al. Method for assuring accuracy of bone biopsy using technetium 99 bone scan. *Cancer* 59:723-725, Feb. 1987.
14. Gibson, Robert S., and Beller, George A. The role of thallium-201 scintigraphy in predicting future cardiac events. In Pohost, Gerald M., ed.-in-chief, *New Concepts in Cardiac Imaging—1987.* Chicago: Year Book Medical Publishers, Inc., 1987, pp. 113-135.
15. Greenberger, Norton, J., and Isselbacher, Kurt J. Disorders of absorption. In Braunwald, Eugene, et al. eds., *Harrison's Principles of Internal Medicine,* 11th ed. New York: McGraw-Hill Book Co., 1987, pp. 1260-1276.
16. Harbert, John C. Radioiodine therapy of hyperthyroidism. In *Nuclear Medicine Therapy.*

New York: Thieme Medical Publishers, Inc., 1987, pp. 1-36.

17. Haynes, Barton F. Enlargement of lymph nodes and spleen. In Braunwald, Eugene, et al. eds., *Harrison's Principles of Internal Medicine*, 11th ed. New York: McGraw-Hill Book Co., 1987, pp. 272-278.

18. Held, Kathryn D. Radiobiology: biologic effects of ionizing radiations. In *Nuclear Medicine Therapy*. New York: Thieme Medical Publishers, Inc., 1987, pp. 257-284.

19. Herbert, Victor. The blood. In Ingbar, Sidney H., and Braverman, Lewis E., eds., *Werner's The Thyroid*, 5th ed. Philadelphia: J.B. Lippincott Co., 1986, pp. 878-884.

20. Ingbar, Sidney H. Diseases of the thyroid. In Braunwald, Eugene, et al. eds., *Harrison's Principles of Internal Medicine*, 11th ed. New York: McGraw-Hill Book Co., 1987, pp. 1732-1752.

21. Kaplan, W.D. et al. Thallium-201 brain tumor imaging: A comparative study with pathologic correlation. *Journal of Nuclear Medicine* 28:47-52, Jan. 1987.

22. Kim, E. Edmund, and Haynie, Thomas P. Radiopharmaceuticals. *Nuclear Diagnostic Imaging: Practical Clinical Applications*. New York: Macmillian Publishing Co., Inc., 1987, pp. 17-44.

23. ———. Instrumentation. Ibid., pp. 45-82.

24. ———. Musculoskeletal imaging. Ibid., pp. 103-152.

25. ———. Cardiovascular imaging. Ibid., pp. 153-197.

26. ———. Endocrine imaging. Ibid., pp. 199-244.

27. ———. Gastrointestinal tract imaging. Ibid., pp. 245-265.

28. ———. Hepatic and biliary imaging. Ibid., pp. 267-308.

29. ———. Hematologic and infectious disease imaging. Ibid., pp. 309-345.

30. ———. Pulmonary imaging. Ibid., pp. 347-379.

31. ———. Genitourinary imaging. Ibid., pp. 381-420.

32. ———. Central nervous system imaging. Ibid., pp. 421-459.

33. ———. Other useful procedures and new technology. Ibid., pp. 463-486.

34. Kowalsky, Richard J., and Perry J. Randolph. Physics of radiopharmaceuticals. In *Radiopharmaceuticals in Nuclear Medicine Practice*. Norwalk, CT: Appleton & Lange, 1987, pp. 13-57.

35. ———. Quality control of radiopharmaceuticals. Ibid., pp. 123-146.

36. ———. Thyroid—Clinical evaluation of the thyroid gland. Ibid., pp. 181-210.

37. ———. Liver, gallbladder, spleen and bone marrow. Ibid., pp. 271-314.

38. ———. Kidney and genitourinary systems. Ibid., pp. 314-349.

39. ———. Total body imaging: Gallium and indium radiopharmaceuticals. Ibid., pp. 379-409.

40. Kramer, Elissa L., et al. Gallium-67 scans of the chest in patients with acquired immunodeficiency syndrome. *Journal of Nuclear Medicine* 28:1107-1114, July 1987.

41. Larsen, P. Reed. Thyroid hormone concentrations. In Ingbar, Sidney H., and Braverman, Lewis E., eds., *Werner's The Thyroid*, 5th ed. Philadelphia: J.B. Lippincott Co., 1986, pp. 479-501.

42. Links, Jonathan M., and Wagner, Henry N., Jr. Radiation physics. In Ingbar, Sidney H., and Braverman, Lewis E., eds., *Werner's The Thyroid*, 5th ed. Philadelphia: J.B. Lippincott Co., 1986, pp. 417-431.

43. Matin, Philip. Brain scintigraphy. In Matin, Philip, ed., *Clinical Nuclear Medicine Imaging*. New York: Elsevier Science Publishing Co., Inc., 1986, pp. 1-13.

44. McCall, Ann, et al. Routine use of thallium-technetium scan prior to parathyroidectomy. *The American Surgeon* 53:380-384, July 1987.

45. McKenzie, J. Maxwell, and Zakarij, Margita. Assays of the thyroid-stimulating antibodies (TSAb) of Graves' disease. In Ingbar, Sidney H., and Braverman, Lewis E., eds., *Werner's The Thyroid*, 5th ed. Philadelphia: J.B. Lippincott Co., 1986, pp. 559-575.

46. Murphy, John E., et al. Evaluation of renal function and water, electrolyte, and acid-base balance. In Henry, John Bernard, ed., *Davidsohn Clinical Diagnosis and Management by Laboratory Methods*, 17th ed. Philadelphia: W.B. Saunders Co., 1984, pp. 118-132.

47. Nalesnik, William, PhD. Personal communications.

48. National Council on Radiation Measurements. *Precautions in the Management of Patients Who Have Received Therapeutic Amounts of Radionuclides*. Report 36. Washington, DC: U.S. Government Printing Office.

49. Ohtake, Tahrum, et al. Evaluation of regurgitant faction of the left ventricular by gated cardiac blood-pool scanning using SPECT. *Journal of Nuclear Medicine* 28:19-24, Jan. 1987.

50. Price, David C. Bone marrow scintigraphy. In Matin, Philip, ed., *Clinical Nuclear Medicine Imaging*. New York: Elsevier Science Publishing Co., Inc., 1986, pp. 92-116.

51. Robertson, James S. Absorbed dose calculations. In Herbert, John C., *Nuclear Medicine Therapy*. New York: Thieme Medical Publishers, Inc., 1987, pp. 285-296.

52. Schafer, Andrew I., and Bunn, H. Franklin. Anemias of iron deficiency and iron over-

load. In Braunwald, Eugene, et al., eds., *Harrison's Principles of Internal Medicine*, 11th ed. New York: McGraw-Hill Book Co., 1987, pp. 1493-1498.

53. Schelbert, Heinrich R. Evaluation and quantification of regional myocardial blood flow with positron emission tomography. In Pohost, Gerald M., ed.-in-chief, *New Concepts in Cardiac Imaging—1987*. Chicago: Year Book Medical Publishers, Inc., 1987, pp. 197-221.

54. Stadius, Michael L., and Ritchie, James L. Gated blood pool tomography. In Pohost, Gerald M., ed.-in-chief, *New Concepts in Cardiac Imaging—1987*. Chicago: Year Book Medical Publishers, Inc., 1987, pp. 137-154.

55. Stratton, John R., and Ritchie, James L. Indium 111-labeled platelet imaging in man. In Pohost, Gerald M., ed.-in-chief, *New Concepts in Cardiac Imaging—1987*. Chicago: Year Book Medical Publishers, Inc., 1987, pp. 139-196.

56. Tucker, Eugene, MD. Personal communications.

57. Utiger, Robert D. Thyrotropin: Assay and secretory physiology in man. In Ingbar, Sidney H., and Braverman, Lewis E., eds., *Werner's The Thyroid*, 5th ed. Philadelphia: J.B. Lippincott Co., 1986, pp. 304-318.

58. ———. Tests of thyroregulatory mechanisms. Ibid., pp. 511-523.

59. Van Herle, Andre J. Measurement and clinical significance of thyroglobulin in serum and body fluids. In Ingbar, Sidney H., and Braverman, Lewis E., eds., *Werner's The Thyroid*, 5th ed. Philadelphia: J.B. Lippincott Co., 1986, pp. 534-545.

60. Woeber, Kenneth A. Tests of thyroid hormone transport. In Ingbar, Sidney H., and Braverman, Lewis E., eds., *Werner's The Thyroid*, 5th ed. Philadelphia: J.B. Lippincott Co., 1986, pp. 502-510.

Selected Terms Pertaining to Physical Therapy

Orientation

Origin of Terms

actino- (G)—ray
arthr-, arthro- (G)—joint
crymo- (G)—cold
cryo- (G)—cold
hydr-, hydro- (G)—water
kine-, kinesio- (G)—movement
my-, myo- (G)—muscle

ortho- (G)—correct, straight
phon-, phono- (G)—voice, sound
phot-, photo-, (G)—light
physio- (G)—physical, nature
rachio- (G)—spine
radio- (L)—ray
therm-, thermo- (G)—heat

General Terms

- *biofeedback*—process by which the physiologic activity of a patient can be translated into electric signals of a visual or auditory system. Myofeedback is a type of biofeedback in which the physiologic process is muscular activity. Electromyographic biofeedback employs the use of instrumentation to transduce muscle potentials into auditory or visual cues for the purpose of increasing or decreasing voluntary activity. (56)
- *electric current*—stream of electrons flowing along a conductor. (1)
  - *alternating current (A/C)*—bidirectional, intermittent, asymmetric current obtained from the secondary winding of an induction coil; also known as faradic, biphasic, and bipolar current.
  - *direct current (D/C)*—unidirection current with distinct polarity; also called constant, galvanic, monophasic, and monopolar currents. Electrical current that flows in one direction for one second or longer is defined as a direct current. A direct current that flows unidirectionally for a few milliseconds or less is termed a "pulsatile current".
  - *alternating current continuous modulation*—refers to constant variation in rate of electron flow at any given intensity.
  - *direct current continuous modulation*—rate of flow that is uniform at any given intensity.
  - *interrupted modulation*—periods of current flow alternating with cessation of current flow.

—*surging modulation*—periods of current flow and cessation of flow, with a gradual increase and decrease in intensity. In surging modulation, the shift from energy flow to no flow is gradual, whereas in interrupted modulation it is abrupt.

- *electrotesting*—the use of electric to test the reaction of muscles and motor nerves. This includes:
  - —*chronaxie*—the minimal time required for a current twice the strength of the rheobase to elicit a muscle contraction. (12)
  - —*electromyography*—the amplification and recording, both visually and audibly, of minute electric potentials generated by muscle contractions. Electromyograms are valuable in the study of neuromuscular disorders. (17, 26)
  - —*nerve conduction velocity*—electric testing to determine the speed of nerve conduction and residual latency.
  - —*reaction of degeneration*—the reaction of a muscle to galvanic but not faradic current. (17)
  - —*rheobase*—the minimal intensity of current required to elicit muscle contraction. (12)
  - —*strength duration curve*—the graphic representation of current strength and duration required to elicit a minimal muscle contraction. (12)
- *orthosis*—correction of defects. Usually refers to a device applied to patients for supportive assistance or for corrective purposes. Such devices include braces, splints, and so on. (39)
- *pathokinesiology*—the study of kinesiology as related to abnormal human motion.
- *physiatrist*—physician who specializes in physical medicine and rehabilitation.
- *physical agents*—active forces such as water, radiant energy, massage, exercise, electricity, and ultrasound energy. (39)
- *physical medicine*—that branch of medical science that uses physical agents in the diagnosis and management of disease.
- *physical therapist*—professional person qualified to provide physical therapy in such areas as direct patient care, consultation, supervision, teaching, administration, research, and community service. (18)
- *physical therapist assistant*—skilled technical worker who administers physical therapy treatments under the supervision of a physical therapist. (39)
- *physical therapy*—profession that uses knowledge and skills pertaining to physical therapy in caring for persons disabled by disease or injury. The primary focus is on the functional restoration of patients affected with skeletal, neuromuscular, cardiovascular, and pulmonary disorders. Steps to achieve and maintain this focus include an assessment of the patient's current level of function and the degree of the patient's dysfunction, coupled with the establishment of long-term and short-term goals supported by an appropriate treatment plan. Therapeutic measures specific to the patient's condition are applied, as well as periodic evaluation of the patient, treatment plan, and physical therapy modalities. (39)
- *prosthetics*—the designing and fitting of an artificial part, for example, to replace a limb. (39)
- *rehabilitation*—treatment process designed to help physically handicapped persons make maximal use of residual capacities and to enable them to obtain optimal satisfaction and usefulness in terms of themselves, their families, and their community.

Terms Related to Physical Therapy Procedures

- *cryotherapy, crymotherapy*—the use of cold, especially cold packs, immersion in water, or ice massage. (40)

- *electrotherapy*—use of electric current in the treatment of disease. Associated terms are:
  - —*high-voltage pulsed galvanic stimulation (HVPGS)*—use of high voltage (greater than 100 volts) interrupted current, providing a series of pulses of fixed duration in the microsecond range. High-voltage pulsed galvanic stimulation has assisted with burn debridement, pain modulation, and in the reduction of edema. (45)
  - —*iontophoresis*—the introduction of medicinal ions into the tissues by means of direct current. (13, 31)
  - —*neuromuscular electrical stimulation (NMES)*—use of high-frequency, low-amplitude neuromuscular electrical stimulation that serves as an adjunct to range-of-motion, strengthening, facilitation, and spasticity management programs. (3, 4)
  - —*transcutaneous electric nerve stimulation (TENS)*—the use of low-voltage or low-amperage current to produce sensory modulation for control of pain. (5, 33, 35)
- *hydrotherapy*—the use of water in its various forms: liquid, solid, and vapor. Included are terms related to the use of heat and cold. (54) Related terms include:
  - —*Archimedes' principle*—a body full or partially immersed in a liquid experiences an upward thrust equal to the weight of the liquid it displaces. (28)
  - —*burn hydrotherapy*—use of water at approximately 37° to 40° C (98° to 100° F) for cleansing of patient, removal of clothing, and burned tissue. The addition of a suitable disinfectant and salt to the solution are helpful in preventing loss of fluids and electrolytes. Hubbard or whirlpool tanks may also be employed. (28)
  - —*contrast bath*—alternate use of hot and cold water. (54)
  - —*underwater exercise*—immersion of the patient in water, a tank, or a pool, to permit free active motion, relaxation, and full abduction of the extremities, and sometimes for gait training. (28, 54)
  - —*whirlpool*—a treatment that offers temperature control in combination with mechanical effects of water in motion. (28, 54)
- *thermotherapy*—treatment of disease using various forms of heat. Associated terms include:
  - —*conduction*—heat transferred from a warmer object to a cooler one when both objects are in contact. (41, 54)
  - —*convection*—heat exchange between a surface and a fluid moving adjacent to the surface. (54)
  - —*diathermy*—the therapeutic use of high-frequency currents to generate heat within parts of the body. Types of diathermy include microwave and short wave units. (34)
  - —*fluidotherapy*—utilizes a dry heat agent that transfers energy by forced convection. The solid particles become suspended as air is forced through them. This type of therapy impacts mechanical as well as thermal stimulus to cutaneous receptors and has been found to be beneficial in the treatment of chronic musculoskeletal pain. (41, 42)
  - —*hot packs*—a moist heat provided from a canvas case usually filled with a bentonite substance. Between applications, the hot packs are kept immersed in water at a temperature between 72° and 79° C. Towels may be wrapped around the hot packs prior to placement at a particular body site. (41, 42)
  - —*paraffin baths*—refers to mixture of paraffin, paraffin oil, or petroleum jelly used in a bath. Paraffin baths have been effective in relieving pain in rheumatoid and osteoarthritis, especially in areas of the joints distal to the elbow and knee. (41, 42)

—paraffin packs—use of hot paraffin for therapeutic purposes. Paraffin packs are used most often for heat application to the lower extremities. (41, 42)

■ *therapeutic ultrasound*—employment of high-intensity, high-frequency sound waves (considerably above the range of hearing) for therapeutic purposes. Therapeutic ultrasound is used in functional restoration and healing of soft tissue conditions as well as for tissue destruction in surgery and hyperthermia for tumor irradiation. Ultrasound may be used as a deep heating agent to increase the temperature of particular structures, especially in the treatment of musculoskeletal disorders. (58)

—phonophoresis—the introduction of medicinal ions such as hydrocortisone into the tissues by means of ultrasound. (58)

■ *massage*—manipulation of the soft tissues of the body, most effectively performed with the hands, and administered to produce effects on the nervous and muscular systems and the local and general circulation of the blood and lymph. (48)

—acupressure—application of pressure to acupuncture sites to relieve pain.

—cryokinetics—ice massage. (40)

—effleurage—superficial or deep stroking movements.

—friction—deep circular or rolling movements.

—percussion—repeated taps or blows differing in force.

—petrissage—kneading or compression or compression movements.

—tapotement—percussion movements, including cupping, hacking, clapping, tapping, and beating.

—thermassage—massage with heat. (48)

—vibratory massage—frequently performed with a mechanical device, especially to increase bronchial drainage.

■ *radiation therapy*—the therapeutic use of radiant energy, especially infrared and ultraviolet rays.

—infrared—an invisible form of radiant energy, ranging from about 760 to 1,500 mμ in the electromagnetic spectrum and producing heat on absorption. (41)

—ultraviolet—an invisible form of radiant energy, ranging from about 180 to 400 mμ and producing chemical actions on absorption. (58)

Related terms are:

—cold quartz—type of ultraviolet lamp used for local irradiation. (34)

—cosine angle law—the intensity is greatest when the surface to be treated is at a right angle to the lamp. (34)

—electromagnetic spectrum (EMS)—graphic representation of the various waves of radiant energy in ascending order of length. (34)

—erythema—a latent inflammatory reaction caused by a chemical action that takes place in the skin.

—heliotherapy—exposure of the body to sunlight or solar radiation.

—inverse square law—the intensity of radiation from any source varies inversely with the square of the distance from the source. (41)

—minimal erythema dose—irradiation insufficient to cause reddening of the skin.

—mottling—irradiation sufficient to produce abnormally white patches on the skin as well as red blotches. (41)

—suberythema dose—irradiation insufficient to cause slight reddening of the skin.

—third-degree erythema dose—irradiation sufficient to cause edema and blister formation. (41)

■ *therapeutic exercise:*

—terms related to muscle action:

—agonist, prime mover—muscle that is considered the principal one used in a specific movement. (27)

—antagonist—muscle that acts on a joint in the opposite direction. (27)

—concentric—muscle contraction in which the external length of the muscle is decreased; the muscle tension overcomes the load.

—eccentric—muscle contraction in which the muscle lengthens as the load overcomes the tension developed by the muscle.

—fixators—muscles that act from the unconscious level to fix the attachments of the action of the agonists, antagonists, and synergists.

—isokinetic exercise—refers to control of speed of muscular performance achieved by an external mechanism that holds the speed of body movements to constant rates regardless of the degree of forces generated by the participating muscles. The isokinetic device allows suitable mechanical methods of receiving the full muscular force of a body segment throughout a range of motion, but without permitting acceleration to occur. (38)

—isometric or static—muscle contraction in which the muscle is not allowed to shorten or lengthen. (48, 55).

—isotonic or dynamic—muscle contraction in which invisible shortening or lengthening of the muscle occurs. (48)

—synergist—muscle that contracts together with another muscle and has an action identical or nearly identical to the agonist. (38)

—terms related to exercise:

—active—exercise done with voluntary muscle contraction.

—active assistive—exercise done with a combination of voluntary muscle contraction and assistance to an external force.

—breathing—exercise to any of the muscles of breathing designed to increase the work of breathing.

—conditioning—exercises to improve the fitness of a system, such as the cardiovascular system.

—facilitation—stimulation designed to increase muscle tone.

—inhibition—stimulation designed to decrease muscle tone.

—mobilization—gentle passive motion used to re-establish joint play between moving parts of joints.

—passive—joint movements performed by an outside force, usually another person, with the patient neither assisting nor resisting the movements. (48)

—resistive—an active exercise carried out by the patient working against resistance produced by either manual or mechanical means.

Terms Related to Evaluation and Measurements

- *ADL testing*—test that serves to outline as accurately as possible how a patient functions in everyday life; how many activities of daily living (ADL) can be performed in the home and/or in connection with work. Associated terms include:

    —*Barthel index*—weighted index for assessing dependence in basic ADLs for chronic disabled patients. Health professionals judge the number of points to be awarded to a patient based on the amount of help that a person needs to perform an activity. This index rates independence in feeding, transfers from wheelchair to bed, getting on and off toilet, controlling bladder and bowels, dressing, walking and ascending/descending stairs. Overall the scores range from zero to one hundred; zero indicates complete dependence and one hundred indicates complete independence in activity performance. (30)

    —*Katz ADL index*—rating assessment in the range of zero to three. 0 = complete independence; 1 = use of a device; 2 = human help, and; 3 = complete dependence. The six ADLs rated by the health professional include: bathing; dressing; going to the toilet; transfers; continence; and feeding. (30)

    —*Kenny self-care index*—standardized protocol for recording the health professional's judgment of the patient's basic physical functions. The basic functions rated include bed activities; transfers; locomotion; dressing; personal hygiene; and feeding. (30)

—*PULSES profile*—a multidimensional evaluation mechanism employed by the health professional to judge physical and functional status of the client. PULSES is defined as: P—physical condition/health status; U—upper limb functions; L—lower limb functions; S—sensory components (sight and communications); E—excretory functions; and S—support factors, such as significant others, psychological, emotional, social, or financial assistance. (30)

■ *developmental testing*—observing a child under five years of age and recording milestones in areas of gross and fine motor reflexes, language, social, emotional, self-care, and cognitive development.

■ *gait analysis*—methods used to detect deviations in gait resulting from pain, weakness, incoordination, or deformities. (6, 11, 21, 29, 52). Examples of gait deviation include:

—*festination gait, Parkinsonian gait*—refers to condition in which patients have a tendency to break into a run or trot. The pattern is slow to begin and may have a propulsive or retropulsive component. The length of steps is decreased and knee movements are diminished, producing a shuffling gait. In the more severe cases, the patient may only cease this gait pattern when he or she encounters an object or wall.

—*hemiplegic gait*—patient's leg is extended at the knee and circumducted at the hip, with the toe brushing the floor. The arm is flexed at the elbow and the wrist and arm-swinging movements are decreased. Hemispheric stroke is the most common cause of hemiplegic gait.

—*scissor gait, spastic gait*—patient walks slowly with knees extended. There are adduction movements of the hips along with pelvic tilting movements. Weight-bearing occurs on the lateral surface of the foot. The thighs scrape each other during adduction, which produces a scissorlike movement. Cerebral palsy and multiple sclerosis cause this type of gait.

—*senile gait*—refers to difficulties with balance that occur with aging. The older adult man develops forward flexion of the upper portion of the body, as well as flexion of the arms and knees. There is decreased arm swinging and shorter step lengths. The older adult woman develops a waddling gait and shorter step lengths. Older individuals often express fear of falling and a sense of imbalance, which frequently makes them housebound.

—*sensory ataxia gait*—refers to loss of joint position sense in which patients are unaware of the position of the lower extremities and usually stand with legs spread widely apart. The legs are lifted higher than necessary and are flung forward and outward in abrupt motions. Steps vary in length and feet make a slapping sound as they make contact with the floor's surface.

—*steppage gait, equine gait*—refers to condition caused by spasticity or contractures of the gastrocnemius and soleus muscles that prevent the heel from touching the ground. The gait is called equine since it is similar to the gait of the prancing horse.

■ *manual muscle testing*—an important tool used to determine the extent and degree of muscle weakness resulting from disuse, injury, or disease. (36, 55)

■ *measurement of joint motion:*

—*goniometry*—testing the range of joint motion with the aid of a goniometer, a protractor-like instrument with one mobile and one stable arm, used manually in the clinical measurement of joint motion. (22, 43)

—*electrogoniometry*—testing the range of motion with the aid of an electrogoniometer. An electrogoniometer usually consists of a goniometer with a linear potentiometer substituted for the protractor at the axis of the goniometer. The potentiometer changes the electric resistance in direct proportion to the change in joint angle that moves the arm of the goniometer. (22, 43)

- *movement assessment of infants*—tests that evaluate muscle tone, primitive reflexes, automatic reactions, and volitional movements in the first year of life. An assessment of risk for motor dysfunction at four months (age corrected for prematurity) can be tabulated. (16)
- *Peabody developmental motor scale*—refers to an instrument designed to assess gross and fine motor skills in children. Balance, locomotion, receipt, and propulsion of objects are measured by the gross motor scale, whereas the fine motor scale assesses grasping, hand use, eye-hand coordination, and finger dexterity. All items are arranged according to a normal developmental sequence. (16, 46)
- *perceptual motor testing*—testing for perceptual motor skills: a response or family of responses in which receptor, effector, and feedback processes show a high degree of spatial and temporal organization.
- *posture evaluation*—evaluating the position in which various parts of the body are held while sitting, walking, and lying.
- *reflex testing*—method by which the patient's involuntary response to a stimulus is tested to determine the status of the nervous system.
- *sensory testing*—using various tools and techniques to test the patient's responses to sensory stimuli. (17)
- *volumetric measurement*—determining the volume of a limb by measuring the water displaced when the extremity is immersed in a container of water.

Symptomatic Terms

- *analgesia*—loss of normal sense of pain. (37)
- *aphasia*—difficulty with the use of understanding of words due to lesions in association areas.
    - —*motor aphasia*—condition in which the verbal comprehension is intact, but the patient is unable to use the muscles that coordinate speech.
    - —*sensory aphasia*—inability to comprehend the spoken word, if the auditory word center is affected, and the written word, if the visual word center is involved. The patient will not understand the spoken or written word if both centers are involved. (44)
- *arthralgia, arthrodynia*—joint pain. (20, 57)
- *astereognosis*—inability to recognize shape and form of objects by feeling or touch. (2)
- *ataxia*—motor incoordination. (27)
- *ballismus*—violent flinging movements. When affecting only one side of the body, it is called hemiballismus. (27)
- *bradykinesia*—slowness in initiating and performing movement. (27)
- *clonic spasm*—rapid, repeated muscular contractions. (15)
- *contracture*—permanent shortening of one or more muscles caused by paralysis, spasm, or scar formation. (25)
- *diplopia*—double vision.
- *hyperkinesia*—purposeless, excessive involuntary movements. (27)
- *hypotonia*—reduced muscle tension associated with muscular atrophy. (27)
- *incoherence in speech*—illogic flow of ideas that is difficult for the listener to comprehend. (44)
- *intention tremor*—trembling when attempting voluntary movement.

- *Kernig's sign*—when the patient is supine and the thigh is flexed on the abdomen, he or she is unable to extend the leg. (48)
- *pallesthesia*—ability to perceive or recognize vibratory stimuli. (2)
- *paraplegia*—paralysis of lower limbs and at varying degrees of the lower trunk. (27)
- *paresis*—partial paralysis. (21)
- *parathesia*—abnormal sensation; heightened sensory response to stimuli.
- *phantom limb pain*—painful sensation felt by amputee that the limb is still intact.
- *Romberg's sign*—person stands erect with feet together and head straight, first with eyes open and then with eyes closed to ascertain whether or not balance can be maintained. If when eyes are closed, the patient sways or begins to fall, Romberg's sign is said to be positive. (21)
- *tonic spasm*—excessive, prolonged, muscular contractions. (15)
- *tremors*—oscillating, rhythmic movements of muscle groups. (27)
- *vasoconstriction*—narrowing of the vascular lumen, resulting in decreased blood supply.
- *vasodilatation*—widening of the vascular lumen, increasing the blood supply to a part. (41)
- *vasomotor*—referring to nerves that control the muscular contractions of blood vessels. (41)
- *vertigo*—illusion of movement of a person in relation to the environment. The person feels that he or she is spinning (subjective type) or that objects are whirling about (objective type).
  - *central vertigo*—present in disorders of vestibular nuclei, cerebellum, or brainstem, characterized by slow onset, prolonged duration, and absence of hearing impairment or tinnitus.
  - *peripheral vertigo*—present in disorders of vestibular nerve and semicircular canals. It is episodic and explosive, marked by sudden, violent attacks, lasting minutes to hours and usually accompanied by tinnitus and impaired hearing. (14)
- *xerophthalmia*—excessive dryness of the eyes resulting from the destruction of mucin-producing goblet cells, lacrimal ducts, and glands, or from other causes. (24)

Abbreviations

General

A°—angstrom unit
AC—alternating current
ACC—anode closing contraction
AD—abdominal diaphragmatic breathing
ADL—activities of daily living
AE—above elbow
AK—above knee
AKO—ankle-knee orthoses
AOC—anode opening contraction
BE—below elbow
BK—below knee
BP—blood pressure
CCC—cathode closing contraction
COC—cathode opening contraction

CPR—cardiac pulmonary resuscitation
DOE—dyspnea on exertion
DTR—deep tendon reflex
EMG—electromyogram, electromyograph
EMS—electromagnetic spectrum
FAO—foot-ankle orthoses
IR—infrared
KJ—knee jerk
LOM—limitation of motion
MBD—minimal brain dysfunction
MED—minimal erythema dose
MFT—muscle function test
MHz—megahertz
NCV—nerve conduction velocity
PFT—pulmonary function test

PR—pulse rate
PRE—progressive resistive exercise
PROM—passive range of motion
RD—reaction of degeneration
ROM—range of motion
SOB—short of breath
TENS—transcutaneous electric nerve
    stimulation

Organizations

AART—American Association of
    Rehabilitation Therapy
ACPMR—American Congress of Physical
    Medicine and Rehabilitation
ACRM—American Congress of
    Rehabilitation Medicine
AFB—American Foundation
    for the Blind
APTA—American Physical Therapy
    Association

Oral Reading Practice

Hemiplegia

Hemiplegia is one of the most common muscular disorders resulting from lesions occurring in the **brain** or upper segments of the **spinal cord** that affects the human population. Individuals afflicted with hemiplegia demonstrate a severe loss of strength in the arm, leg, and occasionally the face, and associated loss of voluntary movement with alteration of muscle tone and sensation throughout one side of the body. **Vascular** disease of the **cerebrum** and **brain stem** rank as the primary causes of hemiplegia. Secondary causes include **brain contusion, epidural,** and **subdural hemorrhage** followed by less frequently occurring causes such as **brain abscess, brain tumor, encephalitis, demyelinative diseases,** and complications of **meningitis, syphilis,** or **tuberculosis.** (7, 27, 50)

Motor neurons, with cell bodies located in the **cortex** and **axons** extending into the cord, are known as **upper motor neurons,** in contrast to those in the **anterior horn** of the cord, called **lower motor neurons,** which extend toward the muscles. A similar division exists for the **cranial nerves** in the regions where their nerve nuclei perform a function corresponding to that of the spinal cord. (10, 14, 27) When paralysis occurs suddenly and rapidly, it is referred to as a **stroke** or a **cerebrovascular accident.** The involvement affects the **corticospinal** and **corticobulbar** fibers. Damage to the corticospinal and corticobulbar tracts in the upper portion of the brainstem will cause paralysis of the face, arm, and leg on the opposite side. Lesions of the lower part of the brainstem, such as in the **medulla,** affect the **tongue** and occasionally the **pharynx** and **larynx** on one side and arm and leg on the other side. This condition is referred to as **"crossed paralysis".** (27, 53)

Approximately, 32 percent of strokes are the result of **cerebral thrombosis.** (8) A cerebral thrombosis tends to devitalize an upper motor neuron, resulting in its degeneration all the way from the thrombotic lesion to the cord. The lower motor neuron remains uninvolved. Following the initial period of shock, the muscles respond to **reflex arcs** mediated by the cord. Since these reflexes tend to be exaggerated, the muscles of the hemiplegic patient become spastic. This **spasticity** may interfere seriously with the exercise of voluntary muscle power that the patient has regained. Drugs and therapies have tried to overcome the unfortunate handicap and, in extreme cases, surgical intervention has been imperative. It consists of a **transection** of the motor nerve to the extremity, resulting in **flaccid** musculature, which is preferred to the incapacitating spasticity. Lower motor neuron paralysis results from the physiologic block or destruction of the anterior horn cells or their axons in anterior roots and nerves. (20, 27)

Hemiplegia that occurs suddenly is usually caused by involvement of the **internal capsule** resulting from a rupture of a small branch of the **middle cerebral artery (MCA).** An occlusion of the main trunk affects a large portion of the **cerebral hemisphere** and causes contralateral hemiplegia. The arterial distribution of the brain provided by the **MCA** is the site of most strokes. It is occluded most frequently by **emboli** rather than by **thrombi.** Small infarcts may produce transient and permanent paralysis. **Vascular occlusion** may also involve the **cervical** segment of the **internal carotid artery.** (8, 32)

It is a well-known fact that hemiplegia occurs on the side opposite to the brain injury. The reason for this is that about 90 percent of upper motor neurons cross over to the contralateral side at the level of the **medulla oblongata.** (20, 25, 32)

The Hemiplegic Patient

The hemiplegic patient may face several significant obstacles. Some of these include:

- **autotopagnosia**—loss of awareness, rejection, or denial of bodily disease or dysfunction. The patient tends to look away from the hemiplegic side, rejecting the implication that there is anything wrong with it. (21, 25)
- **balance and weight shift**—early in the patient's treatment program, problems of balance and weight should be addressed, otherwise these problems may tend to become habit forming and difficult to overcome. When first learning to sit or stand, the patient has a tendency to fall toward the affected side, with no control or stability. If the patient is not helped to overcome balance and weight shift problems, he or she will not acquire the skills to move correctly. (21, 50, 51, 52)
- **confusion**—results in inability to follow directions. The physiotherapist may need to reinforce verbal commands with demonstration and actually involve the patient in the specific demonstration to assist the patient in overcoming the deficit. Simple repetition of movement without the subject knowing whether or not the movement is correct will not result in learning. One of the key effective reinforcers is the patient's own knowledge of the extent of improvement in the performance of a particular task or movement. (19, 50)
- **dysarthria**—inability to speak properly or formulate words due to muscle weakness involved with speech production. Dysarthric patients are able to read, write, and understand what they hear, even though they are unable to utter a single intelligible word.
- **hemiplegic gait**—patient's leg is extended at the knee and circumducted at the hip, with the toe brushing the floor. The arm is flexed at the elbow and wrist, and arm-swinging movement is decreased. Hemispheric stroke is the most common cause of hemiplegic gait. (6, 11, 21, 29, 52)
- **flaccidity**—affects lower extremity when knee is kept extended on standing, thus making standing and walking harder for the patient. Flaccidity in the upper extremity may be demonstrated by a limp arm, which tends to get in the patient's way. (9, 21)
- **spasticity**—may be a great aid to helping the patient stand or walk. It may prove a problem only when it is sufficiently marked to interfere with function, which might result in the presence of secondary soft tissue contractures. Severe spasticity may be helped by drugs or by various surgical procedures. Other

Figure 84   Cerebral hemorrhage in left internal capsule resulting in right-sided hemiplegia because of crossing (decussation) of corticospinal (pyramidal) tracts in medulla oblongata.

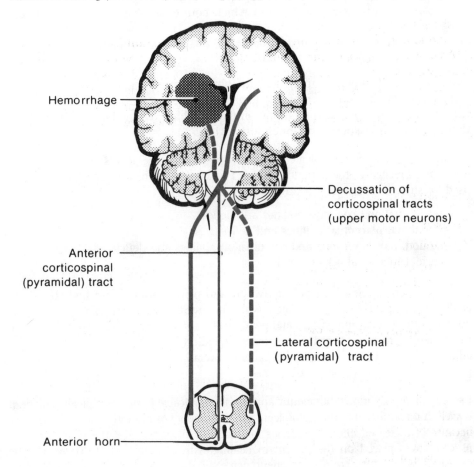

methods to reduce spasticity may include application of heat or cold, deep rhythmical massage over the muscle insertion areas, and rotation of trunk and limbs. Limb rotations have proven effective in providing a more normal control of muscle tone to the patient. (9, 21, 49, 50)

—**speech and language disorders**—inability to conceive thoughts, formulate meaningful sentences or execute purposeful acts represent deficits that can be extremely painful and frustrating for the hemiplegic patient. Some of these conditions are:

—**aphasia**—difficulty with the understanding of words due to lesions in association areas.

—**motor aphasia**—the verbal comprehension is intact, but the patient is unable to use the muscles to coordinate speech.

—**sensory aphasia**—inability to comprehend the spoken word, if the auditory word center is affected, and the written word, if the visual word center is involved. The patient will not understand the spoken or written word if there is involvement of both centers.

—**expressive aphasia**—refers to deficit in logical deduction and communication.

–receptive aphasia—refers to deficit in recognition, understanding, or integration of sensory input, such as speech or symbols.

–mixed aphasia—condition in which both expressive and receptive aspects are present.

–nominal aphasia—inability to name objects but recognition of the object's name when told. (27, 32, 44)

Other associated problems may include physical and emotional conditions that negatively affect the patient's progress. Examples of such condition may be poor lung expansion from **hypotonus,** and relative immobility, **bladder** and **bowel dysfunction, depression, helplessness,** and **loneliness.** (21, 25, 44, 50)

The assessment of the hemiplegic patient by the physical therapist should include key information related to the patient's ability to function with his or her deficits. Criteria used for such an assessment should include:

—intellectual and cognitive abilities and deficits.
—visual and perceptual abilities and deficits.
—motion, motor, sensory, and coordination abilities and deficits.
—current functional activity level.

The assessment findings can be interwoven into planning long-term and short-term goals for the patient and correlated with the overall treatment plan. Therapeutic assessment is an ongoing process and periodically it is important to assess and evaluate the patient's progress toward achievement of indicated goals, so that corresponding adjustments can be initiated in the patient's overall treatment program to meet the patient's current status and needs.

In contemplating various therapeutic approaches applicable to the hemiplegic patient, it is well to remember that the hemiplegic patient cannot sustain long periods of activity because of increased energy demands for motor involvement and the emotional and psychic stress placed on the patient in dealing with a major deficit. There may be occasions when the hemiplegic patient perceives the activity or desired task to be accomplished as beyond his or her control. In such circumstances, especially with the older adult, the patient may show cognitive, motivational, and emotional deficits of helplessness. This type of situation presents a challenge to the physical therapist to prevent or lessen this helplessness. Some approaches to assisting the hemiplegic patient might include providing a series of successful experiences, closely monitoring the patient's expectations of improvement, especially when such expectations cannot be achieved by the patient realistically, and whenever possible allowing the patient to make positive choices.

To ensure that rehabilitation of the hemiplegic patient continues after the physical therapist's treatment session, it is vitally important that other nursing staff and family members and friends be involved in the rehabilitation process. Gradually, the family must be prepared for the termination of the physical therapist's activities and the need to continue the rehabilitation process in the home. (9, 19, 51, 53)

References and Bibliography

1. Alon, Gad. Principles of electrical stimulation. In Nelson, Roger M., and Currier, Dean P., eds., *Clinical Electrotherapy*. Norwalk, CT: Appleton & Lange, 1987, pp. 29-80.

2. Ashbury, Arthur K. Numbness, tingling, and other abnormalities of sensation. In Braunwald, Eugene, et al, eds., *Harrison's Principles of Internal Medicine*, 11th ed. New York: McGraw-Hill Book Co., 1987, pp. 99-104.

3. Baker, Lucinda L. Clinical uses of neuromuscular electrical stimulation. In Nelson, Roger M., and Currier, Dean P., eds., *Clinical Electrotherapy*. Norwalk, CT: Appleton & Lange, 1987, pp. 115-139.

4. Baker, Lucinda L., and Parker, Karen. Neuromuscular electrical stimulation of the muscles surrounding the shoulder. *Physical Therapy* 66: 1930-1937, Dec. 1986.

5. Barr, John O., et al. Transcutaneous electrical nerve stimulation characteristics for altering pain perception. *Physical Therapy* 66:1515-1521, Oct. 1986.

6. Bernat, James L., and Vincent, Frederick M. The neurologic examination. In *Neurology Problems in Primary Care*. Oradell, NJ: Medical Economics Books, 1987, pp. 2-40.

7. ———. Weakness. Ibid., pp. 146-159.

8. ———. Cerebrovascular diseases. Ibid., pp. 260-384.

9. Bohannon, Richard W., and Smith, Melissa B. Assessment of strength deficits in eight paretic upper extremity muscle groups of stroke patients with hemiplegia. *Physical Therapy* 67:522-527, April 1987.

10. Caronna, John J. Neurologic problems. In Samiy, A.H., ed., *Textbook of Diagnostic Medicine*. Philadelphia: Lea & Febiger, 1987, pp. 657-693.

11. Craik, Rebecca L., and Oatis, Carol A. Gait assessment in the clinic: Issues and approaches. In Rothstein, Jules M., ed., *Measurement in Physical Therapy*. New York: Churchill Livingstone, Inc., 1985, pp. 169-205.

12. Cummings, John. Electrical stimulation of healthy muscle. In Nelson, Roger M., and Currier, Dean P., eds., *Clinical Electrotherapy*. Norwalk, CT: Appleton & Lange, 1987, pp. 81-96.

13. Cummings, John. Iontophoresis. In Nelson, Roger M., and Currier, Dean P., eds., *Clinical Electrotherapy*. Norwalk, CT.: Appleton & Lange, 1987, pp. 231-241.

14. Daroff, Robert B. Dizziness and vertigo. In Braunwald, Eugene, et al., eds., *Harrison's Principles of Internal Medicine*, 11th ed. New York: McGraw-Hill Book Co., 1987, pp. 76-79.

15. Dichter, Marc A. The epilepsies and convulsive disorders. In Braunwald, Eugene, et al., eds., *Harrison's Principles of Internal Medicine*, 11th ed. New York: McGraw-Hill Book Co., 1987, pp. 1921-1930.

16. Dietz, Jean C., et al. Relationships between infant neuromotor assessment and preschool motor measures. *Physical Therapy* 67:14-17, Jan. 1987.

17. Echternach, John L. Measurements issues in nerve conduction velocity and electromyographic testing. In Rothstein, Jules M., ed., *Measurement in Physical Therapy*. New York: Churchill Livingstone, Inc., 1985, pp. 281-304.

18. Frantz, Steve, et al. The physical therapist's role in the treatment of diabetes. *Clinical Management in Physical Therapy* 7:30-31, Jan.-Feb. 1987.

19. Frazer, F.W. Stroke care in the home. In Downie, Patricia A., ed., *Cash's Textbook of Neurology for Physiotherapists*, 4th ed. Philadelphia: J.B. Lippincott Co., 1986, pp. 296-313.

20. Gilliland, Bruce C. Miscellaneous arthritides and extraarticular rheumatism. In Braunwald, Eugene, et al., eds., *Harrison's Principles of Internal Medicine*, 11th ed. New York: McGraw-Hill Book Co., 1987, pp. 1465-1469.

21. Gilman, Sid. Ataxia and disorders of equilibrium and gait. In Braunwald, Eugene, et al., eds., *Harrison's Principles of Internal Medicine*, 11th ed. New York: McGraw-Hill Book Co., 1987, pp. 91-96.

22. Gogia, Prem P., et al. Reliability and validity of goniometric measurements of the knee. *Physical Therapy* 67:192-195, Feb. 1987.

23. Golden, Jane C., and Miles, Daniel S. Assessment of peripheral hemodynamics using impedance plethysmography. *Physical Therapy* 66:1544-1547, Oct. 1986.

24. Goldhaber, Paul. Oral manifestations of disease. In Braunwald, Eugene, et al., eds., *Harrison's Principles of Internal Medicine*, 11th ed. New York: McGraw-Hill Book Co., 1987, pp. 163-169.

25. Griggs, Robert C. Muscle pains, spasms, cramps, and episodic weakness. In Braunwald, Eugene, et al., eds., *Harrison's Principles of Internal Medicine*, 11th ed. New York: McGraw-Hill Book Co., 1987, pp. 96-99.

26. Griggs, Robert C., Bradley, Walter G., and Shahani, Bhagwan T. Approach to the patient with neuromuscular disease. In Braunwald, Eugene, et al., eds., *Harrison's Principles of Internal Medicine*, 11th ed. New York: McGraw-Hill Book Co., 1987, pp. 2047-2058.

27. Growdon, John H., and Young, Robert R.

Paralysis and other disorders of movement. In Braunwald, Eugene, et al., eds., *Harrison's Principles of Internal Medicine*, 11th ed. New York: McGraw-Hill Book Co., 1987, pp. 79-91.

28. Haralson, Kathleen M. Therapeutic pool programs. *Clinical Management in Physical Therapy* 5:10-13, March-April 1985.

29. Holden, Maureen C., et al. Gait assessment for neurologically impaired patients: Standards for outcome assessment. *Physical Therapy* 66:1530-1539, Oct. 1986.

30. Jette, Alan M. State of the art in functional status assessment. In Rothstein, Jules M., ed., *Measurement in Physical Therapy*. New York: Churchill Livingstone, Inc., 1985, pp. 137-168.

31. Kahn, Joseph. Non-steroid iontophoresis. *Clinical Management in Physical Therapy* 7:14-15, Jan.-Feb. 1987.

32. Kistler, J. Philip, Ropper, Allan H., and Martin, Joseph B. Cerebrovascular disease. In Braunwald, Eugene, et al., eds., *Harrison's Principles of Internal Medicine*, 11th ed. New York: McGraw-Hill Book Co., 1987, pp. 1930-1960.

33. Klein, Jennifer, and Pariser, David. Transcutaneous electrical nerve stimulation. In Nelson, Roger M., and Currier, Dean P., eds., *Clinical Electrotherapy*. Norwalk, CT: Appleton & Lange, 1987, pp. 209-230.

34. Kloth, Luther. Shortwave and microwave diathermy. In Michlovitz, Susan L., eds., *Thermal Agents in Rehabilitation*. Philadelphia: F.A. Davis Co., 1986, pp. 177-216.

35. Krause, Ann W., et al. Effects of unilateral and bilateral auricular transcutaneous electrical nerve stimulation on cutaneous pain threshold. *Physical Therapy* 67:507-511, April 1987.

36. Lamb, Robert L. Manual muscle testing. In Rothstein, Jules M., ed., *Measurement in Physical Therapy*. New York: Churchill Livingstone, Inc., 1985, pp. 47-55.

37. Maciewicz, Raymond, and Martin, Joseph B. Pain: Pathophysiology and management. In Braunwald, Eugene, et al., eds., *Harrison's Principles of Internal Medicine*, 11th ed. New York: McGraw-Hill Book Co., 1987, pp. 14-17.

38. Mayhew, Thomas P., and Rothstein, Jules M. Measurement of muscle performance with instruments. In Rothstein, Jules M., ed., *Measurement in Physical Therapy*. New York: Churchill Livingstone, Inc., 1985, pp. 57-102.

39. Meyer, Sr. Joan, RPT. Personal communication.

40. Michlovitz, Susan L. Cryotherapy: The use of cold as a therapeutic agent. In Wolfe, Steven L., ed.-in-chief, and Michlovitz, Susan L., ed., *Thermal Agents in Rehabilitation*. Philadelphia: F.A. Davis Co., 1986, pp. 73-98.

41. ———. Biophysical principles of heating and superficial heat agents. Ibid., pp. 99-118.

42. ———. The use of heat and cold in the management of rheumatic diseases. Ibid., pp. 277-294.

43. Miller, Peter J. Assessment of joint motion. In Rothstein, Jules M., ed., *Measurement in Physical Therapy*. New York: Churchill Livingstone, Inc., 1985, pp. 103-136.

44. Mohr, Jay P., and Adams, Raymond D. Disorders of speech and language. In Braunwald, Eugene, et al., eds., *Harrison's Principles of Internal Medicine*, 11th ed. New York: McGraw-Hill Book Co., 1987, pp. 121-127.

45. Newton, Roberta A. High-voltage pulsed galvanic stimulation: Theoretical bases and clinical applications. In Nelson, Roger M. and Currier, Dean P., eds., *Clinical Electrotherapy*. Norwalk, CT: Appleton & Lange, 1987, pp. 165-183.

46. Palisano, Robert J. Concurrent and predictive validities of the Bayley motor scale and the Peabody developmental motor scale. *Physical Therapy* 66: 1714-1719, Nov. 1986.

47. Seitz, Laurence M., and Kleinkort, Joseph A. Low-power laser: Its applications in physical therapy. In Wolfe, Steven L., ed.-in-chief, and Michlovitz, Susan L., ed., *Thermal Agents in Rehabilitation*. Philadelphia: F.A. Davis Co., 1986, pp. 217-238.

48. Shearn, Martin A. Arthritis and musculoskeletal disorders. In Schroeder, Steven A., Krupp, Marcus A., and Tierney, Lawrence M., Jr., eds., *Current Medical Diagnosis & Treatment—1988*. Norwalk, CT: Appleton & Lange, 1988, pp. 496-532.

49. Thurston, Nancy Mathys, et al. Thermographic evaluation of the painful shoulder in the hemiplegic patient. *Physical Therapy* 66:1376-1381, Sept. 1986.

50. Todd, J.M., and Davies, P.M. Hemiplegia—Assessment and approach. In Downie, Patricia A., ed., *Cash's Textbook of Neurology for Physiotherapists*, 4th ed. Philadelphia: J.B. Lippincott Co., 1986, pp. 253-266.

51. Todd, J.M., and Davies, P.M. Hemiplegia—Physiotherapy. In Downie, Patricia A., ed., *Cash's Textbook of Neurology for Physiotherapists*, 4th ed. Philadelphia: J.B. Lippincott Co., 1986, pp. 267-295.

52. Venna, Nagogopal. Dizziness, falling and fainting: Differential diagnosis in the aged. (Part II) *Geriatrics* 41:31-33, 36-37, 41-42, 45, July 1986.

53. Wade, J.P.H. Clinical aspects of stroke. In Downie, Patricia A., ed., *Cash's Textbook of*

Neurology for Physiotherapists, 4th ed. Philadelphia: J.B. Lippincott Co., 1986, pp. 240-252.

54. Walsh, Mark T. Hydrotherapy: The use of water as a therapeutic agent. In Wolfe, Steven L., ed.-in-chief, and Michlovitz, Susan L., ed., *Thermal Agents in Rehabilitation*. Philadelphia: F.A. Davis Co., 1986, pp. 119-139.

55. Watkins, Mary P. Clinical evaluation of thermal agents. In Wolfe, Steven L., ed.-in-chief, and Michlovitz, Susan L., ed., *Thermal Agents in Rehabilitation*. Philadelphia: F.A. Davis Co., 1986, pp. 241-262.

56. Wolf, Steven L. Electromyographic biofeedback: An overview. In Nelson, Roger M. and Currier, Dean P., eds., *Clinical Electrotherapy*. Norwalk, CT: Appleton & Lange, 1987, pp. 259-278.

57. Zarro, Vincent J. Mechanisms of inflammation and repair. In Wolfe, Steven L., ed.-in-chief, and Michlovitz, Susan L., ed., *Thermal Agents in Rehabilitation*. Philadelphia: F.A. Davis Co., 1986, pp. 3-17.

58. Ziskin, Marvin C., and Michlovitz, Susan L. Therapeutic ultrasound. In Wolfe, Steven L., ed.-in-chief, and Michlovitz, Susan L., ed., *Thermal Agents in Rehabilitation*. Philadelphia: F.A. Davis Co., 1986, pp. 3-17.

PART 3

Review Guide

Answers to Multiple Choice Questions

Index

Key Concepts

Several benefits can be derived from *taking words apart* and learning about their makeup. New words are most often not new at all. New words are manufactured from bits and pieces of old words. If we examine these *bits* and *pieces* that make up words in current usage, we can anticipate how some of these components might be utilized to meet new word needs and how they come to be in that particular form. The task of understanding new terms containing many of the old, familiar components will be greatly simplified.

base or root word elements—refer to the main body of the word. It may be accompanied by a prefix and/or a suffix.

> Example: adenoma
> aden- = base or root = gland
> -oma = suffix = tumor
> adenoma = gland tumor

prefix—refers to one or two syllables or word parts placed before a word to modify or alter its meaning.

> Example: hemigastrectomy
> hemi- = prefix = half
> gastr- = base or root = stomach
> -ectomy = suffix = removal or excision of
> hemigastrectomy = removal of half of the stomach

suffix—one or two syllables or word parts attached to the end of a word to modify or alter its meaning.

> Example: hysterectomy
> hyster- = base or root = uterus
> -ectomy = suffix = removal or excision of
> hysterectomy = removal of uterus

"pertaining to" suffix—selected suffixes meaning "pertaining to" include: *-ac, -al, -ic, -eal, -ary,* and *-ous.*

> Example: hemic
> hem = base or root = blood
> -ic = suffix = pertaining to
> hemic = pertaining to blood

"one who" suffix—selected suffixes meaning "one who" include: *-er, -ist*

> Example: pathologist
> -pathy = suffix = disease or morbid condition
> o = combining form element, vowel = o
> -logy = suffix = science or study of
> -ist = suffix = one who
> pathologist = one who studies disease or morbid conditions

combining form—results when a vowel, usually a, i, e, or o, is added to a word base or root. One usually deletes the vowel from a combining form when the next letter that follows is a vowel.

> Example: proctitis
> procto- = combining form denoting relationship to the rectum
> -itis = suffix = inflammation of
> proctitis = correct combination
> proctoitis = incorrect combination (o should be dropped)
> proctitis = inflammation of the rectum

compound word—results when some form of two or more base or root word elements are used to form a word. Usually adjectives or nouns are added to a root word to form compound words, or compound words may include a combining form element, a base or root word element, and a suffix or word ending.

Example: myocardiopathy

myo- = combining form element denoting relationship to muscle

cardio- = combining form element denoting relationship to heart

-pathy = suffix = disease or morbid condition

myocardiopathy = disease of the heart muscle.

Chapter 1. Orientation to Medical Terminology

INSTRUCTIONS: Analyze the terms listed.

Example: ab—away from.

Base or Root Words

arth- _____	derm- _____	ili- _____
blephar- _____	gastr- _____	lith- _____
chir- _____	hyster- _____	proct- _____

Prefixes

an- _____	ec- _____	hypo- _____
ante- _____	em- _____	para- _____
bi- _____	endo- _____	peri- _____
contra- _____	epi- _____	retro- _____

Suffixes

-algia _____	-oma _____	-oid _____
-cele _____	-pathy _____	-osis _____
-ectasis _____	-centesis _____	-plasty _____
-iasis _____	-ectomy _____	-spasm _____
-malacia _____	-lysis _____	-tripsy _____

Combining Form Word Elements

angio- _____	glyco- _____	pyelo- _____
anthropo- _____	kinesio- _____	pyo- _____
carcino- _____	mono- _____	schizo- _____
fibro- _____	neuro- _____	strepto- _____

INSTRUCTIONS: Definitions of medical terms appear in Column 1. In Column 2, write the corresponding medical term that best fits the definition listed in Column 1.

Example: Column 1   Column 2
            Inflammation of the appendix   appendicitis

Column 1   Column 2

1. Softening of the brain   1._____

2. Fixation of undescended testicle   2._____

3. Equality of the size of cells   3._____

4. Enlargement of the spleen   4._____

5. Removal of an ovary   5._____

6. Suture of a cleft palate   6._____

7. Vomiting of blood   7._____

8. Occurring after a meal   8._____

9. Removal of half of the stomach   9._____

10. Swelling of the eyelids   10._____

INSTRUCTIONS: Supply the prefix, suffix, or combining form word element for each of the English words listed below.

Example: behind—post.

across _____   pus _____

all _____   fever _____

enlargement _____   half _____

human being _____   around _____

disease _____   dilatation _____

between _____   scanty _____

INSTRUCTIONS: In Column 1, prefixes, suffixes, roots, and combining form elements are listed. In Column 2, write a medical term that includes the word element listed in Column 1. In Column 3, define the medical term that you have written in Column 2.

Example: Word element   Medical term   Medical term definition
         -itis   appendicitis   Inflammation of the appendix.

Word element	Medical term	Medical term definition
1. -lysis		
2. -osis		
3. enter-		
4. trachel-		
5. hypo-		
6. infra-		
7. sub-		
8. syn-		
9. tri-		
10. cephalo-		
11. oligo-		
12. duodeno-		
13. schizo-		
14. -emia		
15. -desis		

Chapter 2. Disorders of the Skin and Breast

INSTRUCTIONS: Define the following terms.

    Example: cutis (L)—skin.

---

cryo- (G) _____ lacto- (L) _____ papula (L) _____

derma- (G) _____ mama- (L) _____ pyo- (G) _____

-graphy (G) _____ masto- (G) _____ sclero- (G) _____

hidro- (G) _____ melano- (G) _____ thele- (G) _____

kerato- (G) _____ onycho- (G) _____ vesico- (L) _____

INSTRUCTIONS: Take the following words apart and define.

    Example: mastitis—mast = root word = breast; -itis = suffix = inflammation of.
        Note combining element(s) when appropriate.

---

1. alopecia _____

   _____

2. athelia _____

   _____

3. mastopexy _____

   _____

4. mastotomy _____

   _____

5. melanoderma _____

   _____

INSTRUCTIONS: Define abbreviations.

    Example: CC—chief complaint

---

cc _____ FS _____

Dx _____ MH _____

FH _____ PH _____

INSTRUCTIONS: Define the following terms.
Example: fissure of nipple—deep furrow in nipple.

1. carbuncle _____

_____

2. dermabrasion _____

_____

3. areola _____

_____

4. acne _____

_____

5. cellulitis _____

_____

6. decubitus ulcer _____

_____

7. comedo _____

_____

8. ecchymosis _____

_____

9. electrodesiccation _____

_____

10. impetigo contagiosa pyoderma _____

_____

11. Paget's disease of the nipple _____

_____

12. psoriasis _____

_____

Chapter 3. Musculoskeletal Disorders

INSTRUCTIONS: Define the following terms.

Example: coxa (L)—hip bone

---

arthro- (G) _____   ischio- (G) _____   pelvis (L) _____

bursa (L) _____   myelo- (G) _____   rhabdo- (G) _____

fascia (L) _____   myo- (G) _____   scolio- (G) _____

femur (L) _____   osteo- (G) _____   tendo- (L) _____

INSTRUCTIONS: Select the letter that represents the correct answer and place it on the blank line.

Example: Panarthritis is   __A__

    A. inflammation of all joints   B. inflammation of the liver

    C. inflammation of the pancreas   D. inflammation of ankle joints

---

1. The suffix -desis in arthrodesis means   _____
   A. repair   B. removal   C. closure   D. fixation

2. Albers-Schönberg disease may be called   _____
   A. osteogenesis imperfecta congenita
   B. osteogenesis imperfecta tarda
   C. osteopetrosis
   D. osteochondromatosis

3. Removal of lime salts especially from bone is called   _____
   A. demineralization   B. demolase
   C. decalcification   D. crepitation

4. Pseudogout may be called   _____
   A. chondroblastoma   B. coxarthrosis
   C. chondrocalcinosis   D. crepitation

5. Keller operation is performed for   _____
   A. torticollis deformity   B. hallus valgus deformity
   C. talipes valgus deformity   D. none of these

6. Osteoclast refers to   _____
   A. bone-forming cells   B. bone-absorbing cells
   C. bony outgrowth   D. none of these

7. Albright's syndrome may be called   _____
   A. aneurysmal bone cyst   B. fibrous dysplasia of bone
   C. fibrosarcoma of bone   D. avascular necrosis of bone

8. Marie-Strümpell arthritis may also be called   _____
   A. post-traumatic arthritis   B. gouty arthritis
   C. repetitive articular trauma   D. ankylosing spondylitis

9. Talipes valgus refers to _____
   A. forefoot touches ground; walking on toes
   B. arch broken; entire sole rests on ground
   C. foot everted; inner side of sole touches ground
   D. foot inverted; outer side of sole rests on ground

INSTRUCTIONS: Figure 7 from the text is an anterior view of the skeleton. Fill in the anatomic area name as indicated by the line protruding from that particular site. As an example, the first anatomic bone area name, frontal, has been filled in.

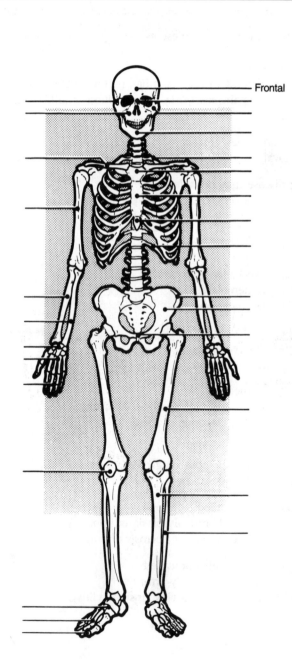

Frontal

Chapter 4. Neurologic and Psychiatric Disorders

INSTRUCTIONS: Define the following terms.

Example: axion (G)—axis

dynamo- (G) _____   phren- (G) _____   schizo- (G) _____

ganglio- (G) _____   plexus (L) _____   soma (G) _____

neuro- (G) _____   psycho- (G) _____   synapse (G) _____

INSTRUCTIONS: Figure 28 from the text is the median section of the brain and spinal cord. Fill in the anatomic area name as indicated by the line protruding from that particular site. As an example, the first anatomic area name, cranium, has been filled in.

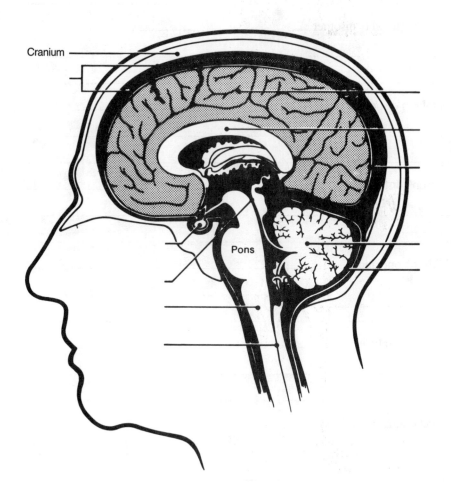

INSTRUCTIONS: Define the following terms.
    Example: dementia—an irreversible impairment of cognitive intellectual capacities.

1. alcohol amnestic disorder _____

    _____

2. anorexia nervosa _____

    _____

    _____

3. bulimia nervosa _____

    _____

    _____

4. profound mental retardation _____

    _____

    _____

5. schizoid personality disorder _____

    _____

    _____

6. somatoform disorders _____

    _____

    _____

7. Parkinson's disease _____

    _____

    _____

8. Torkildsen's operation _____

    _____

    _____

9. Dawson's encephalitis _____

    _____

    _____

10. von Recklinghausen's disease _____

    _____

    _____

Chapter 5. Cardiovascular Disorders

INSTRUCTIONS: Define the following terms.
    Example: cor (L)—heart.

an- (G) _____   brady- (G) _____   myo- (G) _____

angio- (G)_____   cardio- (G) _____   phlebo- (G) _____

arterio- (G)_____   corona (L) _____   tachy- (G) _____

atrio- (L) _____   hemo- (G) _____   thrombo- (G)_____

INSTRUCTIONS: Define the terms listed.
    Example: ischemia—reduced blood supply to an organ, usually due to arterial narrowing.

1. endocardium _____

_____

2. myocardium _____

_____

3. hypertrophic cardiomyopathy _____

_____

4. Ebstein's anomaly _____

_____

5. carotid endarterectomy _____

_____

INSTRUCTIONS: Define the abbreviations.
    Example: Hg—mercury

AMI_____   M _____

ASHD_____   MI_____

BBB_____   MS _____

CVA _____   PAC _____

CVP _____   PAT _____

ESR _____   SBE _____

IVC _____   TIA _____

LVH _____   VCG _____

INSTRUCTIONS: Select the letter that represents the correct answer and place it on the blank line.

Example: The suffix -ectomy in thrombectomy means _____ B ____
      A. repair   B. removal   C. closure   D. fixation

---

1. Aneurysm means _____
   A. shunting of oxygenated blood from the left to right atrium
   B. syndrome characterized by short attacks of precordial pain
   C. node found in the atrioventricular bundle
   D. dilatation or bulging out of the wall of the heart or any other artery

2. Patent ductus arteriosus means _____
   A. persistence of communication between pulmonary artery and aorta after birth
   B. dextroposition of right ventricle after birth
   C. shunting of oxygenated blood to the right ventricle from the left ventricle
   D. none of the above

3. Variant angina may be called _____
   A. Purkinje's angina   B. Prinzmetal's angina
   C. Valsalva's angina   D. none of these

4. Mitral commissurotomy means _____
   A. separation of the stenotic valve at points of fusion
   B. resection of mitral lesions
   C. revision of chordae muscle
   D. all of these

5. Coarctation of aorta _____
   A. constriction of a segment of the aorta
   B. dilatation of a segment of the aorta
   C. both of the above
   D. none of these

6. A strong, jerky beat followed by a sharp decline and collapse of beat is called _____
   A. dicrotic pulse   B. bigeminal pulse
   C. Corrigan's pulse   D. none of the above

7. Cardiac standstill that occurs with certain forms of heart block, causing syncope and possible fatal convulsions is known as _____
   A. Eisenmenger's syndrome
   B. Stokes-Adams syndrome
   C. Wolff-Parkinson-White syndrome
   D. Ebstein's anomaly

Chapter 6. Disorders of the Blood and Blood-Forming Organs

INSTRUCTIONS: Define the following terms.

Example: lien (L)—spleen.

adeno- (G) _____   leuko- (G) _____   -penia (G) _____

aniso- (G) _____   megalo- (G) _____   plasmo- (G) _____

blasto- (G) _____   micro- (G) _____   poikilo- (G) _____

cyto- (G) _____   myelo (G) _____   -poly (G) _____

hemo- (G) _____   -oma (G) _____   reticulum (L) _____

histo- (G) _____   -osis (G) _____   spleno- (G) _____

INSTRUCTIONS: Take the following words apart and define.

Example: splenectomy—splen = root or base word = spleen; -ectomy = suffix = removal.

Note combining form when appropriate.

1. lymphoma _____

_____

2. lymphangitis _____

_____

3. lymphadenotomy _____

_____

4. asplenia _____

_____

5. splenoptosis _____

_____

6. splenomegaly _____

_____

7. splenopexy _____

_____

8. splenorrhexis _____

_____

9. thrombocytopenia _____

_____

10. cytapheresis _____

_____

_____

INSTRUCTIONS: Select the letter that represents the correct answer and place it on the blank line.

   Example: Sideroblasts are   _____B_____
   A. circulating red cells containing stainable iron granules
   B. nucleated erythrocytes containing stainable iron granules
   C. immature red cells in intermediary stage of development between nucleate and anucleate forms
   D. normal non-nucleated red blood cells

1. The misspelled word is   _____
   A. myeloproliferative   B. thrombocytes
   C. plesmacytes   D. leukocytes

2. Variation of red cells, seen in pernicious anemia, is   _____
   A. leukocytosis   B. thrombocytosis
   C. erythrocytosis   D. anisocytosis

3. Cyclic fever in Hodgkin's disease and some other disorders characterized by several days of pyrexia followed by periods of normal body temperature is known as   _____
   A. Cameroon fever   B. Pel-Ebstein fever
   C. Corsican fever   D. none of these

4. The suffix -penia in lymphocytopenia indicates   _____
   A. increase   B. crushing   C. decrease   D. binding

5. The misspelled word is: _____
   A. autologous   B. isogenic   C. alogenic   D. none of these

6. Christmas disease may be called   _____
   A. hemophilia-A, factor VIII deficiency
   B. hemophilia-B, factor IX deficiency
   C. vascular hemophilia
   D. all of the above

7. The liquid portion of blood without cellular elements is called   _____
   A. serum   B. platelets
   C. plasma   D. reticulocytes

8. The name Waldenström is associated with   _____
   A. amyloidosis   B. plasma cell myeloma
   C. myelofibrosis   D. macroglobulinemia

Chapter 7. Respiratory Disorders

INSTRUCTIONS: Select the letter that represents the correct answer and place it on the blank line.

Example: A keeled chest may be called   _____C_____
      A. barrel chest   B. flail chest
      C. pectus carinatum   D. rachitic chest

---

1. Excessive formation of serous fluid within the pleural cavity is termed _____
   A. hydropneumothorax   B. pleural effusion
   C. hemothorax   D. empyema of pleura

2. Caldwell-Luc operation is associated with _____
   A. ethmoidectomy   B. antrotomy
   C. bronchotomy   D. tracheotomy

3. Opening of the nasal cavity into the nasopharynx is called _____
   A. concha   B. choana
   C. carina   D. coryza

4. Excision of nasal septum or part of it is called _____
   A. submucous resection   B. turbinectomy
   C. ethmoidectomy   D. none of these

5. The misspelled word is _____
   A. laryngotracheobronchitis   B. laryngismus
   C. bronchiectasis   D. asthmatecus

6. Disease of the lungs due to injury by dust from any source is _____
   A. histoplasmosis   B. asbestosis
   C. pneumoconiosis   D. atelectasis

INSTRUCTIONS: Define the following terms.
    Example: sinusitis—inflammation of a sinus or sinuses.

---

1. allergic rhinitis _____

   _____

2. bronchoplasty _____

   _____

3. heart lung transplantation _____

   _____

   _____

4. epistaxis _____

   _____

5. pulmonary embolectomy _____

_____

_____

INSTRUCTIONS: Define the following terms and abbreviations.
   Examples: pyo- (G)—pus.   TF—tactile fremitus

1. choane _____

_____

2. osmo- (G) _____

_____

3. antro- (L) _____

_____

4. spheno- (G) _____

_____

5. glottis (G) _____

_____

6. COPD _____

7. LSB _____

8. PND _____

9. TB _____

10. TNM _____

INSTRUCTIONS: Fig. 41 from the text is an anterior view of the larynx. Fill in the anatomic area name as indicated by the line protruding from that particular site. As an example, the first anatomic area name, the epiglottic cartilage, has been filled in.

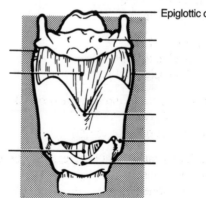

Epiglottic cartilage

Chapter 8. Digestive Disorders

INSTRUCTIONS: Select the letter that represents the correct answer and place it on the blank line.

Example: Tongue-tie may be called   __D__

    A. chilosis   B. herpangina

    C. torus palatinus   D. ankyloglossia

---

1. The misspelled word is   _____
   A. palatoplasty   B. cheilostomatoplasty
   C. choedochoplasty   D. proctoplasty

2. Meckel's diverticulum is associated with   _____
   A. jejunum   B. ascending colon
   C. descending colon   D. ileum

3. Heinecke-Mikulicz procedure may be called   _____
   A. vagotomy   B. pyloroplasty
   C. pyloromyotomy   D. gastrojejunostomy

4. The Fredet-Ramstedt operation may be called   _____
   A. vagotomy   B. pyloroplasty
   C. pyloromyotomy   D. gastrojejunostomy

5. The sphincter of Oddi refers to   _____
   A. pancreatic duct   B. cystic duct
   C. bile duct   D. none of these

6. The misspelled word is   _____
   A. mucoviscidosis   B. cholastasis
   C. hyperammoniemia   D. hyperalimentation

7. A collection of lymphoid tissue lodged in the tonsillar fossa on either side of the oral part of the pharynx is   _____
   A. pharyngeal tonsil   B. both A and C
   C. palatine tonsil   D. none of these

8. The alimentary canal extends from the   _____
   A. mouth to anus   B. ascending colon to anus
   C. mouth to duodenum   D. mouth to cecum

9. Gingivitis is inflammation of the   _____
   A. gum   B. tongue   C. lip   D. cheek

10. Repair of cleft palate is called   _____
    A. palatoplasty   B. cheiloplasty
    C. glossorrhaphy   D. esophagorrhaphy

11. Opening between stomach and duodenum is called   _____
    A. pylorus   B. cardiac orifice
    C. fundus of stomach   D. none of these

12. Parotid gland and duct located below the ear may be called   _____
    A. Wharton's duct   B. Stensen's duct
    C. Bernard's duct   D. none of these

13. Telescoping of intestine may be associated with _____
    A. intussusception   B. steatorrhea
    C. borborygmus   D. none of these

14. Collection of fluid in the peritoneal cavity is _____
    A. hemoperitoneum   B. ascites
    C. melena   D. cholemia

15. Another term for belching is _____
    A. bulimia   B. hypergastrinemia
    C. eructation   D. borborygmus

INSTRUCTIONS: Define the following terms.
    Example: gastrocele—hernia of the stomach

1. cheilostomatoplasty _____

_____

2. sclerosing cholangitis _____

_____

3. choledocholithiasis _____

_____

4. pancreatic pseudocyst _____

_____

5. splenorenal shunt _____

_____

6. esophagojejunostomy _____

_____

7. jejunoileal bypass _____

_____

8. esophagogastroduodenoscopy _____

_____

Chapter 9. Urogenital Disorders

INSTRUCTIONS: Select the letter that represents the correct answer and place it on the blank line.

Example: improperly descended testis is   <u> C </u>
      A. anorchism   B. tenesmus
      C. cryptorchism   D. trabeculation

1. Blood in urine is   _____
   A. glycosuria   B. hematuria
   C. nocturia   D. oliguria

2. Outer portion of the kidney is called   _____
   A. renal medulla   B. renal pelvis
   C. renal cortex   D. none of these

3. Antiglomerular basement membrane nephritis may be called   _____
   A. Goodpasture's syndrome   B. Alport's syndrome
   C. Dietl's crisis   D. none of these

4. Nephroblastoma may be called   _____
   A. Grawitz's tumor   B. Wilms' tumor
   C. both A and B   D. none of these

5. Hereditary nephritis may be called   _____
   A. Grawitz's tumor   B. Alport's syndrome
   C. Wilms' tumor   D. Goodpasture's syndrome

6. Form of nephritis involving the renal glomeruli of both kidneys is known as   _____
   A. glomerulonephritis   B. hereditary nephritis
   C. interstitial nephritis   D. pyelonephritis

7. Separation of kidney from blood supply is termed   _____
   A. ecchymoses   B. rupture
   C. avulsion   D. none of these

8. Renal cell carcinoma may be called   _____
   A. Grawitz's tumor   B. Wilm's tumor
   C. Alport's syndrome   D. Goodpasture's syndrome

9. Meeting point between ureter and renal pelvis is called   _____
   A. ureteric orifice   B. ureteropelvic junction
   C. ureterovesical junction   D. none of these

10. Surgical destruction of renal adhesions is called   _____
   A. nephropexy   B. nephrolysis
   C. nephrostomy   D. nephrotomy

INSTRUCTIONS: Take the following words apart and define.
Example: nephropathy—nephr = root or base word = kidney; o = combining form; -pathy = suffix = disease.
Note appropriate combining form.

1. anorchism _____

_____

2. cystolithotomy _____

_____

3. cystorrhaphy _____

_____

4. epididymitis _____

_____

5. epididymovasostomy _____

_____

6. glomerulonephritis _____

_____

7. nephrolithiasis _____

_____

8. nephrolysis _____

_____

9. nephroureterectomy _____

_____

10. pyelolithotomy _____

_____

11. ureterocystostomy _____

_____

12. ureterolysis _____

_____

13. ureteropyelostomy _____

_____

Chapter 10. Gynecologic Disorders

INSTRUCTIONS: Select the letter that represents the correct answer and place it on the blank line.

Example: Condylomas are   _____C_____
        A. cancer arising from epidermal cells
        B. cancer arising from squamous cells
        C. warty growths scattered over vulva
        D. hobnail cells

---

1. Bartholin's glands are located   _____
   A. deep to the levator ani   B. deep to the clitoris
   C. deep to the bulbocavernosus muscles   D. none of these

2. Stein-Leventhal syndrome may be called   _____
   A. ruptured tubo-ovarian abscess   B. Meigs syndrome
   C. polycystic ovarian syndrome   D. pyosalpingx

3. The cervical canal is the   _____
   A. superior dome-shaped portion of uterus
   B. constriction of uterus between body and cervix
   C. passageway between uterine cavity and vagina
   D. lower part of the uterus extending from isthmus to vagina

4. A panhysterectomy represents removal of the uterus and   _____
   A. includes the ovaries   B. includes ovaries and tubes
   C. excludes the fundus   D. includes the cervix

5. Excessive bleeding during the menstrual period is   _____
   A. amenorrhea   B. dysmenorrhea
   C. oligomenorrhea   D. none of these

6. Wertheim's operation refers to   _____
   A. removal of entire uterus and dissection of regional lymph nodes
   B. tubal implantation
   C. partial removal of the uterus
   D. hysteropexy

7. Skene's glands are   _____
   A. urethral glands in the female
   B. warty growths near the vagina
   C. horny growths of the cervical canal
   D. salivary glands in the female

8. Infrequent menstrual bleeding is   _____
   A. hypomenorrhea   B. cryptomenorrhea
   C. dysmenorrhea   D. oligomenorrhea

9. The term for surgical puncture of the cul-de-sac is   _____
   A. colpoclesis   B. culdoscopy
   C. culdocentesis   D. colposcopy

10. Tracheloplasty may be called _____
    A. Baldy-Webster procedure   B. Sturmdorf procedure
    C. Gilliam procedure   D. none of these

INSTRUCTIONS: Fig. 54 from the text depicts the uterus and related structures. Fill in the anatomic area name as indicated by line protruding from that particular site. As an example, the first anatomic area name, the uterine tube, has been filled in.

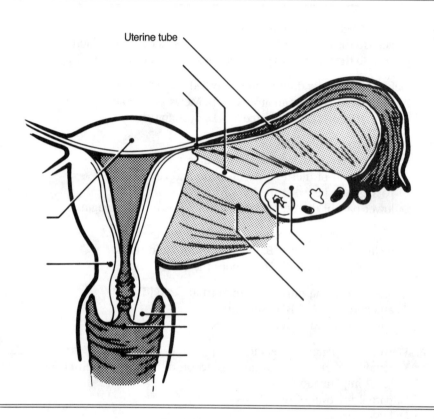

Uterine tube

INSTRUCTIONS: Define the abbreviations.
    Example: PID—pelvic inflammatory disease

FSH _____

GC _____

IUD _____

CIS _____

LMP _____

PMP _____

ACOG _____

Chapter 11. Obstetric, Fetal, and Neonatal Disorders

INSTRUCTIONS: Select the letter that represents the correct answer and place it on the blank line.

Example: Neonate refers to   _____C_____
    A. birth   B. new   C. newborn   D. naval

---

1. Lack of oxygen in the blood of the newborn is   _____
    A. atelectasis neonatorum   B. caput succedaneum
    C. asphyxia neonatorum   D. none of these

2. Down's syndrome may be called   _____
    A. trisomy G_{13} B. trisomy G_{21}
    C. both A and B   D. none of these

3. Fatty substance which covers the newborn at birth is   _____
    A. meconium   B. vernix caseosa
    C. phocomelia   D. none of these

4. Discharge from the birth canal following delivery is   _____
    A. pica   B. colostrum   C. dystocia   D. lochia

5. Softening of the uterine cervix, indicative of pregnancy, is   _____
    A. Chadwick's sign   B. Goodell's sign
    C. Hagar's sign   D. none of the above

6. Couvelaire uterus may be called   _____
    A. hydatidiform mole   B. subinvolution of uterus
    C. involution of uterus   D. uteroplacental apoplexy

7. Fetus dead, but retained in utero for days or weeks is   _____
    A. incomplete abortion   B. missed abortion
    C. septic abortion   D. induced abortion

8. Application of forceps when head is on perineum is called   _____
    A. mid-forceps   B. high forceps
    C. low forceps   D. none of these

9. Deficient amount of amniotic fluid is called   _____
    A. colostrum   B. asphyxia
    C. oligiohydramnios   D. none of these

10. Upper opening into true pelvic cavity is called   _____
    A. pelvic inlet   B. pelvic outlet
    C. promontory of the sacrum   D. both A and B

INSTRUCTIONS: Define the following terms.

Example: cesarean section—removal of the fetus through an incision into the uterus.

---

1. amniocentesis _____

2. Braxton-Hicks sign _____

_____

3. effacement _____

_____

4. engagement _____

_____

5. breech extraction _____

_____

6. Apgar score _____

_____

7. premature infant _____

_____

8. bilirubin _____

_____

9. cephalic version _____

_____

10. TORCH infections _____

_____

INSTRUCTIONS: Define the abbreviations listed.
    Example: FHT—fetal heart tone.

CDC_____   LOA _____

EDC_____   LOP _____

FTND _____   ROT _____

RML _____   RMA_____

LSP _____   RMT _____

Chapter 12. Endocrine and Metabolic Disorders

INSTRUCTIONS: Define the following terms.
   Example: endo- (G)—within

ad- (L) _____   spermato- (G) _____

adreno- (L) _____   thymo- (G) _____

ecto- (G) _____   thyro- (G) _____

meli- (G) _____   tropho- (G) _____

INSTRUCTIONS: Select the letter that represents the correct answer and place it on the blank line.

   Example: Hormone means   __B__
      A. to secrete   B. to excite   C. to swell   D. to shield

1. Graves' disease may be called   _____
   A. hyperthyroidism   B. hyperparathyroidism
   C. hypothyroidism   D. none of these

2. Seminiferous tubule dysgenesis may be called   _____
   A. Noonan's syndrome   B. Edward's syndrome
   C. Klinefelter's syndrome   D. Only A and B

3. Masculinization in women is   _____
   A. ovarian dysgenesis   B. hypogonadism
   C. virilism   D. vitiligo

4. A sudden recurrence after a remission is   _____
   A. progeria   B. paracusis
   C. exacerbation   D. proptosis

5. The name Hashimoto is associated with disease of the   _____
   A. pancreas   B. thyroid
   C. pituitary gland   D. thymus

INSTRUCTIONS: Define the following terms.
   Example: hypercholesterolemia—excessive cholesterol concentration in the circulating blood.

1. autosomal aberration _____

_____

2. chromosome analysis _____

_____

3. chromosomal fragmentation _____

_____

4. cytogenetics _____

_____

5. recessive gene _____

_____

6. mitosis _____

_____

7. mutation _____

_____

8. nondisjunction _____

_____

9. phenotype _____

_____

10. sex chromosomes _____

_____

INSTRUCTIONS: Define the abbreviations listed.
   Example: AD—autosomal dominant.

ACTH _____

ADH _____

BMR _____

GTT _____

HDL _____

NaCL _____

17-OH _____

XX _____

Chapter 13. Disorders Pertaining to the Sense Organ of Vision

INSTRUCTIONS: Define the following terms.

   Example: kerato- (G) —horny

---

cornea (L) _____ iris (G) _____

dacryo- (G) _____ nystagmus (G) _____

cyclo- (G) _____ oculo- (L) _____

cysto- (G) _____ ophthalmo- (G) _____

enucleate (L) _____ phaco-, phako- (G) _____

INSTRUCTIONS: Select the letter that represents the correct answer and place it on the blank line.

   Example: The globe or eyeball is called   __C__

      A. cornea   B. retina   C. bulb of the eye   D. fovea

---

1. Small avascular area of the retina around the fovea is the   _____
   A. orbit   B. ciliary zonule   C. macula lutea   D. iris

2. Inflammation of the iris and ciliary body is   _____
   A. iridodialysis   B. iritis   C. synechia   D. iridocyclitis

3. The name of Wagner is associated with   _____
   A. vitreous hemorrhage   B. vitreoretinal degeneration
   C. vitreous infections   D. vitreous detachment

4. Separation of the retina from the choroid, resulting in blindness
   if not relieved, is known as: _____
   A. edema of the retina   B. detachment of the retina
   C. Coat's disease   D. none of these

5. The name Kelman is associated with   _____
   A. phacoprosthesis   B. thermokeratoplasty
   C. phacoemulsification   D. cyclodialysis

6. The phrase Scheie's operation is associated with   _____
   A. thermal sclerostomy   B. peripheral iridectomy
   C. cryopexy of sclera   D. sclera buckling operation

7. Accessory row of lashes near or in the orifices of meibomian glands is   _____
   A. chemosis   B. macula lutea
   C. distichiasis   D. fovea

INSTRUCTIONS: Read the definition listed, then fill in the blank with the correct medical term.

Example: surgical closure of eyelid—tarsorrhaphy

1. Tissue removal by a high-powered pulsed ultraviolet laser radiation _____

2. Eyes turning inward _____

3. Eyes turning outward _____

4. Procedure for cutting through a tendon _____

5. Inflammation of the iris and ciliary body_____

6. Detachment of outer margin of the iris from ciliary body_____

7. Separation of the retina from the choroid_____

8. Procedure whereby small superior retinal breaks are treated with cryotherapy, intravitreal gas injection, and patient positioning _____

9. Normal vision, no refractive error _____

10. Recession of the eyeball into the orbit _____

11. Inequality in refractive power of right and left eye _____

12. Newly formed capillaries covering the cornea like a film_____

13. Adhesion between the palpebral and bulbar conjunctiva_____

14. Nearsightedness _____

15. Removal of eyeball _____

Chapter 14. Disorders Pertaining to the Sense Organ of Hearing

INSTRUCTIONS: Define the following terms.
Example: acoustic (G) — sound

auricle (L) _____

cochlea (G) _____

myringo- (L) _____

ot-, oto- (G) _____

salpingo- (G) _____

INSTRUCTIONS: Take the following words apart and define.
Example: otitis = ot = ear = base or root word; -itis = inflammation of = suffix.
Note combining elements when appropriate.

1. tympanitis _____

_____

2. otoplasty _____

_____

3. otosclerosis _____

_____

4. mastoidectomy _____

_____

5. myringotomy _____

_____

INSTRUCTIONS: Define the following terms.
Example: decibel — unit expressing intensity of sound.

1. anacusis _____

_____

2. presbycusis _____

_____

3. paracusis of Willis _____

_____

4. ossicles of the tympanic cavity _____

_____

5. helix _____

_____

INSTRUCTIONS: Select the letter that represents the correct answer and place it on the blank line.

Example: The helix is associated with   __A__

A. external ear   B. inner ear   C. middle ear   D. none of these

1. The round window facing the internal ear is   _____
   A. aditus ad antrum   B. fenestra vestibuli
   C. fenestra cochleae   D. pinna

2. Thin, clear amber fluid in middle ear is   _____
   A. serous otitis media   B. secretory otitis media
   C. serous otitis media with hemotympanum   D. all of these

3. Genetic deafness due to aplastic changes in osseous and membranous labyrinth is called   _____
   A. congenital deafness   B. noise deafness
   C. hysteric deafness   D. Mondini's deafness

4. The name Lempert is associated with   _____
   A. mastoid antrotomy   B. fenestration operation
   C. decompression of endolymphatic sac   D. myringotomy

5. Means for determining the type of hearing impairment in relation to sound conduction and sound perception: _____
   A. tone decay test   B. tuning fork tests
   C. short increment sensitivity index   D. none of these

6. Which of the following is *not* part of the ossicles of the tympanic cavity?   _____
   A. malleus   B. cochlea   C. incus   D. stapes

7. Meniere's disease may be called   _____
   A. otospongiosis   B. endolymphatic hydrops
   C. acoustic neuroma   D. vibratory tinnitus

Chapter 15. Multisystem Disorders
INSTRUCTIONS: Define the following terms.
   Example: ameba (G)—change

gono- (G) _____   sapro- (G) _____

lympho- (L) _____   strepto- (G) _____

myco- (G) _____   tricho- (G) _____

INSTRUCTIONS: Define the following terms.
   Example: antitoxin—immune serum that prevents the deleterious action of a toxin.

1. acid-fast bacilli _____

_____

2. acquired immunodeficiency syndrome (AIDS) _____

_____

3. agglutination _____

_____

4. Kawasaki syndrome _____

_____

5. Lyme disease _____

_____

INSTRUCTIONS: Select the letter that represents the correct answer and place it on the blank line.
   Example: An organism that grows on dead matter is called   __B__
      A. parasite   B. saprophyte   C. chlamydiae   D. none of these

1. German measles may be called   _____
   A. variola   B. rubeola   C. varicella   D. rubella

2. Undulant fever may be called   _____
   A. salmonellosis   B. shigellosis   C. brucellosis   D. leptospirosis

3. The name Weil is associated with   _____
   A. salmonellosis   B. shigellosis   C. brucellosis   D. leptospirosis

4. The name Chagas is associated with   _____
   A. African trypanosomiasis   B. American trypanosomiasis
   C. visceral leishmaniasis   D. mucocutaneous leishmaniasis

5. The name Waldenström is associated with   _____
   A. macroglobulinemia   B. agammaglobulinemia
   C. multiple myeloma   D. Wiskott-Aldrich syndrome

6. Lymphadenopathy with hypergammaglobulinemia complicated by
   benign or malignant lymphoma is associated with   _____
   A. Wiskott-Aldrich syndrome   B. Marfan's syndrome
   C. Sjögren syndrome   D. only A and B

7. Hansen's disease is associated with   _____
   A. Mycobacterium leprae   B. Mycobacterium tuberculosis
   C. Hemophilus influenzae, type B D. Histoplasma capsulatum

INSTRUCTIONS: Diseases are listed in Column 1. In Column 2, write the etiologic agents that correspond to each disease.

Example: **Disease**   **Etiologic agent**
         actinomycosis   actinomyces

Disease	**Etiologic Agent**
1. blastomycosis	
2. candidiasis	
3. histoplasmosis	
4. syphilis	
5. hookworm disease	1.
	2.
6. taenia infestation	1.
	2.
	3.
7. whooping cough	
8. legionnaires' disease	
9. diphtheria	
10. meningococcal meningitis	
11. scarlet fever	
12. infectious mononucleosis	1.
	2.

Chapter 16. Selected Terms Pertaining to Anesthesiology
INSTRUCTIONS: Define the following abbreviations.
   Example: PDR—Physicians' Desk Reference.

ACh _____

ADI _____

$CHCl_3$ _____

C_3H_6 _____

C_2HCl_3 _____

He _____

N_2O _____

NF _____

O_2 _____

Pent. _____

SC _____

Vin. _____

USD _____

USP _____

INSTRUCTIONS: Select the letter that represents the correct answer and place it on the blank line.
   Example: What causes low carbon dioxide content and deliberate
            hypertension as an adjunct to general anesthesia?   __B__
      A. hypercarbic anesthesia   B. hypocarbic anesthesia
      C. inhalation anesthesia   D. inhalation therapy

1. Which agent does *not* belong in the group listed below?   _____
   A. halothane   B. ether   C. cyclopropane   D. vinethene

2. Injection of a dilute anesthetic agent under the skin to anesthetize the
   nerve endings and nerve fibers is called   _____
   A. caudal anesthesia   B. infiltration anesthesia
   C. axillary brachial block anesthesia   D. only A and C

3. Which term is *not* related to methods of general anesthesia?   _____
   A. endotracheal anesthesia   B. inhalation anesthesia
   C. topical anesthesia   D. intravenous anesthesia

4. Which agent does *not* belong in the group listed below?   _____
   A. Surital   B. Avertin   C. Trilene   D. Brevital

5. A liquid anesthetic drug dropped on a gauze mask that covers the patient's nose and mouth and permits the inhalation of the vaporized drug is called the _____
   A. semiclosed method   B. open method
   C. closed method   D. none of these

INSTRUCTIONS: Define the following terms.

   Example: General anesthesia—state of unconsciousness accompanied by varying degrees of muscular relaxation and freedom from physical pain.

1. analeptics _____

   _____

2. anesthesiology _____

   _____

3. antiemetic drugs _____

   _____

4. arterial hypotension during anesthesia _____

   _____

   _____

5. lid reflex _____

   _____

6. malignant hyperthermia syndrome _____

   _____

   _____

7. response evaluation to anesthetics _____

   _____

Chapter 17. Selected Terms Pertaining to Gerontology

INSTRUCTIONS: Define the following terms.

Example: presbyopia—defective vision resulting from changes in accommodation in the aging process.

1. gerontology _____

_____

2. hospice _____

_____

3. Alzheimer's disease _____

_____

4. arteriosclerosis obliterans _____

_____

5. transient ischemic attacks _____

_____

6. arcus senilis _____

_____

7. attitude therapy _____

_____

8. Cheyne-Strokes respiration _____

_____

9. enuresis _____

_____

10. Kussmaul breathing _____

_____

11. pain _____

_____

12. Raynaud's disease _____

_____

13. therapy of reminiscence _____

_____

INSTRUCTIONS: Select the letter that represents the correct answer and place it on the blank line _____ .

Example: Using conversation or only a couple of words to stimulate the older adult and bring him or her back to reality is termed   <u>C</u>
A. reality therapy   B. attitude therapy
C. therapy of remotivation   D. supportive psychotherapy

1. The names of Broca and Wernicke are associated with   _____
   A. agnosia   B. aloneness   C. alienation   D. aphasia

2. The behavior of making up tales to fill in memory gaps is associated with   _____
   A. disengagement   B. confabulation   C. dyskinesia   D. fasciculation

3. Billroth II refers to   _____
   A. gastrojejunal anastomosis   B. gastroduodenal anastomosis
   C. colon resection   D. only A and B

4. Rhytidectomy is associated with   _____
   A. thyroid   B. renal pelvis   C. wrinkled skin   D. none of these

5. Paralysis of intestinal muscles and absence of bowel sounds that may be due to electrolyte imbalance or operative handling of the intestines is termed   _____
   A. dynamic (mechanical) ileus   B. adynamic (paralytic) ileus
   C. dynamic (mechanical) ilius   D. adynamic (paralytic) ilius

6. Which term does *not* belong in the following group?   _____
   A. Barthel index   B. Katz index   C. Henry system   D. Kenny system

7. Sensory inability to recognize objects is called   _____
   A. aphasia   B. apraxia
   C. ataxia   D. agnosia

8. The utilization of a modified and controlled environment in the treatment of mental disease represents   _____
   A. reality therapy   B. therapy of remotivation
   C. milieu therapy   D. therapy of reminiscence

9. Hearing loss that occurs with aging may be referred to as   _____
   A. presbylibrium   B. presbyopia
   C. presbycusis   D. progeria of adult

10. Quick, shuffling steps and accelerated gait seen in Parkinson's disease is termed   _____
    A. disengagement   B. fasciculation
    C. festination   D. presbycusis

INSTRUCTIONS: Define the following terms.
　　Example: asthenia (G)—weakness; GSA—Gerontological Society of America

---

geronto- (G) _____　　-logy (G) _____　　presby- (G) _____

AARP _____　　COPD _____　　SDAT _____

Chapter 18. Selected Terms Pertaining to Oncology

INSTRUCTIONS: Define the following terms.

    Example: -oma (G)—tumor

---

astro- (G) _____

carcino- (G)_____

kerato- (G)_____

onco- (G) _____

sarco- (G) _____

INSTRUCTIONS: Select the letter that represents the correct answer and place it on the blank line.

    Example: Wart-like projection, usually occurring in the mouth and cheek areas is   C

    A. sarcoma   B. ulcer   C. verrucous   D. none of these

---

1. Loss in the regularity and normal arrangement of cells is   _____

    A. metaplasia   B. dysplasia   C. hyperplasia   D. only A and C

2. A malignant striated muscle tumor is   _____

    A. leiomyosarcoma   B. Ewing's sarcoma

    C. rhabdomyosarcoma   D. osteosarcoma

3. Clinical appearance of tumor in regression following initial dose of radiation is   _____

    A. radiosensitivity   B. radiocurability

    C. radioresponsiveness   D. remission

4. Which neoplasm does *not* belong in the group of terms listed?   _____

    A. hemangioma   B. ependymoma   C. glioblastoma   D. astrocytoma

5. A histologically primitive cell with the capacity to give rise to a large number of descendants in a process of self-renewal is   _____

    A. stem cell   B. sessile polyp   C. dedifferentiation   D. differentiation

---

INSTRUCTIONS: Define the following terms.

    Example: embryonal, embryonic—pertaining to embryo, also to marked immaturity.

---

1. erythroplakia _____

_____

2. clone _____

_____

3. carcinoma in situ (CIS) _____

_____

4. fractionation _____

_____

5. lymphocyte _____

_____

6. metastasize _____

_____

7. Papanicolaou smear _____

_____

8. chondrosarcoma _____

_____

9. tumor marker _____

_____

10. TNM system _____

_____

11. sessile polyp _____

_____

12. modality _____

_____

13. chemotherapy _____

_____

14. oncogene _____

_____

_____

Chapter 19. Selected Terms Pertaining to the Clinical Laboratory

INSTRUCTIONS: Define measurements of the metric system listed below.
   Example: m—meter.

kg _____	L _____	dm _____
mg _____	ml _____	mm _____
μg _____	nm _____	ng _____
μm _____	pg _____	pm _____

INSTRUCTIONS: Define the following abbreviations.
   Example: molality—moles of solute in one kilogram of solvent.

mmol _____	A _____	mEq _____
nmol _____	Hz _____	mEq/l _____
mol _____	N _____	mIU _____
mol/kg _____	W _____	IU _____

INSTRUCTIONS: Define the following terms.
   Example: coagulant—substance contributing to clot formation.

1. hematocrit _____

_____

2. thrombus _____

_____

3. prothrombin time _____

_____

4. ABO system _____

_____

INSTRUCTIONS: Select the letter that represents the correct answer and place it on the blank line.
   Example: An ion-carrying positive electric charge that travels toward the
            negative pole is called a(n)   __B__
      A. anode   B. cation   C. cathode   D. anion

1. The Gibson-Cooke technique is associated with   _____
   A. liver function tests   B. intestinal absorption tests
   C. gastric exfoliative cytology   D. sweat test

2. The name Bence-Jones is associated with   _____
   A. phenotype   B. insulin tolerance test
   C. basal metabolic rate   D. protein molecule

3. The diagnostic maneuver consisting in compression of one or both
   jugular veins that normally results in a quick brief rise of pressure of
   the cerebrospinal fluid is a test associated with the name   _____
   A. von Gierke   B. Hollander   C. Castle   D. Queckenstedt

4. The use of insulin-induced hypoglycemia to evaluate the outcome of
   vagotomy is associated with the name   _____
   A. von Gierke   B. Hollander   C. Castle   D. Queckenstedt

5. The secretin test is associated with the names   _____
   A. Dreiling and Hollander   B. Hollander and Castle
   C. Dreiling and Castle   D. Hollander and Ham

6. The name Wilson is associated with   _____
   A. hepatolenticular degeneration   B. hemopyelectasis
   C. hidrocystomatosis   D. hypolemmal degeneration

7. The name Ham is associated with   _____
   A. glucose tolerance test   B. insulin tolerance test
   C. acid hemolysis test   D. Wasserman test

8. Phenolsulfonphthalein (PSP) is a dye test for   _____
   A. liver impairment   B. pancreatic impairment
   C. kidney impairment   D. gallbladder impairment

9. Determination of the approximate amount of calcium in the urine is
   determined by   _____
   A. Clinitest   B. Ketostix test
   C. Sensi-tex test   D. Sulkowitch test

10. The polypeptide hormone secreted by the alpha cells of the pancreatic
    islets is called   _____
    A. prolactin   B. glucagon
    C. lutropin   D. estriol

INSTRUCTIONS: Select *one* disease, condition, or syndrome in which the component
mentioned is increased or decreased. Write your selection in the appropriate blank.
    Example: there is an increase of the follicle-stimulating hormone (FSH) in *Kline-felter's syndrome* and a decrease in *panhypopituitarism*.

---

1. serum biocarbonate shows an increase in _____

   and a decrease in _____

2. serum calcium shows an increase in _____

  and a decrease in _____

3. serum chloride shows an increase in _____

  and a decrease in _____

4. serum magnesium shows an increase in _____

  and a decrease in _____

5. plasma potassium shows an increase in _____

  and a decrease in _____

6. plasma sodium shows an increase in _____

  and a decrease in _____

7. 17-ketosteroids (17-KS) shows an increase in _____

  and a decrease in _____

8. plasma testosterone shows an increase in _____

  and a decrease in _____

9. erythrocyte sedimentation rate (ESR) shows an increase in _____

  and a decrease in _____

10. carbon dioxide content in serum of adults shows an increase in _____

  and a decrease in _____

INSTRUCTIONS: Define the abbreviations.
  Example: E_2 = estradiol

1. ACTH _____

2. ADH _____

3. AST _____

4. ELISA _____

5. GTT _____

6. HCG _____

7. HDL _____

8. HLA _____

9. MCV _____

10. TIBC _____

INSTRUCTIONS: Define the following terms.
  Example: pregnanediol—hormone produced in the liver by progesterone metabolism and excreted in the urine.

1. augmented histamine test _____

_____

2. basal metabolic rate _____

_____

3. guaiac test _____

_____

4. ketone bodies _____

_____

5. thromboplastin _____

_____

Chapter 20. Selected Terms Pertaining to Radiology, Diagnostic Ultrasound, and Magnetic Resonance Imaging

INSTRUCTIONS: Define the following abbreviations.
   Example: AP—anterior-posterior

CAT _____   LCA _____

DSA _____   RCA _____

LSB _____   f _____

TNI _____   V _____

TP _____   ACR _____

INSTRUCTIONS: Define the following terms.
   Example: density—mass per unit of volume.

1. absorption of x-rays _____

   _____

2. bit _____

   _____

3. discography _____

   _____

4. arteriography _____

   _____

5. percutaneous transhepatic cholangiography _____

   _____

   _____

   _____

6. magnetic resonance imaging (MRI) _____

   _____

7. transcranial Doppler (TCD) sonography _____

   _____

INSTRUCTIONS: Fill in the blank spaces below with the appropriate term.
    Example: False features in the image produced by the imaging process are termed
            _____artifacts_____

1. Modification of Carr-Purcell RF pulse sequence with 90° phase shift in the rotating frame of reference between the 90° and subsequent 180° pulses is termed _____

2. A technique for studying nuclear magnetic resonance by continuously applying RF radiation to the sample and slowly sweeping either the RF frequency or the magnetic field through the resonance values is termed _____

3. Electrical conductor interposed between transmitter and/or receiver coil and patient to block out electric fields is termed _____

4. The amount and direction of the rate of change in space of some quantity, such as a magnetic field strength, is termed_____

5. Unit of frequency; equal to one thousand Hertz is termed_____

6. Unit of frequency; equal to one million Hertz is termed_____

7. Wave frequency intermediate between auditory and infrared is termed_____

8. Burst of RF magnetic field delivered to object by RF transmitter is termed _____

9. The period of time between the beginning of a pulse sequence and the beginning of the succeeding (essentially identical) pulse sequence is termed _____

10. Spin-lattice or longitudinal relaxation time; the characteristic time constant for spins to tend to align themselves with the external magnetic field is termed _____

Chapter 21. Selected Terms Pertaining to Nuclear Medicine

INSTRUCTIONS: Define the following terms.
   Example: fission (L)—cleft, split

iso- (G) _____   proto- (G) _____

kine- (G) _____   tele- (G) _____

INSTRUCTIONS: Define the following terms.
   Example: electrons—negatively charged particles revolving around the nucleus.

1. atomic weight _____

   _____

2. becquerel (Bq) _____

   _____

   _____

3. beta particle _____

   _____

   _____

4. positron emission tomography (PET) _____

   _____

   _____

5. brain imaging _____

   _____

   _____

6. Iofetamine HCL I-123 (SPECTamine) _____

   _____

   _____

7. infarct-avid myocardial imaging _____

   _____

   _____

INSTRUCTIONS: Define abbreviations.
  Example: RAIU—radioactive iodine uptake

A _____

FTI _____

MPL _____

RIA _____

TBI _____

TRH _____

TSH _____

INSTRUCTIONS: Fill in the blank spaces below with the appropriate term.
  Example: The amount of radioactive material present in the body of human beings
           or animals is termed _____ body burden. _____

1. A sensitive radiation detector composed of a tube filled with gas and a scaler. It is
   used to detect nuclear radiation. It is termed_____

2. The sum of neutrons and protons in a nucleus is termed_____

3. Determination of vitamin B_{12} absorption as an aid in diagnosis of pernicious
   anemia and malabsorption of B_{12} due to other causes is termed _____

INSTRUCTIONS: Define unit of measurement.
  Example: Bev—1 billion electron volts

E_____

erg_____

ev_____

Chapter 22. Selected Terms Pertaining to Physical Therapy

INSTRUCTIONS: Define the following terms.

Example: actino- (G) —ray

---

arthr- (G) _____   ortho- (G) _____

crymo- (G)_____   phono- (G)_____

hydro- (G) _____   physio- (G) _____

INSTRUCTIONS: Fill in the blank listed below with the correct term.

Example: Nerves that control the muscular contractions of blood vessels are termed _____vasomotor_____

---

1. Ability to perceive or recognize vibratory stimuli is termed _____

2. Violent flinging movement is termed _____

3. Muscle contraction is which the muscle is not allowed to shorten or lengthen is termed _____

4. Double vision is termed _____

5. When person stands erect with feet together and head straight, first with eyes open and then with eyes closed to ascertain whether or not balance can be maintained is termed _____

6. Periods of current flow and cessation of flow, with a gradual increase and decrease in intensity is termed _____

7. Rapid, repeated muscular contractions is termed_____

8. Joint pain is termed _____

9. Inability to recognize shape and form of objects by feeling or touch is termed _____

10. Motor incoordination is termed _____

INSTRUCTIONS: Define the abbreviations listed.
  Example: BE—below elbow

AC _____

ADL _____

AE _____

AK _____

BP _____

BK _____

DTR _____

KJ _____

LOM _____

ROM _____

INSTRUCTIONS: Define the following terms.
  Example: Orthosis—correction of defects. Usually refers to a device applied to
         patients for supportive assistance or for corrective purposes, e.g., braces,
         splints, etc.

1. high-voltage pulsed galvanic stimulation (HVPGS) _____

   _____

   _____

2. convection _____

   _____

3. hot packs _____

   _____

4. Barthel index _____

   _____

5. equine gait _____

   _____

Answers to the Multiple Choice Questions in Review Guide

p. 539-540	1-D	p. 551	1-B	p. 562	1-C
	2-C		2-C		2-A
	3-C		3-A		3-D
	4-C		4-B		4-B
	5-B		5-B		5-B
	6-B		6-A		6-B
	7-B		7-C		7-B
	8-D		8-A		
	9-C		9-B	p. 563-564	1-D
			10-B		2-C
p. 544	1-D				3-D
	2-A				4-B
	3-B	p. 553-554	1-D		5-A
	4-A		2-C		6-C
	5-A		3-C		7-A
	6-C		4-D		
	7-B		5-D	p. 565-566	1-C
			6-A		2-B
p. 546	1-C		7-A		3-C
	2-D		8-D		4-C
	3-B		9-C		5-B
	4-C		10-B		
	5-C			p. 568	1-D
	6-B	p. 555	1-C		2-B
	7-C		2-B		3-A
	8-D		3-B		4-C
			4-D		5-B
p. 547	1-B		5-B		6-C
	2-B		6-D		7-D
	3-B		7-B		8-C
	4-A		8-C		9-C
	5-D		9-C		10-C
	6-C		10-A		
				p. 570	1-B
p. 549-550	1-C				2-C
	2-D	p. 557	1-A		3-C
	3-B		2-C		4-A
	4-C		3-C		5-A
	5-C		4-C		
	6-B		5-B	p. 573	1-D
	7-C				2-D
	8-A				3-D
	9-A	p. 559	1-C		4-B
	10-A		2-D		5-A
	11-A		3-B		6-A
	12-B		4-B		7-C
	13-A		5-C		8-C
	14-B		6-A		9-D
	15-C		7-C		10-B

Index

AA. *See* Alcoholics Anonymous (AA)
AABB. *See* American Association of Blood Banks (AABB)
AAMD. *See* American Association on Mental Deficiency (AAMD)
AAMIH. *See* American Association for Maternal and Infant Health (AAMIH)
A&P. *See* Auscultation and percussion (A&P)
AAPA. *See* American Academy of Physicians' Assistants (AAPA)
AARP. *See* American Association of Retired Persons (AARP)
AART. *See* American Association of Rehabilitation Therapy (AART) *and* American Association of Respiratory Therapy (AART)
Ab. *See* Antibody (Ab)
Abdomen
    anatomical division, clinical division, quadrants, regions, 22
    and diagnostic ultrasound, 479-80
Abdominal aortic aneurysm wrapping, 116
Abdominal esophagus, 182
Abdominal imaging, 471-72
Abdominal perineal resection, 191
ABE. *See* Acute bacterial endocarditis (ABE)
Aberrant pancreatic tissue polyps, 186
ABNM. *See* American Board of Nuclear Medicine (ABNM)
Abnormal chest, 171
Abortion, 92, 253
Abortus, 258
ABO system, 426
Above the elbow (AE), 57
Above the knee (AK), 57

ABR. *See* American Board of Radiology (ABR)
Abreaction, 89
Abscess, 181
    brain, 70
    of breast, 31
    of lung, 167
    of meninges, 77
    and peritoneum, 199
    tubo-ovarian, 241
Abuse, cocaine, 91-93
ABVD program of chemotherapy, 155
AC. *See* Air conduction (AC)
ac, and time schedule for medication, 202
Acantholysis bullosa, 27
Accelerator globulin (AcG), 143
Accessory organs of vision, 302-6
Accessory spleens, 153
Accidental hypothermia (AH), 381-82
Accommodation, 307
ACD. *See* Acid citrate dextrose (ACD) *and* Anterior chest diameter (ACD)
ACDK. *See* Acquired cystic disease of kidney (ACDK)
Acetabulum, 47, 58
Acetylcholine (ACh), 375
ACG. *See* Angiocardiography (ACG) *and* Apex cardiogram (ACG)
AcG. *See* Accelerator globulin (AcG)
ACh. *See* Acetylcholine (ACh)
Achalasia, 184
Achlorhydria, 189
Achondroplasia, 49-50
Achylia gastrica, 189
Acid-base imbalance, 276-77
Acid-citrate-dextrose (ACD), 146, 147, 153
Acid-fact bacillus (AFB), 173, 331

Acid hemolysis test, 432
Acidosis, 277
Acid perfusion test, 201
Acitivity therapy, 390-91
Acne, 26
ACNM. *See* American College of Nuclear Medicine (ACNM) *and* American College of Nurse Midwifery (ACNM)
ACNP. *See* American College of Nuclear Physicians (ACNP)
ACOG. *See* American College of Obstetricians and Gynecologists (ACOG)
Acoustic tumors, 77
ACPMR. *See* American Congress of Physical Medicine and Rehabilitation (ACPMR)
Acquired cystic disease of kidney (ACDK), 214
Acquired immunodeficiency syndrome (AIDS), 148, 336, 357, 414
ACR. *See* American College of Radiology (ACR)
ACRM. *See* American Congress of Rehabilitation Medicine (ACRM)
Acrocentric, 280
Acrocyanosis, 118
Acromegaly, 77, 273
ACS. *See* American Cancer Society (ACS) *and* American College of Surgeons (ACS) *and* Association of Clinical Scientists (ACS)
ACTH. *See* Adrenocorticotropic hormone (ACTH)
Actinomycetes, infections caused by, 339
Actinomycosis, 224
Actinomycosis of sinus, 160
Activated water, 495

Activation analysis, 495
Activity therapy, 90
Actuarial method, 119
Acuity, visual, 307
Acupuncture analgesia, 374-75
Acute bacterial endocarditis (ABE), 126
Acute exposure, 495
Acute idiopathic polyneuropathy, 66
Acute leukemia, 144
Acute limb ischemia, 114
Acute lymphocytic leukemia (ALL), 154
Acute myeloblastic leukemia (AML), 154
Acute myocardial infarction (AMI), 126
Acute necrotizing gingivitis, 181
Acute non-lymphocytic leukemia
    (ANLL), 154
Acute respiratory disease (ARD), 173
Acute respiratory failure (ARF), 167, 173
Acute synovitis, 47-48
Acute yellow atrophy of liver, 194
AD. See Autosomal dominant (AD)
ADA. See American Dietetic Association
    (ADA)
Addiction, drug, 259
Addisonian crisis, 273
Addison's disease, 273
Adenocarcinoma, 167, 224-25, 237
Adenoids, 183
Adenomatous polyps, 186
Adenopathy, 202
Adenosine triphosphate (ATP), 287
Adenotonsillectomy, 184
Adenotonsillitis, 183
Adenoviral infections, 333
ADH. See Antidiuretic hormone (ADH)
Adhesive bursitis, 49
Adhesive capsulitis, 49
ADI. See American Drug Index (ADI)
Adjuvant, 399
ADL testing, 519-20
Adnexal tumor, 70
Adnexectomy, 242
Adrenal crisis, 273
Adrenalectomy, 275
Adrenal glands, 272
    and imaging, 488
Adrenal hormones, 440-41
Adrenal neoplasms, 273
Adrenocorticotropic hormone (ACTH),
    271, 287
Adult, older. See Older adults
Adult chorea, 73
Adult hemoglobin (Hb A), 142, 153
Adult respiratory disease syndrome
    (ARDS), 167, 173
Adventitia, 114
Adynamic ileus, 191
AE. See Above the elbow (AE)
Aerobes, 331
AESP. See Applied extrasensory
    projection (AESP)

AFB. See Acid-fact bacillus (AFB) and
    American Foundation for the
    Blind (AFB)
Afferent, position and direction, 23
AFP. See Alpha fetoprotein (AFP)
Afterbirth, 253
AGA. See Appropriate for gestational age
    (AGA)
Aganglionic megacolon, 192
Ageism, 379
Agenesis, 213
Agglutination, 331, 426
Aggression, 86
Aging process, 379
Agitation, 87
Agnosia, 388
Agranulocytosis, 145
Ag. See Antigen (Ag)
A/G ratio. See Albumin/globulin ratio
AH. See Accidental hypothermia (AH)
AHA. See American Heart Association
    (AHA) and American Hospital
    Association (AHA)
AHF. See Antihemophilic factor (AHF)
AHF-A. See Antihemophilic factor A
    (AHF-A)
AHF-B. See Antihemophilic factor B
    (AHF-B)
AHF-C. See Antihemophilic factor C
    (AHF-C)
AHG. See Antihemophilic globulin
    (AHG)
AICD. See Automatic implantable
    cardioverter defibrillator (AICD)
AID. See Automatic implantable
    defibrillator (AID)
AIDS. See Acquired immunodeficiency
    syndrome (AIDS)
AIDS-related complex (ARC), 357
AIHA. See Autoimmune hemolytic
    anemia (AIHA)
AIL. See Angioimmunoblastic
    lymphadenopathy (AIL)
Air arthrogram, 466
Air conduction (AC), 326
AK. See Above the knee (AK)
ALA. See American Lung Association
    (ALA)
Albers-Schonberg disease, 50
Albinism, 26
Albright's syndrome, 50
Albumin/globulin ratio, 227
    protein, 447
Albuminuria, 222
Alcohol amnestic disorder, 80
Alcohol hallucinosis, 80
Alcoholic cardiomyopathy, 105
Alcoholic pancreatitis
Alcoholics Anonymous (AA), 91
Alcohol-induced organic mental
    disorders, 79-80

Alcohol intoxication, 80
Alcoholism, dementia associated with,
    80
Alcohol withdrawal, uncomplicated, 80
Alcohol withdrawal delirium, 80
Aldosteronism, 273
Algorithm, 463
Alienation, 388
Alkalosis, 277
ALL. See Acute lymphocytic leukemia
    (ALL)
Allergen, 331
Allergic rhinitis, 160
Allergy, 331
Allogenic marrow transplantation, 148
Alopecia, 26, 199
Alpha fetoprotein (AFP), 264, 410
Alpha particle, 495
Alport's syndrome, 213
ALT. See Argon laser trabeculoplasty
    (ALT)
Alveolar gland, simple and compound, 29
Alveoli, 165, 179
Alzheimer's disease, 382
AMA. See American Medical Association
    (AMA)
Amastia, 31
Amaurosis fugax, 312
Ambivalence, 87
Amblyopia, 312
Ambulatory electrographic monitoring,
    125
Amebic abscess, 195
Amenorrhea, 240
American Academy of Physicians'
    Assistants (AAPA), 33
American Association for Maternal and
    Infant Health (AAMIH), 265
American Association of Blood Banks
    (AABB), 154, 459
American Association of Rehabilitation
    Therapy (AART), 523
American Association of Respiratory
    Therapy (AART), 33
American Association of Retired Persons
    (AARP), 392
American Association on Mental
    Deficiency (AAMD), 91
American Board of Nuclear Medicine
    (ABNM), 511
American Board of Radiology (ABR),
    489
American Cancer Society (ACS), 392
American College of Nuclear Medicine
    (ACNM), 511
American College of Nuclear Physicians
    (ACNP), 511
American College of Nurse Midwifery
    (ACNM), 265
American College of Obstetricians and
    Gynecologists (ACOG), 244, 265

American College of Radiology (ACR), 489
American College of Surgeons (ACS), 244
American Congress of Physical Medicine and Rehabilitation (ACPMR), 523
American Congress of Rehabilitation Medicine (ACRM), 523
American Dietetic Association (ADA), 33
American Drug Index (ADI), 375
American Foundation for the Blind (AFB), 523
American Heart Association (AHA), 126
American Hospital Association (AHA), 392
American Lung Association (ALA), 173
American Medical Association (AMA), 392
American Medical Record Association (AMRA), 33
American Physical Therapy Association (APTA), 33, 523
American Psychiatric Association (APA), 91
American Society of Clinical Pathologists (ASCP), 154
American Society of Hospital Pharmacists (ASHP), 33
American Society of Law and Medicine (ASLM), 154
American Society of Radiologic Techologists (ASRT), 33
American Thoracic Society (ATS), 173
Ametropia, 312
AMI. *See* Acute myocardial infarction (AMI)
AML. *See* Acute myeloblastic leukemia (AML)
Amnesia, 81
Amniocentesis, 261
Amniography, 472
Amnion, 258
Amniotic fluid, 258
  analysis, 454-55
Ampulla, 241
Amputation, 44
  abbreviations, 57
Amputation neuroma, 66
AMRA. *See* American Medical Record Association (AMRA)
Amyloidosis, 106, 146
Amyotrophic lateral sclerosis, 70
ANA. *See* Antinuclear antibodies (ANA)
Anaclitic, 87
Anacusis, 323
Anaerobes, 331
Analeptics, 369
Anal fistula, 190
Analgesia, 78, 369, 521
  stage of, 372
Anaphylactoid purpura, 143-44

Anaphylaxis, 355
Anaplasia, 402
Anasarca, 112
Anastomose, 58
Anastomosis, 117, 127, 188, 192
  of blood vessels, 116
Anatomic division
  of abdomen, 22
  of back, 23
Anatomic position, 24
Anemia, 141, 154
  radiation, 474
  of blood loss, 141
Anencephalia, 70
Anesthesia, 78, 369
  and arterial hypertension, 370
  dissociative, 374
  general, 372-73
  local, 374-75
  and reflexes, 374
  regional, 374-75
Anesthesiologist, 369
Anesthesiology
  study guide, 565-66
  terms pertaining to, 369-78
Anesthetics, classification of, 377
Aneursymal bone cyst, 42
Aneurysm, 71, 77, 102
  resection of, 116
Aneurysmectomy, 112, 116
Aneurysm of aorta, 114
ANF. *See* Antinuclear factor (ANF)
Angina pectoris, 102, 382
Angiocardiography (ACG), 126
Angioimmunoblastic lymphadenopathy (AIL), 357
Angiosarcoma, 28, 186
Angiospasm, 118
Anion, 434
Anisocytosis, 148
Anisometropia, 312
Ankyloglossia, 180, 260
Ankylosing spondylitis, 47
Ankylosis, 47, 50
ANLL. *See* Acute non-lymphocytic leukemia (ANLL)
Ann Arbor staging classification of Hodgkins' disease, 151
Annihilation reaction, 495
Annular, 30
Anode, 434
Anomalies, congenital, 102
Anorchism, 225
Anorexia nervosa, 81, 92, 189
Anosmia, 160
Anovulation, 243
Anoxemia, 170
Anoxia, 170
ANS. *See* Autonomic nervous system (ANS)
Answers, to review guide questions, 582

Anterior, position and direction, 23
Anterior chest diameter (ACD), 173
Anterior pituitary hormones, 441-42
Anterior-posterior (AP), 173
Anterior superior spine (ASS), 57
Anterolateral, 58
Anteroposterior (AP), 57, 173
Anthracosis, 167
Antianxiety agents, 89
Antibody (Ab), 153, 355
  screen, 427
Anti-D antibody injection, 261-62
Antidepressant, 89, 92
Antidiuretic hormone (ADH), 227, 287
Antiemetic drugs, 369
Antigen (Ag), 153, 355, 427
Antigenic determinants, 174
Antihemophilic factor (AHF), 143, 153
  AHF-A, AHF-B, AHF-C, 143
Antihemophilic globulin (AHG), 143, 153
Antihemophilic human plasma, 147
Antineoplastic drugs, 155
Antinuclear antibodies (ANA), 427, 428
Antinuclear factor (ANF), 427
Antipsychotic agents, 89
Antiseptic, 331
Antisocial personality disorder, 84
Antistreptolysin-O titer, 119
Antitoxin, 331
Antrectomy, 189
  gastric, 188
Antrotomy, 160
Antrum, gastric, 185
Antrum of Highmore, 160
Anular, 30
Anulus fibrosus, 47
Anulus remodeling, 109
Anuria, 216
Anus, 190
  imperforate, 260
Anxiety disorders, 80-81
Aorta, 114
  aneurysm of, 114
  coarctation of, 127
Aortic aneurysm resection, abdominal, 116
Aortic arch syndrome, 114
Aortic atresia, 114
Aortic insufficiency, 107
Aortic lacerations, 116
Aortic sinuses, 101
Aortic stenosis (AS), 107, 126, 127
Aortocoronary artery bypass, 109
Aortofemoral bypass grafting, 116
Aortoiliac disease, 114
Aortoiliac occlusions, 394
Aortoiliac replacement grafting, 116
Aortoplasty, 117
APA. *See* American Psychiatric Association (APA)

APAP. *See* Association of Physician Assistant Programs (APAP)

Apasia, 521

Apex cardiogram (ACG), 124, 126

Apex of lung, 165

Apgar score, 260

Aphagia, 185

Aphasia, 78, 525-26
  motor and sensory, 78

Aphonia, 162

Aphthous stomatitis, 180

Aplasia
  of bronchus, 164
  of lung, 167

Aplastic anemia, 141

Apnea, 170

Aponeurosis, 53

Apoplexy, 71, 274
  uteroplacental, 256

Appendectomy, 192

Appendicitis, 190

Appendix vermiformis, 190

Applied extrasensory projection (AESP), 91

Appropriate for gestational age (AGA), 264

Apraxia, 388

AP. *See* Anterior-posterior (AP) *and* Anteroposterior (AP)

APTA. *See* American Physical Therapy Association (APTA)

Aqueduct, cerebral and ventricles, 69-70

AR. *See* Autosomal recessive (AR)

Arachnodactylia, 286

Arachnodactyly, 359

Arachnoid, 69

Arbovirus encephalitides, 333

ARC. *See* AIDS-related complex (ARC)

Archival storage, 463

Arcus senilis, 388

ARD. *See* Acute respiratory disease (ARD)

ARDS. *See* Adult respiratory disease syndrome (ARDS)

Areola, 31

ARF. *See* Acute respiratory failure (ARF)

Argon laser, 30

Argon laser trabeculoplasty (ALT), 309

Argyll-Robertson pupil, 302

Arrhythmia, 103-4
  cardiac, 92

Arterial blood gases, 432-33

Arterial homograft, 116

Arterial hypertension, and anesthesia, 370

Arterial septal defect, 108

Arterial spiders, 199

Arteries, 113-19
  coats of, 114
  coronary, 99-113
  of heart, 101

Arteriolosclerosis, 114

Arteriosclerosis, 114-15

Arteriosclerosis obliterans (ASO), 115, 126

Arteriosclerotic heart disease (ASHD), 126

Arteriovenous (AV), 121, 126

Arthralgia, 53, 521

Arthritis, 47-48, 429

Arthroclasia, 50

Arthrodesis, 50

Arthrodynia, 53

Arthrolysis, 50

Arthropathy, 48

Arthroplasty, 51-52, 58

Arthroscopy, 52

Arthrotomy, 52

Articular, 53

Articulations, 47
  See also Joints

Artifact, 463

Artificial ankylosis, 50

Artificial pneumothorax, 172

Artificial ventilation, 370

AS. *See* Aortic stenosis (AS)

Asbestosis, 167

Aschoff bodies, 112

Ascites, 154, 197

ASCP. *See* American Society of Clinical Pathologists (ASCP)

ASD. *See* Atrial septal defect (ASD)

Aseptic, 45

ASHD. *See* Arteriosclerotic heart disease (ASHD)

ASHP. *See* American Society of Hospital Pharmacists (ASHP)

Asian, and skin-coloring process, 26

ASLM. *See* American Society of Law and Medicine (ASLM)

ASO. *See* Arteriosclerosis obliterans (ASO)

Asphxia, intrauterine, 258

Asphyxia neonatorum, 259

Asplenia, 153

ASRT. *See* American Society of Radiologic Techologists (ASRT)

Assay, 421

Association of Clinical Scientists (ACS), 154, 459

Association of Physician Assistant Programs (APAP), 33

ASS. *See* Anterior superior spine (ASS)

Asthma, 164, 165

Asthmatic bronchitis, 165

Astrocytoma, 71

Asymptomatic, 57

Asystole, 112

Ataractics, 89

Ataxia, 78, 521
  Friedreich's, 73

Atelectasis, 167

Athelia, 31

Atherogenic index, 119

Atherosclerosis, 71, 114

Atherosclerotic occlusive disease, 392-94

Athetosis, 78

Athlete's foot, 27

Atom, 495

Atomic weight, 495

Atony
  of bladder, 219
  of uterus, 253

Atopic skin disorders, 26

ATP. *See* Adenosine triphosphate (ATP)

Atresia
  of anus, 260
  of choanae, 159
  of vagina and vulva, 233

Atria, of heart, 99, 100

Atrial arrhythmias, 103

Atrial fibrillation, 103

Atrial flutter, 103

Atrial septal defect (ASD), 102, 126

Atrioseptostomy, by balloon catheter, 108

Atrioventricular (AV), 126

Atrioventricular block, 104

Atrioventricular bundle, 99

Atrioventricular nodal arrhythmias, 103

Atrioventricular nodal rhythm, 103

Atrioventricular node (AV node), 99

Atrioventricular orifices and valves, 101

Atrophic candidiasis, 180

Atrophic rhinitis, 160

ATS. *See* American Thoracic Society (ATS)

Attitude, obstetric, 256

Attitude therapy, 391

Audiology, 324

Audiometry, 324

Auditory foramen, 58

Augmented ventilation, 172-73

Aura, 78

Aural vertigo, 68

Auscultation and percussion (A&P), 173

Autism, 87

Autogenous, 116

Autografting of bone, 44

Autoimmune diseases, 357-58

Autoimmune hemolytic anemia (AIHA), 154

Autoimmunization, 355

Autologous marrow transplantation, 148

Autologous transfusions, 146

Automatic implantable cardioverter defibrillator (AICD), 119

Automatic implantable defibrillator (AID), 119

Autonomic nervous system (ANS), 91

Autosomal aberration, 280

Autosomal dominant (AD), 286
  inheritance, 280-82

Autosomal recessive (AR), 286
  recessive inheritance, 280-82

Autosplenectomy, 153
Autotopagnosia, 524
Autotransplantation of bone, 44
AV. *See* Atrioventricular (AV) *and*
    Arteriovenous (AV)
Avascular, 45
AV node. *See* Atrioventricular node (AV
    node)
Avoidant personality disorder, 85
Avulsion, 213
Axial, 463
Axillo-axillary bypass graft, 117
Axon, 65
Azoospermia, 226
Azotemia, 215, 245
Azotemic osteodystrophy, 44

BA. *See* Barium (BA)
Babinski's reflex, 88
Bacille Calmette-Guerin (BCG), 173,
    403
Bacilli, infections caused by, 339
Back, anatomic division of, 23
Background radiation, 495
Back projection, 463
Bacteria, pyogenic, 34
Bacterial diseases, tests, 348-50
Bacterial endocarditis, 127
Bacterial infections, 34
Bacteriologic studies, 306
Bacterium, 331
Baker's cyst, 48
Balanitis, 225
Baldy-Webster procedure, 240
Ballism, 78
Ballismus, 521
Ballistocardiography, 124
Balloon catheter, 108
Balloon tamponade, 200
Ballottement, 256
Banding, 282
Bandl's ring, 256
Banti's syndrome, 153
BAO. *See* Basal acid output (BAO)
Barium (BA), 201
Barrel chest, 171
Barr test for nuclear sex, 283
Barthel index, 381
Bartholin, duct of. *See* Duct of Bartholin
Bartholin's adenitis, 234
Bartholin's glands, 233
Bartholin's retention cysts, 234
bas. *See* Basophils (bas)
Basal acid output (BAO), 201
Basal body temperature (BBT), 251, 264
Basal cell carcinoma, 28, 202
Basal cell papilloma, 28
Basal ganglia, 69
Basal metabolic rate (BMR), 287, 444
Basal nuclei, 69
Base element, 4

Base, of lung, 165
Basilar artery stenosis, 73
Basophils (bas), 140, 153
BBB. *See* Bundle branch block (BBB)
BBT. *See* Basal body temperature (BBT)
BC. *See* Bone conduction (BC)
BCG. *See* Bacille Calmette-Guerin (BCG)
BE. *See* Below the elbow (BE)
Becquerel (Bq), 496
Bedsore, 27
Behavior therapy, 90, 391
Behcet's syndrome, 180
Bell's palsy, 66
Below the elbow (BE), 57
Below the knee (BK), 57
Bence-Jones protein, 447
Benign, 399
Benign bone neoplasms, 42
Benign mesenchymoma, 48
Benign mucous membrane pemphigoid,
    180
Benign neoplasms, 48, 56
Benign prostatic hypertrophy (BPH), 227
Beta particle, 496
Bibliotherapy, 90
Bicuspid valve, 101
bid, and time schedule for medication,
    202
Bifurcation, 163
Bigeminal pulse, 118
Bile duct, 193
Biliary calculi, 196
Biliary encephalopath, 260
Biliary structure, 196
Biliary system, 196, 198-99
Bilirubin, 430
Billings method, 252
Bioassay, 421
Biochemistry, 421
    hormones and metabolism, 440-49
    serum, plasma, and whole blood,
        434-40
Biofeedback, 90, 515-16
Bioprosthesis, 111
Biopsy, 182
    of breast, 32
    and fertility studies, 243-44
    and lungs, 169
    of lympy nodes, 152
    and malignant neoplasms, 202
    micro-. *See* Microbiopsy
    of pericardium, 108
    renal, 216
    and thorax, 172
Biparietal diameter (BPD), 264
Bipedal lymphangiography, 155
Bipolar disorders, 83
Bipolar lead, 124
Birthmark, 28
Bitemporal, 58
Bjork-Shiley prosthesis, 111

BK. *See* Below the knee (BK)
Blackhead, 30
Bladder, 218-22
    and syphilis, 220
Bladder neck obstruction, 219
Blalock-Hanlon operation, 108
Blalock-Taussig total repair, 109
Blast injury, 167
Blebs, 33
Bleeding disorders, 143
Bleeding time, 423
Bleomycin, 155
Blepharectomy, 305
Blepharedema, 306
Blepharochalasis, 387
Blepharoplasty, 387
Blighted ovum, 251
Blister, 33
Blocking, 87
Blood
    disorders of, 139-58
    disorders amenable to surgery, 156
    and radionuclides, 504
    study guide, 545-46
    urea, nitrogen (BUN), 227
    whole, 146-47, 434-40
Blood cells, 147
Blood dyscrasia, 148
Blood-forming organs
    disorders of, 139-58
    disorders amenable to surgery, 156
    study guide, 545-46
Blood gas determinations, 432-33
Blood group, 426
Blood grouping systems, 426
Blood pressure (BP), 33, 114, 126
Blood proteins, 147-48
Blood sugar level, 444
Blood type, 426
Blood urea nitrogen (BUN), 448
BMR. *See* Basal metabolic rate (BMR)
Body
    planes of, 23, 24
    of stomach, 185
Body burden, 496
Body dysmorphic disorder, 86
Body image, 87
Bone, 39-46
    brittle, 50
    cancellous, 39
    compact, 39
    eosinophilic granuloma of, 150
    fibrous dysplasia of, 50
    grafting, 44
    necrosis of, 45
    neoplasms, 42-43
    porous, 44
    supernumerary, 44
Bone conduction (BC), 326
Bone marrow, 39, 145-46
    failure of, 141

transplantation, 148
Bone seeker, 496
Bony palate, 179
Borborygmus, 192
Bougienage for esophageal stricture, 184
Bowel infarction, 191
Bowman's capsule, 211
BP. *See* Blood pressure (BP)
BPD. *See* Biparietal diameter (BPD)
BPH. *See* Benign prostatic hypertrophy (BPH)
Bq. *See* Becquerel (Bq)
Brachiocephalic lacerations, 116
Bradycardia, 112, 174, 388
Bradycardia-tachycardia syndrome, 104
Bradykinesia, 388, 521
Brain, 68-79
    abscess, 70
    decompression of, 77
    deficits, 92
    and diagnostic ultrasound, 477
    excision of lesion, 77
    growth retardation, 92
    marrow, 69
    and MR imaging, 485-86
    stem, 58, 69
    tumors, 70-71
Braxton-Hicks sign, 256
Breast
    cancer, 31-32
    conditions amenable to surgery, 34-36
    disorders of, 31-33
    imaging, 473
    references and bibliography, 36-37
    and skin, 25-37
    study guide, 537-38
Breath sounds (BS), 173
Breech extraction, 261
Breech presentations, 257, 264
Brenner tumor, 241
Brittle bones, 50
Brockenbrough technique, 123
Bromsulphalein (BSP), 201
Bronchi, 163-65
Bronchial breathing, 170
Bronchial carcinoid, 164
Bronchiectasis, 164
Bronchiogenic carcinoma, 164
Bronchioles, 163
Bronchioli, 163
Bronchitis, 164
Bronchofiberoscopy, 169
Bronchoplasty, 165
Bronchopleural fistula, 164
Bronchopneumonia, 168
Bronchopulmonary segment, 167
Bronchopulmonary tree, 167
Bronchoscopy, 165
Bronchotomy, 165
Brucellosis, 148
Brudzinski's sign, 88

Bruit of placenta, 256
BS. *See* Breath sounds (BS)
BSP. *See* Bromsulphalein (BSP)
Buccal mucosa, 34
Budd-Chiari syndrome, 194
Buerger's disease, 116
Bulbourethral glands, 218
Bulimia nervosa, 81, 189
Bullae, 34
Bullous eruption, 33
BUN. *See* Blood, urea, nitrogen (BUN)
Bundle branch block (BBB), 104, 126
Bundle of His, 99
Bunionectomy, 52
Burkitt's lymphoma, 150
Burn, 26
    electrosurgical excision of, 30
    first, second, and third degree, 26
Bursae, 46-53
Bursitis, 48
Bypass graft, 116
Byssinosis, 167

CA. *See* Chronogical age (CA)
Ca. *See* Calcium (Ca) *and* Cancer (Ca)
Cafe-au-lait spots, 30
Calcification, 463
    of tracheal rings, 163
Calcinosis, 114-15
Calcitonin, 58
Calcium (Ca), 57
Calculated day of confinement (CDC), 264
Calculus
    in ureter, 217
    of bladder, 219
Caldwell-Luc operation, 160
Calendar rhythm, 252
Calices, 211
Callositas, 26
Callus, 45
Cancer (Ca), 57, 91, 185, 191, 399
    breast, 31-32
    and elderly, 382
    and environmental causes, 416
    grading and staging systems terms, 402-3, 404
    laryngeal, 162
    nasal skin, 159
    nasopharyngeal, 159
    studies related to, 403, 409-10
    terms related to modalities, 410-13
Candida, 337
Candida albicans, 180
Candidiasis, 180
Canthus, 303
Capillaries, 113-19
Capsular laceration, 53
Caput medusae, 199
Caput succedaneum, 259
Carbohydrate (COH), 201

Carbohydrate tolerance tests, 444-45
Carbon dioxide laser, 30
Carbuncle, 27
Carcinoembryonic antigen (CEA), 201, 410
Carcinogenic agent, 399
Carcinoid, 164
Carcinoidosis, 106
Carcinoid syndrome, 277
Carcinoma, 162, 164, 181, 185, 399
    basal cell, 28, 202
    of cervix, 237
    of esophagus, 184
    of gallbladder, 196
    of liver, 196
    of the lung, 167
    and male genital organs, 224-25
    of a salivary gland, 181
    and uterus, 238-39
    of vagina, 234
    of vulva, 234
Carcinoma in situ (CIS), 244, 399
Cardia, of stomach, 185
Cardiac arrest, 103
Cardiac arrhythmia, 92, 103-4
Cardiac biopsy, 108
Cardiac catheterization, 123-24
Cardiac dysrhythmias, 103-4
Cardiac edema, 112
Cardiac index, 119
Cardiac message, open, 108
Cardiac monitor, 119
Cardiac orifice, 185
Cardiac pacing, electronic and physiologic, 119
Cardiac pressures, 124
Cardiac pulmonary resuscitation (CPR), 522
Cardiac syncope, 112
Cardiac tamponade, 104
Cardiac transplantation, 108
Cardiogenic shock, 112, 118
Cardiomyopathies, 105
Cardioplegia, 120
Cardiopulmonary (CP), 126
Cardiopulmonary arrest, 105
Cardiopulmonary bypass, 120
Cardiopulmonary resuscitation, 120
Cardiovascular disorders, 99-138
    amenable to surgery, 128-33
    and diagnostic ultrasound, 477-79
    study guide, 543-44
Cardiovascular imaging, 469-71, 487
Cardioversion, 120
Caries, dental, 180
Carina, 163
Carotid artery ligation, 76
Carotid compression test, 88
Carotid endarterectomy, 76, 116
Carotid occlusive disease, 115
Carotid pulse, 126

Carotid sinus syncope, vasopressor type, 112
Carotid-subclavian anastomosis, 117
Carotid-subclavian bypass graft, 117
Carpal tunnel syndrome, 49
Carpentier-Edwards bioprosthesis, 111
Carpoptosia, 53
Cartilages, 46-53, 162
    detachment of, 53
Cartilaginous joint, 47
Castle's intrinsic factor, 189
CAT. *See* Child's Apperception Test (CAT)
Catalepsy, 87
Cataracts, 382-83, 387
    operations, 298-99
Catatonic type, schizophrenia, 85
Catharsis, 87
Catheter, balloon, 108
Catheterization, cardiac and coronary artery, 123-24
Cathode, 434
Caucasian, and skin-coloring process, 26
Caudal, position and direction, 23, 24
Causalgia, 66
Cauterization, 412
Cavities, of the heart, 99, 100
Cavity of tooth, 180
CBC. *See* Complete blood count (CBC)
CBF. *See* Cerebral blood flow (CBF)
CBS. *See* Chronic brain syndrome (CBS)
CC. *See* Chief complaint (CC)
CCA. *See* Circumflex coronary artery (CCA)
CCCR. *See* Closed chest cardiopulmonary resuscitation (CCCR)
CCF. *See* Cephalin cholesterol flocculation (CCF)
CCU. *See* Coronary care unit (CCU)
CDC. *See* Calculated day of confinement (CDC) *and* Centers for Disease Control (CDC)
CDH. *See* Congenital dislocation of the hip (CDH)
CEA. *See* Carcinoembryonic antigen (CEA)
Cecectomy, 192
Cecostomy, 192
Cecum, 190
Celiac disease, 191
Cell body, 65
Cells
    blood, 147
    giant, 181
    hairy, 144-45, 154
    oat, 167
    plasma, 140, 146
    red, 140-46
    Reed-Sternberg, 154
    reticulum, 186
    round, 186
    sickle, 142

    small, 167
    squamous, 167, 181
    staff, 139-40
    stem, 144
    white blood, 144-45
Cellulitis, 27
Centers for Disease Control (CDC), 245, 392
Centimeters, 34
Central, position and direction, 23
Central nervous system (CNS), 91
Central venous pressure (CVP), 120, 126
Centromere, 282
Cephalic, position and direction, 23, 24
Cephalic version, 261
Cephalin cholesterol flocculation (CCF), 201
Cerbical rib, 43
Cerebellum, 69
Cerebral aneurysm, 71, 77
Cerebral arteriovenous malformation, 71
Cerebral atherosclerosis, 71
Cerebral blood flow (CBF), 91
Cerebral concussion, 71
Cerebral cortex, 69
Cerebral embolism, 71
Cerebral hemorrhage, 259
Cerebral infarction, 71
Cerebral ischemia, 71, 112
Cerebral localization, 69
Cerebral palsy (CP), 71, 91
Cerebral thrombosis, 71
Cerebrospinal fluid (CSF), 91, 456
Cerebrospinal otorrhea, 78
Cerebrospinal rhinorrhea, 78
Cerebrovascular accident (CVA), 71, 91, 126, 127, 383
Cerebrovascular disease (CVD), 71-73, 91, 126
Cerebrovascular insufficiency syndrome, 73
Cerebrum, 69
Cervical disk disease, 49
Cervical esophagus, 182
Cervical lymph nodes, 202
Cervical mediastinotomy, 172
Cervical region, of back, 23
Cervical rib and scalenus anticus syndrome, 115
Cervical spondylosis, 49
Cervicetomy, 240
Cervicitis, 238
Cervicobrachial pain syndrome, 49
Cervix
    dilatation of, 256
    of uterus, 237
Cervix uteri, disease of, 237
Cesarean section (CS), 256, 264
Cestodes, 342
CF. *See* Christmas factor (CF)

CGL. *See* Chronic granulomatous leukemia (CGL)
Chadwick's sign, 256
Chagas' disease, 105
Cheilitis, 181
Cheiloplasty, 181
Cheilostomatoplasty, 181
Chemosis, 306
Chemosurgery, 305
Chemotherapy, 155, 411, 412-13
Chest, 171
    imaging, 485-87
    radiography of, 471
Cheyne-Stokes respiration, 170, 388
Chickenpox, 333
Chief complaint (CC), 33
Childbirth, natural, 252
Childbirth without fear, 252
Childbirth without pain (CWP), 264
Child's Apperception Test (CAT), 91
Chilitis, 181
Chlamydiae, infections, 335-36
Chloasma, 30
Choana, 159
Cholangitis, 196
Cholecystectomy, 198
Cholecystitis, 196
Cholecystojejunostomy, 198
Choledochoduodenostomy, 198
Choledocholithiasis, 196
Choledochoplasty, 198
Cholelithiasis, 196
Cholemia, 194
Cholestasis, 199
Cholesterol esters, 278
Chondritis, 48
Chondroblastoma, 48
Chondrocalcinosis, 48
Chondroma, 48
Chondroplasty, 52
Chondrosarcoma, 48, 59
Chordal fenestration and resection, 109
Chordal shortening, 109
Chordee, of penis, 225
Chordoma, 48
Chordotomy, 76-77
Chorea, 73, 78
Chorioadenoma destruens, 255
Choriocarcinoma, 226, 255
Chorion, 258
Choroid, 293
Christmas disease (CD), 144
Christmas factor (CF), 143, 153
Chromatid, 282
Chromatin, 154, 282
Chromosomal abnormality, 127
Chromosome, 282
    sex, 281
Chrondrectomy, 52
Chronic asthmatic bronchitis, 165
Chronic brain syndrome (CBS), 91

Chronic congestive splenomegaly, 153
Chronic cystic mastitis, 32
Chronic granulomatous leukemia (CGL), 145, 154
Chronic lymphocytic leukemia (CLL), 144, 154
Chronic myelocytic leukemia (CML), 144, 154
Chronic obstructive bronchitis, 164
Chronic obstructive diseases, 164
Chronic obstructive pulmonary disease (COPD), 168, 173, 383
Chronogical age (CA), 91
Chvostek's sign, 260
Cicatrix of skin, 30
Cicatrization, 30
Cilia, 303
Ciliary zonule, 293
Ciliated columnar, 29
Cingulumotomy, 76
Circumcision, 226
Circumflex coronary artery (CCA), 126
Cirrhosis of the liver, 194
CIS. *See* Carcinoma in situ (CIS)
Classification, of neoplasms, 404-9
Claudication, 53, 118
Cleft lip, 181
Cleft palate, 181
Clinical division, of abdomen, 22
Clinical laboratory
    orientation, 421-23
    study guide, 572-75
    terms pertaining to, 421-62
Clipping, of frenulum linguae, 181, 260
Clitoris, 233
CLL. *See* Chronic lymphocytic leukemia (CLL)
Clone, 399
Clonic spasm, 57, 521
Clonogenic asays, 403
Closed chest cardiopulmonary resuscitation (CCCR), 126
Closed reduction, 45
Clostridium perfringens, 27
Clotlysis, 423
Clot retraction, 423-24
Clubfoot, 50
CML. *See* Chronic myelocytic leukemia (CML)
CMV. *See* Controlled mechanical ventilation (CMV) *and* Cytomegalovirus (CMV)
CNS. *See* Central nervous system (CNS)
Coagulant, 423
Coagulation, 143-44
    factors, 143
Coarctation, of aorta, 115, 116-17, 127
Coats, of arteries, 114
Cocaine, abuse and dependency, 91-93
Cocci, infections caused by, 338-39
Cochlea, 319

Cochlear apparatus, functional tests of, 324-25
COH. *See* Carbohydrate (COH)
Cold anoxic arrest, 121
Cold cardioplegia, 120
Cold conization, 239
Cold-punch transurethral resection of vesical neck, 220
Colectomy, 192
Colic, 192
Colic flexure, 190
Colitis, 190
Collagen, 359
    diseases, 106
Colocystoplasty, 221
Colon, 190
    resection, 192
Colonoscopy, 200
Colostomy, 192
Colostrum, 256
Colphrrhaphy, 235
Colpocleisis, 234
Colpomicroscopy, 234
Colpoperineoplasty, 235
Colpoperineorrhaphy, 235
Colposcopy, 235
Colpotomy, 235
Coma, 78
Combined radiotherapy, 155
Combining form word elements, and definitions, 20-21
Comedo, 30
Commission on Professional Hospital Activities (CPHA), 33
Commissurotomy, 109
Commitment, 79
Common hepatic duct, 193
Common Procedural Terminology (CPT), 33
Compensated heart failure, 105
Compensation, 87
Complement fixation tests, 244
Complete blood count (CBC), 153
Completed stroke (CS), 91
Complete heart block, 104
Complete ovarian oblation, 242
Compound alveolar gland, 29
Compound elements, 6-15, 533-34
Compression, of cervical cord and thoracic or lumbar cord, 76
Compulsion, 80, 87
Computed tomography (CT), 155, 464
Concha, 159
Concussion, 71
Conditioned reflex (CR), 91
Conditioned stimulus (CS), 91
Conduction, 324
    disturbances, 104
    system, of heart, 99, 100
Condylomas, 234
Confabulation, 87

Confinement
    CDC. *See* Calculated day of confinement (CDC)
    EDC. *See* Estimated day of confinement (EDC)
Confluent, 30
Congenital, 261
Congenital anomalies, 102
Congenital dislocation of the hip (CDH), 57
Congenital megacolon, 190
Congenital pancytopenia, 141
Congenital septal defects, correction of, 108
Congenital stridors, 259
Congenital tumor, 70
Congestive dilatated cardiomyopathy, 105
Congestive heart failure, 105, 127, 383-84
Conjunctiva, 303
    disorders of, 304
Connective tissue, diseases of, 359-60
Conn's syndrome, 273
Consolidation, 174
Constrictive pericarditis, chronic, 107
Consumption coagulopathy, 143
Contact activation cofactor, 143
Contact factor, 143
Contact lenses, 307
Contagious, 331
Contamination, 496
Continuous positive airway pressure (CPAP), 172-73
Contour, 58
Contraception, 251
Contrapuncture, 56
    Dupeytren's and Volkmann's, 56
Controlled mechanical ventilation (CMV), 173
Contusions, 213
Conventional values, 421
Conversion, 87
    disorder, 86
Convulsion, 78, 92
Cooley's anemia, 142
COPD. *See* Chronic obstructive pulmonary disease (COPD)
Copectomy, 234
Cordectomy, 76
Cord hemorrhage, 259
Cordotomy, 76-77
    percutaneous and selective, 77
Corium, 25
Cornea, 293
    disorders, 294-95
Corneal operations, 299
Coronal, body plane, 23, 24
Coronary arteries, 101
    and heart, 99-113
Coronary artery
    bypass, 109

catheterization, 123-24
perfusion, 120
Coronary atherosclerosis, 106
Coronary atherosclerotic heart disease,
106
Coronary care unit (CCU), 126
Coronary heart disease (CHD), 384
Coronary risk factors, 112
and Framingham Study, 113
Coronary sinus, 101
Cor pulmonale, acute and chronic, 106
Corpus albicans, 241
Corpus callosum, 69
Corpus luteum, 241
Corpus uteri, diseases and malfunctions
of, 238
Corrigan's pulse, 118
Cortex
of bone, 39
cerebral, 69
Cortical adenoma, 213
Corticotropin-releasing factor (CRF), 287
Cortisone, 34
Cor triatriatum, 102
Cor triloculare, 102
Coryza, 159
Costoclavicular space, 115
Counter, 496
Counterpulsation, 120
Countershock, 120
Couvelaire uterus, 256
Cowper's glands, 218
Coxa plana, 43, 44
Coxarthropathy, destructive, 48
Coxa valga, 43
Coxa vara, 43
CP. See Cardiopulmonary (CP) and
Cerebral palsy (CP)
CPAP. See Continuous positive airway
pressure (CPAP)
CPHA. See Commission on Professional
Hospital Activities (CPHA)
CPR. See Cardiac pulmonary resuscitation
(CPR)
cps. See Cycles per second (cps)
CPT. See Common Procedural
Terminology (CPT)
CR. See Conditioned reflex (CR)
Crack, 92
Cramp, 57
Cranial nerve, 58
Craniectomy, 77
Craniocerebral trauma, 73, 75
Craniotomy, 77
Crepitation, 45
Crepitus, 53
CREST syndrome, 359
CRF. See Corticotropin-releasing factor
(CRF)
Crib death, 92
Cricoid cartilage, 162

Crohn's disease of small intestine, 191
Cross-matching, 426
Crown, of tooth, 180
Cryohypophysectomy, 275
Cryoneurosurgery, 77
Cryoprecipitate (Cryo), 147
Cryosurgery, 412
of skin, 29
Cryotherapy, 516
Cryptomenorrhea, 240
Cryptorchism, 225
Crypts, 182
Crystine stones, 447
CS. See Cesarean section (CS) and
Completed stroke (CS) and
Conditioned stimulus (CS)
CSF. See Cerebrospinal fluid (CSF)
CT. See Computed tomography (CT)
Cul-de-sac, 235
Culdocentesis, 239
Culdoscopy, 239
Culture, for Neisseria gonorrhoeae, 244
Curettage, of skin, 29
Curie, 496
Curie units, multiples of, 510
Curvatures of stomach, 185
Cushing's disease, 273
CVA. See Cerebrovascular accident (CVA)
CVD. See Cerebrovascular disease (CVD)
CVP. See Central venous pressure (CVP)
CWP. See Childbirth without pain (CWP)
Cyanosis, 154, 170
Cycles per second (cps), 91
Cyclic combination chemotherapy, 155
Cyclic vomiting, 189
Cyclothymia, 83
Cyclothymic, 87
Cyclotron, 496
Cylindruria, 286
Cyro. See Cryoprecipitate (Cryo)
Cyst, 42
Cystadenoma of ovary, 241
Cystectomy, 220-21
Cystic duct, 193
Cystic fibrosis, 343
Cystitis, 219
Cysto. See Cystoscopic examination
(cysto.)
Cystolithotomy, 221
Cystometrogram, 222
Cystometry, 223
Cystoplasty, 221
Cystorrhaphy, 221
Cystoscopic examination (cysto.), 227
Cystoscopy, 221
Cystostomy, 221
Cysts, of ovary, 241
Cytapheresis, 147
Cytogenetics, 282-83
and genetics, 286-87
studies, 243, 286

Cytologic studies, 243
of gynecologic conditions, 243
Cytology, exfoliative, 403
Cytomegalovirus (CMV), 148, 334
infections, 260
Cytopathologic studies, 243
Cytoplasm, 154
Cytotoxic, 194

Dacarbazine, 155
Dacryoadenectomy, 305
D&C. See Dilatation and curettage (D&C)
Dark adaptation, 307
Dark-field examination, 244
Dawson's encephalitis, 76
DC. See Direct current (DC)
DCC. See Direct current cardioversion
(DCC)
DCR. See Direct cortical response (DCR)
Debilated patient, 127
Debility, 154
Decalcification, 45, 58
Decompression, of brain and spinal cord,
77
Decontamination, 496
Decortication, 172
Decubitus ulcer, 27
Deep, position and direction, 23, 24
Defibrillator, 121
Definitions, and form work elements,
20-21
Definitive, 169
Deflection of septum, 159
Degenerative, 127
Degenerative joint disease, 58
Deglutition, 185
Deglycerolized red cells, 147
Dehiscence of wound, 241
Delirium, 83, 87
stage of, 372
Delirium tremens (DT), 80, 91
Delivery, 261
Delusional syndrome, organic, 84
Delusions, 87
of grandeur, of persecution, and of
reference, 87
Demand pacing, 119
Demarcation, 58
Dementia, 83, 87
and alcoholism, 80
Demineralization, 45
Dendrite, 65
Dendron, 65
Denial, 87
Density, 464
Dental caries, 180
Denudation, 34
Denuded, 34
Deoxycorticosterone (DOC), 287
Deoxyribonucleic acid (DNA), 264, 283,
399-400

fingerprinting, 264
Department of Health and Human Services (DHHS), 392
Dependence
   cocaine, 91-93
   psychological, 92
Dependent personality disorder, 85
Depersonalization, 87
   disorder, 81
Depigmentation, 30
Depression, 83, 92, 526
   respiratory, 92
Depressive disorders, 83
Depressive episode, 82
Depressive mood syndrome, 82
Derma, 25
Dermabrasion, 29
Dermatitis, 27, 33
Dermatographism, 30
Dermatophytosis, 27
Dermis, 25
Dermographia, 30
Dermoplasty, 160
Descriptive psychiatry, 79
Destructive coxarthropathy, 48
Detachment of cartilage, 53
Dextroposition of the aorta, 103
DFI. See Disease-free environment (DFI)
DHHS. See Department of Health and Human Services (DHHS)
Diabetes insipidus, 277
Diabetes mellitus, 277
Diabetic ketoacidosis (DKA), 277, 287
Diabetic retinopathy, 77
Diagnosis (Dx), 33
   and radionuclides, 507-9
Diagnostic radiology, 488
Diagnostic Related Group (DRG), 392
Diagnostic suffixes, 6-7
Diagnostic tests, and radionuclides, 504-9
Diagnostic ultrasound, 475-81
   studies, 477-81
   study guide, 576-77
Dialysis, 223
Diaphragm, 53
Diaphragmatic hernia, 56
Diaphragmatic infarction, 107
Diaphysis, 39
Diarrhea, 192, 260
Diarthrodial joint, 47
Diastolic augmentation procedure, 121
Diastolic blood pressure, 114
Diastolic murmur (DM), 126
DIC. See Diffuse intravascular coagulation (DIC)
Dicrotic pulse, 118
Diencephalon, 69
Dietl's crisis, 216
Differential leukocyte count, 145
Differentiation, 402

Diffuse intravascular coagulation (DIC), 143, 154
Digestive disorders, 179-210
   and conditions amenable to surgery, 203-6
   study guide, 549-50
Digestive system, tests, 449-51
Digital, 118, 464
Digital blanching, 118
Dilatation
   of aorta, 115
   of cervix, 256
   of esophagus, 184
   of larynx, 162
Dilatation and curettage (D&C), 239, 244
Diopter, 307
DIP. See Distal interphalangeal (joint) (DIP)
Diplegia, 78
Diploe, 39, 58
Direct contact, 331
Direct cortical response (DCR), 91
Direct current (DC), 120
Direct current cardioversion (DCC), 126
Direct current defibrillation, 121
Direction, and position, 23-24
Disc, intervertebral, 47
Discoid, 30
Discrete, 30
Disease, hematologic findings in, 425-34
Disease-free environment (DFI), 401
Disengagement, 388
Dislocation, 48
Disorganized type, schizophrenia, 85
Dispensary of the United States of America, The (USD), 375
Displacement, 87
   of uterus, 238
Disruptive trauma of joint, 48
Dissecting type, aneurysm of aorta, 114
Dissection, 202
Disseminated sclerosis, 75
Dissocial behavior, 87
Dissociation, 88
Dissociative anesthesia, 374
Dissociative disorders, 81
Distal, position and direction, 23, 24
Distal interphalangeal (joint) (DIP), 57
Distress, fetal, 92, 258
Disuse atrophy, 56
Diverticula of esophagus, 184
Diverticulectomy, 192
Diverticulitis, 190
Diverticulosis, 190
DKA. See Diabetic ketoacidosis (DKA)
DM. See Diastolic murmur (DM)
DNA. See Deoxyribonucleic acid (DNA)
DOC. See Deoxycorticosterone (DOC)
Dominant, 283
Dopper techniques, 489
Doppler flood flowmetry, 121

Dorsal, position and direction, 23, 24
Dose, 496
Dosimeter, 496
Double depression, 83
Douglas' pouch, 235
Down's syndrome, 259, 284
Doxorubicin, 155
Dragging inguinal pain, 226
Drainage
   of infected skin lesion, 30
   of meninges for abscess or hematoma, 77
Dressler's syndrome, 112
DRG. See Diagnostic Related Group (DRG)
Drugs
   and fetotoxicity, 258
   interactions, and gerontology, 380-81
   monitoring, 457
   and neonate, 259
   and oncology, 399
DT. See Delirium tremens (DT)
D trisomy, 284
Duct of Bartholin, 180
Ductography, 473
Ducts, lymphatic, 149
Ductus arteriosus, 127
Ductus deferens, 224
Duhamel procedure, 192
Dumping syndrome, 189
Duodenal ulcer, 190
Duodenoscopy, 200
Duodenum, 189
Dura mater, 69
Dwarfism, 273
Dx. See Diagnosis (Dx)
Dynamic ileus, 191
Dynamic psychiatry, 79
Dysarthria, 78
Dyschondroplasia, 49-50
Dyscrasia, 148, 358
Dysentery, 190
Dysgerminoma, 241
Dyskeratosis, 400
Dyskinesia, 78, 388
Dysmenorrhea, 240
Dysmorphophobia, 86
Dyspepsia, 189
Dysphagia, 185
Dysphonia, 162
Dysplasia, 213
   skeletal, 49-50
Dyspnea, 154, 170, 389
Dyspnoea, 170
Dysrhythmia, 103-4
Dysthymia, 83
Dystocia, 256
Dystonia, 78
Dystrophy, 56
Dysuria, 222

Ear, 317-24
    conditions of, 319
    conditions amenable to surgery,
        327-28
Ear, nose, and throat (ENT), 326
Early shock, 118
Eastern equine encephalitis (EEE), 333
Eating disorders, 81
Ebstein's anomaly, 106
Ecchymoses, 213
Ecchymosis, 30
ECG. *See* Electrocardiogram (ECG)(EKG)
    and Electrocardiography (ECG)
Echography, 475
Eclampsia, 254
ECMO. *See* Extracorporeal membrane
        oxygenation (ECMO)
ECT. *See* Electroconvulsive therapy (ECT)
Ectopic polypeptides, 410
Ectopic pregnancy, 254
Ectopy, 213
    of testis, 225
Eczema, 27
Eczematoid, 31
Eczematous, 31
EDC. *See* Estimated day of confinement
        (EDC)
Edema, 112, 168
Edematous swelling, 226
Educational therapy, 90
Edward's syndrome, 284
EEE. *See* Eastern equine encephalitis
        (EEE)
EEG. *See* Electroencephalogram (EEG)
Effacement, 256
Effective renal plasma flow (ERPF), 227
Effective sensory projection (ESP), 91
Effector, 65
Efferent, position and direction, 23, 24
Effusion, hemorrhagic and synovial, 53
Ego, 79
EIA. *See* Enzyme-linked immunoassay
        (EIA)
Eisenmenger's syndrome, 106
Ej. *See* Elbow jerk (Ej)
Ejaculatory duct, 224
EKG. *See* Electrocardiogram (ECG)(EKG)
Elbow jerk (Ej), 91
Elective cardiac arrest, 121
Electric shock therapy (EST), 91
Electrocardiogram (ECG)(EKG), 126
    computer analysis, 124
    fetal. *See* Fetal electrocardiogram
        (FECG)
Electrocardiography (ECG), 124-25
    fetal, 261
    techniques, 125
Electrocauterization, 412
    of endocervix, 239
Electrocochleography, 324
Electroconvulsive therapy (ECT), 90, 91

Electrodesiccation, 30
Electroencephalogram (EEG), 91
Electroencephalography, 88
Electrokymography, 125
Electrolytes, 434-36
    balance, 434
Electromyogram (EMG), 57
Electronarcosis, 90
Electronics, medical, 122
Electronystagmography, 88
Electroshock treatment, 90
Electrosurgical excision of burn, 30
Electrotesting, 516
Electrotherapy, 517
Elements, of medical terms, 4, 6-24
ELISA. *See* Enzyme-linked
        immunosorbent assay (ELISA)
Elliptocytic anemia, 142
Elliptocytosis, 142, 154
Elschnig pearls, 302
Embolectomy, 117, 170
Embolism, 71, 115, 168
Embolization, trancatheter, 224
Embryo, 258
Embryonic period, 251
EMG. *See* Electromyogram (EMG)
Empathy, 87
Emphysema, 164, 168
Empyema
    of gallbladder, 196
    of pleura, 171
Encephalitis, 333
    Dawson's, 76
    lethargica, 73
Encephalocele, 73
Encephalon, 69
Encephalopathy, hypertensive, 75
Enchondromatosis, 49-50
Endarterectomy, 76, 116
Endocarditis, bacterial, 106
Endocardium, 101
Endocrine glands, 271-76
    conditions amenable to surgery, 288
    disorders, 271-91
    and neuroradiography, 468-69
    function studies, 440-44
    study guide, 557-58
Endocrinopathy, 106
Endolaryngeal carcinomas, 162
Endolarynx, 162
Endometrial biopsy, 243-44
Endometriosis, 238
Endometritis, 238
Endorectal ileoanal anastomosis, 192
Endoscopic retrograde
        cholangiopancreatography, 200
Endoscopic sclerotherapy, 201
Endoscopy, gastrointestinal, 200
Endosteum, 39
Endotracheal anesthesia, 372
End-to-end anastomosis, 117, 192

Engagement, 257
Engorgement, 257
ENT. *See* Ear, nose, and throat (ENT)
Enteritis, 191
Enucleation, 299
Enuresis, 222
Environment, and cancer causes, 416
Enzyme
    myocardial, 436-38
    and red cell destruction, 142
    serum, 438-40
Enzyme-linked immunoassay (EIA), 409
Enzyme-linked immunosorbent assay
        (ELISA), 409
EOM. *See* Extraocular muscles (EOM)
eos. *See* Eosinophils (eos)
Eosinophilic granuloma of bones, 150
Eosinophils (eos), 140, 153
Ependymoma, 71
Epicardial pacing, 120
Epicondylalgia, 49
Epicondylitis, 49
Epidemic parotitis, 181
Epidermaphytosis, 27
Epidermis, 25, 33
Epidermoid, 202
    cyst, 42
Epidermolysis bullosa, 27
Epidermophyton, 27
Epididymectomy, 226
Epididymis, 224
Epididymitis, 225
Epididymovasostomy, 226
Epigastric pain, 189
Epigastric regions, 22
Epiglottis, 162
Epiglottitis, 162
Epilepsy, 73, 77
Epiphora, 306
Epiphyseal arrest, 44
Epiphyseal stapling, 44
Epiphysiodesis, 44
Epiphysis, 39
Epiphysistis, acute, 43
Episioplasty, 235
Episiotomy, 256, 264
Epistaxis, 127, 160
Epithalamus, 69
Epithelial polyps, 186
Epithelium, 25, 202
    types of, 29
Epstein-Barr virus, 334
Epulis, 181
Equatorial plane, 283
ERA. *See* Estradiol receptor assay (ERA)
ERPF. *See* Effective renal plasma flow
        (ERPF)
Eructation, 189, 261
Eruption, 31
Erysipelas, 27
Erythema, 31, 199

Erythematous skin, 33
Erythremia, 142
Erythroblastosis fetalis, 141-42, 259
Erythroblasts, 139
Erythrocytes, 139, 141-42
Erythrocytic sedimentation rate (ESR), 126, 153
Erythrocytosis, 148
Erythromycin, 174
Erythropenia, 149
Erythropoiesis, 139, 141
Esophageal diverticulectomy, 184
Esophageal manometric studies, 201
Esophageal perforation, 184
Esophageal reflux ulceration, 184
Esophageal sphincter, 182, 183
Esophageal stricture, 184
Esophageal trauma, 184
Esophageal varices, 184
Esophagitis, 184
Esophagogastroduodenoscopy, 200
Esophagojejunostomy, 184
Esophagomyotomy, 185
Esophagoplasty, 184
  with reversed gastric tube, 184
Esophagorrhaphy, 184
Esophagus, 182-85
Esotropia (ET), 308
ESP. *See* Effective sensory projection (ESP) *and* Extrasensory perception (ESP)
ESR. *See* Erythrocytic sedimentation rate (ESR)
EST. *See* Electric shock therapy (EST)
Estimated day of confinement (EDC), 264
Estradiol receptor assay (ERA), 403, 409
ESWL. *See* Extracorporeal shock wave lithotripsy (ESWL)
ET. *See* Esotropia (ET)
ETF. *See* Eustachian tubal function (ETF)
Ethmoidal sinus, 160
Ethmoidectomy, 160
Etiology, 57, 202
Eunichism, 273
Euphoria, 78
Euploidy, 283
Eustachian tubal function (ETF), 326
Evaluation, and physical therapy, 519-21
Evisceration, 299
Ewing's sarcoma, 42, 401
Exacerbation, 34, 279
Examination, neurologic, 88
Exchange transfusion, 201, 264
Excision
  of Bartholin's gland, 235
  of brain lesion, 77
  of skin lesion, 30
  surgery, 169
Excoriation, 31
Exercise, therapeutic, 518-19

Exfoliative cytology, 403
Exhaled-air ventilation, 121
Exophthalmos, 276
Exostectomy, 44
Exostoses, 50
Exotropia (XT), 308
Expressive aphasia, 525
Exstrophy of bladder, 219
External arteriovenous (AV) shunt, 121
External cardiac compression, 121
External ear, and operative terms, 321-33
Extirpative, 169
Extracorporeal circulation, 121
Extracorporeal membrane oxygenation (ECMO), 262, 264
Extracorporeal shock wave lithotripsy (ESWL), 223, 227
Extrahepatic block, 196
Extranodal, 155
Extraocular muscles (EOM), 308
Extrapleural thoracoplasty, 169
Extrasensory perception (ESP), 91
Extravasation, 118
Extrinsic asthma, 164
Eye, 293-302
  chambers of, 293
  conditions amenable to surgery, 310-12
Eyelid, disorders of, 304

Face presentations, 264
Facial thermography, 88-89
FACOG. *See* Fellow of American College of Obstetricians and Gynecologists (FACOG)
Factor, 421
Factors, coagulation, 143
  deficiencies, 144
Fallopian tubes, 241
Fallot, tetralogy of. *See* Tetralogy of Fallot
False diverticula, 184
Familial hypophosphatemia, 44
Family-Centered Maternity Care (FCMC), 265
Family history (FH), 33
Family planning, natural, 252
Family Service Association of America (FSAA), 265
Fanconi's syndrome, 141
Fascia, 53
Fasciculation, 78, 389
Fascitis, 56
Fasting blood sugar (FBS), 287
Fatigability, 127
Fatty liver, 194
Faucial tonsil, 183
FBS. *See* Fasting blood sugar (FBS)
FCMC. *See* Family-Centered Maternity Care (FCMC)
FDP. *See* Fibrin-fibrinogen degradation products (FDP)

Fear, childbirth without, 252
Fecal fistula, 190
Fecalith, 192
FECG. *See* Fetal electrocardiogram (FECG)
FEF. *See* Forced expiratory flow (FEF)
Fellow of American College of Obstetricians and Gynecologists (FACOG), 265
Femoral pulse, 127
Femoropopliteal arterial reconstruction, 117
Femoropopliteal occlusions, 394-95
Femorortibial bypass grafting, 117
Femur, 58
Fenestration, 109
Fertility studies, 243-44
Festination, 78, 389
Fetal, obstetrical, and neonatal conditions, 251-69
  See also other fetal listings and Fetus
Fetal anomaly, 258
Fetal anoxia, 258
Fetal development, 261
Fetal disorders, study guide, 555-56
Fetal distress, 92, 258
Fetal electrocardiogram (FECG), 262, 264
Fetal electrocardiography, 261
Fetal heart rate (FHR), 264
Fetal heart tone (FHT), 264
Fetal hemoglobin (Hb F), 153
Fetal hemolytic disease, 258
Fetal monitoring, 261
Fetal period, 251, 257-59
Fetal phonocardiography, 262
Fetal tests, 429-33
Fetography, 473
Fetor hepaticus, 199
Fetotoxicity, 258
Fetus, 258
  and fetotoxicity, 258
  immature, 251
  See also listings under Fetal
FEV. *See* Forced expiratory volume (FEV)
FFP. *See* Fresh frozen plasma (FFP)
FH. *See* Family history (FH)
FHR. *See* Fetal heart rate (FHR)
FHT. *See* Fetal heart tone (FHT)
Fiberoptic gastroscopy, 200
Fibrillation, 103, 104
Fibrinase, 143
Fibrin-fibrinogen degradation products (FDP), 143, 153
Fibrin-fibrinogen related antigens (FR-antigens), 143, 153
Fibrin-fibrinogen split products (FSP), 153
Fibrinogen, 143
Fibrinolysis, 149
Fibrin-stabilizing factor, 143

Fibromas, 186
Fibroplastic endocarditis, 106
Fibrosarcoma, 59
    of bone, 43
Fibrosis, 58, 464
Fibrous dysplasia of bone, 50
Fibrous histiocytoma, 59
Fibrous joint, 47
FIGO. See International Federation of
        Gynecology and Obstetrics
        (FIGO)
Filariasis, 148
Fingerprinting, Genetic and DNA, 264
Fission, nuclear, 497
Fissure, 213
    anal, 190
    of nipple, 32
Fissure in ano, 190
Fistula, 163, 164, 190, 234
Fistulo in ano, 190
Fixation, internal, 45
Fixed-rate pacing, 120
Flaccid, 33
Flail chest, 171
Flapping chest cage, 171
Flapping tremor, 199
Fletcher factor, 143
Flexures of colon, 190
Flocculation tests, 244
Floppy disk, 464
Fluorescent treponemal antibody
        absorption (FTA-ABS) test, 244
Fluoroscopy, 464
Flutter, 103
Follicle-stimulating hormone (FSH), 244
Fontanel, 259
Footling presentation, 257
Foramen ovale, 101
Forced expiratory flow (FEF), 173
Forced expiratory volume (FEV), 173
Forceps applications, 261
Fornix, 303
Fossa of Rosenmuller, 183
Fovea, 294
Foveolate type gastritis, 187
Fractionation, 400
Fractions, plasma, 147-48
Fracture (Fx), 43, 45, 57
Framingham Study, and coronary risk
        factors, 113
Frank breech, 257
FR-antigens. See Fibrin-fibrinogen related
        antigens (FR-antigens)
FRC. See Functional residual capacity (FRC)
Freckles, and skin-coloring process, 26
Fredet-Ramsteat operation, 188
Free cholesterol, 278
French language, 3
Frenulum, 180, 181
Frenulum linguae, 180
    clipping of, 260

Frequency, 324
Fresh frozen plasma (FFP), 147
Freud, Sigmund, 90
Friedreich's ataxia, 73
Frontal, body plane, 23, 24
Frontal sinus, 160
Frozen section (FS), 32, 33
Frozen shoulder, 49
FS. See Frozen section (FS)
FSAA. See Family Service Association of
        America (FSAA)
FSH. See Follicle-stimulating hormone
        (FSH)
FSP. See Fibrin-fibrinogen split products
        (FSP)
FTA-ABS test. See Fluorescent
        treponemal antibody absorption
        (FTA-ABS) testE FTND. See Full-
        term normal delivery (FTND)
Fugue, 81
Fulguration of skin, 30
Full-term normal delivery (FTND), 264
Functional residual capacity (FRC), 173
Functional tests
    of cochlear apparatus, 324-25
    of vestibular apparatus, 325
    of vision, 307-8
Fundic patch operation, 184
Fundoplication, 184
Fundus
    of stomach, 185
    of uterus, 237
Fungating, 202
Fungi, and infections, 339-40
Fungoides, 152
Furunculosis, 28
Fusiform type, aneurysm of aorta, 114
Fx. See Fracture (Fx)

Gait analysis, 520
Galactosemia, 278
Gallbladder, 193, 196
    carcinoma of, 196
Gallstone pancreatitis
Gamete, 283
Gamma globulin (IgC), 147
Gammaphotography, 500
Gamma ray, 497
Ganglion, 65
    basal, 69
    cyst of bone, 42
Ganglionectomy, 68
Ganglioneuroma, 66
Gangrene, 27
Gantry, 464
Gas, blood, 432-33
Gastrectomy, 188
Gastric analysis, 449
Gastric malignant neoplasms, 185-86
Gastric polyps, 186
Gastric resection, 188, 387

Gastric types, 188
Gastric ulcers, 186
Gastritis, 187
Gastrocele, 187
Gastrocolitis, 187
Gastroduodenal anastomosis, 188
Gastroduodenitis, 187
Gastroenteritis, 187
Gastrointestinal (GI), 201
    endoscopies, 200
    studies, and radionuclides, 504-5
    tract, 449-54
Gastrojejunal anastomosis, 188
Gastrojejunostomy, 188
Gastropathy, 187
Gastroptosis, 187
Gastrostomy, 188
Gaucher's disease, 278
GBM. See Glomerular basement
        membrane (GBM)
GC. See Gonorrhea (GC)
Geiger-Muller counter, 497
Gene, 283
General anesthesia, 372-73
General anesthetics, classification of, 377
Generalized anxiety disorder, 80
Genetics
    and cytogenetics, 286-87
    fingerprinting, 264
Genital organs, male. See Male genital
        organs
Genitourinary (GU), 227
Genome, 283
Genotype, 283
Genu valgum, 43
Genu varum, 43
Geriatrics, 381
German language, 3, 4
German measles, 334
Gerontologist, 381
Gerontology, 381
    study guide, 567-69
    terms pertaining to, 379-98
Gerontoxon, 388
Gestation, 251, 257
GFR. See Glomerular filtration rate (GFR)
GI. See Gastrointestinal (GI)
Giant cell epulis, 181
Giant cell tumor, 42
Giantism, 273
Gibson-Cooke technique, 451
Gillespie, N.A., 372
Gingivae, 180
Gingivitis, 181
Glands
    endocrine, 271-76
    salivary, 179-82
    types of, 29
Glass factor, 143
Glaucoma, 296, 308-10
    operations, 300-301

Glioblastoma multiforme, 71
Glomerular basement membrane
        (GBM), 227
Glomerular capsule, 211
Glomerular filtration rate (GFR), 227
Glossectomy, 181
Glossitis, 181
Glossodynia, 182
Glossorrhaphy, 181
Glottis, 162
Glucagon, 445
Glucose-6-phosphate dehydrogenase
        (G6PD) deficiency, 142, 154
Glucose tolerance test (GTT), 287
Glycogenoses, 278
Glycosuria, 222, 279
Goblet cell, 29
Goiter, 273
Goldschneider's disease, 27
Gonioscopy, 307
Gonorrhea (GC), 244, 336
Gonorrheal vaginitis, 234
Gonosome, 283
Goodell's sign, 257
Goodpasture's syndrome, 213
Grading systems. See Cancer
Grafting, 116
    bone, 44
    skin, 30
Graft-versus-host disease (GvH)(GVHD),
        148, 154
Grandeur, delusions of, 87
Granulation, 31
Granulocyte transfusion, 147
Granulocytic series, 139-40
Granulocytopenia, 145, 155
Granuloma fungoides, 152
Granulomatous colitis, 190
Graphospasm, 56
Gravida, 251
Gravidarum, 254
Gray matter, 70
Great vessel, imaging, 487
Greek language, 3
Grief reaction, 389
Group psychotherapy, 90
G6PD. See Glucose-6-phosphate
        dehydrogenase (G6PD) deficiency
GTT. See Glucose tolerance test (GTT)
GU. See Genitourinary (GU)
Guedel, A.E., 372
Guillain-Barre syndrome, 66
Guilt, 92
Gums, 180
Guttate, 31
GvH. See Graft-versus-host disease
        (GvH)(GVHD)
GVHD. See Graft-versus-host disease
        (GvH)(GVHD)
Gyn. See Gynecology (Gyn)
Gynecology (Gyn), 244

amenable to surgery, 246-47
and diagnostic ultrasound, 480-81
disorders, 233-49
conditions, cytologic studies of, 243
study guide, 553-54

HAA. See Hepatitis Australia antigen
        (HAA) and Hepatitis associated
        antigen (HAA)
Hagemann factor (HF), 143
HAI. See Hemagglutination-inhibition
        immunoassay (HAI)
Hair glands, 28
Hairy cell leukemia (HCL), 144-45, 154
Half-life, radioactive, 497
Halitosis, 182
Hallucinations, 87
Hallucinogens, 89
Hallucinosis, 80
Hallux malleus, 48
Hallux valgus, 48
Hallux varus, 48
Ham test, 432
Hancock bioprosthesis, 111
Hand-Schuller-Christian disease, 150
Hand-shoulder syndrome, 49
Hard palate, 179
Harelip, 181
Harrington instrumentation and fusion,
        53
Hashish, 92
Hb. See Hemoglobin (Hb) and
        Hemoglobin concentration (Hb)
Hb A. See Adult hemoglobin (Hb A)
HBE. See His bundle electrocardiogram
        (HBE) and His bundle
        electrography (HBE)
Hb F. See Fetal hemoglobin (Hb F)
Hb S. See Sickle cell hemoglobin (Hb S)
HCD. See Heavy-chain disease (HCD)
HCFA. See Health Care Financing
        Administration (HCFA)
HCG. See Human chorionic gonadotropin
        (HCG)
HCL. See Hairy cell leukemia (HCL)
Hct. See Hematocrit (Hct)(Ht)
HD. See Hip disarticulation (HD)
HDL. See High-density lipoproteins
        (HDL)
HDN. See Hemolytic disease of newborn
        (HDN)
HE. See Hereditary elliptocytosis (HE)
Head injury, 73, 75
Health Care Financing Administration
        (HCFA), 392
Hearing
    conditions amenable to surgery,
        327-28
    disorders, 317-30
    imaging, 474
    loss, 321

loss deficits, 58
study guide, 561-62
Heart
    action, recordings of, 124-26
    block, degrees of, 104
    cavities of, 99, 100
    conduction system of, 99, 100
    and coronary arteries, 99-113
    failure, 105, 383-84
    orifices and valves, 101
    transplantation, 108
    wall and covering, 101
Heart-lung machine, 121
Heart-lung resuscitation (HLR), 126
Heart-lung transplantation, 170
Heavy-chain disease (HCD), 154, 358
Heberden's nodes, 53
Hegar's sign, 257
Heller esophagomyotomy, 185
Helminthic diseases, tests, 353-55
Helminthic parasites, and infections,
        342-43
Helplessness, 526
Hemagglutination-inhibition
        immunoassay (HAI), 153
Hemangioma, 42
Hemangiopericytoma, 186
Hemapheresis, 147
Hemarthrosis, 48
Hemartoma, 48, 186
Hematemesis, 189
Hematocrit (Hct)(Ht), 153, 424
Hematology, 421
    abbreviations related to, 153
    and disease findings, 425-34
    disorders, abbreviations related to, 154
    and immunohematology, 423-25
Hematoma, 213
    of meninges, 77
Hematopoiesis, 139
Hematuria, 222
Hemiblock, 104
Hemiglossectomy, 181, 202
Hemilaryngectomy, 162
Hemiparesis, 78
Hemipelvectomy (HP), 57
Hemiplegia, 78, 523-26
Hemochromatosis, 149, 194
Hemodialysis, 223
Hemodilution, 121
Hemodynamics, 124
Hemoglobin (Hb), 139, 153, 424
    Hb A. See Adult hemoglobin (Hb A)
    Hb F. See Fetal hemoglobin (Hb F)
    Hb S. See Sickle cell hemoglobin
        (Hb S)
Hemoglobin concentration (Hb), 424
Hemoglobinuria, 142
Hemogram, Schilling's, 145
Hemolysis, 149
Hemolytic anemias, 141

Hemolytic disease of newborn (HDN), 141-42, 154, 264
Hemoperitoneum, 198
Hemophilia-A, 144
Hemophilia-B, 144
Hemopoiesis, 139
Hemoptysis, 170
Hemorrhage
    cerebral, 259
    cord, 259
    and pregnancy, 257
Hemorrhagic effusion, 53
Hemorrhoidectomy, 192
Hemorrhoids, 191
Hemothorax, 171
Henoch-Schonlein syndrome, 143-44
Heparinized whole blood, 146
Hepatic bruit, 199
Hepatic calculi, 194
Hepatic coma, 194
Hepatic encephalopathy, 194
Hepatic failure, fulminant, 194
Hepatic flexure, 190
Hepatic function, tests, 452-54
Hepatic injury, drug-induced, 194
Hepatic necrosis, 194
Hepatic trauma, 194
Hepatitis, 148, 335
    viral, 194
Hepatitis associated antigen (HAA), 201
Hepatitis Australia antigen (HAA), 201
Hepatobiliary tract, 449-54
Hepatolienal fibrosis, 153
Hepatoma, 195
Hepatomegaly, 154
Hepatomy, 198
Hepatorenal syndrome, 195
Hereditary elliptocytosis (HE), 142, 154
Hereditary hemorrhagic telangiectasia, 144
Hereditary multiple exostoses, 50
Hereditary spherocytosis (HS), 142, 154
Hermaphrodite, 284
Hernia, 56, 198
    hiatal, 187, 189
    hiatus, 56, 187, 189
    umbilical, 260
Hernioplasty, 199
Herniorrhapy, 199
Herpangina, 181
Herpes, 334, 336, 260
Herpes zoster, 360-61
Hesitancy, 222
Heterotopic, 58
HF. See Hagemann factor (HF)
Hg. See Mercury (Hg)
Hiatal hernia, 187, 189
Hiatus hernia, 56, 187, 189
Hiccough, 170
Hiccup, 170
High-density lipoproteins (HDL)

High-molecular-weight (HMW) kininogen, 143
Highmore, antrum of. See Antrum of Highmore
High-output gastrointestinal fistula, 190
Hilus, 167, 211
Hip
    fracture of, 43
    joint, arthroplasties of, 51-52
Hip disarticulation (HD), 57
Hirschsprung's disease, 190, 192
Hirsutism, 276
His, bundle of. See Bundle of His
His bundle electrocardiogram (HBE), 126
His bundle electrography (HBE), 125
Histiocytes, 149
Histiocytosis X, 150
Histocompatibility, 355
Histocytes, 149
Histoincompatibility, 148
Histologic study, 243-44
Histoplasmosis, 168
Histrionic personality disorder, 85
HIV. See Human immunodeficiency virus (HIV)
Hives, 29
HLR. See Heart-lung resuscitation (HLR)
HMW. See High-molecular-weight (HMW) kininogen
Hodgkin's disease, 151, 154-55
Hodgkin's lymphoma, 186
Hofmeister technique, 188
Hollander insulin hypoglycemia test, 450
Holter monitoring, 125
Homograft, 111, 116
    of bone, 44
Homologous transfusions, 146
Homotransplantation of bone, 44
Horizontal, body plane, 23, 24
Hormones, 271, 287
    adrenal, 440-41
    anterior pituitary, 441-42
    assays, 403
    biochemistry, 440-49
    placental, 442
    steroid, 442-43
    studies, 243
Hospice, 381
Howard test, 448
HP. See Hemipelvectomy (HP)
HPL. See Human placental lactogen (HPL)
HPO. See Hypothalamic-pituitary-ovarian (HPO)
HR interval, 125
HS. See Hereditary spherocytosis (HS)
hs, and time schedule for medication, 202
HSG. See Hysterosalpingography (HSG)
Ht. See Hematocrit (Hct)(Ht)
Human chorionic gonadotropin (HCG), 264, 410

Human immunodeficiency virus (HIV), 360, 414
Human placental lactogen (HPL), 264, 410
Hunner's ulcer, 220
Huntington's chorea, 73
HVD. See Hypertensive vascular disease (HVD)
Hyaline membrane disease, 265-66
Hydatiform mole, 256
Hydramnios, 254
Hydrocele, 225
Hydrocephalus, 75, 78, 259
    surgical shunts for, 78
Hydrogen ion concentration (pH), 227
    measurements, 201
Hydronephrosis, 227-28
Hydropheumothorax, 171
Hydrophobia, 334
Hydrops of gallbladder, 196
Hydrosalpinx, 241
Hydrotherapy, 517
Hydroureter, 217
Hymen, 233
Hyperaeration, 170
Hyperaliminatation, 201
Hyperammoniemia, 199
Hyperbilirubinemia, 259
Hypercalcemia, 58, 214
Hypercalcemic syndrome, 273
Hypercalciuria, 58
Hypercapnia, 170
Hypercarbia, 170
Hypercarbic anesthesia, 372
Hyperchloremia, 279
Hyperchlorhydria, 189
Hypercholesterolemia, 279
Hyperchylomicronemia, 279
Hyperemesis gravidarum, 254
Hyperemia, 306
Hyperesthesia, 79
Hypergastrinemia, 189
Hyperglycemia, 279
Hyperinsulinism, 274
Hyperkalemia, 279
Hyperkeratosis, 28
Hyperkinesia, 57, 521
Hypermastia, 32
Hypermenorrhea, 240
Hypernatremia, 279
Hyperpigmentation, 31, 34
Hyperplasia, of breast, 32
Hyperplastic gastropathy, 187
Hyperplastic polyps, 186
Hyperpnea, 170
Hypersensitivity, 355
Hypersplenic syndrome, 153
Hypersplenism, 153
Hypertension, 92, 115, 276, 384
    arterial, 370
    renal, 215

Hypertensive encephalopathy, 75
Hypertensive vascular disease (HVD), 115, 126
Hypertriglyceridemia, 280
Hypertrophic cardiomyopathy, 105
Hypertrophic pyloric stenosis, 187
Hypertrophic rhinitis, 160
Hypertrophy
    of right ventricle, 103
    of tonsils, 183
Hyperuricemia, 214
Hyperventilation, 170, 370
    syndrome, 170
Hypnosis, 90
Hypocarbonic anesthesia, 374
Hypochlorhydria, 189
Hypochondriacal neurosis, 86
Hypochondriac regions, 22
Hypochondriasis, 86
Hypogastric region, 22
Hypoglycemic states, 278
Hypomanic episode, 82
Hypomastia, bilateral and unilateral, 32
Hypomenorrhea, 240
Hypophosphatemia, familial, 44
Hypophysectomy, 276
Hypophysis, 271
Hypoplasia
    of breast, 32
    of epiglottis, 162
Hypospadias, 219
Hypothalamic-pituitary-ovarian (HPO), 244
Hypothalamus, 69
Hypothermia
    accidental. *See* Accidental hypothermia (AH)
    induced, 121
Hypothyroidism, 287
Hypotonia, 57, 521
Hypovolemic shock, 118
Hypoxia, 170, 370
    of newborn, 259
Hysterectomy, 239
Hysterical neurosis, conversion type, 86
Hysterosalpingography (HSG), 244, 264
Hysteroscopy, 239

IABP. *See* Intra-aortic balloon pump (IABP)
IACP. *See* Intra-aortic counterpulsation (IACP)
IASD. *See* Interatrial septal defect (IASD)
ICD-9-CM. *See* International Classification of Diseases, 9th Revision, Clinical Modification (ICD-9-CM)
ICF. *See* Intracellular fluid (ICF)
ICM. *See* International Confederation of Midwives (ICM)
ICS. *See* Intercostal space (IS)(ICS)

ICSH. *See* Interstitial cell-stimulating hormone (ICSH)
ICT. *See* Insulin coma therapy (ICT)
Icterus, 199
ICU. *See* Intensive care unit (ICU)
IDDM. *See* Insulin-dependent diabetes mellitus (IDDM)
Identification, 88
Idiogram, 283
Idiopathic myelofibrosis (IMF), 154
Idiopathic respiratory distress syndrome, 260
Idiopathic thrombocytopenia purpura (ITP), 154
IDK. *See* Internal derangement of the knee (IDK)
IE. *See* Intracardiac electrography (IE)
IF. *See* Interstitial fluid (IF)
IgC. *See* Gamma globulin (IgC)
Igs. *See* Immunoglobulins (Igs)
Ileitis, 191
Ileostomy, 192
Ileum, 189
Ileus, 191
Illinois Test of Psycholinguistic Ability (ITPA), 91
Illusions, 87
IM. *See* Intramuscular (IM)
IMAG. *See* Internal mammary artery graft (IMAG)
Image intensifier, 465
Imaging
    abdominal, 471-72
    and adrenal glands, 488
    breast, 473
    cardiovascular, 469-71, 487
    great vessel, 487
    and hearing, 474
    and kidney, 488
    magnetic resonance, 481-85
    musculoskeletal, 467-68
    obstetric, 472-73
    radionuclide, 501-4
    urogenital, 472
    and vision, 473-74
IMF. *See* Idiopathic myelofibrosis (IMF)
Immature fetus, 251
Immobilization, simple, 45
Immune response, 355
Immunity, 379
    transplantation, 357
    tumor, 409
Immunofluorescent staining, 174
Immunogen, 356
Immunoglobulins (Igs), 356
Immunohematology, and hematology, 423-25
Immunoincompetence, 148
Immunologic deficiency states, 358
Immunologic diseases, 355-58
Immunologic tests, 426-29

Immunology, 356
Imperforate anus, 260
Impetigo contagiosa, 28, 260
Implantation, 400
IMV. *See* Intermittent mandatory ventilation (IMV)
Incision, of infected skin lesion, 30
Incisional biopsy, 32
Incoherence, in speech, 87
Incontinence, stress, 220
Induced hypothermia, 121
Induration, 202
Infaction, 71
Infant
    mature, 251
    postmature and premature, 252
    term, 264
Infarction, 107
Infection, 331-55
    and actinomycetes, 339
    and bacilli, 34, 339
    and chlamydiae, 335-36
    and cocci, 338-39
    and fungi, 339-40
    and helminthic parasites, 342-43
    laboratory tests for, 345-55
    and Legionellacea, 337
    and mycoplasmas, 337
    of newborn, 260
    ocular, 298
    and protozoa, 341-42
    and Rickettsiae, 337-38
    and sexually transmitted diseases, 336-37
    and spirochetes, 340-41
    TORCH, 260
    and viruses, 34, 333-35
    and yeasts, 339-40
Inferior, position and direction, 23, 24
Inferior vena cava (IVC), 126, 154
Inferior wall infarction, 107
Infertility, female, 241-42
Infiltration, 154, 202
Inflammatory pseudotumors, 186
Infundibular resection, 109
Inhalation therapy, 371
Inner ear
    conditions of, 320-21
    operative terms, 322-23
Inoculation, 332
Insertion of muscle, 53
Insomnia, 92
Insufficiency, 107, 108
Insufflation, 243
    tubal, 244
Insulin, 274
Insulin coma therapy (ICT), 91
Insulin-dependent diabetes mellitus (IDDM), 287
Integument, 25
Intelligence quotient (IQ), 91

Intelligence tests, 89
Intensive care unit (ICU), 227
Interactions, drug, 380
Interatrial septal defect (IASD), 126
Interbrain, 69
Intercostal arteries, 127
Intercostal space (IS)(ICS), 57, 173
Intermediate, position and direction, 23, 24
Intermittent mandatory ventilation (IMV), 173
Intermittent positive-pressure breathing (IPPB), 173
Intermittent positive pressure ventilation (IPPV), 173
Internal carotid ischemia, 73
Internal carotid stenosis, 73
Internal carotid syndrome, 73
Internal derangement of the knee (IDK), 48, 57
Internal fixation, 45
Internal mammary arteries, 101
Internal mammary artery graft (IMAG), 109, 126
Internal mammary-coronary artery anastomoses, 109
Internal thoracic arteries, 101
International Classification of Diseases, 9th Revision, Clinical Modification (ICD-9-CM), 33
International Confederation of Midwives (ICM), 265
International Federation of Gynecology and Obstetrics (FIGO), 244, 403, 404
International Society for the Study of Vulvar Disease, 234
International System of Units, 421
Interpupillary distance (PD), 308
Interstitial cell-stimulating hormone (ICSH), 287
Interstitial cystitis, 220
Interstitial fluid (IF), 287
Interstitial nephritis, 213
Intertriginous, 31
Interventricular septal defect (IVSD), 126
Intervertebral disc, 47
Intestinal malabsorption syndromes, 191
Intestinal obstruction, 191
Intestines, small and large, 189-93
Intoxication, 80, 84
Intra-aortic balloon counterpulsation, 122
Intra-aortic balloon pump (IABP), 126
Intra-aortic counterpulsation (IACP), 126
Intracardiac electrography (IE), 125
Intracellular fluid (ICF), 287
Intracranial aneurysm, 71
Intracranial hematoma, 73
Intracranial hemorrhage, 73
Intracranial tumor, 70

Intrahepatic block, 196
Intramuscular (IM), 57
Intraocular pressure (IOP), 308
    disorders of, 296
Intraoperative autologous transfusion, 146
Intrapelvic, 58
Intrauterine, 92
Intrauterine asphyxia, 258
Intrauterine device (IUD), 244
Intrauterine pressure (IUP), 264
Intrauterine transfusion, 262
Intravenous pyelogram (IVP), 227
Intrinsic asthma, 164
Intrinsic factor, 189
Intussusception, 191, 192
Invasion, 400
Inversion, of uterus, 254
Inverted Y field irradiation, 155
Involution, of uterus, 254
Ion, 434, 497
Ionescu-Shiley bioprosthesis, 111
Ionization, 497
IOP. *See* Intraocular pressure (IOP)
IPPB. *See* Intermittent positive-pressure breathing (IPPB)
IPPV. *See* Intermittent positive pressure ventilation (IPPV)
IQ. *See* Intelligence quotient (IQ)
Iridodonesis, 302
Iris, 293
Iron deficiency anemia, 141
IS. *See* Intercostal space (IS)(ICS)
Ischemia, 45, 71, 73, 112, 118
Ischemic colitis, 190
Ischemic heart disease, 106
Islets of Langerhans, 193
Isobars, 499
Isoenzymes, 436-38
Isogenic marrow transplantation, 148
Isoimmunization, Rh. *See* Rhesus factor isoimmunization
Isolated pulmonic stenosis, 102
Isomers, 499
Isotones, 499
Isotopes, 500
Isthmus, of uterus, 237
ITP. *See* Idiopathic thrombocytopenia purpura (ITP)
ITPA. *See* Illinois Test of Psycholinguistic Ability (ITPA)
IUD. *See* Intrauterine device (IUD)
IUP. *See* Intrauterine pressure (IUP)
IVC. *See* Inferior vena cava (IVC)
IVP. *See* Intravenous pyelogram (IVP)
IVSD. *See* Interventricular septal defect (IVSD)

Jaundice, 154, 199
    nuclear, 260
Jejunoileal bypass, 192

Jejunum, 189
Joint motion, measurement, 520
Joints, 46-53
    disruptive trauma of, 48
    See also Articulations
Judkins' technique, 124
Jugular venous pulse (JVP), 126
Junge kernige, 139
Juvenile chorea, 73
JVP. *See* Jugular venous pulse (JVP)

K. *See* Potassium (K)
Kaposi's sarcoma, 186
Karyotype, 283
Katz index, 381
Kawasaki's disease, 245
Kawasaki syndrome, 343
KB. *See* Knee bearing (KB)
KD. *See* Knee disarticulation (KD)
Keloid, 28
Kenny system, 381
Keratinization, 202
Keratocanthoma, 28
Keratometry, 307
Keratosis, 26
    seborrheic, 28
Kernicterus, 260
Kernig's sign, 88, 522
Ketatotic, 31
Ketone bodies, 445
Ketosis, 280
Kidney, 211-17
    and imaging, 488
    infections, 213
    injuries, 213
    neoplasms of, 213-14
    ureter, bladder (KUB), 227
Kinetocardiography, 125
Kininogen, 143
Kj. *See* Knee jerk (Kj)
Klinefelter's syndrome, 281, 284
Knee, arthroplasties of, 52
Knee bearing (KB), 57
Knee disarticulation (KD), 57
Knee jerk (Kj), 91
Kohler, 409
Kolmer test, 244
Korsakoff's disease, 80
Kraurosis of vulva, 234
KUB. *See* Kidney, ureter, bladder (KUB)
Kuhnt-Junius disease, 297
Kussmaul breathing, 280, 389
Kyphosis, 48, 58

LA. *See* Left atrium (LA)
Label compound, 497
Labia majora, 233
Labia minora, 233
Labia oris, 180
Labile factor, 143
Labor, stages of, 257

Laboratory, clinical. *See* Clinical laboratory
Laboratory tests, for infectious diseases, 345-55
Lacerations, 53, 213
Lacrimal apparatus, disorders of, 304-5
Lacrimation, 306
LAD. *See* Left anterior descending (coronary artery)(LAD)
Lagging, 283
Laki-Lorand factor (LLF), 143
Lamaze method, 252
Laminectomy, 77
Langerhans, islets. *See* Islets of Langerhans
Languages, 3
LAP. *See* Leucine aminopeptidase (LAP)
Laparoscopy, 239, 244
Laparotomy, 155, 199
   staging, 412
Large for gestational age (LGA), 264
Large intestine, 189-93
Laryngeal cancer, 162
Laryngeal stridor, 162
Laryngectomy, 162
Laryngismus, 162
Laryngitis, 162
Laryngoplasty, 162
Laryngoscopy, 162
Laryngospasm, 162
Laryngostomy, 162
Laryngotracheobronchitis, 162
Larynx, 161-62
Laser
   excision of laryngeal cancer, 162
   surgery, 30
Lassitude, 154
Last menstrual period (LMP), 244, 264
Lateral, position and direction, 23, 24
Lateral heart failure, 105
Lateral wall infarction, 107
Late shock, 118
Latex tests, 428
Latin language, 3, 4
LATS. *See* Long-acting thyroid stimulator (LATS)
Lavage, of sinus, 160
Law of tangents, 465
LBW. *See* Low birth weight (LBW)
LCP. *See* Legg-Calve-Perthes disease (LCP)
LDL. *See* Low-density lipoproteins (LDL)
Leaflet resection, 109
Left anterior descending (coronary artery)(LAD), 126
Left atrium (LA), 126
Left iliac fossa (LIF), 57
Left lower extremity (LLE), 57
Left mentoanterior (LMA), 264
Left mentoposterior (LMP), 264
Left mentotransverse (LMT), 264

Left occipitoanterior (LOA), 264
Left occipitoposterior (LOP), 264
Left occipitotransverse (LOT), 264
Left sacroanterior (LSA), 264
Left sacroposterior (LScP), 264
Left sacroposterior (LSP), 264
Left scapuloanterior (LScA), 264
Left-sided heart failure (LHF), 126
Left sternal border (LSB), 173
Left upper extremity (LUE), 57
Left ventricle (LV), 126
Left ventricular hypertrophy (LVH), 126
Legg-Calve-Perthes disease (LCP), 44, 57
Legionellacea, infections caused by, 337
Legionella pneumophila, 168, 174
Legionnaires' disease, 168, 174, 337
Leiomyoblastoma, 186
Leiomyomas, 186
Leiomyosarcoma, 186
Lens, disorders of, 296
Leptospirosis, 340
Leriche's syndrome, 114
LES. *See* Lower esophageal sphincter (LES)
Lesions, 154
   brain, 77
Lethal pyrexia, 92
Letterer-Siwe disease, 151
Leucine aminopeptidase (LAP), 201
Leukapheresis, 147
Leukemia, 144-45
Leukemic reticuloendotheliosus, 144-45
Leukemoid reaction, 144
Leukocyte, 139
   of granulocytic series, 139-40
   transfusion, 147
Leukocytosis, 149
Leukoderma, 27
Leukopenia, 145, 149
Leukoplakia, 202
   of mouth, 182
   of vulva, 234
Leukorrhea, 235
LGA. *See* Large for gestational age (LGA)
LGV. *See* Lymphogranuloma venereum (LGV)
Lhermitte's syndrome, 155
LHF. *See* Left-sided heart failure (LHF)
Libido, 87
Libman-Sacks endocarditis, 106
Lichen planus, 27
Lidocaine, 92
Lie, or presentation, 257
Lienitis, 153
LIF. *See* Left iliac fossa (LIF)
Ligamentous, 127
Ligaments, 46-53
   of uterus, 235
Light reaction (LR), 308
Limb pain, phantom, 45
Limitation of motion (LOM), 57

Linear accelerators, 465
Linitis plastica, 186
Linton flap procedure, 30
Lip, 180, 181
   reconstruction, 182
Lipid, 445-46
Lipid metabolism disorders, 278
Lipidosis, 279
Lipomas, 186, 213
Lipoproteins, 279, 446
Liposarcoma, 186
Lipping, 53
Lithium, 92
Littre, urethral glands of. *See* Urethral glands of Littre
Liver, 193, 194-96, 198, 451-54
   abscess, 195
   carcinoma of, 196
Liver palms, 199
LLE. *See* Left lower extremity (LLE)
LLF. *See* Laki-Lorand factor (LLF)
LMA. *See* Left mentoanterior (LMA)
LMC. *See* Lymphocytic choriomeningitis (LMC)
LMP. *See* Last menstrual period (LMP) *and* Left mentoposterior (LMP)
LMT. *See* Left mentotransverse (LMT)
LOA. *See* Left occipitoanterior (LOA)
Lobar pheumonia, 168
Lobe, of lung, 167
Lobectomy, 169
Lobocytes, 140
Local anesthesia, 374-75
Local excision, of skin lesion, 30
Lochia, 257
Locomotor ataxia, 76
Loffler's endocarditis, 106
LOM. *See* Limitation of motion (LOM)
Loneliness, 526
Long-acting thyroid stimulator (LATS), 287
Longitudinal, body plane, 23, 24
LOP. *See* Left occipitoposterior (LOP)
Lordosis, 48
LOT. *See* Left occipitotransverse (LOT)
Low birth weight (LBW), 264
Low-density lipoproteins (LDL)
Lower esophageal sphincter (LES), 182, 201
LP. *See* Lumbar puncture (LP)
LR. *See* Light reaction (LR)
LSA. *See* Left sacroanterior (LSA)
LSB. *See* Left sternal border (LSB)
LScA. *See* Left scapuloanterior (LScA)
LScP. *See* Left sacroposterior (LScP)
LSD. *See* Lysergic acid diethylamide (LSD)
LSP. *See* Left sacroposterior (LSP)
LUE. *See* Left upper extremity (LUE)
Lumbago, 53
Lumbar puncture (LP), 91

Lumbar region, 22, 23
Lumbosacral pain, 227
Lumen, aortic, 127
Lung, 165-71
  biopsy, 169
  resection, 169
  transplantation, 169-70
Lupus vulgaris, 27
LV. *See* Left ventricle (LV)
LVH. *See* Left ventricular hypertrophy
    (LVH)
Lyme disease, 340
lymph. *See* Lymphocytes (lymph)
Lymphacytosis, 152
Lymphadenectomy, 152
Lymphadenitis, 152
Lymphadenopathy, 152
Lymphadenotomy, 152
Lymphangiography, 155
Lymphangioma, 152
Lymphangitis, 152
Lymphatic channels, 149-52
Lymphatic duct, 149
Lymphedema, 152
Lymph node, 149-52
  biopsy, 169
Lymphocyte (lymph), 140, 149, 153,
    356, 400
  dyscrasias, 358
Lymphocytic choriomeningitis (LMC),
    152
Lymphocytopenia, 152
Lymphogranuloma venereum (LGV),
    336
Lymphoma, 152, 186
Lymphosarcoma, 186
Lysergic acid diethylamide (LSD), 91

M. *See* Murmur (M)
Macrocytosis, 149
Macroglobulinemia, 146
Macronodular cirrhosis, 194
Macrophages, 140
Macule, 31
Magnetic resonance imaging, 481-85
  study guide, 576-77
Major depression, 82, 83
Major salivary glands, 180
Malaria, 148, 195-96
Male genital organs, 224-27
Malignant, 400
Malignant bone neoplasms, 42-43
Malignant hyperthermia syndrome
    (MHS), 371, 375-76
Malignant neoplasms, 48-49, 56
  and oral cavity, 202
Malignant smooth muscle tumors of the
    stomach, 186
Malingering, 87
Mallory-Weiss syndrome, 187

Mammaplasty, augmentation and
    reduction, 32
Mammary abscess, 31
Mammary arteries, 101
Mammary gland, 31
Mammectomy, 32-33
Mammoplasty, 32
Mandibulectomy, 202
Manic depressive reactions, 77
Manic episode, 82
Manic mood syndrome, 82
Mantle field irradiation, 155
Manual delivery, of placenta, 261
Manual muscle testing, 520
MAO. *See* Maximal acid output (MAO)
    and Monoamine oxidase (MAO)
Mar, 283
Marble bones, 50
Marfan's syndrome, 359
Marie-Strumpell arthritis, 47
Marijuana, 92
Marital history (MH), 33, 244
Marker, tumor, 409
Marker chromosome, 283
Marrow
  bone, 141, 145-46, 148
  red, 39
  transplantations, 146-48
  yellow, 39
Marrow brain, 69
Marshall-Marchett repair, 221
Marsupialization of Bartholin's gland
    cyst, 235
Massage, 518
Mass number, 497
Mastalgia, 33
Mastectomy, 32-33
Master's test, 123
Mastitis, 32
Mastodynia, 33
Mastopexy, 33
Mastoplasty, 32
Mastotomy, 33
Matrix, of bone, 39
Matter, white and gray, 70
Mature infant, 251
Maxillary sinus, 160
Maximal acid output (MAO), 201
Maximum breathing capacity (MBC), 173
MBC. *See* Maximum breathing capacity
    (MBC)
MCH. *See* Mean corpuscular hemoglobin
    (MCH)
MCL. *See* Midcostal line (MCL)
MCT. *See* Mean circulation time (MCT)
MCTD. *See* Mixed connective tissue
    disease (MCTD)
MCV. *See* Mean corpuscular volume (MCV)
MDAA. *See* Muscular Dystrophy
    Association of America, Inc.
    (MDAA)

Mean circulation time (MCT), 153
Mean corpuscular hemoglobin (MCH),
    153, 424
Mean corpuscular volume (MCV), 153
Measles, 334
Measurements
  and diagnostic ultrasound, 475-76
  and metric system, 421, 422
  and nuclear medicine, 510-11
  and physical therapy, 519-21
  and radiology, 489
  traditional, 423
  volumetric, 521
Meatotomy, 221
Mechanical ileus, 191
Mechanical prosthesis, 111
Meckel's diverticulum, 191
Meconium, 261
Medial, position and direction, 23, 24
Medial calcinosis, 114-15
Median
  body plane, 23, 24
  position and direction, 23, 24
Mediastinal imaging, 485-87
Mediastinal node biopsy, 172
Mediastinal spread, 154
Mediastinitis, 171
Mediastinoscopy, 172
Mediastinum, 171-73
Medical electronics, 122
Medical terminology
  concepts, 3-6
  elements of, 4, 6-24
  objectives and values, 3
  orientation to, 3-24
  study guide, 534-36
Medications, and time schedule
    abbreviations, 202
Medicine, nuclear. *See* Nuclear medicine
Medulla, 39
Medulla oblongata, 69
Medullary cavity, 39
Megabladder, 220
Megacolon, 192
Megaloblastic anemia, 141
Megaloblastosis, 149
Megalocystis, 220
Megavoltage radiotherapy, 155
Meig's syndrome, 242
Meiosis, 284
Melanoderma, 27
Melena, 192
MEN. *See* Multiple endocrine neoplasia
    (MEN)
Menetrier's disease, 187
Meninges, 69
  abscess and hematoma, 77
Meningitis, 75
  otitis, 326
Meningocele, 75, 76, 260
Meningomyelocele, 76

Menopause, 243
Menorrhagia, 240
Mental Health Association (MHA), 91
Mental mechanism, 87-88
Mental retardation, 82
Mercury (Hg), 126
Mesencephalon, 69
Mesenchymal polyps, 186
Mesenchymoma, benign, 48
Mesenteric artery thrombosis, 191
Mesentery, 190
Mesocolon, 190
Mesothelial polyps, 186
Mesothelioma of the pleura, 171
Metabolic disorders, 271-91
    study guide, 557-58
Metabolic studies, 444-48
Metabolism, biochemistry, 440-49
Metabolite, 446
Metacarpal-phalangeal (MP), 57
Metaphase, 284
Metaphysis, 39
Metastatic tumor, 70
Metathalamus, 69
Metric system, 421, 422
Metrorrhagia, 240
MH. *See* Marital history (MH)
MHA. *See* Mental Health Association
    (MHA)
MHS. *See* Malignant hyperthermia
    syndrome (MHS)
MI. *See* Myocardial infarction (MI)
Microbiopsy, 243
Microcephalus, 75
Microcytosis, 149
Microneurosurgery, 77
Micronodular cirrhosis, 194
Microphages, 140
Microphthalmia, 286
Microsporum, 27
Microsurgery, and hearing, 321
Micturition, 222
Midbrain, 69
Midcostal line (MCL), 173
Middle ear
    conditions of, 320
    operative terms, 322
Midsternal line (MSL), 57, 173
Milia, 31
Milieu therapy, 90
Millicurie, 497
Millimeter, 34
Millimeter of mercury (mm Hg), 126
Milstein, 409
Miniscus, 47
Minnesota Multiphasic Personality
    Inventory (MMPI), 89, 91
Minor salivary glands, 180
Mital insufficiency, 107
Mitosis, 284
Mitral commissurotomy, 109

Mitral stenosis (MS), 107, 126
Mitral valve, 101
    prolapse, 106
    reconstruction, 109
    valvotomy, 111
Mixed aphasia, 526
Mixed connective tissue disease (MCTD),
    359
mm Hg. *See* Millimeter of mercury
    (mm Hg)
MMPI. *See* Minnesota Multiphasic
    Personality Inventory (MMPI)
MN system, 426
Modalities, cancer, 410-13
Modality, 155, 400
Modified Gilliam procedure, 240
Mohs' chemosurgery, 305
Molality, 434
Molarity, 435
Molds, 332
Mole, 28
Monckeberg's medial calcific sclerosis,
    114-15
Mongolism, 259
Moniliform, 31
Monitoring, 497
    therapeutic drug, 457
Monoamine oxidase (MAO), 91
Monoclonal antibodies, 409
Monocytes, 140
Mononucleosis, 148, 334, 428-29
Mood disorders, 83
    types of, 83
Mood episode, 82
Mood swings, rapid, 92
Mood syndrome, depressive and manic,
    82
MOPP program of chemotherapy, 155
Moro reflex, 261
Mosaicism, 284
MOSES. *See* Multidimensional
    observation scale for elderly
    subjects (MOSES)
Motility, ocular, 305
Motor aphasia, 78, 525
Motor areas, 69
Mouth, 179, 182
MP. *See* Metacarpal-phalangeal (MP)
MS. *See* Mitral stenosis (MS) *and*
    Multiple sclerosis (MS)
MSL. *See* Midsternal line (MSL)
Mucocutaneous lymph node syndrome,
    245, 343
Mucopurulent discharge, 227
Mucosal neuroma syndrome, 274
Mucous colitis, 190
Multidimensional observation scale for
    elderly subjects (MOSES), 392
Multiform, 31
Multilobar, 174
Multipara, 252

Multiple choice questions, answers, 582
Multiple endocrine neoplasia (MEN),
    274
Multiple lymph node excision, 152
Multiple myeloma, 146
Multiple personality, 81
Multiple polyposis, 191
Multiple sclerosis (MS), 75, 91
Multiples of curie units, 510
Multisystem disorders, 331-65
    study guide, 563-64
Mumps, 181, 334
Murmur (M), 112, 126
Muscles, 53-57
    anterior view and posterior view,
        54-55
Muscular dystrophy, 56
Muscular Dystrophy Association of
    America, Inc. (MDAA), 57
Musculoskeletal disorders, 39-63
    study guide, 539-40
Musculoskeletal imaging, 467-68,
    485-87
Music therapy, 90
Mustard, 155
Mustard's operation, 108
Mutation, 284
Myasthenia gravis, 56
Mycology, 332
Mycoplasmas, infections, 337
Mycosis fungoides, 152
Mycotic diseases, tests, 351
Mycotic vaginitis, 234
Myelencephalon, 69
Myelin sheath, 65
Myelitis, 75
Myelocytes, 139
Myelofibrosis, 146
Myeloma, 43, 146
    multiple and solitary, 43
Myelopoiesis, 140
Myeloproliferative, 140
    disorders, 145
Myelosclerosis, 146
Myelosuppression, 155
Myocardial disease, primary and
    secondary, 106
Myocardial enzymes, 436-38
Myocardial infarction (MI), 126, 384
    acute, 107
Myocardial ischemia, 112
Myocardial revascularization, 109
Myocardial sinusoids, 101
Myocarditis, 106
Myocardium, 101
Myocardosis, 106
Myomectomy, 239
Myometrium, 235
Myoplasty, 56
Myorrhaphy, 56
Myositis, 56

Myotasis, 56
Myxedema, 274

NAACOG. *See* Nurses' Association of the
    American College of Obstetricians
    and Gynecologists (NAACOG)
NAMH. *See* National Association of
    Mental Health (NAMH)
NARC. *See* National Association for
    Retarded Children (NARC)
Narcissistic personality disorder, 84
Narcoanalysis, 90
Naris, 159
Nasal meatus, 159
Nasal polyp, 159
Nasal septum, 159
Nasal skin cancer, 159
Nasopharyngeal cancer, 159
Nasopharyngitis, 160
Nasopharynx, 159
Nasotracheal (NT), 375
National Association for Retarded
    Children (NARC), 91
National Association of Mental Health
    (NAMH), 91
National Cancer Institute (NCI), 155
National Center for Health Statistics
    (NCHS), 392
National Council on Aging (NCOA), 392
National Council on Radiation Protection
    and Measurements, 498
National Formulary, The (NF), 375
National Health Insurance (NHI), 392
National Institute of Health (NIH), 146,
    392
National Institute of Mental Health
    (NIMH), 91
National Institute on Drug Abuse
    (NIDA), 92
National Safety Council (NSC), 392
National Society for Crippled Chidren
    and Adults (NSCCA), 57
Natural childbirth, 252
Natural family planning, 252
NB. *See* Newborn (NB)
NCHS. *See* National Center for Health
    Statistics (NCHS)
NCI. *See* National Cancer Institute (NCI)
NCOA. *See* National Council on Aging
    (NCOA)
Near point of convergence (NPC), 308
Neck
    of tooth, 180
    whiplash injury of, 44
Necrosis, of bone, 45
NED. *See* No evidence of disease (NED)
Negroid, and skin-coloring process, 26
Neisseria gonorrhoeae, 244
Nematodes, 342-43
Neobladder, 221

Neonatal
    chlamydial infections, 260
    disorders, study guide, 555-56
    obstetrical, and fetal conditions,
        251-69
    period, 259-61
    tests, 429-33
    See also Neonate *and* Newborn (NB)
Neonate, 92, 262-64
    conditions amenable to surgery
    and drug addiction, 259
    high-risk, 251
    hypoxia of, 259
    infections of, 260
    See also Neonatal *and* Newborn (NB)
Neoplasms, 48-49, 56
    adrenal, 273
    and bladder, 220
    bone, 42-43
    classification of, 404-9
    gastric malignant, 185-86
    of kidney, 213-14
    leiomyoma, 56
    malignant, 202
    myoma, 56
    myosarcoma, 56
    rhabdomyoma, 56
    rhabdomyosarcoma, 56
    thyroid, 275
    of uterus, 238-39
Neoplastic, 202
    growth pattern, 402
Nephrectomy, 216
Nephritis, 213
Nephrolithiasis, 58, 214
Nephrolithotomy, 216
Nephrolithotripsy, 223
Nephrolysis, 216
Nephron, 211
Nephropathy, 214
Nephropexy, 216
Nephroptosis, 214
Nephrorrhaphy, 216
Nephrosclerosis, 213
Nephrostomy, 216
Nephrotic syndrome, 214
Nephroureterectomy, 216
Nerves, 65-68
    cell, 65-66
    cranial, 65
    fiber, 66
    of heart, 101
    spinal, 65, 66
Nettle rash, 29
Neuralgia, 68
Neurectomy, 68
Neurilemma, 65-66
Neurilemoma, 66
Neuroanastomosis, 68
Neurofibrils, 66

Neurofibromatosis, 75
Neurogenic bladder, 220
Neurogenic tumors, 186
Neurolemma, 65-66
Neurolemoma, 66
Neurologic disorders, 65-79, 106
    and conditions amenable to
        neurosurgery, 93-94
    examination, 88
    studies, 88-89
    study guide, 541-42
    See also Neurosurgery
Neurology. *See* Neurologic disorders
Neuroma, 66
    amputation, 66
Neurons, 65-66
    classification by function, 66
    structure of, 65-66
Neuroplasty, 68
Neuroradiography, 468-69
Neurorrhaphy, 68
Neurosurgery
    neurologic conditions amenable to,
        93-94
    psychiatric conditions amenable to,
        93-94
    stereotaxic, 77
    See also Neurologic disorders
Neurotomy, 68
Neutralization tests, 428
Neutropenia, 145, 149
Neutrophilia, 149
Neutrophilic band, 139-40
Neutrophilic lobocytes, 140
Neutrophilic metamyelocytes, 139
Neutrophilic myelocytes, 139
Neutrophils, 139, 140
Nevus, 28
Newborn (NB), 264
    See also Neonatal *and* Neonate
NF. *See National Formulary, The* (NF)
NHI. *See* National Health Insurance
    (NHI)
NHL. *See* Non-Hodgkin's lymphoma
    (NHL)
NIDA. *See* National Institute on Drug
    Abuse (NIDA)
Nidus, 45
NIH. *See* National Institute of Health
    (NIH)
Nikolsky sign, 34
NIMH. *See* National Institute of Mental
    Health (NIMH)
Nissl bodies, 66
Nitrogen mustard, 155
Nocturia, 222
No evidence of disease (NED), 401
Nominal aphasia, 526
Nondisjunction, 284
Non-Hodgkin's lymphoma (NHL), 152,
    154, 186

Noninvasive techniques, 465
Noonan's syndrome, 284, 286
No rapid eye movements (sleep)(NREM), 91
Normablasts, 140
Normal pressure hydrocephalus (NPH), 385
Normocytes, 140
Normothermia, 122
Nose, 159-60
Nosology, 332
Nothing by mouth (NPO), 227
NPC. *See* Near point of convergence (NPC)
NPH. *See* Normal pressure hydrocephalus (NPH)
NPO. *See* Nothing by mouth (NPO)
NRC. *See* Nuclear Regulatory Commission (NRC)
NREM. *See* No rapid eye movements (sleep)(NREM)
NSC. *See* National Safety Council (NSC)
NSCCA. *See* National Society for Crippled Chidren and Adults (NSCCA)
NT. *See* Nasotracheal (NT)
Nuclear fission, 497
Nuclear jaundice, 260
Nuclear medicine, 495-514
    study guide, 578-79
    and symbols, 510
    tests, 510
Nuclear Regulatory Commission (NRC), 511
Nuclear transformation, 498
Nucleoli, 154
Nucleon, 498
Nucleus, 69, 154, 332
    of atom, 498
    basal, 69
Nucleus pulposus, 47
Nuclide, 498, 499
Nurses' Association of the American College of Obstetricians and Gynecologis (NAACOG), 265
Nystagmus, 79, 323

Oat cell carcinoma, 167
OB. *See* Obstetrics (OB)
Obesity, 279
Obliterated, 127
OBS. *See* Organic brain syndrome (OBS)
Obsession, 80, 88
Obsessive compulsive disorder, 80
Obsessive compulsive neurosis, 80
Obsessive-compulsive personality disorder, 85
Obstetrical
    fetal, and neonatal conditions, 251-69
    disorders, study guide, 555-56
    period, 251-57
    tests, 429-33
    See also Obstetrics (OB)

Obstetric-gynecologic-neonatal (OGN), 264
Obstetrics (OB), 264
    conditions amenable to surgery and diagnostic ultrasound, 480-81
    imaging, 472-73
    See also Obstetrical
Obstipation, 192
Obstructive jaundice, 154
Occlusion of lactiferous ducts, 32
Occupational therapy, 90
Ocular infections, 298
Ocular motility, disorders of, 305
Ocular tumors, 298
Oddi, sphincter of. *See* Sphincter of Oddi
ODM. *See* Ophthalmodynamometry (ODM)
OGN. *See* Obstetric-gynecologic-neonatal (OGN)
Oil glands, 28
Older adults
    disorders affecting, 381-90
    and psychotherapy, 390-91
Old tuberculin (OT), 173
Oligodendroglioma, 71
Oligohydramnios, 254
Oligomenorrhea, 240
Oligospermia, 227
Oliguria, 222
Ollier's disease, 49-50
Omenta, 185
Omphalocele, 260
Oncofetal antigens, 410
Oncogene, 401
Oncogenesis, 401
Oncology
    defined, 413-15
    study guide, 570-71
    terms pertaining to, 399-419
Oncovin, 155
Onychia, 27
Onychomycosis, 28
Oophorectomy, 242
Oophoritis, 242
Oophoropexy, 242
Oophoroplasty, 242
Open reduction, 45
Operative suffixes, 7-9
Ophthalmia neonatorum, 260
Ophthalmodynamometry (ODM), 308
Optic nerve, disorders of, 297-98
Oral cavity, 34, 179-82
    cancer resection, 182
    and malignant neoplasms, 202
Oral mucosa, 202
Orbit, 294
Orchiectomy, 226
Orchiopexy, 226
Orchioplasty, 226
Orchitis, 225
Organic brain syndrome (OBS), 91, 385

Organic delusional syndrome, 84
Organic mental disorders, alcohol-induced, 79-80
Organic mental syndromes, 83-84
Organic personality syndrome, 84
Organs
    blood-forming, 139-58
    male genital. *See* Male genital organs
Orifices, of heart, 101
Origin, of muscle, 53
Ortho. *See* Orthopedics (Ortho)
Orthopedics (Ortho), 57
    conditions amenable to surgery, 59-61
Orthopnea, 170
Orthosis, 516
Oscillation, 122
Oscillometer, 122
Oscilloscope, 124
Osmolality, 447
Osseous tissue, 39
Ossicles, 58
Ossification, 39
Ostealgia, 45, 58
Ostectomy, 44
Osteitis deformans, 43-44, 57, 385
Osteoarthritis, 47
    post-traumatic, 48
Osteoblast, 42, 58
Osteoblastoma, 42
Osteochondritis deformans juvenile, 44
Osteochondromas, 42
Osteochondromatosis, 50
Osteoclasia, 44
Osteoclasis, 44
Osteoclastic, 58
Osteoclastoma, 59
Osteoclasts, 42
Osteocytes, 42
Osteodynia, 45
Osteodystrophy, 44
Osteogenesis imperfecta, 50
Osteogenesis imperfecta congenita, 50
Osteogenesis imperfecta tarda, 50
Osteogenic sarcoma, 43, 59
Osteoid, 42
Osteoid osteoma, 42
Osteolysis, 44, 58
Osteolytic, 154
Osteomalacia, 44
Osteomyelitis, 44
Osteopetrosis, 50
Osteophyte, 45
Osteoplastic, 154
Osteoplasty, 44
Osteoporosis, 44, 58, 385
Osteoporosis circumscripta, 58
Osteoporotic, 58
Osteotomy, 45
OT. *See* Old tuberculin (OT)
Otalgia, 323
Otitis meningitis, 326

Otoplasty, 321
Ova, 240
Ovalocytosis, 142
Ovarian biopsies, bilateral, 244
Ovarian follicle, 240
Ovarian lesions, and ultrasound, 480
Ovarian wedge resection, 242
Ovariectomy, 242
Ovaries, 240-43
    cyst of, 241
    and uterine tubes, 240-43
Overirradiation, 474
Oviducts, 241
Ovulation, 243
Ovulation method, 252
Oxymetry, 122
Oxytocin challenge tests, 262

PA. *See* Pernicious anemia (PA) *and*
        Posterior-anterior (PA) *and*
        Posteroanterior (PA) *and* Prostate
        antigen (PA) *and* Pulmonary
        artery (PA)
Pa. *See* Pascal (Pa)
PAC. *See* Premature atrial contractions
        (PAC)
Pacing
    methods of, 120
    types of, 119-20
Packed cell volume (hematocrit)(PCV),
        147, 153
Paget's disease,
    of bone, 43-44, 57-59, 385
    of nipple, 32
PAHO. *See* Pan American Health
        Organization (PAHO)
Pain, 381
    cervicobrachial syndrome, 49
    dragging inguinal, 226
    epigastric, 189
    lumbosacral, 227
    paroxysmal, 68
    phantom limb, 45
    pleuritic, 172
    prodromal, 227
    psychogenic, 77
    renal, 217
    shoulder, 49
    somatoform disorder, 86
    ureteral, 222
Palate, 179, 181
Palatine tonsil, 183
Palatoplasty, 182
Palliative, 59, 202
Pallidectomy, 77
Pallidotomy, 77
Pallor, 154
Palmar erythema, 199
Palpitation, 112
Palsy, 71

Pan American Health Organization
        (PAHO), 392
Pancreas, 193, 196-97, 199, 271-72,
        449-54
    and tumors
Pancreatectomy, 199
Pancreatic duct, 193
Pancreatic islets, 193
Pancreatic juice, 193
Pancreatitis, 196-97
Pancreatoduodenectomy, 199
Pancreatojejunostomy, 199
Pancytopenia, 141, 149, 155
Panendoscopy, 221
Panhysterectomy, 239, 242
Panic disorder, 80-81
Pannus, 306
Pansinusitis, 160
PAP. *See* Prostatic acid phosphatase (PAP)
Papanicolaou's method (Pap smear), 243
Papillae, of tongue, 179
Papilla mammae, 31
Papillary, 401
Papilloma, 401
    basal cell, 28
Pap smear. *See* Papanicolaou's method
        (Pap smear)
Papule, 31
Paracusis of Willis, 323
Paralysis, flaccid and spastic, 56
Paralysis agitans, 75
Paralytic ileus, 191
Parametritis, 238
Paranasal sinuses, 160
Paranoid personality disorder, 84
Paranoid type, schizophrenia, 86
Paraparesis, 79
Paraphimosis, 225
Paraplegia, 79, 389
Parasites, 332
    and infections, 342-43
Parasympathetic fibers, 101
Parathyroidectomy, 276
Parathyroid hormone (PTH), 287
Parathyroidism, 274
Parathyroids, 272
Parenchyma, 154
    of lung, 167
Parenchymatous amyloidosis, 146
Paresis, 79
Paresthesia, 79
Parietal pleura, 171
Parkinson's disease, 75, 77, 385
    operations for, 77
Paronychia, 27
Parotid duct, 180
Parotidectomy, 182
Parotid gland, 180
Parotitis, 181
Paroxysmal atrial tachycardia (PAT), 103,
        126

Paroxysmal digitan cyanosis, 118
Paroxysmal nocturnal dyspnea (PND),
        171, 173
Paroxysmal nocturnal hemoglobinuria
        (PHN), 142, 432
Paroxysmal pain, 68
Parrot fever, 335
Partial heart block, 104
Parturient, 252
Pascal (Pa), 435
Passive-aggressive personality disorder,
        85
Past history (PH), 33
PAT. *See* Paroxysmal atrial tachycardia
        (PAT)
Patch, ventricular, 108
Patellar tendon bearing (prosthesis)
        (PTB), 57
Patellofemoral joint replacement, 52
Patent ductus arteriosus (PDA), 102, 126
Pathogenic, 333
Pathokinesiology, 516
pc, and time schedule for medication,
        202
PCT. *See* Plasmacrit test (PCT)
PCV. *See* Packed cell volume
        (hematocrit)(PCV)
PD. *See* Interpupillary distance (PD)
PDA. *See* Patent ductus arteriosus (PDA)
PDR. *See* *Physician's Desk Reference* (PDR)
PE. *See* Plasma exchange (PE)
Peabody developmental motor scale, 521
Peak inspiratory pressure (PIP), 173
Peau d'orange, 33
Pectus carinatum, 171
Pedal circulation, 118
Pediculosis, 27
PEEP. *See* Positive and end-expiratory
        pressure (PEEP)
Peer Review Organization (PRO), 392
PEG. *See* Pneumoencephalogram (PEG)
Pel-Ebstein pyrexia, 152
Pelvic inflammatory disease (PID), 242,
        244, 337
Pelvimetry, 473
Pelvis, 253
Pemphigus, 27, 33-34
    vulgaris, 33
Pemphix, 33
Penis, 224
Pepsin, 450
Percutaneous angiographic embolization,
        122
Percutaneous cordotomy, 77
Percutaneous needle biopsy, 169
Percutaneous nephrolithotomy (PNL),
        227
Percutaneous transluminal angioplasty,
        122
Perforated viscus, 191
Perfusion in intracardiac surgery, 122

Periapical abscess, 181
Periapical tissue biopsy, 182
Periarthritis, of shoulder joint, 49
Pericardial tamponade, 104
Pericardiectomy, 109
Pericarditis, 107
Pericardium, 101
   biopsy of, 108
Perichondritis, 162
Perimetritis, 238
Perimetry, 307
Perinatology, 252
Perineum, 233
Periodontal disease, 181
Periosteum, 42
Peripartum cardiomyopathy, 105
Peripheral, position and direction, 23, 24
Peripheral arterial insufficiency of
      extremities, 115
Peripheral nervous system (PNS), 91
Peripheral vascular disease, 115
Peritoneal dialysis, 223
Peritoneoscopy, 200
Peritoneum, 193, 197-98, 199
Peritonitis, 198
Peritonsillar abscess, 183
Permanent threshold shift (PTS), 326
Pernicious anemia (PA), 141, 154
Persecution, delusions of, 87
Personality, multiple, 81
Personality disorder, 84-85
Personality syndrome, organic, 84
Persuasion, 90
PET. See Positron emission tomography
      (PET)
Petechiae, 31
Peutz-Jeghers polyps, 186
Peutz-Jeghers syndrome, 187
PH. See Past history (PH)
pH. See Hydrogen ion concentration (pH)
Phagocytes, 140
Phantom limb pain, 45
Pharmacology
   psycho-. See Psychopharmacology
   texts, 375
Pharyngeal flap augmentation, 184
Pharyngeal flap operation, 184
Pharyngeal recess, 183
Pharyngeal tonsil, 183
Pharyngitis, 183
Pharynx, 182-85
Phenolsulfonphthalein (PSP), 227
Phenotype, 447
Phenyketonuria, 279
Phenylalanine, 431
Phenylpyruvic acid positive (PPA pos),
      264
Pheresis, 147
Philadelphia chromosome, 284
Phimosis, 225
PH interval, 125

Phlebitis, 115
Phleborrhapy, 117
Phlebosclerosis, 115
Phlegmasia alba dolens, 254
PHN. See Paroxysmal nocturnal
      hemoglobinuria (PHN)
Phobia, 88
Phocomelia, 260
Phonocardiography, 125
   fetal, 262
   intracardiac, 125
Phospholipids, 278
Phthisis, 168
Phylebotomy, 117
Physical therapy, 515-29
   and evaluation and measurement,
      519-21
   study guide, 580-81
Physician's Desk Reference (PDR), 375
PI. See Present illness (PI)
Pia mater, 69
Pica, 81, 257
PID. See Pelvic inflammatory disease
      (PID)
Pigment, 25
Piles, 191
Pilosebaceous, 25
   apparatus, 28
PIP. See Peak inspiratory pressure (PIP)
   and Proximal interphalangeal
      (joint) (PIP)
Pituitary tumor, 70, 77
PK. See Pyruvate kinase (PK) deficiency
Placenta, 253, 254, 261
   albatio, 254
   abruption, 254
   accreta, 254
   bruit of, 256
   hormones, 442
   previa, 254
   proteins, 410
Planes, of body, 23, 24
Plasma, 140
   biochemistry, 434-40
Plasma cell, 140
   dyscrasias, 358
   myeloma, 146
Plasmacrit test (PCT), 153
Plasmacytes, 140
Plasmacytoma, 43, 186
Plasma exchange (PE), 147-48
Plasma fractions, 147-48
Plasmapheresis, 148
Plasma protein factor (PPF), 148
Plasma renin activity (PRA), 227
Plasma thromboplastic component
      (PTC), 143
Plasma thromboplastin antecedent
      (PTA), 143, 153
Plasmodium falciparum, 196
Plasmodium malariae, 195

Plasmodium ovale, 196
Plasmodium vivax, 196
Plastic operation, on skin, 30
Platelet concentration, 147
Plateletpheresis, 147
Platelets, 140
Platybasia, 58
Play therapy, 90
Plethysmography, 126
Pleura, thorax, 171-73
Pleural adhesions, 172
Pleural biopsy, 172
Pleural cavity, 171
Pleural effusion, 171, 172, 174
Pleural exudate, 172
Pleural peel, 172
Pleurectomy, 172
Pleurisy, 171
Pleuritic pain, 172
Pleuritis, 171
Pleurocentesis, 173
Pleurodynia, 172
Pleuropneumonia-like organisms
      (PPLO), 168, 173
Plexus, brachial, sacral, and of spinal
      nerves, 66
PMN. See Polymorphonuclear neutrophils
      (PMN)
PMS. See Premenstrual syndrome (PMS)
PNC. See Premature atrioventricular
      nodal contractions (PNC)
PND. See Paroxysmal nocturnal dyspnea
      (PND)
Pneumocele, 168
Pneumoconiosis, 168
Pneumoencephalogram (PEG), 91
Pneumonectomy, 169
Pneumonia, 168, 385
Pneumonitis, 168
Pneumonocele, 168
Pneumophila, 174
PNL. See Percutaneous nephrolithotomy
      (PNL)
PNS. See Peripheral nervous system
      (PNS)
po, and time schedule for medication,
      202
Podalic version, 261
Podiatrist, 381
Poikilocytosis, 149
Polcystic liver disease, 196
Poliomyelitis, 75-76
Polya technique, 188
Polycystic ovarian syndrome, 242
Polycythemia, 142
Polycythemia rubra vera, 142
Polydactylia, 286
Polyhydramnios, 254
Polymenorrhea, 240
Polymorphnuclear, 140
Polymorphonuclear basophils, 140

Polymorphonuclear eosinophils, 140
Polymorphonuclear neutrophils (PMN), 139, 140, 153
Polymyositis, 56
Polyneuritis, 68
Polyneuropathy, 68
  acute idiopathic, 66
Polyorchidism, 225
Polyorchism, 225
Polyp, 186
  nasal, 159
Polyphagia, 189
Polyuria, 222
Pons, 69
Porphyria, 279
Portal circulation, 193
Portal hypertension, 196
Position, and direction, 23-24
Positive and end-expiratory pressure (PEEP), 167, 173
Positron emission tomography (PET), 496
Posterior, position and direction, 23, 24
Posterior-anterior (PA), 173
Posterior wall infarction, 107
Posteroanterior (PA), 173
Postinfarction syndrome, 112
Postlobectomy, 169
Postmature infant, 252
Postoperative pancreatitis
Postperfusion syndrome (PPS), 126
Postpneumonectomy, 169
Postpradial (PP), 201, 287
Post-transfusion disorders, 148
Post-traumatic stress disorder, 81
Potassium (K), 287
  depletion, 214
PP. *See* Postpradial (PP)
PPA pos. *See* Phenylpyruvic acid positive (PPA pos)
PPD. *See* Purified protein derivative (PPD)
PPF. *See* Plasma protein factor (PPF)
PPLO. *See* Pleuropneumonia-like organisms (PPLO)
PPS. *See* Postperfusion syndrome (PPS) *and* Prospective Payment System (PPS)
PRA. *See* Plasma renin activity (PRA)
Preanesthetic medication, 371
Precordial cardiography, 125
Precordial shock, 122
Predeposit autologous transfusion, 146
Prednisone, 155
Preeclampsia, 254
Prefixes, 4, 16-20, 533-34
Pregnancy
  ectopic, 254
  and hemorrhage, 257
  hypertensive disorder of, 254
  trimester of, 253

Pregnancy urine (PU), 264
Prekallikrein, 143
Preleukemia, 145
Premature atrial contractions (PAC), 126
Premature atrioventricular nodal contractions (PNC), 103
Premature infant, 252
Premature ventricular contractions (PVC), 103, 126
Premedication, 371
Premenstrual syndrome (PMS), 240
Presbyacusia, 389
Presbyatrics, 381
Presbylibrium, 389
Presbyopia, 389
Presentations, 257, 264
Present illness (PI), 33
Pressor effect, 276
Pressure sore, 27
Primary atypical pneumonia, 168
Primary brain tumor, 70
Primipara, 252
PR interval, 124, 125
Prinzmetal's angina, 102
prn, and time schedule for medication, 202
PRO. *See* Peer Review Organization (PRO)
Proaccelerin, 143
Procaine, 92
Procarbazine, 155
Proconvertin, 143
Proctitis, 191
Proctocolectomy, 192
Proctoplasty, 192
Proctosigmoidoscopy, 200
Prodromal pain, 227
Profile, 465
Profundaplasty, 117
Profundoplasty, 117
Progesterone receptor assay, 403, 409
Prognosis, 34, 58
Progressive stroke, 71
Projection, 88
Projective tests, 89
Prolapse
  of bladder, 220
  of cord, 259
  of rectum, 191
Proliferation, 31, 149
Prophylactic dialysis, 223
Proprietary urine studies, 448-49
Proptosis, 276
Prospective Payment System (PPS), 392
Prostate, 224, 225
Prostate antigen (PA), 409
Prostatectomies, 226
Prostatic acid phosphatase (PAP), 409
Prostatism, 227
Prostatitis, 225
Prosthesis, 117

abbreviations, 57
Prosthetics, 516
Proteins
  blood, 147-48
  placental, 410
Proteinuria, 222
Prothrombin, 143, 424
Prothrombin time (PT), 424
Protozoa
  and infections, 341-42
  diseases, tests, 352-53
Prower factor, 143
Proximal, position and direction, 23, 24
Proximal interphalangeal (joint) (PIP), 57
Proximal subclavian stenosis, 73
Pruritus ani, 193
Pruritus vulvae, 235
Pseudoagglutination, 149
Pseudogout, 48
Pseudohemophilia, 144
Pseudomembranous candidiasis, 180
Pseudoneruoma, 66
Psittacosis, 335
Psoriasis, 28
PSP. *See* Phenolsulfonphthalein (PSP)
Psychedelics, 89
Psychiatric disorders, 79-88
  and conditions amenable to neurosurgery, 93-94
  study guide, 541-42
Psychiatry, descriptive and dynamic, 79
Psychoanalysis, 90
Psychodynamics, 79
Psychogenic amnesia, 81
Psychogenic fugue, 81
Psychogenic pain, 77
Psychogerontology, 381
Psychological dependence, 92
Psychometric tests, 89
Psychometry, 79
Psychopharmacology, 89
Psychosocial milieu, 91
Psychotherapy, 89-90
  and older adults, 390-91
Psychotogens, 89
PT. *See* Prothrombin time (PT)
PTA. *See* Plasma thromboplastin antecedent (PTA)
PTB. *See* Patellar tendon bearing (prosthesis) (PTB)
PTC. *See* Plasma thromboplastic component (PTC)
PTH. *See* Parathyroid hormone (PTH)
PTS. *See* Permanent threshold shift (PTS)
Ptyalism, 182
Ptyalith, 181
PU. *See* Pregnancy urine (PU)
Pudendum, 233
Puerperal hematoma, 254
Pulmonary artery (PA), 126

balloon counterpulsation, 122
Pulmonary banding, 109
Pulmonary decortication, 172
Pulmonary edema, 168
Pulmonary embolectomy, 170
Pulmonary embolism, 168
Pulmonary emphysema, 168
Pulmonary hypertension, 168
Pulmonary infarction, 168
Pulmonary pleura, 171
Pulmonary resection, 169
Pulmonary thrombosis, 168
Pulmonary tuberculosis, 168
Pulmonary valvotomy, 109, 112
Pulmonary wedge pressure (PWP), 122, 126
Pulmonic stenosis, 102
Pulse, 118
    analysis, 126
    deficit, 118
Pulseless disease, 114
PULSES profile, 520
Pulsion diverticula, 184
Pupil, 313
Pure pulmonary stenosis, 102
Purified protein derivative (PPD), 173
Purkinje fibers, 99, 101
Purpura, 144
Purulent pericarditis, 107
Pustule, 31
PVC. See Premature ventricular contractions (PVC)
P wave, 124, 125
PWP. See Pulmonary wedge pressure (PWP)
Pyelonephritis, 213
Pyeloplasty, 216
Pyelotomy, 216
Pylolithotomy, 216
Pyloric, part of stomach, 185
Pyloric sphincter, 185
Pyloromyotomy, 188
Pyloroplasty, 188
Pylorospasm, 261
Pylorus, 185
Pyoderma, 28
    faciale, 28
Pyogenic abscess, 195
Pyogenic bacteria, 34
Pyopheumothorax, 171
Pyosalpinx, 242
Pyothorax, 171
Pyoureter, 217
Pyrexia, lethal, 92
Pyrosis, 189
Pyruvate kinase (PK) deficiency, 142, 154
Pyuria, 222

QA. See Quality Assurance (QA)
qh, and time schedule for medication, 202

qid, and time schedule for medication, 202
QRS complex, 124, 125
Quadrants, of abdomen, 22
Quality Assurance (QA), 392
Quickening, 257
Quinsy, 183
Q wave, 125

RA. See Right atrium (RA)
Rabies, 334
Rachitic chest, 171
Rachitis, 44
RAD. See Radiation absorbed dose (RAD)
Radial neck dissection, 182
Radiation
    anemia, 474
    and cancer modalities, 410-11
    injury, 474-75
    pericarditis, 155
    protection guide, 498
    therapy, 518
Radiation absorbed dose (RAD), 511
Radical resection of esophageal cancer, 185
Radiculitis, 68
Radioassay, 498
Radioautograph, 498
Radiobiology, 499
Radiocurability, 401
Radiodermatitis, 474-75
Radiograph, 465
Radioimmunoassay (RIA), 499
Radioiodine, and thyroid gland, 506, 511-12
Radioisotopes, 58, 499
Radiologic studies, 466-75
Radiologist, 466
Radiology
    diagnostic, 488
    study guide, 576-77
    terms pertaining to, 463-75
    therapeutic, 488-89
Radionecrosis, 475
Radionuclide diagnostic tests, 504-9
Radionuclide imaging, 501-4
Radionuclides, 499-500
    and diagnosis, 507-9
    symbols, 510
    in therapy, 509-10
Radionuclidic imaging devices, 500
Radio-opaque, 412
Radiotherapy, 154, 155
Radium, 466
Radner method, 123
Radon, 466
Rales, 171
Range of motion (ROM), 57
Rapid eye movements (deep sleep)(REM), 91

Rapid mood swings, 92
Rapid plasma reagin (RPR) test, 244
Rarefied, 58
Rash, nettle, 29
Rashkind's operation, 108
Rational-emotive therapy, 90
Raynaud's disease, 115, 118, 385-86
Raynaud's phenomenon, 359
RBC. See Red blood count (RBC)
RBE. See Relative biologic effectiveness (RBE)
RCA. See Right coronary artery (RCA)
RD. See Respiratory disease (RD)
RDS. See Respiratory distress syndrome (RDS)
Reactor, 500
Read's method, 252
Reality therapy, 391
Receptive aphasia, 526
Receptor, 66
Recordings, of heart action, 124-26
Recreational therapy, 90
Rectocele, 191
Rectouterine pouch, 235
Rectum, 191
    cancer, 191
Red blood count (RBC), 153
Red cells, conditions affecting, 140-46
Reduction
    closed and open, 45
    of intussusception, 192
    of volvulus, 192
Reed-Sternberg cell, 154
Reference, delusions of, 87
Reference interval, 422
Reference values, 422
    and CVP, 120
Reflexes
    and anesthesia, 374
    testing, 521
Regenerative polyps, 186
Regional anesthesia, 374-75
Regional irradiation, 411
Regions, of abdomen, 22
Regression, 88, 390
Regurgitation, 185
Rehabilitation, 516
Reiter's syndrome, 49
Rejection phenomenon, 356
Relative biologic effectiveness (RBE), 500
REM. See Rapid eye movements (deep sleep)(REM) and Roentgen equivalent man (REM)
Reminiscence, therapy of, 391
Remission, 280, 401
Remotivation, therapy of, 391
Renala corpuscle, 211
Renal artery, occlusions, 395
Renal calculi, 58, 214
Renal cortex, 211
Renal cystic disease, 214

Renal excretion rate (RER), 227
Renal failure, 215
Renal function studies, 448
Renal hypertension, 215
Renal medulla, 211
Renal medullary necrosis, 215
Renal osteodystrophy, 44
Renal pain, 217
Renal papillae, 211
Renal pelvis, 211
Renal plasma flow (RPF), 227
Renal transplantation, 216
Renal tuberculosis, 215
Renal tubule, 211
Renal vein thrombosis, 215
Rendu-Osler-Weber syndrome, 144
Repetitive articular trauma, 48
Replanation of an extremity, 45
Repression, 88
RER. *See* Renal excretion rate (RER)
RES. *See* Reticuloendothelial system (RES)
Resection, 109
    for esophageal stricture, 185
    of coarctation, 117
Residual type, schizophrenia, 86
Resolution, 466
Respiratory depression, 92
Respiratory disease (RD), 173
Respiratory disorders, 159-78
    amenable to surgery, 174-75
    study guide, 547-48
Respiratory distress syndrome (RDS), 265-66
Respiratory movement (RM), 173
Respiratory volume (RV), 173
Response intensity, evaluation of, 373
Restrictive cardiomyopathy, 105
Resuscitation, CPR. *See* Cardiac pulmonary resuscitation (CPR)
Retardation
    in brain growth, 92
    mental. *See* Mental retardation
Reticulocytes, 140
Reticulocytosis, 149
Reticuloendothelial system (RES), 149-50, 153
Reticuloendotheliosus, 144-45
Reticulum cell lymphosaroma, 186
Retina, 293
    disorders of, 296-97
    repairs of, 301
Retinopathy, 296
Retinoscopy, 307
Retraction
    clot, 423-24
    skin, 33
Retrograde method, 124
Retrolental fibroplasia, 260
Retroperitoneal lymph node, 154
Review guide, 533-81

answers, 582
Reye's syndrome, 334
RF. *See* Rheumatic fever (RF)
Rheoencephalography, 89
Rhesus factor isoimmunization, 431
Rhesus factor negative (Rh neg), 264
Rhesus factor positive (Rh pos), 264
Rheumatic fever (RF), 126
Rheumatic heart disease, 107
Rheumatoid arthritis, 429
Rheumatoid nodules, 53
RHF. *See* Right-sided heart failure (RHF)
Rh-Hr system, 426
Rhinitis, 160
Rhinolith, 160
Rhinophyma, 28
Rhinoplasty, 160
Rhinorrhea, 160
Rh isoimmunization. *See* Rhesus factor isoimmunization
Rh neg. *See* Rhesus factor negative (Rh neg)
Rh pos. *See* Rhesus factor positive (Rh pos)
Rhythm method, 252
Rhytidectomy, 387
Rhytidoplasty, 387
RIA. *See* Radioimmunoassay (RIA)
Rib, 43
Richettsial diseases, tests, 348
Rickets, 44
Rickettsiae, infections caused by, 337-38
Rickettsial isolation techniques, 174
Rickettsial stains, 174
RIF. *See* Right iliac fossa (RIF)
Rifampin, 174
Right atrium (RA), 126
Right coronary artery (RCA), 126
Right iliac fossa (RIF), 57
Right lower extremity (RLE), 57
Right mediolateral (episiotomy)(RML), 264
Right mentoanterior (RMA), 264
Right mentoposterior (RMP), 264
Right mentotransverse (RMT), 264
Right occipitoanterior (ROA), 264
Right occipitoposterior (ROP), 264
Right occipitotransverse (ROT), 264
Right sacroanterior (RSA), 264
Right sacroposterior (RSP), 264
Right scapuloanterior (RScA), 264
Right scapuloposterior (RScP), 264
Right-sided heart failure (RHF), 126
Right upper extremity (RUE), 57
Right ventricle (RV), 126
Right ventricular hypertrophy (RVH), 126
Rigidity, 57, 390
Rigor, 57
Rima glottidis, 162
RLE. *See* Right lower extremity (RLE)

RM. *See* Respiratory movement (RM)
RMA. *See* Right mentoanterior (RMA)
RML. *See* Right mediolateral (episiotomy)(RML)
RMP. *See* Right mentoposterior (RMP)
RMT. *See* Right mentotransverse (RMT)
ROA. *See* Right occipitoanterior (ROA)
Rocky Mountain spotted fever, 337
Roentgen equivalent man (REM), 511
Roentgenographic, 58
Roentgenography, 155, 465-66
ROM. *See* Range of motion (ROM)
Romberg's sign, 88, 522
Romberg test, 325
Root
    of tooth, 180
    element, 4, 10-15
    of spinal nerves, 66
ROP. *See* Right occipitoposterior (ROP)
Rorschach Personality Test, 89
Rosenmuller, fossa of. *See* Fossa of Rosenmuller
ROT. *See* Right occipitotransverse (ROT)
Rouleaux formation, 149
Round cell lymphosarcoma, 186
Roux-en-Y procedures, 198
RPF. *See* Renal plasma flow (RPF)
RPR test. *See* Rapid plasma reagin (RPR) test
RSA. *See* Right sacroanterior (RSA)
RScA. *See* Right scapuloanterior (RScA)
RScP. *See* Right scapuloposterior (RScP)
RSP. *See* Right sacroposterior (RSP)
Rubella syndrome, 260
Rubells, 334
Rubin test, 243, 244
RUE. *See* Right upper extremity (RUE)
Rugae, 185
Rupture, 127, 213
    of aneurysm, 115
    of uterus, 254
RV. *See* Respiratory ventricle (RV) *and* Right volume (RV)
RVH. *See* Right ventricular hypertrophy (RVH)
R wave, 125
Rye histopatholic classification of Hodgkins' disease, 151

SA. *See* Sinoatrial (node)(SA)
Sacculated type, aneurysm of aorta, 114
SACH. *See* Solid ankle cushion heel (foot prosthesis) (SACH)
Sacral region, of back, 23
SAFP. *See* Serum alpha-fetoprotein (SAFP)
Sagittal, body plane, 23, 24
St. Anthony's fire, 27
St. Jude Medical prosthesis, 111
St. Louis encephalitis (SLE), 91, 333
Saline abortion, 261

Salivary glands, 179-82
Salivation, 182
Salpingectomy, 242
Salpingitis, 242, 337
Salpingolysis, 242
Salpingo-oophorectomy, 242
Salpingoplasty, 243
SA node. *See* Sinoatrial node (SA node) *and* Sinus node (SA node)
Saphenous vein graft (SVG), 109, 126
Saprophyte, 333
Sarcoidosis, 106, 343
Sarcoma, 401
Saturation index (SI), 153
SBE. *See* Subacute bacterial endocarditis (SBE)
SC. *See* Semiclosed (SC)
SCA. *See* Sickle cell anemia (SCA)
Scabies, 28
Scalenus anticus syndrome, 115
Scanning, nuclear medicine, 500
Scanning speech, 79
Schiller test, 244
Schilling's Hemogram, 145
Schizoid personality disorder, 84
Schizophrenia, 85-86
Schizotypal personality disorder, 84
Schwann, sheath of. *See* Sheath of Schwann
Sciatica, 68
Sciatic neuritis, 68
Scintiphotography, 500
Scirrhous, 401
Sclera, disorders, 294-95
Scleroderma, 359
Sclerosing cholangitis, 196
Sclerosis, 70, 75, 297
Sclerotherapy, 201
Scoliosis, 49
Scotoma, 302
Scrotum, 224
SD. *See* Shoulder disarticulation (SD)
Sebaceous glands, 25
Seborrheal, 31
Seborrheic, 31
  keratosis, 28
Sebum, 25
Secretin test, 450
Sectioning, 155
Secundines, 253
Sedimentary rate (SR), 126
Segmental resection, 169
Seizures, 92
Selective cordotomy, 77
Semiclosed (SC), 375
Semilunar valves, 101
Seminal fluid, 455
Seminoma, 226
Senescent psychiatric disorders, 386
Senescent skin disorders, 386
Senescent tumor, 390

Senescent visual disorders, 386
Senescent. *See also* Senile
Senile macular degeneration (SMD), 392
Senile vaginitis, 234
Senile. *See also* Senescent
Senning's operation, revised technique, 109
Sensitivity, 355, 422
Sensory aphasia, 78, 525
Sensory areas, 69
Sensory deprivation, 88
Sensory testing, 521
Septal dermoplasty, 160
Septectomy, 160
Septic shock, 118, 243
Septum, 159
Sequelae, 58
Sequential vein graft, 109
Sequestration, 45
Sequestrectomy, 45
Sequestrum, 44
Serologic tests, 426-29
  for syphilis, 244
Serum, 33, 140
  albumin, 148
  biochemistry, 434-40
  enzyme, abnormalities, 438-40
  iron level, 434
Serum alpha-fetoprotein (SAFP), 201, 451
Serum prothrombin conversion accelerator (SPCA), 143
Sex chromosomes, 281
Sexually transmitted diseases, and infections, 336-37
SGA. *See* Small for gestational age (SGA)
Sheath of Schwann, 65-66
Shirey technique, 123
Shock, 112, 118, 122
Shock lung, 168
Shock therapy, 90
Short bowel syndrome, 191
Short gut syndrome, 191
Short-increment sensitivity index (SISI), 326
Shoulder, painful, 49
Shoulder disarticulation (SD), 57
Shunts, 78
  and liver, 198
SI. *See* Saturation index (SI)
Sialadenectomy, 182
Sialadenitis, 181
Sialolith, 181
Sialolithiasis, 181
Sialolithotomy, 182
Sickle cell anemia (SCA), 142, 154
Sickle cell disease screening tests, 431-32
Sickle cell hemoglobin (Hb S), 153
Sick sinus syndrome, 104
Sideroblastic anemia, 141
Sideroblasts, 140

Siderocytes, 140
Siderosis, 169
SIDS. *See* Sudden infant death syndrome (SIDS)
Sigmoid bladder, 221
Silicosis, 169
Simmond's disease, 274
Simple alveolar gland, 29
Simple chronic bronchitis, 164
Simple columnar epithelium, 29
Simple immobilization, 45
Simple rosacea, 26
SIMV. *See* Synchronized intermittent mandatory ventilation (SIMV)
Single photon emission computed tomography (SPECT), 496
Singultus, 170
Sinoatrial (node)(SA), 99, 126
Sinus
  of heart, 101
  paranasal, 160
  rhythm, 112
Sinuses of Valsalva, 101
Sinusitis, 160
Sinus node (SA node), 99, 126
Sipple's syndrome, 274
SISI. *See* Short-increment sensitivity index (SISI)
Size of term infant, 264
Sjogren's syndrome, 359
Skeletal dysplasias, 49-50
Skeletal muscle ischemia of arm, 73
Skeleton, anterior view and posterior view, 40-41
Skene's gland, 233
Skin
  and breast, 25-37
  cancer, nasal, 159
  cicatrix of, 30
  -coloring process, 26
  conditions amenable to surgery, 34-36
  cryosurgery of, 29
  curettage of, 29
  disorders of, 25-31
  drainage, 30
  fulguration of, 30
  grafting, 30
  incision, 30
  and plastic operation on, 30
  references and bibliography, 36-37
  retraction, 33
  study guide, 537-38
  tumors of, 28
Skull, and MR imaging, 485-86
SLE. *See* St. Louis encephalitis (SLE) *and* Systemic lupus erythematosus (SLE)
Slice, 466
Slit-beam radiography, 466
Small airways disease, 164
Small cell carcinoma, 167

Small for gestational age (SGA), 264
Small intestine, 189-93
Smallpox, 335
SMD. *See* Senile macular degeneration (SMD)
Smeloff-Cutter prosthesis, 111
SNDO. *See* Standard Nomenclature of Diseases and Operations (SNDO)
SNM. *See* Society of Nuclear Medicine (SNM)
SNS. *See* Sympathetic nervous system (SNS)
Soave procedure, 192
Society of Nuclear Medicine (SNM), 511
Soft palate, 179
Solid ankle cushion heel (foot prosthesis) (SACH), 57
Somatization disorder, 86
Somatoform disorders, 86
Somatoform paid disorder, 86
Somnambulism, 88
Sones' technique, 124
Spasm, 57
SPCA. *See* Serum prothrombin conversion accelerator (SPCA)
Specificity, 422
SPECT. *See* Single photon emission computed tomography (SPECT)
Speech
    incoherence in, 87
    scanning, 79
Spermatic cord, 225
Sphenoidal sinus, 160
Spherocytic anemia, 142
Spherocytosis, 142, 154
Sphincter
    of bile duct, 193
    nepatopancreatic ampulla, 193
Sphincter of Oddi, 193
Sphincteroplasty, 199
Sphincterotomy, lateral internal, 192
Sphygmomanometer, 122
Spider nevi, 199
Spina bifida, 76
Spinal cord, 68-79
    decompression of, 77
    injury, 76
    and MR imaging, 485-86
    tumors, 77
Spinal shock, 222
Spincteroplasty, 199
Spirochetal diseases, tests, 352-53
Spirochetes, infections caused by, 340-41
Spleen, 152-53, 155
Splenectomy, 153, 155
Splenic infarcts, 153
Splenic sequestration crisis, 153
Splenitis, 153
Splenomegalia, 153
Splenomegaly, 153, 154
Splenopexy, 153

Splenoptosis, 153
Splenorrhaphy, 153
Splenorrhexis, 153
Splenotomy, 153
Spondylitis, 47
Spondyloepiphyseal dysplasia, 50
Spondylolisthesis, 50
Spondylosis, 50
Spontaneous abortion, 92
Spontaneous pneumothorax, 171
Sprain, 50
Spur, 53
Squamous cell carcinoma, 167, 181
SR. *See* Sedimentary rate (SR) *and* Stimulus response (SR)
SSPE. *See* Subacute sclerosing panencephalitis (SSPE)
Stable factor, 143
Staff cells, 139-40
Stage of analgesia, 372
Stage of delirium, 372
Stage of toxicity, 372
Staging laparotomies, 412
Staging laparotomy, 155
Staging systems. *See* Cancer
Stains
    immunofluorescent, 174
    rickettsial, 174
Standard Nomenclature of Diseases and Operations (SNDO), 33
Stanford-Binet, 89
Stangury, 227
Staphylococcic folliculitis, 28
Staphylococcus aureus, 28
Starr-Edwards prosthesis, 111
Startle reflex, 261
stat, and time schedule for medication, 202
Status asthmaticus, 165
Steatoma, 28
Steatorrhea, 193, 280
Stein-Leventhal syndrome, 242
Stem cell leukemia, 144
Stenosis, 102, 107, 108
    aortic. *See* Aortic stenosis (AS)
    mitral. *See* Mitral stenosis (MS)
    of larynx, 162
    of trachea, 163
Stensen's duct, 180
Stereotaxic neurosurgery, 77
Stereotaxy, 77
Sterility, 257
Steroid hormones, 442-43
Stethoscope, 122
Stickiness, 284
Still's disease, 50
Stimulation, tactile, 68
Stimulus response (SR), 91
STLI. *See* Subtotal lymphoid irradiation (STLI)
STNI. *See* Subtotal nodal irradiation (STNI)

Stokes-Adams syndrome, 104
Stomach, 185-89
Stomatoplasty, 182
Stool examination, 451
Strabismus, repairs of, 305
Stratified squamous, 29
Stress
    disorder, post-traumatic, 81
    erosive gastritis, 187
    incontinence, 220
    ulcer, 187
Stridor, 154, 162, 259
Stroke, 71, 383
ST segment, 125
Stuart factor, 143
Studies, neurologic, 88-89
Sturmdorf procedure, 240
Subacute bacterial endocarditis (SBE), 126
Subacute sclerosing panencephalitis (SSPE), 76
Subarachnoid hemorrhage, 73
Subclavian flap angioplasty, 116
Subclavian steal syndrome, 73, 115
    operations, 117
Subclavian-subclavian bypass, 117
Subcoma insulin therapy, 91
Subcutaneous tissue, 25
Subinvolution, 254
Sublimation, 88
Sublingual duct, 180
Subluxation, 50
Submandibular duct, 180
Submandibular gland, 180
Submaxillary gland, 180
Submaxillary lymph nodes, 202
Submucous resection, 160
Subsegmental resection, 169
Subthalamus, 69
Subtotal lymphoid irradiation (STLI), 155
Subtotal nodal irradiation (STNI), 155
Subtotal parotidectomy, 182
Subtrochanteric, 58
Sudden cardiac death, 107
Sudden infant death syndrome (SIDS), 92
Sudoriferous glands, 25
Suffixes, 5, 6-16, 533-34
    diagnostic, 6-7
    operative, 7-9
    symptomatic, 9
Sulkowitch test, 447
Superficial, position and direction, 23, 24
Superior, position and direction, 23, 24
Superior vena cava (SVC), 126
Superior vena cava syndrome (SVCS), 115, 402
Supernumerary bone, 44
Supervoltage, 202
Supportive psychotherapy, 90

Supraclavicular nerve entrapment syndrome, 49
Suprapubic vesicourethral suspension, 221
Suprarenals, 272
Supraspinatus syndrome, 49
Suprasternal cardiac catheterization, 123
Surgery
  blood disorders amenable to, 156
  blood-forming disorders amenable to, 156
  breast conditions amenable to, 34-36
  and cancer modalities, 411-12
  cardiovascular conditions amenable to, 128-33
  and digestive disorders amenable to, 203-6
  ear conditions amenable to, 327-28
  endocrine conditions amenable to, 288
  excisional, 169
  and fractures, 45
  gynecologic disorders amenable to, 246-47
  and hydrocephalus, 78
  laser, 30
  neonate conditions amenable to, 266-67
  neuro-. See Neurosurgery
  obstetric conditions amenable to, 266-67
  orthopedic conditions amenable to, 59-61
  respiratory disorders amenable to, 174-75
  and shunts for hydrocephalus, 78
  skin conditions amenable to, 34-36
  thyroid, 276
  urogenital disorder amenable to, 228-30
  and valgus deformity, 52
  vascular, 395
  vision conditions amenable to surgery, 310-12
Susceptibility, 422
Suspension of uterus, 239
Sutter prosthesis, 111
SVC. See Superior vena cava (SVC)
SVCS. See Superior vena cava syndrome (SVCS)
SVG. See Saphenous vein graft (SVG)
Swan-Ganz pulmonary artery catheterization, 122
S wave, 125
Sweat test, 451
Symbols
  and nuclear medicine, 510
  and radiology, 489
Sympathectomy, 68
Sympathetic fibers, 101
Sympathetic nervous system (SNS), 91
Symptomatic suffixes, 9

Synapse, 66
Synchronized direct current countershock, 122
Synchronized intermittent mandatory ventilation (SIMV), 173
Synchronized pacing, 120
Syncope, 79, 112, 127
Syndenham's chorea, 73
Syngenic marrow transplantation, 148
Synovectomy, 53
Synovial effusion, 53
Synovial joint, 47
Synovial membrane, 47
Synovial sarcoma, 49
Synovioma, 49
Synovitis, acute and traumatic, 47-48
Syphilis, 336
  of bladder and urethra, 220
  and male genital organs, 226
  serologic tests for, 244
Syringomyelocele, 76
Systematic chemotherapy, 411
Systemic amyloidosis, 146
Systemic lupus erythematosus (SLE), 360, 429
Systemic muscular and neurologic disorders, 106
Systole, 112
Systolic blood pressure, 114

TAA. See Tumor-associated antigen (TAA)
Tabes dorsalis, 76
Tachycardia, 112, 390
Tachypnea, 171
Tactile fremitus (TF), 173
Tactile stimulation, 68
Takayasu's syndrome, 114
Talipes, 50
Talipes equinus, 50
Talipes planus, 50
Talipes valgus, 50
Talipes varus, 50
Tamponade, 104
Tarsal glands, 303
Tarsal plate, 303
TAT. See Thematic Apperception Test (TAT)
Taxonomy, 333
TB. See Tuberculosis (TB)
TCD. See Transcranial Doppler (TCD) sonography
TDT. See Tone decay test (TDT)
Tearing apart terms, 4-5, 533-34
TEA. See Thromboendarterectomy (TEA)
Teeth, 180
Telangiectasia, 144
Teletherapy, 500
Temperature, pulse, and respiration (TPR), 33
Temperature method, 252
Temporal lobe epilepsy, 77

Temporary threshold shift (TTS), 326
Tendons, 53-57
Tendoplasty, 56
Tendosynovitis, 56
Tenesmus of vesical sphincter, 222
Tennis elbow, 49
Tenodesis, 56
Tenoplasty, 56
Tenosynovectomy, 56
Tenosynovitis, 56
Tension pneumothorax, 172
Teratocarcinoma, 226
Teratogens, 252
Teratology, 253
Teratoma, 226
Term infant, 264
Terminology, medical. See Medical terminology
Terms, tearing apart, 4-5, 533-34
TES. See Treadmill exercise score (TES)
Testes, 224
Testicular tumors, 226
Testing methods, 457-58
Tests
  abbreviations related to, 458-59
  hepatic function, 452-54
  immunologic, 426-29
  laboratory. See Laboratory tests
  nuclear medicine, 510
  psychometric, 89
  and radionuclides, 504-9
  serologic, 426-29
Tetany, 274
Tetracaine, 92
Tetralogy of Fallot, 102, 109, 111
Texts, pharmacology, 375
TF. See Tactile fremitus (TF)
TGA. See Transposition of great arteries (TGA)
Thalamectomy, 77
Thalamotomy, 77
Thalamus, 69
Thalassemia major, 142
Thalassemia minor, 142
Thalassemias, 142
Thayer-Martin (TM) medium, 244
Thelitis, 7
Thematic Apperception Test (TAT), 89, 91
Therapeutic drug monitoring, 457
Therapeutic exercise, 518-19
Therapeutic index, 411
Therapeutic pneumothorax, 172
Therapeutic radiology, 488-89
Therapeutic ultrasound, 518
Therapy
  for older adults, 390-91
  physical. See Physical therapy
  psycho-. See Psychotherapy
  and radionuclides, 509-10
  shock. See Shock therapy